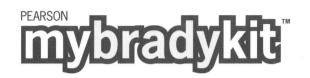 PEARSON **mybradykit**™

 ☑ **W9-CNC-285**

Use the registration code below to gain access to this online study companion. This is a single source for all your student resources that support the textbook. By following the registration instructions below you will link to a wealth of opportunities to further your understanding of your course material. Use this Website in conjunction with your textbook for a multidimensional learning experience. Enjoy!

STEP 1: Register

All you need to get started is a valid email address and the access code below. To register, simply:

1. Go to **www.bradybooks.com**, then click on **mybradykit**. Choose **myemskit**.
2. Click "**Students**" under "**First-time users**."
3. Find the appropriate book cover. Cover must match the textbook edition being used for your class.
4. Click "**Register**" beside your book cover.
5. Read the **License Agreement** and **Private Policy**. If you accept, click "**I Accept**."
6. Leave "**No**" selected under "**Do you have a Pearson account?**"
7. Using a coin scratch off the silver coating below to reveal your access code. Do not use a knife or other sharp object, which can damage the code.
8. Enter your access code in lowercase or uppercase, without the dashes.
9. Follow the on-screen instructions to complete registration.

During registration, you will establish a personal login name and password to use for logging into the Website. You will also be sent a registration confirmation email that contains your login name and password. Be sure to save this email.

Your Access Code is:

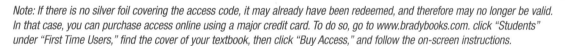

Note: If there is no silver foil covering the access code, it may already have been redeemed, and therefore may no longer be valid. In that case, you can purchase access online using a major credit card. To do so, go to www.bradybooks.com. click "Students" under "First Time Users," find the cover of your textbook, then click "Buy Access," and follow the on-screen instructions.

STEP 2: Log in

1. Go to **www.bradybooks.com** and click on **mybradykit**. Choose **myemskit**. Click on "**Students**" under "**Returning Users**."
2. Find the appropriate book cover. Click on "**Login**" next to your book cover.
3. Enter the login name and password that you created during registration. If unsure of this information, refer to your registration confirmation email.
4. Click "**Login**."

Instructors

For premium-level access that includes testing and lecture support materials, please go to **www.bradybooks.com** and click on **mybradykit** (choose myems or myfirekit). Then go to your individual text book, and click Request Access under the Instructor's bar. You may also click on the Instructor Registration and Student Handout documents for additional information. For further assistance contact your local Brady representative or call 800-852-4508

Got technical questions?

Customer Technical Support: To obtain support, please visit us online anytime at http://247pearsoned.custhelp.com where you can search our knowledgebase for common solutions, view product alerts, and review all options for additional assistance.

SITE REQUIREMENTS

For the latest updates on Site Requirements, go to **www.bradybooks.com** and click on **myemskit**. Click "**Students**" under "**Returning Users**." Pick your book and click "**Login**." Click on "**Need help**" at bottom of page for site requirements and other frequently asked questions.

Important: Please read the Subscription and End-User License agreement, accessible from the book Website's login page, before using the *mybradykit* Website. By using the Website, you indicate that you have read, understood, and accepted the terms of this agreement.

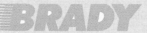

Paramedic Care

Principles & Practice

Patient Assessment

Third Edition

BRYAN E. BLEDSOE, DO, FACEP, EMT-P

Emergency Physician
Midlothian, Texas
and
Professor, Health Sciences
University of Nevada, Las Vegas
Las Vegas, Nevada

ROBERT S. PORTER, MA, NREMT-P

Senior Advanced Life Support Educator
Madison County Emergency Medical Services
Canastota, New York
and
Flight Paramedic
AirOne, Onondaga County Sheriff's Department
Syracuse, New York

RICHARD A. CHERRY, MS, NREMT-P

Clinical Assistant Professor of Emergency Medicine
Technical Director for Medical Simulation
Upstate Medical University
Syracuse, New York

Upper Saddle River, New Jersey 07458

Library of Congress Cataloging-in-Publication Data

Bledsoe, Bryan E., 1955–
   Paramedic care: principles & practice / Bryan E. Bledsoe, Robert S. Porter, Richard A. Cherry. — 3rd ed.
     p. ; cm.
   Includes bibliographical references and index.
   ISBN 978-0-13-513703-1
   1. Emergency medicine. 2. Emergency medical technicians. I. Porter, Robert S., 1950– II. Cherry, Richard A. III. Title.
   [DNLM: 1. Emergencies. 2. Emergency Medical Technicians. 3. Emergency Treatment. WB 105 B646pa 2008]
   RC86. 7. B5964 2008
   616.02′ 5 — dc22

2007036867

Publisher: Julie Levin Alexander
Publisher's Assistant: Regina Bruno
Executive Editor: Marlene McHugh Pratt
Senior Managing Editor for Development: Lois Berlowitz
Project Manager: Sandra Breuer
Managing Photography Editor: Michal Heron
Director of Marketing: Karen Allman
Executive Marketing Manager: Katrin Beacom
Marketing Specialist: Michael Sirinides
Managing Editor for Production: Patrick Walsh
Production Liaison: Faye Gemmellaro
Production Editor: Heather Willison S4Carlisle Publishing Services
Manufacturing Manager: Ilene Sanford
Manufacturing Buyer: Pat Brown
Senior Design Coordinator: Christopher Weigand
Cover Image: Ray Kemp/911 Imaging
Cover and Interior Design: Jill Little
Interior Photographers: Michal Heron, Richard Logan, Scott Metcalfe
Interior Illustrations: Rolin Graphics
Media Product Manager: John J. Jordan
Media Project Manager: Stephen J. Hartner
Composition: S4Carlisle Publishing Services
Media Editor: Joseph Saba
Printing and Binding: Courier/Kendallville
Cover Printer: Phoenix Color

Pearson Education Ltd., London
Pearson Education Singapore, Pte. Ltd.
Pearson Education Canada, Inc.
Pearson Education—Japan
Pearson Education Australia Pty, Limited
Pearson Education North Asia Ltd., Hong Kong
Pearson Educación de Mexico, S.A. de C.V.
Pearson Education Malaysia, Pte. Ltd.
Pearson Education, Upper Saddle River, New Jersey

Notices

It is the intent of the authors and publishers that this textbook be used as part of a formal paramedic education program taught by a qualified instructor and supervised by a licensed physician. The care procedures presented here represent accepted practices in the United States. They are not offered as a standard of care. Paramedic-level emergency care is to be performed only under the authority and guidance of a licensed physician. It is the reader's responsibility to know and follow local care protocols as provided by medical advisors directing the system to which he or she belongs. Also, it is the reader's responsibility to stay informed of emergency care procedure changes.

Notice on Drugs and Drug Dosages

Every effort has been made to ensure that the drug dosages presented in this textbook are in accordance with nationally accepted standards. When applicable, the dosages and routes are taken from the American Heart Association's *Advanced Cardiac Life Support Guidelines.* The American Medical Association's publication *Drug Evaluations,* the *Physicians' Desk Reference,* and the *Prentice Hall Health Professional's Drug Guide* are followed with regard to drug dosages not covered by the American Heart Association's guidelines. It is the responsibility of the reader to be familiar with the drugs used in his or her system, as well as the dosages specified by the medical director. The drugs presented in this book should only be administered by direct order, whether verbally or through accepted standing orders, of a licensed physician.

Notice on Gender Usage

The English language has historically given preference to the male gender. Among many words, the pronouns "he" and "his" are commonly used to describe both genders. Society evolves faster than language, and the male pronouns still predominate in our speech. The authors have made great effort to treat the two genders equally, recognizing that a significant percentage of paramedics and patients are female. However, in some instances, male pronouns may be used to describe both male and female paramedics and patients solely for the purpose of brevity. This is not intended to offend any readers of the female gender.

Notice on Photographs

Please note that many of the photographs contained in this book are taken of actual emergency situations. As such, it is possible that they may not accurately depict current, appropriate, or advisable practices of emergency medical care. They have been included for the sole purpose of giving general insight into real-life emergency settings.

Notice on Case Studies

The names used and situations depicted in the case studies throughout this textbook are fictitious.

10 9 8 7 6 5 4 3 2
ISBN 0-13-513703-9
ISBN 978-0-13-513703-1

Dedication

This text is respectfully dedicated to all EMS personnel who have made the ultimate sacrifice. Their memory and good deeds will forever be in our thoughts and prayers.

BEB, RSP, RAC

Content Overview

VOLUME 1 INTRODUCTION TO ADVANCED PREHOSPITAL CARE

Below is a brief content description of each chapter in Volume 1, *Introduction to Advanced Prehospital Care.*

Chapter 1 Introduction to Advanced Prehospital Care 1

▶ Introduces the world of paramedicine and the DOT paramedic curriculum
▶ Summarizes the expanding roles of the paramedic
▶ Emphasizes the importance of professionalism in paramedic practice

Chapter 2 The Well-Being of the Paramedic 14

▶ Presents material crucial to the survival of the paramedic in EMS
▶ Addresses physical fitness, nutrition, and personal protection from disease
▶ Details the role of stress in EMS and important coping strategies

Chapter 3 EMS Systems 47

▶ Reviews the history of EMS and provides an overview of EMS today
▶ Details the various, integrated aspects of EMS design and operation
▶ Explains the importance of medical direction in prehospital care

Chapter 4 Roles and Responsibilities of the Paramedic 81

▶ Discusses expectations and responsibilities of the modern paramedic
▶ Emphasizes the importance of ethical behavior, appearance, and patient advocacy

Chapter 5 Illness and Injury Prevention 102

▶ Addresses the importance of illness and injury prevention in EMS, emphasizing scene safety and the safety of all rescuers
▶ Emphasizes the importance of paramedic participation in illness and injury prevention programs in the community

Chapter 6 Medical/Legal Aspects of Advanced Prehospital Care 117

▶ Provides an overview of civil law as it applies to prehospital care and the paramedic
▶ Discusses steps the paramedic can take to protect against malpractice action and liability

Chapter 7 Ethics in Advanced Prehospital Care 149

▶ Presents the fundamentals of medical ethics
▶ Discusses the interrelationships among ethics, morals, the law, and religious beliefs

continued

Content Overview

VOLUME 1 INTRODUCTION TO ADVANCED PREHOSPITAL CARE (continued)

Chapter 8 General Principles of Physiology and Pathophysiology 169

▶ Presents an overview of basic pathophysiology relevant to advanced prehospital care
▶ Is presented in three parts: Part 1—the normal cell and the cellular environment; Part 2—disease causes and pathophysiology; Part 3—the body's defenses against disease and injury

Chapter 9 General Principles of Pharmacology 289

▶ Presents an overview of basic pharmacology relevant to advanced prehospital care
▶ Is presented in two parts: Part 1—basic pharmacology; Part 2—drug classifications

Chapter 10 Intravenous Access and Medication Administration 391

▶ Details the skill of medication administration in advanced prehospital care
▶ Presents an overview of medical mathematics and drug dose calculation

Chapter 11 Therapeutic Communications 487

▶ Discusses skills and techniques of communication between the paramedic and the patient and between the paramedic and other health care providers

Chapter 12 Life Span Development 507

▶ Discusses physiological and psychosocial characteristics of developmental stages from infancy through late adulthood

Chapter 13 Airway Management and Ventilation 529

▶ Details the skills of airway management and ventilation at the level of advanced prehospital care

Appendix: Research in EMS 647

▶ Discusses the importance of research in EMS
▶ Explains how to read and evaluate published research
▶ Describes how to undertake or to participate in a research project

Content Overview

VOLUME 2 PATIENT ASSESSMENT

Below is a brief content description of each chapter in Volume 2, *Patient Assessment.*

Chapter 1   **The History**   1

▶ Provides the basic components of a complete health history
▶ Discusses how to effectively conduct an interview
▶ Provides suggestions for communicating with difficult patients, hostile patients, and patients with language barriers

Chapter 2   **Physical Exam Techniques**   27

▶ Presents the techniques of conducting a comprehensive physical exam
▶ Includes in each section a review of anatomy and physiology

Chapter 3   **Patient Assessment in the Field**   183

▶ Offers a practical approach to conducting problem-oriented history and physical exams

Chapter 4   **Clinical Decision Making**   246

▶ Provides the basic steps for making clinical decisions
▶ Discusses how to think critically in emergency situations

Chapter 5   **Communications**   262

▶ Discusses communication, the key component that links every phase of an EMS run
▶ Includes several examples of typical radio medical reports

Chapter 6   **Documentation**   286

▶ Describes how to write a prehospital care report (PCR)
▶ Offers examples of the various narrative writing styles

Content Overview

VOLUME 3 MEDICAL EMERGENCIES

Below is a brief content description of each chapter in Volume 3, *Medical Emergencies.*

Chapter 1   Pulmonology   1

▶ Discusses respiratory system anatomy, physiology, and pathophysiology
▶ Discusses respiratory system emergencies
▶ Emphasizes recognition and treatment of reactive airway diseases such as asthma

Chapter 2   Cardiology   64

▶ Discusses cardiovascular system anatomy, physiology, and pathophysiology
▶ Presents material crucial to advanced prehospital cardiac care
▶ Is presented in three parts: Part 1—essential cardiac anatomy, physiology, and electrophysiology; Part 2—cardiac and peripheral vascular system emergencies; Part 3—12-lead ECG monitoring and interpretation

Chapter 3   Neurology   265

▶ Discusses nervous system anatomy, physiology, and pathophysiology
▶ Discusses recognition and management of neurologic emergencies

Chapter 4   Endocrinology   323

▶ Discusses endocrine system anatomy, physiology, and pathophysiology
▶ Discusses recognition and management of endocrine emergencies, with emphasis on diabetic emergencies

Chapter 5   Allergies and Anaphylaxis   356

▶ Reviews the immune system and the pathophysiology of allergic and anaphylactic reactions
▶ Discusses recognition and treatment of allergic reactions, with emphasis on anaphylactic reactions

Chapter 6   Gastroenterology   375

▶ Discusses gastrointestinal system anatomy, physiology, and pathophysiology
▶ Discusses recognition and management of gastrointestinal emergencies

Chapter 7   Urology and Nephrology   410

▶ Discusses genitourinary system anatomy, physiology, and pathophysiology
▶ Discusses recognition and management of urinary system emergencies in males and females and male reproductive system emergencies

Content Overview

VOLUME 3 MEDICAL EMERGENCIES (continued)

Chapter 8 Toxicology and Substance Abuse 444

▶ Discusses basic toxicology and both common and uncommon causes of poisoning
▶ Discusses overdose and substance abuse, including drug and alcohol abuse
▶ Discusses recognition and management of poisoning, overdose, and substance abuse emergencies

Chapter 9 Hematology 510

▶ Discusses the anatomy, physiology, and pathophysiology of the blood, blood-forming organs, and the reticuloendothelial system
▶ Discusses recognition and management of hematological emergencies

Chapter 10 Environmental Emergencies 544

▶ Details the impact of the environment on the body, emphasizing physical, chemical, and biological aspects
▶ Discusses recognition and management of heat disorders, cold disorders, drowning emergencies, diving emergencies, high-altitude emergencies, and radiation emergencies

Chapter 11 Infectious Disease 591

▶ Addresses specific infectious diseases and modes of transmission
▶ Emphasizes prevention of disease transmission, especially the protection of prehospital personnel
▶ Discusses recognition and management of specific infectious diseases

Chapter 12 Psychiatric and Behavioral Disorders 660

▶ Presents an overview of psychiatric disorders and behavioral problems
▶ Discusses recognition and management of psychiatric and behavioral emergencies

Chapter 13 Gynecology 691

▶ Discusses female reproductive system anatomy, physiology, and pathophysiology
▶ Discusses recognition and management of gynecological emergencies

Chapter 14 Obstetrics 712

▶ Discusses the anatomy and physiology of pregnancy
▶ Discusses how to assist a normal delivery
▶ Discusses recognition and management of complications of pregnancy and delivery

Content Overview

VOLUME 4 TRAUMA EMERGENCIES

Below is a brief content description of each chapter in Volume 4, *Trauma Emergencies*.

Chapter 1   Trauma and Trauma Systems   1

▶ Discusses the nature of trauma and its costs to society
▶ Introduces the concept of trauma care systems
▶ Outlines the role of the paramedic in trauma care
▶ Introduces trauma triage protocols

Chapter 2   Blunt Trauma   20

▶ Describes the kinetics and biomechanics of blunt trauma
▶ Outlines how to evaluate the mechanism of injury in cases of blunt trauma in order to determine likely injuries

Chapter 3   Penetrating Trauma   60

▶ Describes the physics of penetrating trauma and the effects of penetrating trauma on the body
▶ Outlines how to evaluate the mechanism of injury of penetrating trauma in order to determine likely injuries

Chapter 4   Hemorrhage and Shock   83

▶ Describes the anatomy, physiology, and pathophysiology of the cardiovascular system as they apply to hemorrhage and shock
▶ Discusses the assessment and management of hemorrhage and shock

Chapter 5   Soft-Tissue Trauma   134

▶ Reviews the anatomy and physiology of the integumentary system
▶ Discusses the pathophysiology of soft-tissue trauma
▶ Discusses the assessment and management of soft-tissue trauma, including a discussion of bandaging

Chapter 6   Burns   182

▶ Describes the anatomy, physiology, and pathophysiology of burn injuries
▶ Discusses the assessment and management of burns

Chapter 7   Musculoskeletal Trauma   221

▶ Reviews the anatomy and physiology of the musculoskeletal system
▶ Discusses the various types of injuries and conditions that can affect the musculoskeletal system
▶ Discusses the assessment and management of musculoskeletal trauma, including discussions of realignment, splinting, and pain control

Content Overview

VOLUME 4 TRAUMA EMERGENCIES (continued)

Chapter 8   Head, Facial, and Neck Trauma   280

▶ Reviews the anatomy and physiology of the head, face, and neck
▶ Describes the common results of trauma to these regions
▶ Discusses the assessment and management of trauma to the head, face, and neck, with special emphasis on early recognition of injuries and early protection of the airway

Chapter 9   Spinal Trauma   344

▶ Reviews the anatomy and physiology of the spine
▶ Discusses common mechanisms of spinal injury
▶ Discusses the assessment and management of spinal injuries and suspected spinal injuries

Chapter 10   Thoracic Trauma   404

▶ Reviews the anatomy and physiology of the thorax
▶ Discusses common mechanisms of thoracic injury
▶ Discusses the assessment and management of thoracic injuries

Chapter 11   Abdominal Trauma   452

▶ Reviews the anatomy and physiology of the abdomen
▶ Describes abdominal trauma pathology by organ and organ systems
▶ Discusses the assessment and management of abdominal injuries, with special emphasis on the need for maintaining a high index of suspicion when there is potential internal injury

Chapter 12   Shock Trauma Resuscitation   484

▶ Reviews the process of assessment for the trauma patient
▶ Describes the basic elements and steps of shock trauma resuscitation
▶ Reviews methods of improving the delivery of care to trauma patients, including good communications, use of air medical transport, and participation in research programs

Content Overview

VOLUME 5 SPECIAL CONSIDERATIONS/OPERATIONS

Below is a brief content description of each chapter in Volume 5, *Special Considerations/Operations.*

Chapter 1 Neonatology 1

▶ Introduces the specialized world of neonatology
▶ Discusses how size and anatomy affect assessment and treatment
▶ Emphasizes neonatal resuscitation in the field setting

Chapter 2 Pediatrics 40

▶ Provides an overview of common and uncommon pediatric emergencies encountered in a field setting
▶ Emphasizes that children are not "small adults"
▶ Presents specialized pediatric assessment techniques and field emergency procedures

Chapter 3 Geriatrics 146

▶ Reviews the anatomy and physiology of aging
▶ Discusses the assessment and treatment of emergencies commonly seen in the elderly

Chapter 4 Abuse and Assault 218

▶ Provides information about detecting abusive or dangerous situations
▶ Discusses the special needs of victims of abuse or assault

Chapter 5 The Challenged Patient 238

▶ Addresses the special needs of patients with physical, mental, or cultural challenges
▶ Emphasizes strategies that can be used to reduce challenged patient stress
▶ Describes methods to conduct a thorough and accurate assessment of a challenged patient

Chapter 6 Acute Interventions for the Chronic Care Patient 263

▶ Discusses the role of EMS personnel in treating home care patients and patients with chronic medical conditions
▶ Provides an overview of equipment commonly found in a home care setting
▶ Examines strategies for working with the family and caregivers encountered in most home care situations

Chapter 7 Assessment-Based Management 306

▶ Discusses the diagnostic skills involved in assessment-based management
▶ Provides scenarios that illustrate comprehensive patient assessment

Content Overview

VOLUME 5 SPECIAL CONSIDERATIONS/OPERATIONS (continued)

Chapter 8 Ambulance Operations 335

▶ Reviews the medical equipment aboard most ambulances and stresses the need for safe driving procedures
▶ Emphasizes the need for a constant state of readiness for every call

Chapter 9 Medical Incident Management 360

▶ Discusses the National Incident Management System
▶ Shows how the incident management system can be used in daily operations

Chapter 10 Rescue Awareness and Operations 399

▶ Details the varying involvement of EMS personnel in rescue operations
▶ Emphasizes the importance of scene safety and the early request for specialized rescue teams

Chapter 11 Hazardous Materials Incidents 446

▶ Emphasizes the danger of hazmat situations and the fundamental procedures in identifying hazardous materials
▶ Details the procedures in assessing and treating contaminated patients

Chapter 12 Crime Scene Awareness 478

▶ Provides an overview of crime scene operations
▶ Discusses the importance of preserving evidence while providing effective patient care

Chapter 13 Rural EMS 500

▶ Goes beyond the DOT curriculum to enhance the awareness of the special needs of rural residents and wilderness recreation participants and of the EMS personnel who serve them
▶ Emphasizes the importance of distance in decision making at most rural emergencies

Chapter 14 Responding to Terrorist Acts 524

▶ Provides information on explosive, nuclear, chemical, and biological agents
▶ Emphasizes scene safety
▶ Discusses how to recognize a terrorist attack
▶ Details responses to terrorist attacks

Detailed Contents

Series Preface xxiii ▸ Preface xxix ▸ Acknowledgments xxxi ▸ About the Authors xxxv

Chapter 1   The History 1

INTRODUCTION   3

ESTABLISHING PATIENT RAPPORT   4
Setting the Stage 4 ▸ The First Impression 4 ▸ Introductions 5 ▸ Asking
Questions 6 ▸ Language and Communication 8 ▸ Taking a History on Sensitive Topics 9

THE COMPREHENSIVE PATIENT HISTORY   10
Preliminary Data 10 ▸ The Chief Complaint 11 ▸ The Present Illness 11 ▸ The Past
History 13 ▸ Current Health Status 14 ▸ Review of Systems 17

SPECIAL CHALLENGES   19
Silence 19 ▸ Overly Talkative Patients 20 ▸ Patients with Multiple Symptoms 20
▸ Anxious Patients 20 ▸ Patients Needing Reassurance 21 ▸ Anger and Hostility 21
▸ Intoxication 21 ▸ Crying 21 ▸ Depression 22 ▸ Sexually Attractive or Seductive Patients
22 ▸ Confusing Behaviors or Histories 22 ▸ Limited Intelligence 22 ▸ Language Barriers
23 ▸ Hearing Problems 23 ▸ Blindness 23 ▸ Talking with Families or Friends 23

Chapter 2   Physical Exam Techniques 27

PHYSICAL EXAMINATION APPROACH AND OVERVIEW   30
Examination Techniques 31 ▸ Equipment 35 ▸ The General Approach 38

OVERVIEW OF A COMPREHENSIVE EXAMINATION   39
The General Survey 39

ANATOMICAL REGIONS   51
The Skin 52 ▸ The Hair 55 ▸ The Nails 58 ▸ The Head 60 ▸ The Eyes 62 ▸ The Ears 72
▸ The Nose 76 ▸ The Mouth 78 ▸ The Neck 82 ▸ The Chest and Lungs 84
▸ The Cardiovascular System 92 ▸ The Abdomen 97 ▸ The Female Genitalia 103 ▸ The
Male Genitalia 106 ▸ The Anus 107 ▸ The Musculoskeletal System 108 ▸ The Peripheral
Vascular System 136 ▸ The Nervous System 142

PHYSICAL EXAMINATION OF INFANTS AND CHILDREN   167
Building Patient and Family Rapport 167 ▸ General Appearance and Behavior 167
▸ Anatomy and the Physical Exam 169

RECORDING EXAMINATION FINDINGS   175

Chapter 3   Patient Assessment in the Field 183

INTRODUCTION   186

SCENE SIZE-UP   187
Standard Precautions 188 ▸ Scene Safety 190 ▸ Location of All Patients 195 ▸ Mechanism
of Injury 196 ▸ Nature of the Illness 197

THE INITIAL ASSESSMENT 198
Forming a General Impression 198 ▶ Mental Status 200 ▶ AVPU Levels 200 ▶ Airway Assessment 201 ▶ Breathing Assessment 206 ▶ Circulation Assessment 207 ▶ Priority Determination 210

THE FOCUSED HISTORY AND PHYSICAL EXAM 211
The Major Trauma Patient 211 ▶ The Isolated-Injury Trauma Patient 221 ▶ The Responsive Medical Patient 222 ▶ The Unresponsive Medical Patient 230

THE DETAILED PHYSICAL EXAM 231
Components of the Comprehensive Exam 232 ▶ Vital Signs 238 ▶ Recording Exam Findings 238

ONGOING ASSESSMENT 238
Mental Status 238 ▶ Airway Patency 238 ▶ Breathing Rate and Quality 239 ▶ Pulse Rate and Quality 240 ▶ Skin Condition 240 ▶ Transport Priorities 240 ▶ Vital Signs 240 ▶ Focused Assessment 240 ▶ Effects of Interventions 241 ▶ Management Plans 241

Chapter 4   Clinical Decision Making 246

INTRODUCTION TO CRITICAL THINKING 248

PARAMEDIC PRACTICE 248
Patient Acuity 249 ▶ Protocols and Algorithms 250

CRITICAL THINKING SKILLS 250
Fundamental Knowledge and Abilities 251 ▶ Useful Thinking Styles 253

THINKING UNDER PRESSURE 255
Mental Checklist 255

THE CRITICAL DECISION PROCESS 256
Form a Concept 256 ▶ Interpret the Data 257 ▶ Apply the Principles 257 ▶ Evaluate the Results 257 ▶ Reflect on the Incident 258 ▶ Putting It All Together 258

Chapter 5   Communications 262

INTRODUCTION TO COMMUNICATION 264

BASIC COMMUNICATION MODEL 265

VERBAL COMMUNICATION 266

WRITTEN COMMUNICATION 267
Terminology 268

THE EMS RESPONSE 269

COMMUNICATION TECHNOLOGY 276
Radio Communication 276 ▶ Alternative Technologies 278 ▶ New Technology 279

REPORTING PROCEDURES 280
Standard Format 280 ▶ General Radio Procedures 281

REGULATION 282

Chapter 6   Documentation   286

INTRODUCTION   288

USES FOR DOCUMENTATION   288
Medical 288 ▶ Administrative 289 ▶ Research 289 ▶ Legal 289

GENERAL CONSIDERATIONS   290
Medical Terminology 292 ▶ Abbreviations and Acronyms 292 ▶ Times 297
▶ Communications 298 ▶ Pertinent Negatives 298 ▶ Oral Statements 298
▶ Additional Resources 298

ELEMENTS OF GOOD DOCUMENTATION   299
Completeness and Accuracy 299 ▶ Legibility 299 ▶ Timeliness
301 ▶ Absence of Alterations 301 ▶ Professionalism 302

NARRATIVE WRITING   302
Narrative Sections 302 ▶ General Formats 305

SPECIAL CONSIDERATIONS   307
Patient Refusals 307 ▶ Services Not Needed 309 ▶ Multiple-Casualty
Incidents 309

CONSEQUENCES OF INAPPROPRIATE DOCUMENTATION   311

CLOSING   311

Precautions on Bloodborne Pathogens and Infectious Disease   317
Suggested Responses to "You Make the Call"   319
Answers to "Review Questions"   323
Glossary   325
Index   329

Photo Scans/Procedures

2-1   Taking Vital Signs   43

2-2   Examining the Head   64

2-3   Examining the Eyes   67

2-4   Examining the Ears   74

2-5   Examining the Nose   79

2-6   Examining the Mouth   81

2-7   Examining the Neck   85

2-8   Examining the Chest   89

2-9   Assessing the Cardiovascular System   96

2-10   Examining the Abdomen   104

2-11   Examining the Wrist and Hand   114

2-12   Examining the Elbow   118

2-13   Examining the Shoulder   122

2-14   Examining the Ankle and Foot   125

2-15   Examining the Knee   129

2-16   Examining the Hip   133

2-17   Assessing the Spine   135

2-18   Assessing the Peripheral Vascular System   140

2-19   Assessing the Cranial Nerves   155

2-20   Assessing the Motor System   158

2-21   Testing the Reflexes   165

3-1   Circulation Assessment   208

3-2   Rapid Trauma Assessment—The Head and Neck   215

3-3   Rapid Trauma Assessment—The Chest   217

3-4   Rapid Trauma Assessment—The Pelvis and Extremities   219

3-5   Detailed Physical Exam—The Head and Neck   233

3-6   Detailed Physical Exam—The Torso   236

3-7   Ongoing Assessment   239

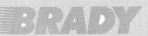

It's Your Profession

Dear Student:

Congratulations on your decision to undertake the EMT-Paramedic educational program. Your desire to further your education and to help your community is indeed noble. As authors, we welcome you to the *Paramedic Care: Principles & Practice* program, which will provide the core foundation for your paramedic education. This series of five volumes will serve as a guide through the educational process. Your instructor will lead you through the materials contained in these books and help you to integrate what you have learned into clinical practice.

Rest assured that the *Paramedic Care: Principles & Practice* series contains accurate, state-of-the-art information. The author team, collectively, has over 75 years of pre-hospital care experience. All three authors hold graduate or professional college degrees and are experienced educators in their own right. Our author team is intimately involved in EMS on a daily basis either in a local EMS system, an educational program, or at a national level. The Brady EMS texts have long been regarded as a respected leader in prehospital educational materials. We are proud to be a part of the Brady team and to continue the legacy.

The author team is backed by a team of publishing professionals whose only acceptable standards are quality and accuracy. Every person involved in the writing and production of this text has made a commitment to quality. Publisher, editors, artists, compositors, and support staff have invested thousands of hours in the books you will be reading to assure that you are provided with the best educational materials available. In addition to the core textbooks, Brady has prepared myriad support materials to assist you and your instructors. These include instructional CDs, a companion website, companion workbooks, review manuals, and an online test preparation program. Brady provides the entire package—all prepared with the same commitment to accuracy and quality.

Textbooks constitute only a part of the educational process. You will be led through this challenging yet rewarding process by your instructors. They are experienced EMS personnel and educators who will clarify the art and science of prehospital care and answer questions you will have. Textbooks can only illustrate the performance of psychomotor skills. Your instructors will guide you through mastery of these essential skills prior to entering the clinical setting. As part of your educational program, you will observe and practice these skills on living patients, to prepare you for the realities of prehospital emergencies.

Welcome to the world of paramedicine. Be safe. Have fun. We wish you all the best in your education and in the practice of EMS.

Sincerely,

Bryan E. Bledsoe, DO, FACEP   Robert S. Porter   Richard A. Cherry

Series Preface

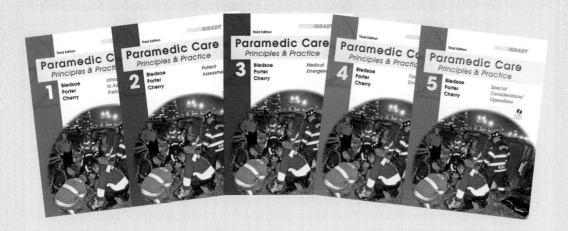

Congratulations on your decision to further your EMS career by undertaking the course of education required for certification as an Emergency Medical Technician–Paramedic! The world of paramedic emergency care is one that you will find both challenging and rewarding. Whether you will be working as a volunteer or a paid paramedic, you will find the field of advanced prehospital care very interesting.

This textbook, **the 3rd edition of *Paramedic Care: Principles & Practice,*** will serve as your guide and reference to advanced prehospital care. It is based on the U.S. Department of Transportation's *Emergency Medical Technician–Paramedic National Standard Curriculum* and is divided into five volumes:

Volume 1 *Introduction to Advanced Prehospital Care*
Volume 2 *Patient Assessment*
Volume 3 *Medical Emergencies*
Volume 4 *Trauma Emergencies*
Volume 5 *Special Considerations/Operations*

Volume 1, *Introduction to Advanced Prehospital Care,* presents the foundations of paramedic practice as well as an introduction to pathophysiology, pharmacology, medication administration, and airway management and ventilation. **Volume 2, *Patient Assessment,*** adds the cognitive and psychomotor skills of patient assessment, communications, and documentation. This knowledge base expands as the series applies it to the medical patient in **Volume 3, *Medical Emergencies,*** and to the trauma patient in **Volume 4, *Trauma Emergencies.*** **Volume 5, *Special Considerations/Operations,*** enriches these general patient care concepts and principles with applications to special patients and circumstances we commonly see as paramedics. The product of this complete and integrated series is a set of principles of care you will be required to practice as a paramedic.

Your paramedic education program should include ample classroom, practical laboratory, in-hospital clinical, and prehospital field experience. These educational experiences must be guided by instructors and preceptors with special training and experience in their areas of participation in your program.

DEVELOPING ADVANCED SKILLS

The psychomotor skills of fluid and medication administration, advanced airway care, ECG monitoring and defibrillation, and advanced medical and trauma patient care are best learned first in the classroom and the skills laboratory and then in the clinical and field settings. Commonly required advanced prehospital skills are discussed in the text as well as outlined in the procedure photo summaries. Review these before and while practicing each skill.

It is important to underscore that neither this nor any other text can teach skills. Care skills are learned only under the watchful eye of a paramedic instructor and perfected during your clinical and field internship.

CONTENT OF THE FIVE VOLUMES

It is intended that your program coordinator will assign reading from *Paramedic Care: Principles & Practice* in preparation for each classroom lecture and discussion session. The knowledge gained from reading this text will form the foundation of the information you will need in order to function effectively as a paramedic in your EMS system. Your instructors will build on this information to strengthen your knowledge and understanding of advanced prehospital care so that you may apply it in your practice.

The content of each volume of *Paramedic Care: Principles & Practice* is summarized below, with an emphasis on "what's new" in this 3rd edition. All volumes have been updated to conform to the *2005 American Heart Association Guidelines for Cardiopulmonary Resuscitation and Emergency Cardiovascular Care.*

Volume 1 Introduction to Advanced Prehospital Care

Volume 1 addresses the fundamentals of paramedic practice, including paramedic roles and responsibilities, pathophysiology, pharmacology, medication administration, and advanced airway management.

What's New in Volume 1?

- In Chapter 1, "Introduction to Advanced Prehospital Care," there is a new emphasis on **overlapping responsibilities in three areas: health care, public health, and public safety.**
- In Chapter 2, "The Well-Being of the Paramedic," there is additional emphasis on **safe driving habits and avoiding ambulance collisions.** Critical Incident Stress Debriefings are no longer recommended, the new emphasis among mental health practitioners being **resiliency-based care** to promote emotional strength. Special "Legal Notes" discuss **substance abuse in EMS** and **field pronouncements regarding not resuscitating pulseless victims of blunt trauma.**
- In Chapter 3, "EMS Systems," a section is added on the new **National EMS Scope of Practice** and the **four new levels of EMS licensure (Emergency Medical Responder, Emergency Medical Technician, Advanced EMT, and Paramedic)** that will be recognized as the new Scope of Practice is adopted. A new section, "Twenty-First Century," discusses **post 9/11 changes, problems, and challenges such as coordination among agencies, communications,** and others.
- Chapter 6, "Medical/Legal Aspects of Advanced Prehospital Care," contains a new section on the **duty to report** (e.g., abuse), and a discussion of **terminating resuscitaiton of pulseless blunt-trauma patients**.
- Chapter 8, "General Principles of Pathophysiology," includes a new section on **natriuretic peptides** and their effects on the circulatory system.

- Chapter 13, "Airway Management and Ventilation," discusses **continuous waveform capnography** as the best way to monitor endotracheal tube placement and ventilation status, and an important new section on **approaches to the difficult airway** has been added.

Volume 2: Patient Assessment

Volume 2 builds on the assessment skills taught in the basic EMT course, emphasizing advanced-level patient assessment and clinical decision making at the scene.

What's New in Volume 2?

- Chapter 2, "Physical Exam Techniques," and Chapter 3, "Patient Assessment in the Field" include twenty-one new **Assessment Pearls** features.
- Chapter 3, "Patient Assessment in the Field," includes new information on **hemostatic agents** (e.g., HemCon and QuickClot) used by the military to stop uncontrolled hemorrhage, that may soon be used by civilian EMS responders. A discussion is included of new **hemoglobin-based oxygen-carrying solutions** (e.g., PolyHeme and HemoPure) that show promise for prehospital use.
- Chapter 5, "Communications," includes new information on **event data recorders (EDRs)** that auto makers may install in some vehicles. A discussion is also included of the **need to update the current analog 911 system to adopt newer technologies** that could handle digital text, data, photos, and videos and improve EMS response capabilities.

Volume 3: Medical Emergencies

Volume 3 addresses the paramedic level of care in medical emergencies. Particular emphasis is placed on respiratory and cardiovascular emergencies, which are the most common EMS medical calls.

What's New in Volume 3?

- Chapter 1, "Pulmonology," now includes discussions of **continuous positive airway pressure (CPAP) devices** in the treatment of **obstructive sleep apnea,** adult respiratory distress syndrome (ARDS), chronic bronchitis, and carbon monoxide inhalation. **New-generation pulse oximeters (CO-oximeteres)** that can distinguish carbon monoxide saturation from oxygen saturation are discussed.
- Chapter 2, "Cardiology," has added discussion of the following dysrhythymias not included in prior editions: **sinus block, sinus pause, sick sinus syndrome, supraventricular tachycardia, 2:1 AV block, junctional bradycardia, torsades de pointes, agonal rhythm,** and **P wave asystole.** New information is included on **ECG changes due to hypokalemia, hyperkalemia, hypocalcemia, hypercalcemia, and digitalis.** Discussion has been added on **distinguising ST-segment elevation myocardial infarction (STEMI) and non-ST-segment elevation myocardial infarction (NSTEMI).** A new section on **reperfusion therapies** has been included with new sections on **percutaneous intervention (PCI), coronary arteriogram/angiogram, percutaneous transluminal coronary angioplasty (PTCA), primary coronary stenting,** and **coronary artery bypass grafting (CABG).** Various uses of CPAP are dicussed, including **CPAP for management of congestive heart failure.** New information is included on **three phases of cardiac arrest—electrical, circulatory, and metabolic phases—with implications for emergency care** of an arrest. **Field termination of resuscitation** is also discussed.
- Chapter 3, "Neurology," has added information on the **CO-oximeter** as an assessment tool to detect carbon monoxide poisoning as a possible cause of altered

mental status. A new section on **prehospital stroke scoring systems—Los Ange-les Prehospital Stroke Screen (LAPSS) and Cincinnati Prehospital Stroke Scale (CPSS)** has been added.

▶ Chapter 6, "Gastroenterology," now includes discussion of **hepatitis G** in addition to the other forms of hepatitis.

▶ Chapter 8, "Toxicology and Substance Abuse," includes entirely revised and updated sections on **carbon monoxide and cyanide poisonings (and their co-occurrence)** and new treatments. New sections are included on **"Serotonin Syndrome," "Africanized Honey Bees,"** and **"Ciguatera Poisoning."**

▶ Chapter 10, "Environmental Emergencies" features an extensively revised and updated section on **drowning.**

▶ Chapter 11, "Infectious Disease" includes new information on **postexposure pro-phylaxis for AIDS, hepatitis G,** and **avian influenza.**

▶ Chapter 12, "Psychiatric and Behavior Disorders," has a new section on **excited delirium.**

Volume 4: Trauma Emergencies

Volume 4 discusses advanced prehospital care of the trauma patient, from mechanism-of-injury analysis to care of specific types of trauma to general principles of shock/trauma resuscitation.

What's New in Volume 4?

▶ Chapter 1, "Trauma and Trauma Systems," discusses an important **public-health approach to trauma** in the new section **"Trauma as a Disease,"** with subsections on surveillance, risk analysis, intervention development, implementation, and evaluation.

▶ Chapter 2, "Blunt Trauma," includes extensively revised and updated sections on **blunt trauma, kinetics of impact,** and **biomechanics of trauma.**

▶ Chapter 4, "Hemorrhage and Shock," includes a new section on **topical hemostatic agents** to promote clotting.

▶ Chapter 8, "Head, Facial, and Neck Trauma," has an added discussion of the **Monroe Kelly doctrine** explaining the factors that can increase intracranial pressure to the point of brain herniation. There is a new emphasis on monitoring ventilation levels through **capnography and pulse oximetry to avoid both hyperventilation and hypoventilation** and to keep ventilation within optimal ranges.

▶ Chapter 9, "Spinal Trauma," has been **extensively revised and updated through-out** to include new information on spinal anatomy and physiology and spinal syndromes (including **pediatric spinal injuries**) and to reflect **current guidelines on spinal clearance and spinal care.**

▶ Chapter 10, "Thoracic Trauma," has added a section on **commotio cordis,** which is ventricular fibrillation induced by a direct blow to the chest, as a (rare) cause of **sudden death in young athletes.**

Volume 5: Special Considerations/Operations

Volume 5 addresses such topics as neonatal, pediatric, and geriatric care; home health care; challenged patients; as well as incident command, ambulance service, rescue, hazardous materials incidents, crime scene operations, and responding to terrorist acts.

What's New in Volume 5?

◗ Chapter 1, "Neonatology," notes structures needed for intrauterine life that change after birth and includes new illustrations of **congenital anomalies.** Included are **new guildelines on treatment of vigorous and nonvirgorous newborn infants when meconium is present.** There are also **new guidelines for administration of naloxone in cases of maternal narcotic use.**

◗ Chapter 2, "Pediatrics," includes a new section on **rescue airways** (e.g., pediatric LMA). The Trauma section includes a new segment on **multiple casualty incidents involving children** with discussion of the **JumpSTART** pediatric triage system.

◗ Chapter 3, "Geriatrics," features a new section on **ankylosing spondylitis** (severe spinal deformity).

◗ Chapter 4, "Abuse and Assault," features a new section on **maternal drug abuse.**

◗ Chapter 8, "Ambulance Operations," includes new information on the **importance of specific response times.**

◗ In Chapter 9, "Medical Incident Management," the section on the **U.S. Department of Homeland Security National Incident Management System (NIMS) has been extensively updated.**

◗ Chapter 10, "Rescue Awareness and Operations," includes a new section on **hybrid vehicles** and the dangers to rescuers of hybrid vehicles' **high-voltage electrical systems.**

◗ In Chapter 11, "Hazardous Materials Incidents," there is new information on a safer and less toxic antidote for cyanide poisoning, the **Cyanokit.**

Preface to Volume 2

Today's paramedics are professional health care clinicians and practitioners of emergency field medicine. The present paramedic curriculum provides both a broad-based medical education and a specific intensive training program designed to prepare paramedics to perform their traditional role as providers of emergency field medicine. The curriculum also provides a broad foundation in anatomy and physiology, patient assessment, pathophysiology of disease, and pharmacology that allows paramedics to expand their roles in the health care industry. The five-volume *Paramedic Care: Principles & Practice* and, in particular, *Volume 2, Patient Assessment*, reflect these broad and specific purposes.

This volume provides paramedic students with the principles of patient assessment. The first two chapters present the techniques of conducting a comprehensive history and physical exam. The remaining chapters discuss ways to apply the techniques learned in the first two chapters to real patient situations.

OVERVIEW OF THE CHAPTERS

Chapter 1, "The History" provides the basic components of a complete health history. These components include the chief complaint, the present history, the past history, the current health status, and the review of systems. This constitutes a comprehensive history and is not meant to be used in its entirety in emergency field situations. Elements of the comprehensive history will be used, as appropriate, in the field. Chapter 1 also discusses how to effectively conduct an interview and use nonverbal communication skills to elicit vital information from your patients. In addition, it provides suggestions for communicating with difficult patients, communicating with hostile patients, and overcoming language barriers.

Chapter 2, "Physical Exam Techniques" presents the techniques of conducting a comprehensive physical exam. Like the history, the comprehensive physical exam taught in this volume is not intended for all situations. With time and clinical experience, you will learn which components of the history and physical exam are appropriate to assess and manage each particular patient and situation. If you are hired to conduct pre-employment physical exams, for example, you may use the history and physical exam in their entirety. If you are assessing and managing a critical patient in the field, you will select those components most appropriate for that situation. Topics in this chapter include assessing the skin, the head, the neck, the chest (along with the respiratory and cardiovascular systems), the abdomen and digestive system, the extremities and musculoskeletal system, and the peripheral vascular system as well as how to conduct a comprehensive neurologic exam. Included in each section is a review of the anatomy and physiology relevant to those areas of the exam.

Chapter 3, "Patient Assessment in the Field" offers a practical approach to conducting problem-oriented history and physical exams. It deals with ways to use your new skills to assess patients in the field. With time and clinical experience, you will learn which components are appropriate for different situations. Topics include scene safety, the initial assessment, the focused history and physical exam (for the responsive medical patient, the unresponsive medical patient, the trauma patient with significant mechanism of injury, and the trauma patient with an isolated injury), the detailed physical exam, and the ongoing assessment.

Chapter 4, "Clinical Decision Making" provides the basic steps for making clinical decisions. It describes each step in detail and discusses how to think critically in emergency situations. Topics include forming a concept, interpreting the data, applying principles of emergency medicine, evaluating your treatment plan, and reflecting on your care after the emergency response. The approaches discussed in this chapter are unique to emergency medical services textbooks.

Chapter 5, "Communications" deals with verbal communication. Communication is the key component that links all phases of an EMS response and helps ensure continuity of care. Topics include the principles of communication, communication during the different phases of an EMS response, communication technology, and giving an oral medical report. The chapter provides several examples of typical radio medical reports.

Chapter 6, "Documentation" concerns writing a prehospital care report, or PCR. Topics include the use of medical terminology and abbreviations, the elements of a good report, writing the narrative, and dealing with patient refusals. The chapter provides examples of the various narrative writing styles.

SUMMARY OF VOLUME 2

This volume, *Patient Assessment,* describes how to conduct a comprehensive history and physical exam and how to document your findings appropriately. It also describes how to perform a problem-oriented patient assessment on a real patient in the field, report your findings to your medical direction physician as well as to personnel of the receiving facility, and document the response on your PCR.

Acknowledgments

REVIEW BOARD

Our special thanks to Joseph J. Mistovich, Chairperson and Professor, Department of Health Professions, Youngstown State University, Youngstown, Ohio, for his review of the first edition of *Patient Assessment*. His knowledge of the paramedic curriculum, experience, and high standards proved to be significant contributions to text development.

Our special thanks also to Dr. Howard A. Werman, Professor, Department of Emergency Medicine, The Ohio State University College of Medicine and Public Health, Columbus, Ohio. Dr. Werman's reviews of the first edition were carefully prepared, and we appreciate the thoughtful advice and keen insight he shared with us.

INSTRUCTOR REVIEWERS

The reviewers of this edition of *Paramedic Care: Principles & Practice* have provided many excellent suggestions and ideas for improving the text. The quality of the reviews has been outstanding, and the reviews have been a major aid in the preparation and revision of the manuscript. The assistance provided by these EMS experts is deeply appreciated.

Mike Dymes, NREMT-P
EMS Program Director
Durham Technical Community College
Durham, NC

Ginger K. Floyd, BA, NREMT-P
Assistant Professor
Austin Community College EMS Professions
Austin, TX

Darren P. Lacroix
Del Mar College
Emergency Medical Service Professions
Corpus Christi, TX

Greg Mullen, MS, NREMT-P
National EMS Academy
Lafayette, LA

Deborah L. Petty, BS, EMT-P I/C
Training Officer
St. Charles County Ambulance District
St. Peter's, MO

B. Jeanine Riner, MHSA, BS, RRT, NREMT-P
GA Office of EMS and Trauma
Atlanta, GA

Aaron Weitzman, BS, NREMT-P
Lieutenant (ret.)
Faculty, Emergency Medical Services
Baltimore City Community College
Baltimore, MD

Brian J. Wilson, BA, NREMT-P
Education Director
Texas Tech School of Medicine
El Paso, TX

We also wish to express appreciation to the following EMS professionals who reviewed the second edition of *Paramedic Care: Principles & Practice.* Their suggestions and perspectives helped to make this program a successful teaching tool.

Brenda M. Beasley, RN, BS, EMT-P
Department Chair, Allied Health
Calhoun Community College
Decatur, AL

Shannon Bruley, BAS, EMT-P, I/C
Program Manager
EMS, Firefighter/Paramedic, Fire Science
Henry Ford Community College
Dearborn, MI

Jeff Fritz, BS, NREMT-P
Temple College
Temple, TX

Melissa Kendrick, RN, BSN, BS, NREMT-P
Memorial Hermann Life Flight
Houston, TX

David M. LaCombe, NREMT-P
National EMS Academy
Lafayette, LA

Lawrence Linder, BA, NREMT-P
EMS Faculty
St. Petersburg College
Pinellas Park, FL

Keith A. Monosky, MPM, EMT-P
Assistant Professor
The George Washington University
Washington, DC

Allen O. Patterson
Holmes Community College
Ridgeland, MS

Randy Perkins, CEP
Paramedic Program Director
Scottsdale Community College
Scottsdale, AZ

Janet L. Schulte, BS, AS, NR-CCEMT-P
IHM Health Studies Center
St. Louis, MO

John Todaro, REMT-P, RN, TNS
Director
Emergency Medicine Learning
* and Resource Center*
Orlando, FL

Andrew R. Turcotte, NREMT-P, EMS I/C
Old Orchard Beach Fire Department
Old Orchard Beach, ME

PHOTO ACKNOWLEDGMENTS

All photographs not credited adjacent to the photograph or in the photo credit section below were photographed on assignment for Brady/Prentice Hall/Pearson Education.

Organizations

We wish to thank the following organizations for their valuable assistance in creating the photo program for this edition:

Flower Mound Fire Department
Flower Mound, TX

Tyco Health Care/Nellcor Puritan Bennet
Pleasanton, CA

Models

Thanks to the following people from the Flower Mound Fire Department, Flower Mound, Texas, who provided locations and/or portrayed patients and EMS providers in our photographs.

FAO/Paramedic Wade Woody
FF/Paramedic Tim Mackling
FF/Paramedic Matthew Daniel
FF/Paramedic Jon Rea
FF/Paramedic Waylon Palmer
FF/EMT Jesse Palmer
Captain/EMT Billy McWhorter

About the Authors

BRYAN E. BLEDSOE, DO, FACEP, EMT-P

Dr. Bryan Bledsoe is an emergency physician with a special interest in prehospital care. He received his B.S. degree from the University of Texas at Arlington and his medical degree from the University of North Texas Health Sciences Center/Texas College of Osteopathic Medicine. He completed his internship at Texas Tech University and residency training at Scott and White Memorial Hospital/Texas A&M College of Medicine. Dr. Bledsoe is board certified in emergency medicine.

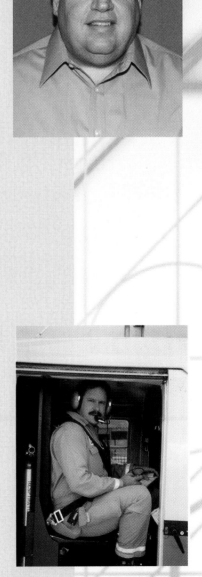

Prior to attending medical school, Dr. Bledsoe worked as an EMT, a paramedic, and a paramedic instructor. He completed EMT training in 1974 and paramedic training in 1976 and worked for 6 years as a field paramedic in Fort Worth, Texas. In 1979, he joined the faculty of the University of North Texas Health Sciences Center and served as coordinator of EMT and paramedic education programs at the university. Dr. Bledsoe is active in emergency medicine and EMS research. He is a popular speaker at state, national, and international seminars and writes regularly for numerous EMS journals. Dr. Bledsoe is on the faculty of the University of Nevada, Las Vegas. He is active in educational endeavors with the United States Special Operations Command (USSOCOM) and co-chairs their Certification and Evaluation Board (CEB).

Dr. Bledsoe has authored several EMS books published by Brady, including *Paramedic Care: Principles & Practice, Essentials of Paramedic Care, Intermediate Emergency Care: Principles & Practice, Critical Care Paramedic, Anatomy & Physiology for Emergency Care, Prehospital Emergency Pharmacology,* and *Pocket Reference for ALS Providers.* He is married to Emma Bledsoe. They have two children, Bryan and Andrea, and a grandson, Andrew, and live on a ranch south of Dallas, Texas. He enjoys saltwater fishing and warm latitudes.

ROBERT S. PORTER, MA, NREMT-P

Robert Porter has been teaching in emergency medical services for 30 years and currently serves as the Senior Advanced Life Support Educator for Madison County, New York, and as a Flight Paramedic with the Onondaga, New York, County Sheriff's Department helicopter service, AirOne. Mr. Porter is a Wisconsin native and received his bachelor's degree in education from the University of Wisconsin. He completed his paramedic training at Northeast Wisconsin Technical Institute in 1978 and earned a master's degree in health education at Central Michigan University in 1990.

Mr. Porter has been an EMT and EMS educator and administrator since 1973 and obtained his national registration as an EMT-Paramedic in 1978. He has taught both basic and advanced EMS courses in the states of Wisconsin, Michigan, Louisiana, Pennsylvania, and New York. Mr. Porter served for more than 10 years as a paramedic program accreditation-site evaluator for the American Medical Association and is a past chair of the National Society of EMT Instructor/Coordinators. He has authored Brady's *Paramedic Care: Principles & Practice, Essentials of Paramedic Care, Intermediate Emergency Care: Principles & Practice, Tactical Emergency Care,* and *Weapons of Mass Destruction: Emergency Care,* as well as the workbooks accompanying this text, *Paramedic Emergency Care,* and *Intermediate Emergency Care.* When not writing or teaching, Mr. Porter enjoys offshore sailboat racing and historic home restoration.

RICHARD A. CHERRY, MS, NREMT-P

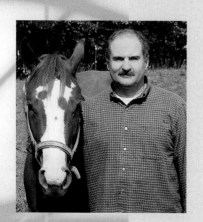

Richard Cherry is Clinical Assistant Professor of Emergency Medicine and Technical Director for Medical Simulation at Upstate Medical University in Syracuse, New York. His experience includes years of classroom teaching and emergency fieldwork. A native of Buffalo, Mr. Cherry earned his bachelor's degree at nearby St. Bonaventure University in 1972. He taught high school for the next 10 years while he earned his master's degree in education from Oswego State University in 1977. He holds a permanent teaching license in New York State.

Mr. Cherry entered the emergency medical services field in 1974 with the DeWitt Volunteer Fire Department, where he served his community as a firefighter and EMS provider for more than 15 years. He took his first EMT course in 1977 and became an ALS provider 2 years later. He earned his paramedic certificate in 1985 as a member of the area's first paramedic class.

Mr. Cherry has authored several books for Brady. Most notable are *Paramedic Care: Principles & Practice, Essentials of Paramedic Care, Intermediate Emergency Care: Principles & Practice,* and *EMT Teaching: A Common Sense Approach.* He has made presentations at many state, national, and international EMS conferences on a variety of teaching topics. He regularly teaches in the paramedic program he helped establish and is Regional Faculty for ACLS and PALS. Mr. Cherry is currently Technical Director for MedSTAR, the center for medical simulation, training, and research at SUNY Upstate. He and his wife, Sue, run a horse-riding camp for children with cancer and other life-threatening diseases on their property in West Monroe, New York. He also plays guitar in a Christian band.

Welcome to Paramedic Care

Brady
Pearson Health Sciences
Upper Saddle River, NJ 07458

Dear Instructor:

Brady, your partner in education, is pleased to present the 3rd edition of our best-selling *Paramedic Care: Principles & Practice.* Like its preceding editions, *PCPP 3* was developed to stay ahead of current trends and practices in Paramedic education and practice. Changes in cardiac care guidelines and equipment, spinal trauma, neonatology, pediatrics, and incident management necessitated one of the most extensive revisions yet. Hundreds of photos and illustrations were updated. We integrated our media—student CD and Companion Website—into each chapter. More visuals are used to explain and reinforce concepts. The Workbooks were updated to include even more critical thinking. A "map" to the new Education Standards will be provided, making transition to these easier and faster.

PCPP's history remains rich and long, and it's changing. A new set of Standards will soon replace the DOT curriculum. Scope of practice will continue to evolve. More research is emerging every day. And EMS is becoming an integral part in the overall chain of care. Brady understands that in times of change, our customers want to be able to rely on us to provide solutions that are accurate, current, and dynamic. Our author team is active and accessible; our editorial, marketing, and sales teams have many years of experience in EMS publishing; and we are backed by the largest and most successful textbook publishing company in the world.

We also know that our customers have unique and different needs. Not all of you will transition to the Standards at the same time. Your scope of practice and protocols are different, depending on where you work. You teach out of firehouses, ambulance services, or colleges. Your students are 18, 35, and 60. You need tools that enable you to teach and learn in your particular environment. Because of this, we will:

- Continue to strive to create products that are flexible, engaging, and relevant;
- Keep our DOT-curriculum products—such as *PCPP*—current for some time, while at the same time offering new solutions for Standards-based education;
- Offer more ways in which to assess students' performance;
- Create curriculum to assist in the Standards transition;
- Provide the largest and most comprehensive Custom solutions in the publishing business.

We continue to believe we have an obligation to provide the best possible product, so that you can teach students to provide the best possible care. After all, it's they who may help us in an emergency some day. You've given us your trust, and for this we thank you.

Sincerely,

Julie Levin Alexander
VP/Publisher

Katrin Beacom
Executive Marketing Manager

Marlene McHugh Pratt
Executive Editor

Thomas Kennally
National Sales Manager

Lois Berlowitz
Senior Managing Editor

Emphasizing Principles

Objectives

Part 1: Cardiovascular Anatomy and Physiology, ECG Monitoring, and Dysrhythmia Analysis (begins on p. 73)

After reading Part 1 of this chapter, you should be able to:

1. Describe the incidence, morbidity, and mortality of cardiovascular disease. (p. 71)
2. Discuss prevention strategies that may reduce the morbidity and mortality of cardiovascular disease. (pp. 71–72)
3. Identify the risk factors most predisposing to coronary artery disease. (pp. 71–72)

◄ **Chapter Objectives with Page References.** List the objectives that form the basis of each chapter, in addition to the page(s) on which each objective is covered.

One of your most important skills as a paramedic will be obtaining and interpreting ECG rhythm strips.

rhythm strip
electrocardiogram printout.

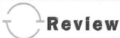**Review**

Factors Affecting Stroke Volume

- Preload
- Cardiac contractility
- Afterload

▲ **Key Points.** Help students identify and learn fundamental points.

▲ **Key Terms.** Located in margins near the paragraphs in which they first appear, these help students master new terminology.

▲ **Content Review.** Summarizes important content, giving students a format for quick review.

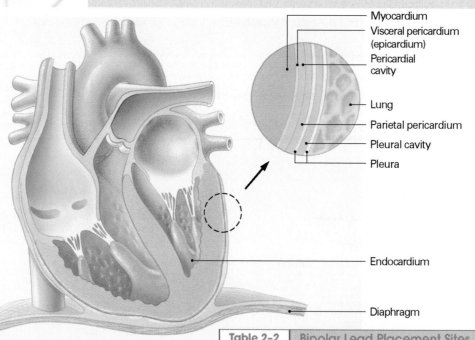

- Myocardium
- Visceral pericardium (epicardium)
- Pericardial cavity
- Lung
- Parietal pericardium
- Pleural cavity
- Pleura
- Endocardium
- Diaphragm

◄▼ **Tables and Illustrations.** Provide visual support to enhance understanding.

▶ **Figure 2-2** Layers of the heart.

Table 2-2	Bipolar Lead Placement Sites	
Lead	**Positive Electrode**	**Negative Electrode**
I	Left arm	Right arm
II	Left leg	Right arm
III	Left leg	Left arm

◗ Summary

Cardiovascular disease is the number-one cause of death in the United States and Canada. Many deaths from heart attack occur within the first 24 hours—frequently within the first hour. With the advent of fibrinolytic therapy, time is of the essence when managing the patient with suspected ischemic heart disease. EMS plays an ever-increasing role in the early recognition of patients suffering coronary ischemia. In certain areas, EMS provides definitive care by initiating fibrinolytic therapy in the field. This is especially important in cases where transport times can be long. With cardiovascular disease, EMS can truly mean the difference between life and death.

▶ **Summary.** Provides students with a concise review of important chapter information.

◗ Review Questions

1. The _____ is a protective sac surrounding the heart and consists of two layers, visceral and parietal.
   a. myocardium
   b. pericardium
   c. mesocardium
   d. endocardium

2. The outermost lining of the walls of arteries and veins is the _____ _____, a fibrous tissue covering that gives the vessel strength to withstand the pressures generated by the heart's contractions.
   a. tunica media
   b. tunica intima
   c. tunica adventitia
   d. visceral media

◀ **Review Questions.** Ask students to recall information and to apply the principles they've just learned.

◗ Further Reading

American Heart Association. *2005 American Heart Association Guidelines for Cardiopulmonary Resuscitation and Emergency Cardiovascular Care.* Dallas, Tex.: American Heart Association, 2005.

Beasley, B. M. *Understanding 12-Lead EKGs: A Practical Approach.* 2nd ed. Upper Saddle River, N.J.: Pearson/Prentice Hall, 2001.

Beasley, B. M. *Understanding EKGs: A Practical Approach.* 2nd ed. Upper Saddle River, N.J.: Pearson/Prentice Hall, 2003.

▶ **Further Reading.** Recommendations for books and journal articles.

◗ Media Resources

See the Student CD at the back of this book for quizzes, animations, videos, and other features related to this chapter. In particular, take a look at the Virtual Tours of the Heart and of the Cardiovascular System as well as the videos and animations on MI and dysrhythmia pathophysiology and a variety of normal cardiac functions and cardiac diseases. Also, visit the Companion Website for Brady's paramedic series at **www.prenhall.com/bledsoe,** where you will find additional reinforcement and links to other resources.

◀ **NEW! Media Resources.** Refer students to resources on the accompanying Student CD and on the book's Companion Website (accessed through **www.prenhall.com/ bledsoe**), where additional activities and information can be found on the chapter's topics. Also, provides links to other topic-specific websites.

Emphasizing Practice

Case Study

As soon as they complete the morning equipment check, Paramedic Unit 4 is dispatched to a difficulty-breathing call in a suburb of the city they serve. The response time is approximately 5 minutes. They arrive on scene at the same time as BLS first responders from the Pine Hill Fire Protection District. The house is a typical suburban residence, and a woman is on the front porch waving at the rescuers. Paramedics Chris Clark and Kim Jones grab the equipment and head for the residence. First responders from the fire department get the stretcher from the ambulance and go

◀ **Case Study.** Draws students into the reading and creates a link between the text content and real-life situations and experiences.

▶ You Make the Call

You and your partner on Medic 3 are dispatched to a well-kept residence about three blocks from the station. The dispatch information relates the nature of the call as a medical emergency. On your arrival at the residence, the patient's wife meets you and shows you to a back room. The patient is a male who appears to be in his late 60s. He is complaining of severe back pain that began approximately 30 minutes ago. He thinks it may be due to some light yard work he did earlier in the day. The patient appears in severe distress, however, and is sweaty and diaphoretic.

▶ **You Make the Call.** Promotes critical thinking by requiring students to apply principles to actual practice.

Procedure 2–6   12-Lead Prehospital ECG Monitoring

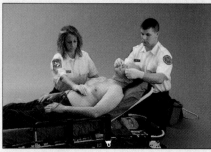

2-6a   Prep the skin.

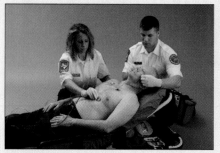

2-6b   Place the four limb leads according to the manufacturer's recommendations.

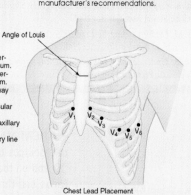

Lead V₁ The electrode is at the fourth intercostal space just to the right of the sternum.
Lead V₂ The electrode is at the fourth intercostal space just to the left of the sternum.
Lead V₃ The electrode is at the line midway between leads V₂ and V₄.
Lead V₄ The electrode is at the midclavicular line in the fifth interspace.
Lead V₅ The electrode is at the anterior axillary line at the same level as lead V₄.
Lead V₆ The electrode is at the midaxillary line at the same level as lead V₄.

Angle of Louis

Chest Lead Placement

2-6c   Proper placement of the precordial leads.

◀ **Procedure Scans.** Provide step-by-step visual support on how to perform skills.

▶ **Patient Care Algorithms.**
Provide graphic "pathways" that
integrate assessment and care
procedures.

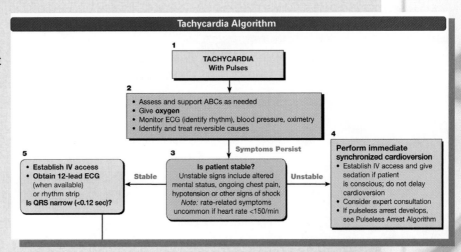

Tachycardia Algorithm

1
TACHYCARDIA
With Pulses

2
• Assess and support ABCs as needed
• Give **oxygen**
• Monitor ECG (identify rhythm), blood pressure, oximetry
• Identify and treat reversible causes

Symptoms Persist

4
Perform immediate
synchronized cardioversion
• Establish IV access and give
  sedation if patient
  is conscious; do not delay
  cardioversion
• Consider expert consultation
• If pulseless arrest develops,
  see Pulseless Arrest Algorithm

5
• Establish IV access
• Obtain 12-lead ECG
  (when available)
  or rhythm strip
Is QRS narrow (<0.12 sec)?

Stable

3
Is patient stable?
Unstable signs include altered
mental status, ongoing chest pain,
hypotension or other signs of shock
Note: rate-related symptoms
uncommon if heart rate <150/min

Unstable

Patho Pearls

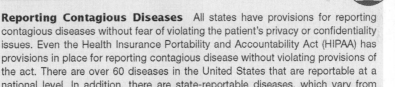

The Best Treatment for Stroke Because strokes are so debilitating, a
tremendous amount of research has been devoted to acute stroke care. Initially,
fibrinolytic therapy was proposed—similar to treatment for ST segment elevation
MI (STEMI). However, strokes are harder to diagnose, and fibrinolytic therapy is only
useful for some causes of stroke.

◀ **Patho Pearls.** Offer a
snapshot of pathological
considerations students will
encounter in the field.

▶ **Legal Notes.**
Present instances in
which legal or ethical
considerations should
be evaluated.

Legal Notes

Reporting Contagious Diseases All states have provisions for reporting
contagious diseases without fear of violating the patient's privacy or confidentiality
issues. Even the Health Insurance Portability and Accountability Act (HIPAA) has
provisions in place for reporting contagious disease without violating provisions of
the act. There are over 60 diseases in the United States that are reportable at a
national level. In addition, there are state-reportable diseases, which vary from
state to state. Some illnesses, including anthrax, brucellosis, diphtheria, pertussis,
plague, and others, must be immediately reported. Others, including AIDS, gonorrhea, leprosy, and syphilis, must be reported within 1 week. Some require reporting of individual cases and others require reporting of numbers only.

Cultural Considerations

Culture and Cardiovascular Disease Cardiovascular disease remains the
number one cause of death in the United States and Canada. The incidence of
cardiovascular disease increased steadily during the twentieth century, although it
has stabilized somewhat over the last decade or so.

◀ **Cultural Considerations.**
Provide an awareness of beliefs
that might affect patient care.

▶ **NEW! Assessment Pearls.**
Highlight important assessment
considerations and techniques.

Assessment Pearls

Crossover Test Have you ever had a patient tell you that one side of his body
was cold? Have you had trouble determining whether one foot was cooler than the
other (indicative of peripheral vascular disease)? A simple trick to help with this is
the crossover test.

Student CD

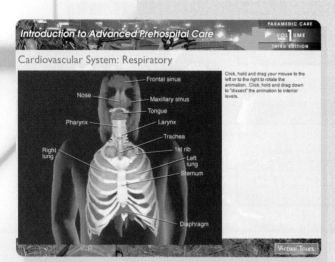

◄ **3D Animation.** Interactive 3D models encourage a deeper understanding of the body and its processes. 360° rotation and virtual dissection reinforce the concepts presented in each volume.

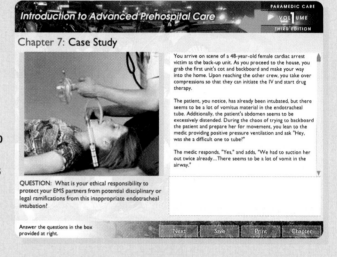

► **Case Study.** Designed to develop critical thinking skills, each case study offers questions and rationales that help to hone the student's assessment skills.

◄ **Drug Guide.** A valuable reference tool, this hotlinked PDF allows quick access to important information regarding the drugs most commonly used by today's paramedic.

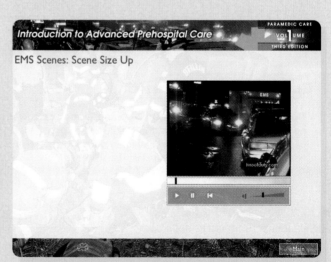

► **EMS Scenes.** Video clips of real-life situations put you in the action. See what you might encounter at an actual emergency scene.

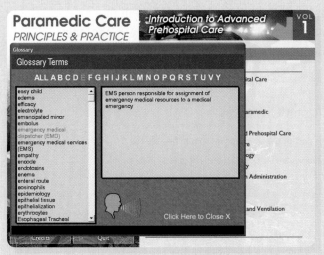

Glossary. This interactive, indexed glossary contains the definitions and audio pronunciations of the key terms presented in each volume.

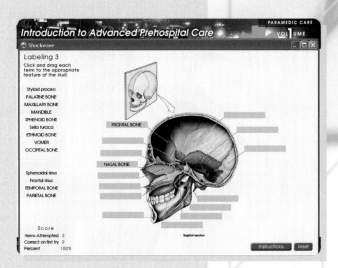

▶ **Interactives.** From Bone Structure to Body Cavities, drag-and-drop interactive exercises make learning both engaging and fun.

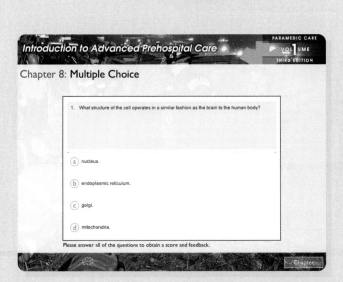

◀ **Multiple Choice.** Each chapter offers self-testing in a multiple-choice format. Upon completion, a score and feedback are provided for post-assessment.

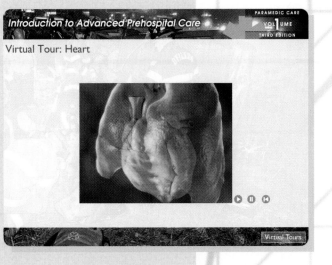

▶ **Virtual Tours.** Including the airway, cardiovascular system, muscle-skeletal system, nervous system, and heart, these narrated tours guide you through the intricate workings of the body systems in an easy-to-understand presentation.

Student Workbook

A student workbook with review and practice activities accompanies each volume of the Paramedic Care series. The workbooks include multiple-choice questions, other exercises, case studies, and special projects, along with an answer key with text page references. Flash Cards are also provided in each volume.

Review of Chapter Objectives

After reading this part of the chapter, you should be able to:

1. **Describe the incidence, morbidity, and mortality of cardiovascular disease.**

   Cardiovascular disease (CVD) is serious and extremely common, with more than 60 million Americans affected. Morbidity is considerable: An American has a nonfatal heart attack (myocardial infarction, MI) roughly every 29 seconds. Coronary heart disease (CHD), one type of CVD, is the single largest killer of Americans and Canadians. Roughly 466,000 Americans die annually from CHD, half of them before reaching a hospital. Many deaths from CHD are sudden and involve lethal cardiac dysrhythmias. Many deaths from MI occur within the first 24 hours, frequently within the first hour.

▶ **Review of Chapter Objectives.** Reviews important content elements addressed by chapter objectives.

Case Study Review

Reread the case study in Chapter 2 of Paramedic Care: Medical Emergencies *before reading the discussion below.*

This case study demonstrates how paramedics react to a typical medical emergency involving chest pain. In addition to observing how the team conducts the patient's initial assessment, note how they respond as the situation quickly changes into a more complex and urgent one.

◀ **Case Study Review.** Reviews and points out essential information and applied principles.

▶▼ **Content Self-Evaluation.** Multiple-choice, matching, and short-answer questions to test reading comprehension.

Content Self-Evaluation

MULTIPLE CHOICE

_____ 1. From innermost to outermost, the three tissue layers of the heart are:
   A. the endocardium, the pericardium, and the myocardium.
   B. the endocardium, the myocardium, and the syncytium.
   C. the endocardium, the myocardium, and the pericardium.
   D. the myocardium, the epicardium, and the pericardium.
   E. the epicardium, the myocardium, and the endocardium.

MATCHING

Write the letter of the ECG leads in the space provided next to the type of leads they are.

A. I, II, III

B. V_1, V_2, V_3, V_4, V_5, V_6

C. aVR, aVL, aVF

_____ 9. unipolar (augmented)

_____ 10. bipolar

_____ 11. precordial

Fill-in-the-Blanks

56. The _____ valves lie between the atria and ventricles, whereas the _____ valves lie between the ventricles and the arteries into which they open.

57. The four properties of cells in the cardiac conductive system are _____ , _____ , _____ , and _____ .

Special Project

Assessing Respiratory Emergencies

Read the assessment written for each of three patients evaluated in a prehospital setting and identify the probable cause for each emergency. Check the Assessment section of the textbook for each disorder to refamiliarize yourself with characteristic findings on history and physical examination.

Scenario 1: You are called to an elementary school where a student has become "suddenly ill" during a class birthday party. You find a distressed seven-year-old child who is breathing rapidly and shallowly and whose skin tone is becoming dusky. The use of accessory muscles to breathe is evident. The school nurse offers you a box containing an inhaler that she says the child uses on an "as needed" basis and states she isn't sure what ingredients were in the cupcakes brought for the party. She adds that the boy has several severe food allergies.

Probable cause: _____

Scenario 2: You are called to a home where an elderly man is "short of breath." On arrival, you find a thin, elderly man with a broad chest whose breathing is labored despite use of a home supplemental oxygen setup. His daughter tells you that he has had a cold recently, and he suddenly became "shorter of breath" this morning. On exam, the man has a fever of

◀ **Special Projects.**
Experiences designed to help students remember information and principles.

▶ **Patient Scenario Flash Cards.** Present scenarios with signs and symptoms and information to make field diagnoses.

CARD 1 PATIENT HISTORY

Dispatch Information: Responding to a residence for a patient complaining of chest pain.

Scene Size-Up: Small but clean home with the patient seated on the couch, in obvious pain, and clutching his chest; no hazards noted.

Medical History
A—anesthetic at the dentist's office ("caine" family)
M—nitroglycerin and calcium supplements
P—sees his doctor yearly but doesn't have any medical problems
L—breakfast an hour ago, 2 eggs, toast, and coffee
E—watching television, nothing unusual

Name/Class: ACETAMINOPHEN (Tylenol, Anacin-3)/Analgesic, Antipyretic

Description: Acetaminophen is a clinically proven analgesic/antipyretic with little effect on platelet function.
Indications: For mild to moderate pain and fever when aspirin is otherwise not tolerated.
Contraindications: Hypersensitivity, children under 3 years.
Precautions: Patients with hepatic disease; children under 12 years with arthritic conditions; alcoholism; malnutrition; and thrombocytopenia.
Dosage/Route: 325 to 650 mg. PO/4 to 6 hours. 650 mg PR/4 to 6 hours.

◀ **Drug Flash Cards.**
Represent drugs commonly used in paramedic care.

Teaching and Learning Package

FOR THE INSTRUCTOR

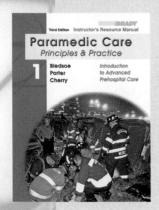

Instructor's Resource Manual. The Instructor's Resource Manual for each volume contains everything needed to teach the U.S. DOT National Standard Curriculum for Paramedics. It fully covers the DOT curriculum with:

- Time estimates for various topics
- Listing of additional resources
- Lecture outlines
- Student activities handouts
- Answers to student review questions
- Case study discussion questions

This manual is also available for download in Word and PDF format so instructors can customize resources to their individual needs.

 TestGen. Thoroughly updated and reviewed. Contains more than 2,000 exam-style questions, including DOT objectives and book page references.

PowerPoints. Updated to include additional illustrations, photos, animations, video clips, and sound. Includes all images from the textbooks.

FOR THE STUDENT

Student CD. In-text CD contains quizzes, a virtual tours, animations, case study exercises, video skills clips, on-scene video footage, and audio glossary.

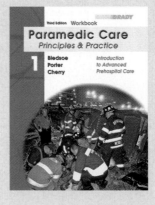

Workbook. Contains review of chapter objectives with summary information; case study review; content self-evaluation that includes multiple-choice, matching, and short-answer questions; special projects; content review; and patient scenario flash cards.

ONLINE RESOURCES

Companion Website. Contains quizzes, labeling exercises, state EMS directories, *New York Times* link, Weblinks, and trauma gallery.

OneKey. A distance learning program to support the series, offered on one of three platforms: Course Compass, Blackboard, or WebCT. Includes the IRM, PowerPoints, Test Manager, and Companion Website for instruction. Features include:

- Course outline
- Online gradebook, which automatically keeps track of students' performance on quizzes, class participation, and attendance
- Ability to upload questions authored offline and to randomize question order for each student
- Ability to add your own URLs and course links, set up discussion boards, and modify navigation features
- A virtual classroom for real-time sessions and communication with students
- Weblinks
- Ability to include your teaching assistants in course creation/management

Other Titles of Interest

SKILLS

Brady Skills Series: Advanced Life Support Skills CD
(0-13-119326-0)
More than 20 skills presented in step-by-step format with introduction, equipment, overview, and close-up, including assessment.

Advanced Life Support Skills (0-13-093874-2)
More than 20 skills presented in full color, with step-by-step photos and rationales.

REVIEW & REFERENCE

Beasley, Mistovich, *EMT Achieve: Paramedic Test Preparation* (0-13-119269-8)
Online test preparation, with full-length exams and quizzes, rationales and supporting text, artwork, and video.

Cherry, *Success! for the Paramedic*, 4th edition
(0-13-238550-3)
Best-selling review, containing test questions with DOT and text page references and rationales.

Miller, *Paramedic National Standards Self-Test*,
5th edition (0-13-199987-7)
Based on the DOT curriculum, uses self-test format to target areas students need to study further. Includes multiple-choice and scenario-based questions.

Bledsoe, Clayden, *Pocket Reference for ALS Providers*, 3rd edition (0-13-170728-0)
Drugs, dosages, algorithms, tables and charts, pediatric emergencies, advanced skills, and home medications provided in an easy-to-use field guide.

Cherry, Bledsoe, *Drug Guide for Paramedics*,
2nd edition (0-13-193645-X)
Handy field resource for accurate, easily accessed information about patient medication.

Cherry, *Patient Assessment Handbook* (0-13-061578-1)
Concise, illustrated, step-by-step procedures for assessment techniques.

ANATOMY & PHYSIOLOGY

Martini, Bartholomew, Bledsoe, *Anatomy & Physiology for Emergency Care*, 2nd edition
(0-13-234298-7)
EMS-specific applications integrated within chapters to provide an emergency care focus to A&P discussions.

CARDIAC/EKG

Walraven, *Basic Arrhythmias*, 6th edition
(0-13-117591-2)
Classic best-seller covers all the basics of EKG interpretation and includes a new student CD. Also contains appendices on clinical implications, cardiac anatomy & physiology, 12-lead EKG, basic 12-lead interpretation, and pacemakers.

Beasley, *Understanding EKGs: A Practical Approach*,
2nd edition (0-13-045215-7)
A direct approach to EKG interpretation that presents all the essential concepts for mastering the basics of this challenging field, while assuming no prior knowledge of EKGs.

Page, *12-Lead ECG for Acute and Critical Care Providers* (0-13-022460-X)
This full-color text presents ECG interpretation in a practical, easy-to-understand, and user-friendly manner.

Beasley, *Understanding 12-Lead EKGs: A Practical Approach*, 2nd edition (0-13-170789-2)
This comprehensive, reader-friendly text teaches beginning students basic 12-lead EKG interpretation.

Mistovich, et al., *Prehospital Advanced Cardiac Life Support*, 2nd edition (0-13-110143-9)
Straightforward and easy to follow, this text offers clear explanations, a colorful design, and includes all of the core concepts covered in an advanced cardiac life support course.

MEDICAL

Dalton, et al., *Advanced Medical Life Support*,
3rd edition (0-13-172340-5)
This groundbreaking text offers a practical approach to adult medical emergencies. Each chapter discusses realistic methods that a seasoned EMS practitioner would use.

Other Titles of Interest

MEDICAL TERMINOLOGY

Turley, *Medical Language* (0-13-094009-7)
Organized by medical specialty, this resource teaches medical language through immersion. It uses clear writing and engaging visuals to draw students into the culture and environment of medical language.

PHARMACOLOGY

Bledsoe, Clayden, *Prehospital Emergency Pharmacology*, 6th edition (0-13-150711-7)
This text and handy reference is a complete guide to the most common medications used in prehospital care.

TRAUMA

Campbell, *International Trauma Life Support*, 6th edition (0-13-237982-1)
Best-selling ITLS text provides a complete course that covers all the skills necessary for rapid assessment, resuscitation, stabilization, and transportation of the trauma patient.

The History

Objectives

After reading this chapter, you should be able to:

1. Describe the techniques of history taking. (pp. 4–10)
2. Discuss the importance of using open- and closed-ended questions. (pp. 6–7)
3. Describe the use of, and differentiate between, facilitation, reflection, clarification, empathetic responses, confrontation, and interpretation. (pp. 8–9)
4. Describe the structure, purpose, and how to obtain a comprehensive health history. (pp. 4–23)
5. List the components of a comprehensive history of an adult patient. (pp. 10–19)

Key Terms

active listening, p. 8
chief complaint, p. 3
closed-ended
    questions, p. 6
delirium, p. 22
dementia, p. 22
depression, p. 22
differential field
    diagnosis, p. 3
diuretic, p. 14
dysmenorrhea, p. 18

dyspnea, p. 17
HEENT, p. 17
hematemesis, p. 18
hematuria, p. 18
hemoptysis, p. 17
intermittent claudication,
    p. 19
nocturia, p. 18
open-ended
    questions, p. 6

orthopnea, p. 17
paroxysmal nocturnal
    dyspnea, p. 18
polyuria, p. 18
primary problem, p. 11
referred pain, p. 12
review of systems, p. 17
tenderness, p. 12
tinnitus, p. 17

Case Study

En route to a call, paramedic supervisor John Bigelow reviews the key elements of a medical interview in his head. John is precepting paramedic student Maryann Conrad and wants to be a positive role model. As they approach the scene, John quickly sizes it up. Nothing seems unusual. To the best of his knowledge, the scene is safe.

According to the dispatch information, John and Maryann are responding to evaluate an elderly man with abdominal pain. Upon first meeting his patient, John notices that he is in no real distress and appears stable. John does an initial assessment and then demonstrates taking a comprehensive patient history for Maryann. He introduces himself and Maryann and asks for his patient's name, which he will use throughout the interview.

John begins with a general question. "What seems to be the problem today, Mr. O'Donnell?"

"My stomach hurts," Mr. O'Donnell replies.

John begins exploring the history of the present illness with questions like "What were you doing when it started? Did it come on suddenly? Does anything make it worse or better? Can you describe how it feels? Can you point to the area that hurts? Does the pain travel anywhere else? How bad is it? On a scale of one to ten, with ten being the worst pain you have ever felt, how would you rate this pain? When did it start? Is it constant or does it come and go? Are you nauseous and have you vomited? Have you experienced a change in your bowel habits? Do you have any difficulty breathing?"

It seems that Mr. O'Donnell's pain came on suddenly after he ate this afternoon. He describes it as a sharp pain in the upper right quadrant that radiates to the right shoulder area. As Mr. O'Donnell answers John's questions, John leans forward, listening intently and often repeating Mr. O'Donnell's words. Maryann watches and learns.

John begins forming his differential field diagnosis, which includes hepatitis, acute myocardial infarction, pneumonia, aneurysm, cholecystitis, gastritis, pancreatitis, and peptic ulcer disease. He continues with the history. "Mr. O'Donnell, have you ever been treated for this problem in the past? Are you being treated for any other problems right now? Do you have diabetes, heart disease, breathing problems, kidney problems, stomach problems? Have you been injured recently? Have you had any surgeries? Does this problem usually happen right after eating? Are you taking any medications for it right now? Are you allergic to any medications? Do you smoke? Do you drink? How often do you drink? Did you drink any alcohol today? Does this problem get worse when you drink? What did you eat today?"

John learns that Mr. O'Donnell commonly has experienced pain after eating fatty foods. When John learns that his patient also drinks moderately every other day, he begins thinking about gallbladder disease. He decides to proceed to the review of body systems, beginning with the gastrointestinal system. He learns that Mr. O'Donnell often has indigestion and protracted episodes of pain and that his stools are clay colored. He also has noticed a yellowish tint to Mr. O'Donnell's eyes and that he feels feverish. Mr. O'Donnell denies vomiting blood or having blood in his stools. Hearing this, John suspects that his patient has cholecystitis. He conducts a focused physical exam and directs Maryann to take vital signs.

En route to St. Joseph's Hospital, John has Maryann conduct a detailed physical exam while he watches. At the hospital John reports to the ED attending, Dr. Zehner, who agrees with his preliminary diagnosis of gallbladder disease. Following an assessment that includes labs and an ultrasound, Dr. Zehner calls for the surgical service. After the call, John reviews the key points of taking a comprehensive patient history with Maryann. He explains how it helped him obtain important pieces of information that allowed him to focus the physical exam and led to his correct field diagnosis.

INTRODUCTION

In the majority of medical cases, you will base your field diagnosis on the patient history. Clearly, how you conduct the patient interview and the questions you ask will determine how much relevant medical information your patient reveals. In medical cases, obtaining an adequate history of your patient's **chief complaint**, recent illnesses, and significant past medical history is as important as, if not more important than, the physical exam. The information you gather will direct the physical exam and reveal clues to your patient's problem. Although we present the history by itself in this chapter, you will most likely conduct it simultaneously with parts of the physical exam.

The ability to elicit a good history is the foundation for providing good care to patients you have never met before. To conduct a good interview, you must gain your patient's trust in just a very short time. Then you must ask the right questions, listen intently to your patient's answers, and respond accordingly. In this chapter we will discuss both the verbal and nonverbal components of taking a comprehensive medical history.

We present the medical history in its entirety, as a well-structured, yet flexible, tool having several component procedures that are conducted in order. In reality, your patient's answers will alter the sequence of your questioning, and some of the information in this chapter will not readily adapt itself to prehospital emergency medicine. As you gain clinical experience, you will learn which components of the history are appropriate to the particular situations you encounter. Whether your patient is critical or stable, the situation determines the length and completeness of the interview. For example, complicated medical cases require a close investigation of your patient's chief complaint and past history. Trauma cases, on the other hand, are generally sudden events not precipitated by medical conditions and require only a modified approach to history taking.

The interview is the focal point of your relationship with your patients. It establishes the bonding necessary for effective and efficient patient care. By asking a series of well-designed questions you begin to build a profile of your patients. You also should have a good understanding of their problems and a list of causes (**differential field diagnosis**) to explain their signs and symptoms. Often, learning about your patient's history, medications, and even his lifestyle will reveal clues to your final field diagnosis.

chief complaint
the reason the ambulance was called.

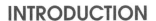

The ability to elicit a good history lays the foundation for good patient care.

differential field diagnosis
the list of possible causes for your patient's symptoms.

ESTABLISHING PATIENT RAPPORT

Your patients will form an opinion about you within the first few minutes, so you must establish a positive rapport quickly. This is not always easy. The situation, the patient, and the conditions will determine your ability to establish rapport. You can do several things, however, to facilitate this task. By asking your patients the right questions you will discover their chief complaint and their symptoms. By responding to them with empathy, you will win their trust and encourage them to discuss freely their problems with you. Their answers will also help you decide which areas require in-depth investigation and which body systems to focus on.

Setting the Stage

Sometimes you will assess a patient from a long-term care facility. If your patient's chart is available, as in a nursing home or extended care facility, review it before conducting the interview. Quickly note his age, sex, race, marital status, address, and occupation. The insight into your patient's life experiences that you begin developing with this information may provide subtle clues to help steer your questioning. Determine any past medical problems or previous referrals for the same condition. Note any treatments rendered and their effects. On emergency scenes, review the first responder's run sheet. Look for the chief complaint, a brief history including a current medication list, and vital signs. Be careful not to let your patient's chart, his past medical history, or someone else's first impression bias your possible field diagnosis. Always accept such information gratefully, but briefly reconfirm it with the patient and conduct your interview with an open mind.

If possible, conduct the interview in a quiet room, alone, with no distractions. Because you are asking your patient to divulge very intimate information, privacy encourages open communication. It should be a place where you and your patient can sit down and comfortably talk about his current problem and past experiences. Unfortunately, on emergency runs, you conduct the patient interview in a variety of settings beyond your control, from the kitchen floor to a busy street corner or a crowded bus. Often the back of your ambulance is where your patient will disclose important personal information to you. Some patients, however, will still be reluctant to reveal intimate information to a nonphysician in the emergency setting. Paramedics are often surprised at the hospital when their patients tell a different story to the physician in the emergency department, but this is common. To maximize your chances of obtaining a good history, practice the following techniques for developing better patient rapport.

The First Impression

When you arrive on the scene, your patient, his family, and bystanders will form an impression of you. You have only a few precious minutes to make that impression a positive one. If you expect your patient to trust you with very private information, you must establish a positive, trusting relationship. Present yourself as a caring, compassionate, competent, and confident health care professional. Because this first impression will be based largely on your appearance, your dress and grooming will play an important role in the paramedic–patient relationship. Your appearance should suggest neatness, cleanliness, pride, and professionalism. Your uniform should be clean and pressed, your shoes or boots polished, your hands and nails clean, and your hair well groomed.

Your voice, body language, gestures, and especially eye contact should communicate that you care about your patient's problems. Your questioning process should

Present yourself as a caring, compassionate, competent, and confident health care professional.

make the patient comfortable, confident in your care, and supportive of your control of the situation. Position yourself at his eye level and focus your attention on him. Give his requests and concerns high priority, even if they are not medically significant. For example, if your patient complains of being cold, cover him with a blanket. Beyond making him feel warmer, it may also increase his confidence in your desire and ability to help. If you cannot care for a complaint immediately, express your concern and assure him that you will either take care of it shortly or get him to a setting where it can be cared for.

A calm, reassuring voice and demeanor can put even the most apprehensive patient at ease. Remember that while his problems may not seem extraordinary to you, they may be extremely disturbing to him. You are accustomed to handling emergency situations; he is not. You are not horrified by a gory scene; he probably is. You deal with life-threatening emergencies every day; he probably never does. Understanding these differences helps you to display an appropriate demeanor and begin your interview.

A calm, reassuring voice and demeanor can put even the most apprehensive patient at ease.

Introductions

As you enter, immediately make eye contact with your patient and maintain it as you conduct the interview. Eye contact is the most important form of nonverbal communication. It tells your patient, "I am sincerely interested in you and your problems." Always keeping in mind that your personal safety takes the highest priority in any emergency, quickly determine whether you should enter your patient's personal space (18 inches to 3 feet). Then kneel, crouch, or sit beside him and address him from eye level or lower to reassure him that he still has some control. Avoid standing over him, which appears threatening or indifferent.

Eye contact is the most important form of nonverbal communication.

Wear an identification badge. Introduce yourself by name, title, and agency. For example, "Hi, my name is Jay. I'm a paramedic with Brewerton Ambulance. What's your name?" Use your patient's name frequently during the interview. Ask him how he wishes to be called—for instance, "Mr. MacCormack," "Nicholas," or "Nick"—and respect his wishes. Avoid using slang terms such as *honey, toots, dude, chief, pops,* or *babe* that your patient might construe as disrespectful and demeaning. This short verbal exchange reveals a wealth of information about your patient's respiratory status, level of consciousness, hearing and speech abilities, and any language barriers.

Be aware of other forms of nonverbal communication. Your job is to gain your patient's trust and cooperation in order to assess and care for him effectively. You do so by demonstrating sincerity through both verbal and nonverbal communication. Patients will detect inconsistencies in what you say and how you say it. Your tone of voice, facial expressions, and body language convey your true attitudes. Your actions must match your words. Touch is a powerful communication tool. Used properly, it conveys compassion, caring, and reassurance to your already apprehensive patient. Make contact by shaking hands or offering a comforting touch (Figure 1-1 ▶). This yields the additional benefit of enabling you to begin your assessment. For example, touching your patient's wrist allows you to make personal contact while quietly assessing his pulse and skin condition. Of course, you should try to get a sense of how your patient reacts to touch. It may make some patients feel threatened or uncomfortable. Avoid touching hostile, paranoid, or combative patients.

Make contact by shaking hands or offering a comforting touch.

Unless your patient is critical, work efficiently but don't rush. As you ask questions, you can delegate other personnel to conduct a focused physical exam, take vital signs, place oxygen, set up an IV, and get the stretcher. Your role as interviewer is to establish patient contact and learn the history.

Be aware of your patient's comfort. If the setting does not lend itself to personal questions, move your patient to a more suitable location. For example, teenage girls

Figure 1-1 When you introduce yourself to your patient, shaking hands or offering a comforting touch will help build trust.

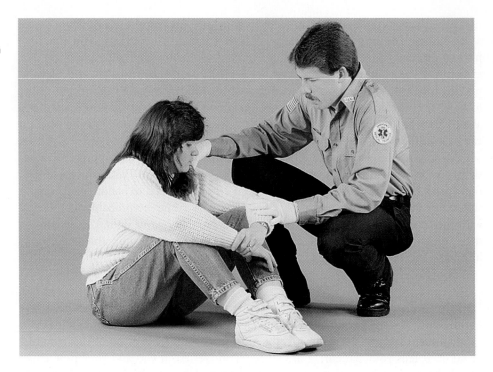

usually will not truthfully answer questions about pregnancy with their parents nearby. Other patients may not reveal relevant items about their medical history with bystanders listening. Sometimes moving your patient to the ambulance offers the needed privacy. If your patient is in obvious distress, try to alleviate his pain or discomfort while you interview him. For example, you may control minor bleeding and cover a wound that causes your patient distress. You might also immobilize a painful fracture site while you conduct the interview. Watch also for subtle signs of discomfort such as squirming, grimacing, and wincing.

Asking Questions

Remembering everything your patient tells you is impossible. Taking notes is acceptable, and most patients will not mind your doing so. If your patient becomes concerned about the notes, simply explain why you are taking them and reassure him that your interactions are confidential. Make sure you maintain contact with your patient. Avoid focusing so closely on the clipboard questionnaire that you ignore your patient, with whom you are trying to establish a caring rapport. Jot down pieces of information crucial to your verbal and written reports such as past history, medications, and vitals.

Asking questions in a way that elicits accurate information from your patients is an art. To gather the patient history, you can use a combination of open-ended and closed-ended questions. Paramedics must understand these two very different types of questions. **Open-ended questions** allow your patient to explain how he feels in detail, in his words, instead of giving "yes" or "no" answers. His responses are usually more accurate and complete. "Can you describe the pain in your chest?" and "Where do you hurt?" are open-ended questions. They deal in generalizations, allowing your patient to respond freely and without limits. Some patients may wander off course when answering open-ended questions, and occasionally you will need to refocus the interview.

Closed-ended questions elicit a short answer to a very direct question. They limit your patient's response to one or two words. They are appropriate when time or your

To gather the patient history, you can use a combination of open-ended and closed-ended questions.

open-ended questions
questions that allow your patient to answer in detail.

closed-ended questions
questions that elicit a one- or two-word answer.

patient's mental status or condition does not allow open-ended questions. For example, if your patient is gasping for breath while you are trying to determine the cause, phrase your questions for one-word answers or yes–no nods: "Does your pain radiate to the shoulder?" or "Do you take diuretics?" Closed-ended questions may be the most effective and efficient way to get your patients to describe their symptoms in exact terms. Their disadvantages are that you may inadvertently lead your patient toward certain answers and that they elicit only the limited information they ask for.

Some patients have difficulty describing their symptoms. In these cases, ask questions with multiple-choice options; for example, "Is your pain sharp, dull, burning, pressure-like, stabbing, or like something else?" Other patients may become confused, especially when more than one person is asking them questions. Avoid this by limiting the interview to one person, asking one question at a time, and allowing time for your patient to answer. Do not rush. You can become an efficient history taker by knowing which questions will elicit the most important information and by maintaining your patient's attention.

Patho Pearls

Listen to the Patient It was the renowned Canadian physician Sir William Osler who said, "Listen to the patient, and he will tell you what is wrong." This advice is as true today as it was 100 years ago. A great deal of information can be determined from a skillful history taking. As you listen to a patient's medical history, try to understand the underlying pathophysiological processes that might cause the symptoms the patient describes. This will help you to fully comprehend the disease process or processes affecting the patient. For example, consider the following case.

Mrs. J. Franklin is a 72-year-old pensioner, twice widowed, who lives in an older section of town. She summons EMS with what initially seem like vague complaints. She reports to the dispatcher, when queried, that she is "just sick." You arrive and begin an assessment starting with a pertinent history. The patient reports that her symptoms began about 2 weeks ago after several family members came to her house with dinner, which included a baked ham. Since that time, she has developed some fatigue, progressive dyspnea, and occasional chest pain. She now reports that she often wakes up at 3:00 A.M. with breathing trouble that resolves when she walks around the room or sleeps with three pillows. She also cannot tie her shoes, and she missed church last Sunday for this very reason. Her medications have remained unchanged and include furosemide, nitroglycerin paste, digoxin, aspirin, and lisinopril.

Clearly, there are physiological cues in the patient's medical history. The symptoms began with a ham dinner. You learn that she kept the ham and has been eating it daily. The ham is salt cured. Thus, her sodium intake may have increased. Her medications have remained unchanged. Her symptoms seem to indicate worsening heart failure with episodes consistent with both left and right ventricular failure. Her nighttime dyspnea and orthopnea are consistent with left heart failure, whereas her inability to tie her shoes could be due to peripheral edema from right heart failure. The fatigue could be attributed to both. Thus, your physical examination should either support or contradict your history findings.

In fact, it was learned later that the patient's heart failure had always been somewhat tenuous and the sodium load she received from the ham was all that was necessary to cause congestive heart failure. She did well with 2 days of hospitalization, diuretic administration, and sodium restriction.

Dr. Osler was correct. The history is often the most important part of patient assessment.

Language and Communication

Use appropriate language. Nothing distances you from your patient more quickly than sophisticated medical terminology. "Have you ever had a heart attack?" is better than "Have you ever had an MI?" Effective communication means connecting with your patient. Most of your patients will not understand medical terms. Use an appropriate level of questions, but do not appear condescending. Other barriers to communication include cultural differences, language differences, deafness, speech impediments, and even blindness. When you encounter such obstacles, try to enlist someone who can communicate with your patient and act as an interpreter. An alternative is to adopt a conservative approach toward assessment, field diagnosis, and treatment, concentrating on just the crucial items.

Listening is an important part of the interview. The old saying "Listen to your patient; he will tell you what is wrong" explains why it is crucial for a skilled clinician to be a good listener. Listen closely to what your patients tell you. Be careful not to develop tunnel vision from dispatch information. Begin your assessment without any preconceived notions about your patient's injuries or illnesses. Also watch for subtle clues that your patient may not be telling the truth. For example, your patient tells you that his chest pain went away, but his facial expressions and body language suggest otherwise. Developing good communication skills takes time and practice.

Avoid working your way in strict order down any prearranged list of questions (such as those in this chapter). Use these lists as a guide only. Listen to your patients and watch for clues to important signs, symptoms, emotions, or other factors. Then modify your questions to follow those clues. The following practices promote **active listening**.

Facilitation   Maintain sincere eye contact, use concerned facial expressions, and lean forward while you listen. Cues such as "Mm-hmm," "Go on," or "I'm listening" all help your patient open up. Sometimes strategic silence is also helpful.

Reflection   Repeat your patient's words. This encourages him to provide more details. Just make sure not to disturb his train of thought. For example:

Patient:	I can't breathe.
You:	You can't breathe?
Patient:	No, it feels like I can't take in a full breath because my chest hurts.
You:	Your chest hurts, too?
Patient:	Yes, it started this morning when I was working in the yard. I usually take a nitro but I'm all out.

This simple reflection encouraged the patient to reveal facts about his history of heart disease. If the paramedic had merely investigated the chief complaint of dyspnea, discovering its true cause may have taken longer. Because the primary problem is not always the chief complaint, allowing your patient to take the lead is sometimes advantageous.

Clarification   In crisis, patients often cannot clearly describe what they feel. They will use vague, general words. Do not hesitate to ask for clarification. For example:

You:	Do you have any allergies?
Patient:	Yes, the last time I took penicillin I had a bad reaction.
You:	Can you describe the reaction?
Patient:	Well, I got itchy all over with a rash.
You:	Did you have any difficulty breathing or feel like you were choking?
Patient:	Oh, no, just the itching and rash.

active listening
the process of responding to your patient's statements with words or gestures that demonstrate your understanding.

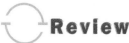

Review

Content

Active Listening Skills

- Facilitation
- Reflection
- Clarification
- Empathy
- Confrontation
- Interpretation

By asking for clarification you distinguish between a simple allergic reaction and life-threatening anaphylaxis.

Empathy   Your patients may be telling you very personal and sometimes embarrassing information about themselves. They may feel frightened, ashamed, and upset to have to tell a stranger these things. Show empathy by responding with "I understand" or "That must have been very difficult" or "I can't imagine having open heart surgery." Sometimes just a gesture like handing someone a tissue or patting him on the shoulder conveys empathy.

Confrontation   Sometimes patients will hide the truth or mask it with other symptoms. Often you will detect inconsistencies in your patient's story. In these cases, you should confront your patient with your observations. For example, "You say your chest doesn't hurt, but you keep rubbing it." Confrontation may help your patient bring his hidden feelings into the open.

Interpretation   Interpretation takes confrontation a step further. Here you interpret your observations and question your patient about what you believe may be the problem. For example, "You say your chest doesn't hurt but you keep rubbing it. Are you afraid you are having a heart attack but don't want to admit it?" Interpretation can backfire if your patient feels you are unjustly accusing him; however, if your patient trusts you and you use interpretation cautiously, it can demonstrate empathy and enhance your rapport.

Asking about Feelings   Your patients are people, not clinical subjects. Ask them how they feel about what they are experiencing. Let them know you are interested in them as people, not just as patients. Showing genuine interest in their problems may unlock the door to key information that they otherwise might not have shared with you.

Taking a History on Sensitive Topics

Paramedic students normally have difficulty questioning their patients about embarrassing, sensitive, or very personal topics such as sexual activities, death and dying, physical deformities, bodily functions, and domestic violence. Even though you may feel uneasy discussing these matters, they can help you learn important information about your patient's illness. To become more comfortable dealing with these subjects, watch experienced clinicians discuss them with their patients. Familiarize yourself with and practice some opening questions on sensitive topics that both put your patient at ease and encourage him to talk about it. If a particular area makes you most uncomfortable, attend a lecture or seminar and learn how professionals deal with this subject daily. Make the unfamiliar familiar and it will seem less imposing.

Let's look at two sensitive topics—physical violence and the sexual history. Your patient may not want to reveal a history of physical abuse. You should consider it when any of the following conditions is present:

- Injuries that are inconsistent with the story given
- Injuries that embarrass your patient
- A delay between the time of the injury and seeking help
- A past history of "accidents"
- Suspicious behavior of the supposed abuser

To earn your patient's trust, try to make him or her feel that the problem is not uncommon and that you understand the reasons for what has occurred. For example, you can ask your female patient, "Sometimes when husbands and wives argue a lot, it leads to physical fighting. I noticed you have some bruises on your arms and legs. Can you tell me what happened? Did someone hit you?" With active listening techniques, such questioning will help establish a rapport that encourages open communication.

Taking a sexual history can be the most embarrassing and uncomfortable topic for an inexperienced health care provider. The sexual history is normally taken later during the history but can be a part of the present illness or past history, depending on your patient's chief complaint. For example, if your patient complains of a genitourinary problem, the sexual history becomes important during the present illness questioning. If your patient has a history of sexually transmitted disease, then the sexual history is relevant to the past history. Whenever you begin the sexual history, it is helpful to prepare your patient with introductory statements and questions like "Now I need to ask you some questions about your sexual health and activity. It may help me determine the cause of your problem and provide better care for you. This information will be strictly confidential. May I begin?" If your patient consents, proceed as follows: "Are you sexually active? Have you had sex with anyone in the last 6 months? Do you have more than one partner? Do you have sex with men or women, or both? Do you take precautions to avoid infection or unwanted pregnancy? Do you have any problems or concerns about your sexual function?" This may seem very uncomfortable for the beginning paramedic, but with time and clinical experience you will develop a sense of where and when these questions are appropriate. It is critical that you remain calm, objective, and nonjudgmental regardless of how your patient answers.

THE COMPREHENSIVE PATIENT HISTORY

This section presents the components of a comprehensive patient history in a systematic order. In practice, you will ultimately select only those components that apply to your patient's situation and status. For example, if you conduct preemployment physical exams for a company, you may use the entire form. On the other hand, if you respond to a gasping patient in acute pulmonary edema, you will focus on the present illness. Common sense and clinical experience will determine how much of the following history to use.

Common sense and clinical experience will determine how much of the history to use.

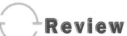

Review

Elements of the Patient History

- Preliminary data
- Chief complaint
- Present illness/injury
- Past history
- Current health status
- Review of systems

Preliminary Data

For documentation, always record the date and time of the physical exam. Determine your patient's age, sex, race, birthplace, and occupation. This provides a starting point for the interview and establishes you as the interviewer. Who is the source of the information you receive about your patient? Is it the competent patient himself, his spouse, a friend, or a bystander? Are you receiving a report from a first responder, the police, or another health care worker? Do you have the medical record from a transferring facility? After you have gathered the information, you should establish its reliability, which will vary according to the source's knowledge, memory, trust, and motivation. Again, reconfirm the information with the patient, if possible. This is a judgment call based on your experience. For example, if the patient information you received from a particular EMT first responder has been accurate in the past, you probably will trust it again. On the other hand, if the nurse at a physician's office has repeatedly provided you with erroneous information, you probably will doubt her accuracy.

The Chief Complaint

The history begins with an open-ended question about your patient's chief complaint. The chief complaint is the pain, discomfort, or dysfunction that caused your patient to request help. In a medical case, it may be a woman's call for help because she has chest pain. In a trauma case, it may be a bystander's call for assistance to a "man down" or a police officer's reporting an injury in an auto collision. Your patient may have called for more than one symptom. It is important to begin with a general question that allows your patient to respond freely. Ask, for example, "Why did you call us today?" or "What seems to be the problem?" Avoid the tunnel vision that often biases paramedics who focus on dispatch information that may or may not accurately describe the situation. As you interview and assess your patient, the chief complaint becomes more specific.

The chief complaint differs from the **primary problem**. Whereas the chief complaint is a sign or symptom noticed by the patient or a bystander, the primary problem is the principal medical cause of the complaint. For example, your patient's chief complaint may be leg pain, while the primary problem is a tibia fracture. When possible, report and record the chief complaint in your patient's own words. For example, "I am having a hard time breathing" is better than "the patient has dyspnea." For the unconscious patient, the chief complaint becomes what someone else identifies or what you observe as the primary problem. In some trauma situations, for instance, the chief complaint might be the mechanism of injury such as "a penetrating wound to the chest" or "a fall from 25 feet."

primary problem
the underlying cause for your patient's symptoms.

The Present Illness

Once you have determined the chief complaint, explore each of your patient's complaints in greater detail. Be naturally inquisitive when exploring the events surrounding these complaints. A practical template for exploring each complaint follows the mnemonic OPQRST–ASPN, an acronym for *Onset, Provocation/Palliation, Quality, Region/Radiation, Severity, Time, Associated Symptoms,* and *Pertinent Negatives.* This line of questioning provides a full, clear, chronological account of your patient's symptoms.

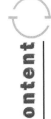

Review

Present Illness—OPQRST—ASPN

- **O**nset of problem
- **P**rovocative/**P**alliative factors
- **Q**uality
- **R**egion/**R**adiation
- **S**everity
- **T**ime
- **A**ssociated **S**ymptoms
- **P**ertinent **N**egatives

Assessment Pearls

Determining the Origin of Chest Pain Chest pain is a common reason people summon EMS. However, the causes of chest pain are numerous. In emergency medicine or EMS, we often look to exclude the most serious causes before determining if chest pain is of a benign origin. Internal organs don't have as many pain fibers as do such structures as the skin and other areas. Pain arising from an internal organ tends to be dull and vague. This is because nerves from various spinal levels innervate the organ in question. The heart, for example, is innervated by several thoracic spinal nerve segments. Thus, cardiac pain tends to be dull and sometimes described as pressure. It also tends to cause referred pain (i.e., pain in an area somewhat distant to the organ), such as pain in the left arm and jaw.

Dull pain that is hard to localize (or to reproduce with palpation) may be due to cardiac disease. One sign often seen with patients suffering cardiac disease is Levine's sign. With Levine's sign, the patient will subconsciously clench his fist when describing the chest pain. Levine's sign is associated with pain of a cardiac origin (e.g., angina or acute coronary syndrome).

Onset   Did the problem develop suddenly or gradually? What was your patient doing when the symptoms started? In medical emergencies, investigate your patient's activities at the time of, or shortly before, the signs or symptoms developed. In some cases, especially trauma, you may have to gather information from a few weeks before the onset of symptoms. For example, the signs and symptoms of a subdural hematoma may not appear until weeks following an injury. Was the patient exercising or exerting himself, or at rest or sleeping? Was he eating or drinking? If so, what? In trauma cases, ensure that a medical problem did not cause the incident. For example, the sudden onset of an illness such as a seizure or syncope may have caused a fall.

Provocation/Palliation   What provokes the symptom (makes it worse)? Does anything palliate the symptom (make it better)? In many illnesses, certain factors such as motion, pressure, and jarring may increase or decrease pain, discomfort, or dysfunction. Does eating, movement, exertion, stress, or anything else provoke the current problem? Positioning also may be a factor. Your patient may wish to curl up and lie on his side to reduce abdominal pain. Your congestive heart failure patients will sit bolt upright to ease respiration. They also may sleep with several pillows raising their upper body to relieve paroxysmal nocturnal dyspnea (PND), a sleep-disturbing breathing difficulty caused by fluid that accumulates in the lungs when they are supine. Ask your patient how breathing affects the discomfort. Deep breathing may increase the acute abdomen patient's pain. A patient with pleuritic or rib-fracture pain will not breathe deeply, whereas breathing may not affect the pain of angina. Any patient with respiratory pain will breathe with shallower but more frequent breaths.

If your patient took a medication shortly before you arrived, its effect or lack of effect may help determine the problem. Drugs such as bronchodilators, hypoglycemic agents, antihypertensives, and anticonvulsants are commonly prescribed and taken at home. Investigate any medication used to relieve a problem and note its effectiveness. Ask about any activity, medication, or other circumstance that either alleviates or aggravates the chief complaint.

Quality   How does your patient perceive the pain or discomfort? Ask him to explain how the symptom feels, and listen carefully to his answer. Does your patient call his pain crushing, tearing, oppressive, gnawing, crampy, sharp, dull, or otherwise? Quote his descriptors in your report.

Region/Radiation   Where is the symptom? Does it move anywhere else? Identify the exact location and area of pain, discomfort, or dysfunction. Does your patient complain of pain "here," while holding a clenched fist over the sternum, or does he grasp the entire abdomen with both hands and moan? If your patient has not done so, ask him to point to the painful area. Identify the specific location, or the boundary of the pain if it is regional.

tenderness
pain that is elicited through palpation.

Determine if the pain is truly pain (occurring independently) or **tenderness** (pain on palpation). Also determine if the pain moves or radiates. Localized pain occurs in one specific area, whereas radiating pain travels away from the source, in one, many, or all directions. Evaluate moving pain's initial location and progression and any factors that affect its movement.

referred pain
pain that is felt at a location away from its source.

Note any pain that may be referred from other parts of the body. **Referred pain** is felt in a part of the body away from the source of the disease or problem. The heart and diaphragm are two areas that most commonly produce referred pain. Cardiac problems such as myocardial infarction or anginal pain are usually referred to the left arm, with occasional referral to the neck, jaw, and back. Pain associated with irritation of the diaphragm (most commonly caused by blood in the abdomen of the supine patient) generally is referred to the clavicular region.

Severity   How bad is the symptom? Severity is the intensity of pain or discomfort felt by your patient. Ask him how bad the pain feels, and then have him compare it to other painful problems he has experienced. Sometimes a patient can describe the severity of the pain on a scale from one to ten, with ten being the worst pain he has ever felt. Also notice the amount of discomfort your patient's condition causes. How easy is it to distract your patient from his concern over the pain? Is your patient very still and resistive to your touch? Is he writhing about? The answers should give you a good idea of the intensity of your patient's pain.

Time   When did the symptoms begin? Is a symptom constant or intermittent? How long does it last? How long has this symptom affected your patient? For several days, hours, or just a few minutes or seconds? When did any previous episodes occur? How does this episode's length vary from earlier ones?

Associated Symptoms   What other symptoms commonly associated with the chief complaint in certain diseases can help rule in your field diagnosis? For example, if the chief complaint is chest pain, ask, "Are you short of breath? Are you nauseous? Have you vomited? Are you dizzy or light-headed?" The presence of these symptoms would help support a field diagnosis of cardiac chest pain.

Pertinent Negatives   Are any likely associated symptoms absent? Their absence is as important to the field diagnosis as their presence, because they help rule out a particular disease or injury. Note any element of the history or physical exam that does not support a suspected or possible field diagnosis. For example, it is significant if your patient who complains of chest pain denies shortness of breath, nausea, and light-headedness.

The Past History

The past medical history may provide significant insights into your patient's chief complaint and your field diagnosis. Look in depth at your patient's general state of health, childhood and adult diseases, psychiatric illnesses, accidents or injuries, surgeries, and hospitalizations. They may reveal general or specific clues that will help you to correctly assess his current problem. Your patient's condition, the situation, and time constraints will determine how much information you can and should gather on the scene. For example, asking about childhood diseases may not be relevant for your acute cardiac or trauma patient.

> The past medical history may provide significant insights into your patient's chief complaint and your field diagnosis.

General State of Health   How does your patient perceive his general state of health?

Childhood Diseases   What childhood diseases did your patient have? Did he have mumps, measles, rubella, whooping cough, chickenpox, rheumatic fever, scarlet fever, or polio? Again, this line of questioning's relevance depends on the patient and the situation.

Adult Diseases   Is your patient a diabetic? Does he have a history of heart disease, breathing problems, high blood pressure, or similar conditions? A preexisting medical problem may contribute to your patient's current problem or influence his care during the next few hours. To discover significant preexisting medical problems, ask if your patient has recently seen a physician or been hospitalized. If so, for what conditions? If you discover a preexisting problem, investigate its effects on your patient. When did the problem last affect him? Is your patient on any special diets or prescribed medications or restricted in activity? Even with the trauma patient, do not forget that a medical problem may have led to an accident or may complicate the effects of trauma. Also, obtain the name of your patient's physician since it may be helpful to the emergency department staff.

Psychiatric Illnesses   Does your patient have a history of mental illness? Has he ever been diagnosed with depression, mania, schizophrenia, or other problems? Is he being treated for a mental illness? If so, what medications is he taking? Has he ever had thoughts of suicide? Has he ever attempted suicide? Tailor these questions for patients you suspect of having a mental illness.

Accidents or Injuries   Has your patient ever had a serious accident or injury requiring hospitalization? Has he had a previous injury that could be a factor in his current problem? For example, a seemingly minor head injury 1 week ago may present now as a subdural hematoma in your unconscious elderly patient. Keep this line of questioning to relevant information only. An old football injury or childhood laceration is probably not influencing your patient's chest pain and respiratory distress today. But his pneumonectomy (surgical removal of a lung) probably is the reason for the absence of lung sounds on his right side.

Surgeries or Hospitalizations   Has your patient had any other hospitalizations or surgeries not already mentioned. Again, these may offer some insight into your suspected field diagnosis. For example, your patient is an 85-year-old man with a long history of congestive heart failure and no history of chronic lung disease. He suddenly presents with severe difficulty in breathing and audible wheezing. You should suspect the obvious—a cardiac problem. Don't look for the five-legged cat.

Current Health Status

The current health status assembles all the factors in your patient's present medical condition. Here, you try to gather information that completes the puzzle surrounding your patient's primary problem. Look for clues and correlations among the various sections of this part of the history. For example, your patient is a heavy smoker, has many allergies to inhaled particles, works in a coal mine, and frequently uses bronchodilating medications. He now complains of shortness of breath and expiratory wheezing. He is probably experiencing an exacerbation of his chronic lung disease.

Current Medications   Is your patient taking any medications? These include over-the-counter drugs, prescriptions, home remedies, vitamins, and minerals. If so, why? Your patient's explanation may not be medically accurate, but it may help to determine underlying conditions. For example, your 65-year-old patient tells you she takes a "water pill." You can safely assume she takes a **diuretic**, and has a history of renal or cardiac problems. A medication not taken as prescribed may be responsible for the current medical problem—possibly by under- or overmedication. A recently prescribed medication may cause an allergic or untoward (severe and unexpected) reaction. It also may be out of date and no longer effective. Even for trauma, emergency department personnel will need to know what medications your patient is taking. For example, if your patient takes warfarin, an anticoagulant, it would interfere with the normal clotting process and actually promote bleeding. If practical, bring your patient's medications to the hospital (Figure 1-2 ▶).

diuretic
a medication that stimulates the kidneys to excrete water.

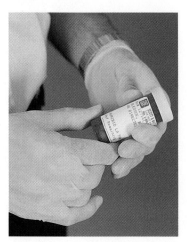

▶ **Figure 1-2**   You should take your patient's medications with you to the hospital, when practical.

Allergies   Does your patient have any known allergies, especially to penicillin, the "caine" family (local anesthetics), tetanus toxoid, or narcotics? These agents are occasionally given in emergency situations. What type of reaction did your patient have to the medication? For example, was it just a mild allergic reaction with a rash and itching or localized swelling or anaphylactic shock? Knowledge of your patient's allergies may prevent additional complications during the emergency department visit, especially if he becomes disoriented or unconscious during transport. If your patient is short of breath with wheezing, ask about environmental allergies. In cases of possible anaphylaxis, ask about allergies to drugs; to foods such as shellfish, nuts, and dairy products; and to insect bites and stings.

Tobacco   Does your patient use tobacco? If so, what type (cigarettes, cigars, pipe, smokeless, or other), how much, and for how long? To quantify his smoking history, multiply the number of packs smoked per day by the number of years he has smoked. The result is his pack/year history. For example, if your patient smoked two packs of cigarettes per day for 25 years, he is a 50 pack/year smoker. Anything over 30 pack/years is considered significant.

Alcohol, Drugs, and Related Substances   Alcohol and drugs are often contributing factors in, if not the primary cause of, your patient's medical problems. Your job is not to pass judgment but to gather data that will help direct your patient's medical treatment. Remaining nonjudgmental will aid you in your questioning. Start with a general question such as "How much alcohol do you drink?" If you suspect a drinking problem may be a factor, you can use the CAGE questionnaire (an alcoholism screening instrument) to determine the presence of alcoholism. Reserve this line of questioning for the chronic patient in a controlled setting. It would be inappropriate in a bar with an unruly, intoxicated patient.

> *The CAGE Questionnaire*
> Have you ever felt the need to **C**ut down on your drinking?
> Have you ever felt **A**nnoyed by criticism of your drinking?
> Have you ever had **G**uilty feelings about drinking?
> Have you ever taken a drink first thing in the morning as an **E**ye-opener?

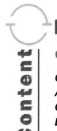

Review

CAGE Questionnaire

Cut down
Annoyed
Guilty
Eye-opener

Content

Two or more "yes" answers suggest alcoholism and further lines of inquiry.

Ask about blackouts, accidents, or injuries that happened while drinking. Also ask about alcohol-related job losses, marital problems, and arrests while under the influence of alcohol. Similarly, ask about drug use: "Do you use marijuana, cocaine, heroin, sleeping pills, or painkillers? How much do you take? How do these drugs make you feel? Have you had any bad reactions?" As your patients realize you are not judging their substance abuse, they may feel more comfortable telling you about their patterns of use.

Diet   Ask about your patient's normal daily intake of food and drink. Perhaps your 78-year-old retiree just moved to the Arizona desert and underestimated the increased fluid loss due to sweating. He does not realize he needs to increase his daily fluid intake, and now he presents weak and dizzy from dehydration. Are there any dietary restrictions or supplements? Ask specifically about his use of foods with stimulating effects such as coffee, tea, cola drinks, and other beverages containing caffeine. For example, your 23-year-old patient with a rapid heartbeat (200 beats per minute) drinks continuous cups of coffee each morning at her highly stressful job.

Screening Tests   Ask about certain screening tests that may have been done for your patient. Some examples include a purified protein derivative (PPD) test for suspected tuberculosis, Pap smears and mammograms for female problems, stool testing for occult blood, and cholesterol tests. Record the dates of the tests and their results.

Immunizations   Ask your patient about his immunizations for diseases such as tetanus, pertussis, diphtheria, polio, measles, rubella, mumps, influenza, hepatitis B, and pneumococcal vaccine. For example, ask the parent of a child suspected of epiglottitis if he had the *Haemophilus influenzae* B vaccine. *Haemophilus influenzae* B is a common cause of epiglottitis and meningitis in children.

Sleep Patterns   Ask your patient what time he normally goes to bed and arises. Does he take daytime naps? Does he have problems falling asleep or staying asleep?

Exercise and Leisure Activities   Does your patient exercise regularly or lead a sedentary existence? Sometimes your patient's lifestyle will support your field diagnosis.

Environmental Hazards   Ask about possible hazards in the home, in school, and at the workplace. For example, your patient may live or work in an area with high levels of toxic substances. Many health problems can be traced to these environmental causes.

Use of Safety Measures   In an auto crash, did your patient use a seat restraint system? Were all passengers belted in? Did the air bag deploy? Such information aids you and the emergency department staff in determining the extent of damage caused by a particular mechanism of injury. For bicycle, in-line skate, and skateboard injuries, ask about the use of helmets and knee and elbow pads.

Family History   Because many disease processes are hereditary, the medical history of immediate family members is important. In the nonemergency setting you may explore deep into the family tree and chart the medical history of grandparents, parents, aunts, and uncles. In the emergency setting, learning that your 45-year-old patient with chest pain had a father and brother who both died of heart attacks in their late 40s is important information. Look for a family history of diabetes, heart disease, hypercholesterolemia, high blood pressure, stroke, kidney disease, tuberculosis, cancer, arthritis, anemia, allergies, asthma, headaches, epilepsy, mental illness, alcoholism, drug addiction, and any symptoms like your patient's.

Home Situation and Significant Others   Who lives at home with your patient? Ask him about his home life—or lack of one. Ask about friends, family, support groups, loved ones. Find out if he has a support network and whom it includes. Who takes care of him when he needs help? Loneliness and isolation may complicate your patient's physical symptoms.

Daily Life   Ask your patient to describe his typical day. When does he get up? What does he do first? Then what? Such questions reveal a lot about your patient's state of mind and general wellness. Is he busy, active, and motivated to get up in the morning? Does he merely exist from the time he awakens and go through life with no purpose or direction? Is he under high levels of stress from morning to night in a job that requires him to take his problems home with him? Find out what kind of life your patient leads. It may reveal a lot about his illness.

Important Experiences   Ask about your patient's upbringing and home life growing up. How much schooling does he have? Was he in the military? What kinds of jobs has he held? What is his financial situation? Is he married, single, divorced, or widowed? What does he do for fun and relaxation? Is he retired or looking forward to retirement? Again, the answers give you a broader picture of your patient.

Religious Beliefs   Some religions forbid certain treatments and have guidelines regarding the management of illness and injury. For example, some forbid whole-blood transfusions. Knowing if your patient is guided by these beliefs can help you understand and care for him better. These questions require some expression of sensitivity, or it might be best to ask broadly if he has any limitations in medical care.

The Patient's Outlook   Find out what your patient thinks and how he feels about the present and future.

Review of Systems

The **review of systems** is a series of questions designed to identify problems your patient has not already mentioned. It is a system-by-system list of questions that are more specific than those asked during the basic history. Again, the patient's chief complaint, condition, and clinical status determine how much, if any, of the review of systems you will use. For example, if your patient complains of chest pain, you may want to review the respiratory, cardiac, gastrointestinal, and hematological systems. If your patient complains of a headache, you may want to review the **HEENT** (head, eyes, ears, nose, and throat), neurologic, peripheral vascular, and psychiatric systems. Let your patient lead you through the history. The following sampling includes a few of the many questions that you might ask.

General   What is your patient's usual weight, and have there been any recent weight changes? Has he had weakness, fatigue, or fever?

Skin   Has your patient noticed any new rashes, lumps, sores, itching, dryness, color change, or changes in nails or hair? Could cosmetics or jewelry have caused these problems?

Head, Eyes, Ears, Nose, and Throat (HEENT)   Has your patient had headaches or recent head trauma? How is his vision? Does he wear glasses or contact lenses? When was his last eye exam? Has he experienced any of the following: pain, redness, excessive tearing, double vision, blurred vision, spots, specks, flashing lights? Has he ever had glaucoma or cataracts? How is his hearing? Does he use hearing aids? Has he ever experienced ringing in the ears (**tinnitus**), vertigo, earaches, infection, or discharge? Does he have frequent colds, nasal stuffiness, nasal discharge, hay fever, nosebleeds, sinus problems? Does he wear dentures? When was his last dental exam? Describe the condition of his teeth and gums. Do his gums bleed? Does he get a sore tongue, dry mouth, frequent sore throats, or hoarseness? Does he have lumps or swollen glands? Has he ever had a goiter, neck pain, difficulty swallowing, or stiffness?

Respiratory   Has your patient ever had wheezing, coughing up of blood (**hemoptysis**), asthma, bronchitis, emphysema, pneumonia, TB, or pleurisy? When was his last chest X-ray? Is he coughing now? If so, can you describe the sputum?

Cardiac   Has your patient ever had heart trouble, high blood pressure, rheumatic fever, heart murmurs, chest pain or discomfort, palpitations, shortness of breath (**dyspnea**), shortness of breath while lying flat (**orthopnea**), or peripheral edema? Has

review of systems
a list of questions categorized by body system.

HEENT
head, eyes, ears, nose, and throat.

tinnitus
the sensation of ringing in the ears.

hemoptysis
coughing up of blood.

dyspnea
the sensation of having difficulty breathing.

orthopnea
difficulty breathing while lying supine.

paroxysmal nocturnal dyspnea
sudden onset of shortness of breath at night.

hematemesis
vomiting of blood.

polyuria
excessive urination.

nocturia
excessive urination at night.

hematuria
blood in the urine.

dysmenorrhea
difficult or painful menstruation.

he ever been awakened from sleep with shortness of breath (**paroxysmal nocturnal dyspnea**)? Has he ever had an ECG or other heart tests?

Gastrointestinal Has your patient ever had trouble swallowing, heartburn, loss of appetite, nausea/vomiting, regurgitation, vomiting of blood (**hematemesis**), indigestion? How often does he move his bowels? Describe the color and size of his stools. Have there been any changes in his bowel habits? Has he had rectal bleeding or black, tarry stools, hemorrhoids, constipation, diarrhea? Has he had abdominal pain, food intolerance, or excessive belching or passing of gas? Has he had jaundice, liver or gallbladder problems, or hepatitis?

Urinary How often does your patient urinate? Has he ever had excessive urination (**polyuria**), excessive urination at night (**nocturia**), burning or pain while urinating, blood in the urine (**hematuria**), urgency, reduced caliber or force of urine flow, hesitancy, dribbling, or incontinence? Has he ever had a urinary tract infection or stones?

Male Genital Has your patient ever had a hernia, discharge from or sores on the penis, testicular pain or masses? Has he ever had a sexually transmitted disease? If so, how was it treated?

Female Genital At what age did your patient have her first menstrual period? Describe the regularity, frequency, duration, and amount of bleeding of her periods. When was her last menstrual period? Does she bleed between periods or after intercourse? Has she ever had difficulty with her period (**dysmenorrhea**) or premenstrual tension? At what age did she become menopausal? Were there symptoms or bleeding? Has she ever had any vaginal discharge, lumps, sores, or itching? Has she ever had a sexually transmitted disease? If so, how was it treated? How many times has she been pregnant? How many deliveries? Any abortions (spontaneous or induced)? Some health care personnel use the G-P-A-L system to document a patient's history of pregnancy:

Gravida	How many times pregnant?
Para	How many viable births?
Abortions	How many abortions (including miscarriages)?
Living	How many living children?

Has she ever had complications of pregnancy? Does she use birth control? If so, what type? If postmenopausal, is she on hormone replacement therapy?

Assessment Pearls

Estimating Gestational Age Occasionally, you'll encounter a pregnant patient who can't provide information that will help you determine the approximate gestational age (e.g., last menstrual period or sonogram). One way to estimate the gestational age is to measure the fundal height. To do this, get a cloth or soft tape measure marked in centimeters. Place the start of the tape on the symphysis pubis bone and measure the distance to the topmost part of the uterus (the fundal height). On average, every centimeter is approximately 1 week of gestation. Thus, a reading of 24 cm correlates to 24 weeks. Please note, however, that this measurement is least accurate early in pregnancy and at the very end of pregnancy when the fetus's head descends into the pelvis.

Peripheral Vascular   Has your patient ever had intermittent calf pain while walking (**intermittent claudication**), leg cramps, varicose veins, or blood clots?

intermittent claudication
intermittent calf pain while walking that subsides with rest.

Musculoskeletal   Has your patient ever experienced muscle or joint pain, stiffness, arthritis, gout, or backache? Describe the location or symptoms.

Neurologic   Has your patient ever experienced any of the following: fainting, blackouts, seizures, speech difficulty, vertigo, weakness, paralysis, numbness or loss of sensation, tingling, "pins and needles," tremors, or other involuntary movements?

Hematologic   Has your patient ever been anemic? Has he ever had a blood transfusion? If so did he have a reaction to it? Does he bruise or bleed easily?

Endocrine   Has your patient ever had thyroid trouble? Did he ever experience heat or cold intolerance, or excessive sweating? Does he have diabetes? Has he ever had excessive thirst, hunger, or urge to urinate?

Psychiatric   Is he nervous? Is he under much stress and tension? Has he ever been depressed? Has he ever thought of committing suicide?

SPECIAL CHALLENGES

No matter how long you practice as a paramedic, some patients will present with special circumstances that challenge your skills. Your ability to deal with them will improve with time and practice.

Silence

Silence can become very uncomfortable if you are impatient. Why has your patient suddenly become silent? This question has no single answer. His silence can have many meanings and many uses. It may result from an organic brain condition that prevents him from forming thoughts. Or it may be due to dysarthria (difficulty in speaking due to muscular impairment). Maybe he is just collecting his thoughts or trying to remember details. Or maybe he is deciding whether he trusts you. He might be clinically depressed or, perhaps, he simply deals with situations by being quiet.

Assessment Pearls

Interviewing the Abused Patient   Remember that abuse can be physical, sexual, or emotional. The abused victim may be a husband or wife, a child or elderly parent, a boyfriend or girlfriend. If you suspect abuse, ask your patients when they feel safe or unsafe at home and watch their reaction. Are they frightened to answer? Do they act defensive and hostile? Do they seem withdrawn or show other inappropriate behaviors? If your gut tells you that your patient may have been abused, follow your local protocols about reporting your objective findings and make sure your patient remains safe while in your care.

What do you do during the silence? Stay calm and observe your patient's non-verbal clues. Is he in pain? Is he scared? Is he on the verge of becoming hysterical or combative, or is he about to cry? You can encourage him to continue speaking by confronting him with your perceptions. For example, "I see you are obviously very upset about this. Do you want to talk about it?" If you sense your patient is not responsive to your questions, perform a brief orientation exam. Speak to him in a loud voice and call him by name. Shake him gently if he does not respond. If this does not elicit a response, assume a neurologic problem and proceed accordingly.

Sometimes your behavior might have caused the silence. Are you asking too many questions too quickly? Have you offended your patient? Have you frightened him? Have you been insensitive? Have you failed to respond to your patient's needs? If your patient suddenly becomes silent, try to determine why, what is happening, and what you should do about it.

Overly Talkative Patients

The patient who rambles on can be just as frustrating to deal with as the one who will not talk at all. Why is your patient talking so fast and so much? Some patients react to stress this way. Maybe he has a lot to say. Maybe he needs someone to talk to; some lonely patients will take any opportunity to communicate with another human being. What can you do in the emergency setting when time is scarce? This problem has no perfect solution. You can lower your goals and accept a less comprehensive history. You can briefly give your patient free reign. You can focus on the important areas and ask closed-ended questions about them. You can interrupt him frequently and summarize what he says. Above all, try not to become impatient.

Patients with Multiple Symptoms

Patients often present with multiple complaints. For example, your elderly patient may present you with a barrage of symptoms from an extensive medical history. Your challenge is to discover the chief complaint and why she called for help today. If she complains of symptoms that suggest multiple disease states, the challenge is compounded. In these types of cases, you must sort through a multitude of information quickly and recognize patterns that lead you to a correct field diagnosis.

Some patients will answer "Yes" to every question you ask. They have every symptom you mention; although possible, this phenomenon is not probable. Your patient might simply misunderstand or be trying hard to cooperate; more than likely he has an emotional problem and requires a psychosocial assessment. Document your findings on your prehospital care report and request a psychological referral. Asking the patient what single complaint led him to call for help today often helps.

Anxious Patients

Anxiety is a natural reaction to stress. People who face serious illness or injury can be expected to exhibit some degree of anxiety. Sometimes this manifests itself as simple nervousness, tenseness, sweating, or trembling. Some patients will fall silent, while others will ramble. Still others may exhibit anxiety attacks marked by a rapid heart rate, nausea and vomiting, chest pain, and shortness of breath. When you detect signs of anxiety, encourage your patient to speak freely about it. For example, you can say, "I see you are concerned about this. Do you want to talk about it?"

Patients Needing Reassurance

Appropriate reassurance is a cornerstone of patient care. You must be careful, however, not to be overly reassuring or to prematurely reassure your anxious patient. It is natural to say, "Relax, everything is going to be all right. We are going to take care of you and get you to the hospital. Just relax and you will be all right." But your patient may have anxiety about something of which you are not aware. For instance, if your chest pain patient is anxious, you might naturally assume he is apprehensive about dying. In reality, he may be anxious about something entirely different. He may be embarrassed about his anxieties, and instead of helping him deal with them, you have helped him cover them up. Now he may decide you are not interested in what is really bothering him and block further communication. Listen carefully to your patient before offering reassurance.

Anger and Hostility

You will often encounter angry patients or their families. They might be angry for many reasons. Your patient is sick, perhaps dying. Family members are anticipating their future loss. Often they will lash out at the easiest target—you. Sometimes you cannot do anything quickly enough or well enough for them. Understand that their anger is a natural part of the grieving process and they may be merely venting their frustration—unfortunately, you are at the receiving end of their outbursts. Try to accept their feelings without getting defensive or angry in return.

Intoxication

Dealing with belligerent, intoxicated patients challenges even the most experienced paramedic. These patients are irrational, they disrupt your control of the scene, and they rarely allow you to examine them. First and foremost, make sure your environment is safe. If your patient acts violently, call for the police before attempting any interaction. As you approach your patient, introduce yourself and offer a handshake. Avoid any challenging body language or remarks. Appear friendly and nonjudgmental, but always stay alert for a potential violent outburst. If your patient is shouting or cursing, do not try to get him to stop or to lower his voice. Listen to what he says, not how he says it, and try to understand his situation before making a clinical judgment. Sometimes a genuine offer of a place to sit will help calm an agitated, intoxicated person. Then you can begin your assessment.

Crying

Sometimes your patients will cry. This can make any paramedic uncomfortable. Crying is just another form of venting, an important clue to your patient's emotions. Accept it as a natural release and do not try to suppress it. Be patient, allow your patient to cry, and then offer a supportive remark. Quiet acceptance and supportive remarks will open the lines of communication once your patient composes himself.

Depression

depression
a mood disorder characterized by hopelessness and malaise.

Depression is a common problem in medicine. It is also commonly misdiagnosed or ignored. It often presents with symptoms such as insomnia, fatigue, weight loss, or mysterious aches and pains. Depression is potentially lethal, so you must recognize its signs and evaluate its severity just as you would chest pain or shortness of breath. Ask your patient if he has ever thought about committing suicide; if he is currently thinking about suicide; if he has the means to commit suicide; and if he has ever attempted it. The more exact and precise his suicide plan, the more apt he is to carry it out.

Sexually Attractive or Seductive Patients

Occasionally you will encounter a patient who is attracted to you or to whom you are attracted. These feelings are natural. The key is not to allow these feelings to affect your behavior. Always keep your relationship professional. If necessary, clearly tell any patient who behaves seductively that you are there on a professional basis, not a personal one. Afterward, determine if how you dressed, what you did, or what you said helped your patient get the wrong impression about your relationship. Did you send the wrong signals? Whenever possible, always have a partner with you to avoid any accusations of improper behavior or touching.

Confusing Behaviors or Histories

You may encounter a patient whose story you just cannot follow. No matter what you ask, the answers leave you confused and frustrated. You cannot seem to develop a clear picture about your patient's problems. In fact, his answers don't even seem to make any sense. For example, you ask, "When did your headache begin?" and he answers, "My head feels like a squirrel." In these cases, the problem is most likely psychotic (mental illness) or organic (**dementia** or **delirium**). Also consider head injury or other physiological conditions such as stroke.

Many psychotic patients live and function in their communities, with varying degrees of success. Some will provide an accurate past history, others will not. If your patient's behavior seems distant, aloof, inappropriate, or even bizarre, suspect a mental illness such as schizophrenia. It may be helpful to focus your assessment on this patient's mental status, with special emphasis on thought, perceptions, and mood.

Delirium and dementia are disorders relating to cognitive function. Delirium is common in the acutely ill or intoxicated patient; dementia occurs more frequently in the elderly. These patients often cannot provide clear, accurate histories. Their descriptions of their symptoms and their accounts of how things happened will be vague and inconsistent. They may appear inattentive to your questions and hesitant in their answers. They may even make up stories to fill in the gaps in their memories. In these cases, do not spend too much time trying to get a detailed history, because you will only become more frustrated. Focus on the mental status exam, with special emphasis on level of response, orientation, and memory. For a more detailed discussion of these problems, see Volume 3, Chapter 12.

dementia
a deterioration of mental status that is usually associated with structural neurologic disease.

delirium
an acute alteration in mental functioning that is often reversible.

Limited Intelligence

You can usually obtain an adequate history from a patient with limited intelligence. Do not assume that he will not be able to provide accurate information concerning his current or past medical status. Also, do not overlook obvious omissions because your patient appears to be giving you a good story. Try to evaluate your patient's education and mental abilities. If you suspect severe mental retardation, obtain the patient's history from family or friends. Above all, show a genuine interest in your patient and try to establish a positive relationship. Then, communication can still happen.

Language Barriers

Few things are more frustrating than responding to an automobile collision with several patients who speak a language you do not understand. It is almost impossible to get an accurate history of the event. In these cases, try to locate an interpreter. Sometimes a family member speaks both languages and is willing to translate for you. Often, however, family members cause more confusion by paraphrasing what the patient and you are saying. Instead of hearing your patient's exact words, you hear the translator's version, and the true meanings become vague. However, do not waste time using your broken foreign language from high school, because you will invariably confuse everyone involved. Instead, ask the translator to provide an exact as possible translation to the patient and to you.

Hearing Problems

The challenge of communicating with a person with a hearing impairment is much like that of overcoming a language barrier. Some options, however, afford a degree of flexibility. You can try handwritten questions, but they can be time consuming. Sign language is effective if the patient practices it and you find a proficient interpreter. If your patient reads lips, you must modify your communication techniques accordingly. Always face him directly in a well-lit setting and speak slowly in a low-pitched voice. Avoid covering your mouth and trailing off at the ends of your sentences. If your patient has one good ear, use that to your advantage. If he wears a hearing aid, make sure it is working. If he has eyeglasses, make sure he wears them. Augment your speech with hand gestures and facial expressions.

Blindness

Blind patients present special problems. You must identify yourself immediately, because they cannot see your uniform. Always announce yourself and explain who you are and why you are there. If possible, take your patient's hand to establish personal contact and to show him where you are. Remember that nonverbal communications such as hand gestures, facial expressions, and body language are useless in these cases. Your voice is your only tool for effective communication.

Talking with Families or Friends

You will often encounter patients who cannot give you any useful information. In these cases, find a third party who can augment the patient history and offer a useful adjunct to the patient's answers (Figure 1-3). The typical case is the postictal patient who cannot describe his seizure activity to you. Another example is learning from his friend that your patient's wife died in an automobile crash just 3 weeks ago. Now you better understand why your patient appears depressed and suicidal. Make sure that patient confidentiality is a priority when you accept personal information from a family member, friend, or bystander.

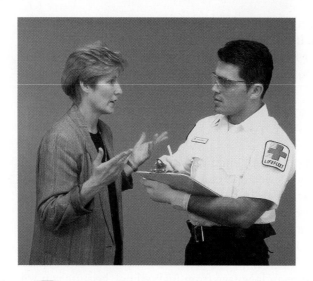

Figure 1-3 If the patient cannot provide useful information, gather it from family members or bystanders. (© Craig Jackson/In the Dark Photography)

▶ Summary

Patient assessment is a comprehensive history and physical exam process. This chapter dealt with taking a good history. While it presented the patient history in its entirety, common sense will determine which parts are appropriate for a given situation. Most of a paramedic's work is patient contact. It is making a connection with people in crisis. Patients most often comment on the attitudes of their paramedics. How well did they relate to them? Did they make them feel at ease? Did they care for them? Patients rarely comment on a paramedic's technical skills. Top-notch paramedics are technically skillful and treat all their patients with dignity and compassion. This begins with the history.

Good patient interaction can lead to good patient outcomes, improved patient satisfaction, and better adherence to treatment. As a paramedic you may be your patient's first contact when he enters the health care world. Let his first impression of the health care industry be your caring, compassionate, professional demeanor. Conducting effective and efficient interviews and communicating with your patient are essential to good medical practice. Medical interviewing is a basic clinical skill that must be learned and practiced, much like airway management.

▶ You Make the Call

You are at lunch when the call comes in to respond to an ill man at the baseball field. A large, midsummer crowd is at the multifield park complex. Upon arrival you meet Mr. George Harmon, a middle-aged man who sits in the bleachers in mild distress. You introduce yourself and begin an initial assessment. Your patient complains of chest pain. You rapidly assess mental status, airway patency, breathing, and circulation. His skin color, mental status, and ability to speak clearly in full sentences suggest he is hemodynamically stable. His strong, regular pulse and warm, dry skin confirm your initial impression. You are ready to elicit the history.

1. List some nonverbal communication techniques that will facilitate open discussion of your patient's problems.

2. Outline the components of the interview you would use for this patient in the following categories:
   a. History of present illness
   b. Past history
   c. Current health status
   d. Review of systems

See Suggested Responses at the back of this book.

▶ Review Questions

1. As you gather the elements of your patient's history, you understand that the list of possible causes for your patient's symptoms is called the:
   a. clinical diagnosis.
   b. field prognosis.
   c. chief complaint.
   d. differential field diagnosis.

2. Your ability to establish rapport with your patient is determined by all of the following EXCEPT the:
   a. situation.
   b. patient.
   c. conditions.
   d. equipment.

3. Your patient is a 65-year-old gentleman whose name is John Berry. Unless otherwise directed by the patient, you should address him as:
   a. honey.
   b. pops.
   c. chief.
   d. Mr. Berry.

4. By simply touching your patient's wrist you can:
   a. make personal contact.
   b. assess pulse.
   c. assess skin condition.
   d. all of the above.

5. Open-ended questions:
   a. allow your patient to explain how he feels in detail.
   b. require only a "yes" or "no" answer.
   c. usually threaten the patient.
   d. limit your patient's responses.

6. A disadvantage of closed-ended questions is that they:
   a. elicit a short answer to a direct question.
   b. are inappropriate when time is limited.
   c. may lead your patient toward certain answers.
   d. are difficult for a mentally challenged patient.

7. Which of the following practices could help you figure out the cause of your patient's complaint?
   a. clarification
   b. reflection

  c. interpretation

  d. any of the above

8. Which of the following is most likely to help if your patient seems to be hiding the truth?

  a. facilitation

  b. reflection

  c. confrontation

  d. interpretation

9. Referred pain is felt in a part of the body away from the source of the disease or problem. The heart and the _____ are two areas that most commonly produce referred pain.

  a. liver

  b. spleen

  c. diaphragm

  d. urinary bladder

10. Blind patients present special problems in history taking. As you gather the history from a blind patient, you should do all of the following EXCEPT:

  a. identify yourself immediately.

  b. explain who you are and why you are there.

  c. speak in a loud, clear voice directly into the patient's ear.

  d. gently take your patient's hand to show him where you are standing.

See Answers to Review Questions at the back of this book.

▶ Further Reading

Bates, Barbara, Lynn S. Bickley, and Robert A. Hoekelman. *A Guide to Physical Examination and History Taking.* 9th ed. Philadelphia: Lippincott, Williams & Wilkins, 2005.

Bledsoe, B.E., R.A. Porter, and R.A. Cherry. "Twenty-five Tricks and Pearls of Physical Examination." *Journal of Emergency Medical Services (JEMS),* March 2005.

Coulehan, John L., and Marian R. Block. *The Medical Interview: Mastering Skills for Clinical Practice.* 5th ed. Philadelphia: F.A. Davis, 2006.

Epstein, Owen, et al. *Clinical Examination.* 3rd ed. St. Louis: Mosby, 2003.

Lipkin, Mack Jr., Samuel M. Putnam, and Aaron Lazare. *The Medical Interview: Clinical Care, Education, and Research.* New York: Springer, 1996.

Seidel, Henry M. *Mosby's Guide to Physical Examination.* 6th ed. St. Louis: Mosby, 2006.

Willms, Janice L., Henry Schniederman, and Paula S. Algranati. *Physical Diagnosis: Bedside Evaluation of Diagnosis and Function.* Baltimore: Williams & Wilkins, 1994.

▶ Media Resources

See the Student CD at the back of this book for quizzes, animations, videos and other features related to this chapter. Also, visit the Companion Website for Brady's paramedic series at **www.prenhall.com/bledsoe**, where you will find additional reinforcement and links to other resources.

Physical Exam Techniques

Objectives

After reading this chapter, you should be able to:

1. Define and describe the techniques of inspection, palpation, percussion, auscultation. (pp. 31–35)
2. Describe the evaluation of mental status. (pp. 142–146)
3. Evaluate the importance of a general survey. (pp. 39–51)
4. Describe the examination of the following body regions, differentiate between normal and abnormal findings, and define the significance of abnormal findings:
   - Skin, hair, and nails (pp. 52–60)
   - Head, scalp, and skull (pp. 60–62)
   - Eyes, ears, nose, mouth, and pharynx (pp. 62–82)
   - Neck (pp. 82–84)
   - Thorax (anterior and posterior) (pp. 84–92)
   - Arterial pulse including rate, rhythm, and amplitude (pp. 92–97)
   - Jugular venous pressure and pulsations (pp. 92–97)
   - Heart and blood vessels (pp. 92–97)
   - Abdomen (pp. 97–103)
   - Male and female genitalia (pp. 103–107)
   - Anus and rectum (pp. 107–108)
   - Musculoskeletal system (pp. 108–136)
   - Peripheral vascular system (pp. 136–142)
   - Nervous system (pp. 142–167)
   - Cranial nerves (pp. 146–154)
5. Describe the assessment of visual acuity. (pp. 62–71)

6. Explain the rationale for the use of an ophthalmoscope and otoscope. (pp. 37, 70–71, 75–78)
7. Describe the survey of respiration. (pp. 42–44, 84–92)
8. Describe percussion of the chest. (pp. 88, 91)
9. Differentiate the percussion notes and their characteristics. (pp. 33–34)
10. Describe special examination techniques related to the assessment of the chest. (pp. 84–92)
11. Describe the auscultation of the chest, heart, and abdomen. (88–92, 97, 101, 103)
12. Distinguish between normal and abnormal auscultation findings of the chest, heart, and abdomen and explain their significance. (pp. 88–92, 97, 101, 103)
13. Describe special techniques of the cardiovascular examination. (pp. 92–97)
14. Describe the general guidelines of recording examination information. (pp. 175–178)
15. Discuss the examination considerations for an infant or child. (pp. 167–174)

Key Terms

ascites, p. 101
auscultation, p. 34
Babinski's response, p. 164
blood pressure, p. 44
borborygmi, p. 103
bradycardia, p. 41
bradypnea, p. 42
bronchophony, p. 91
Broselow tape, p. 40
bruit, p. 95
capnography, p. 49
cardiac monitor, p. 50
cardiac output, p. 94
crackles, p. 88
crepitus, p. 111
Cullen's sign, p. 101
diastole, p. 93
diastolic blood pressure, p. 45
egophony, p. 91
end-tidal carbon dioxide (ETCO$_2$) detector, p. 49
glucometer, p. 51

Grey Turner's sign, p. 101
hypertension, p. 45
hyperthermia, p. 48
hypotension, p. 46
hypothermia, p. 48
inspection, p.31
Korotkoff sounds, p. 45
lesion, p. 54
manometer, p. 36
ophthalmoscope, p. 37
otoscope, p. 37
palpation, p. 32
percussion, p. 33
perfusion, p. 45
pitting, p. 141
pleural friction rub, p. 90
priapism, p. 106
pulse oximeter, p. 48
pulse pressure, p. 45
pulse quality, p. 41
pulse rate, p. 41
pulse rhythm, p. 41
quality of respiration, p. 44

respiration, p. 42
respiratory effort, p. 42
respiratory rate, p. 42
rhonchi, p. 90
sphygmomanometer, p. 36
stethoscope, p. 35
stridor, p. 90
stroke volume, p. 94
systole, p. 93
systolic blood pressure, p. 44
tachycardia, p. 41
tachypnea, p. 42
thrill, p. 95
tidal volume, p. 44
turgor, p. 54
visual acuity wall chart/card, p. 63
vital statistics, p. 39
wheezes, p. 90
whispered pectoriloquy, p. 91

Case Study

The overnight crew at Station 51 tonight consists of paramedic Dale Monday and his EMT-Basic partner, Pam True. Early into their shift they are called to a "man down" at Cirrincione's, a popular Italian restaurant featuring Sicilian cuisine. Upon arrival they find Robert Dalton, an agitated male in his early 70s who just can't seem to stand up. Mr. Dalton is alert and oriented. He complains of general weakness and of being unable to stand without wobbling or to walk a straight line.

Dale begins to elicit a history from Mr. Dalton's wife. She claims he has been having these problems off and on for the past few days but that this is worse. Mr. Dalton denies any chest pain, shortness of breath, dizziness, or nausea. His past history includes coronary artery disease, hypertension, and congestive heart failure. He takes nitroglycerin as needed, furosemide, aspirin, digoxin, captopril, and a potassium supplement. He and his wife have not yet eaten tonight. Dale tells his partner to get the stretcher and continues his assessment, which includes a focused physical exam and vital signs.

Because they have a 35-minute ride to McGivern General Hospital, Dale decides to perform a detailed physical exam en route. His patient appears to be an otherwise healthy 72-year-old man. He is well dressed and well groomed. His vital signs are blood pressure—150/86; heart rate—88, strong and regular; respirations—18; skin—warm, dry, and pink. Dale finds no evidence of head trauma. His patient's ears, nose, and throat are normal. He shows no facial drooping or slurred speech. His pupils are equal and reactive to light and accommodation. Visual acuity is normal. Extraocular muscles are intact. Dale notes nystagmus with his patient's left lateral gaze. He finds no palpable nodes. His patient's trachea is midline, and his chest and abdomen appear normal. His distal extremities are warm and pink. Deep tendon reflexes are 2+ in the upper extremities and 1+ in the lower. His peripheral pulses are strong.

Dale decides to conduct a complete neurologic examination. His patient's mental status is normal. He is alert and oriented to person, place, and time. His responses are appropriate and timely, and he does not drift off the topic or lose interest. His posture is somewhat slumped, and he has trouble maintaining his balance when standing. He also complains of difficulty buttoning his shirt. He has no tremors or fasciculations. His facial expressions are appropriate for the situation. His speech is inflected, clear and strong, fluent and articulate, and he can vary his volume. He expresses his thoughts clearly and speaks spontaneously with a clear and distinct voice. His present state of uncoordinated movement and imbalance agitates him, yet he organizes his thoughts and speaks logically and coherently.

Satisfied that Mr. Dalton's mental status is normal, Dale continues with the motor function exam. Mr. Dalton's general posture is slumped to the left. He has no tremors except at the very end of fine motor movements. His overall muscle bulk, tone, and strength appear normal.

Dale then asks his patient to perform a series of tests aimed at evaluating coordination. First, he asks him to tap the distal joint of his thumb with the tip of his index finger as rapidly as possible. Next he asks him to place his hand palm-up on his thigh, quickly turn it over palm-down, and then repeat this movement as rapidly as possible for 15 seconds. Mr. Dalton cannot perform these tests with his left hand. Nor can he perform point-to-point testing on his left side, and he has tremors at the far point. Finally, he cannot perform the heel-to-shin movement on his left side.

Convinced that his patient is having a left cerebellar infarct, Dale contacts McGivern General Hospital and gives his report to Dr. Hunt, a very impressed emergency physician. Computed tomography and magnetic resonance imaging results confirm Dale's report.

PHYSICAL EXAMINATION APPROACH AND OVERVIEW

Although assessment of a medical patient formally starts with the history, the physical examination actually begins when you first set eyes on your patient. Upon meeting him you immediately assess his general appearance, level of consciousness, breathing effort, and skin color. If you initially use touch as a reassuring gesture, you can also assess skin condition and peripheral pulses. Your physical assessment continues throughout the history as you ask questions and observe your patient's body language, facial expressions, and general demeanor. Thus, you cannot draw an exact dividing line between the history and the physical exam. In emergency street medicine, the two usually occur simultaneously.

Although patient assessment formally starts with the history, the physical examination actually begins when you first set eyes on your patient.

Assessment Pearls

Have a Standard Examination System, and Follow It Every Time When we do something repetitively, we tend to develop patterns. This is true with physical exams. You should establish a personal system or order in which you assess patients. Following your own personal system or pattern will help ensure that you don't leave out part of the exam. In fact, having a system or established pattern is often a medico-legal defense. If you document that you always perform your physical exam the same way, it shows to a jury or judge that there is less of a chance you missed something during your assessment. However, this is not to say that you should never modify your exam. Everyone modifies their exam for children and special situations. But even then, you tend to develop a subroutine that you follow. Again, such a system ensures that an important part of the physical examination is not missed.

Cultural Considerations

A Matter of Respect The physical exam process often includes viewing parts of the body generally shielded from the view of strangers. Because of this, some patients may be particularly sensitive about revealing various aspects of the body to a stranger—even a paramedic.

The way in which you approach a patient for physical assessment must take into consideration the patient's cultural beliefs or customs. In some cultures, especially certain Arab cultures, it is forbidden for a woman to reveal her face or body to a man who is not her husband. This constraint certainly makes a detailed physical exam difficult. Sometimes, in fact, an examination cannot be completed because of patient refusal. In some instances, an examination may be allowed only if the examiner is of the same gender as the patient. Likewise, seemingly innocent comments by rescuers—such as "You have a pretty face. Let me take a look at your head"—can be insulting or offensive. It implies that flattery can convince these patients to consent to something that is not allowed by their culture or religion, or both.

If you work in an area where there is considerable cultural diversity, it is important to understand the cultural beliefs and practices of the groups you may encounter. More important, you must respect these beliefs and customs. In turn, the patients will respect you.

The purpose of the physical exam is to investigate areas that you suspect are involved in your patient's primary problem. Just as we covered the entire history in Chapter 1, we present the entire physical exam in this one. Again, if you practice in a setting other than a prehospital one, such as conducting preemployment physicals for a company, you might perform the entire physical examination outlined here. On an emergency run, you limit the exam to only those aspects that you decide are appropriate. Practice and clinical experience will dictate your ability to apply the skills you learn in this chapter to real situations.

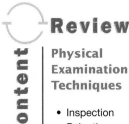

The purpose of the physical exam is to investigate areas that you suspect are involved in your patient's primary problem.

Examination Techniques

Four techniques—inspection, palpation, percussion, and auscultation—are the foundation of the formal physical exam. Each can reveal information essential to a comprehensive patient assessment.

Inspection

Inspection is the process of informed observation (Figure 2-1). A simple, noninvasive technique that clinicians often take for granted, it is also one of their most valuable tools in appraising patient condition. With a keen eye, you can evaluate your patient's condition in great detail.

Inspection begins when you first meet your patient and continues while you take his history. Often, this first impression forms the basis for your history because you will judge your patient's clinical status immediately. Notice how he presents himself. Is he conscious and alert or unconscious and flaccid? Is he lying on the floor, sitting upright, or limping badly on one foot? Is he breathing normally or gasping for each breath? You can learn a great deal about your patient's neurologic, musculoskeletal, and respiratory systems just by careful observation. Watch for changes in his emotional and mental status throughout the history and physical exam.

During the formal physical exam, consciously evaluate each body area, looking for discoloration, unusual motion, or deformity. Pay special attention to areas where you most expect to find signs and where the patient complains of symptoms. For example, if your patient struck his chest against a bent steering wheel, you would

Review

Physical Examination Techniques

- Inspection
- Palpation
- Percussion
- Auscultation

inspection
the process of informed observation.

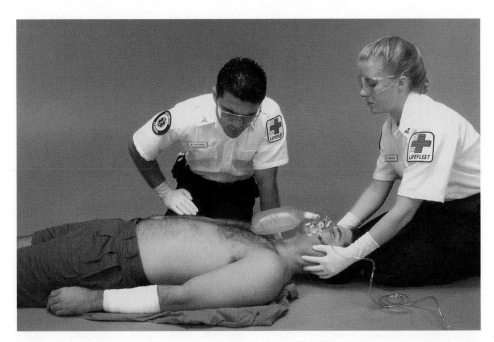

 Figure 2-1 Inspect your patient's body for signs of injury or illness.

expect to see chest wall abnormalities. Remember that you may not notice the skin color changes that follow a significant contusion until after your patient arrives at the emergency department.

Effective inspection depends on good lighting, adequate time, and a curiosity for looking beyond the obvious. During your inspection, draw on your past clinical experiences to identify the signs of illness and injury. Knowing what you are looking for is essential. Do not hurry. Give yourself enough time to inspect and then to process what you see. Inspection is an ongoing process that should not end until you transfer your patient to emergency department staff. Finally, although you must respect your patient's modesty and dignity, never allow clothing to obstruct your examination.

Palpation

palpation

using your sense of touch to gather information.

Palpation is usually the next step in assessing your patient, although sometimes you will inspect and palpate your patient simultaneously. **Palpation** involves using your sense of touch to gather information. With your hands and fingers you can determine a structure's size, shape, and position. You also can evaluate its temperature, moisture, texture, and movement. You can check for growths, swelling, tenderness, spasms, rigidity, pain, and crepitus. When you become skilled at this procedure, you can detect a distended bladder, an enlarged liver, a laterally pulsating abdominal aorta, or the position of a fetus.

Certain parts of your hands and fingers are better than others for specific types of palpation. For example, the pads of your fingers are more sensitive than the tips for detecting position, size, consistency, masses, fluid, and crepitus; therefore, you would use them to palpate lymph nodes or rib fractures (Figure 2-2 ▶). The palm of your hand is better for sensing vibrations such as fremitus. Because its skin is thinner and more sensitive, the back of your hand or fingers is better for evaluating temperature.

Palpation may be either deep or light. You control its depth by applying pressure with your hand and fingers. Since deep palpation may elicit tenderness or disrupt tissue or fluid, you should always perform light palpation first. Use light palpation to assess the skin and superficial structures. Press in approximately 1 centimeter. Apply the same gentle pressure you use to feel a pulse. Too much pressure dulls your sensitivity and can injure your patient.

▶ **Figure 2-2** Palpate with the pads of your fingers to detect masses, fluids, and crepitus.

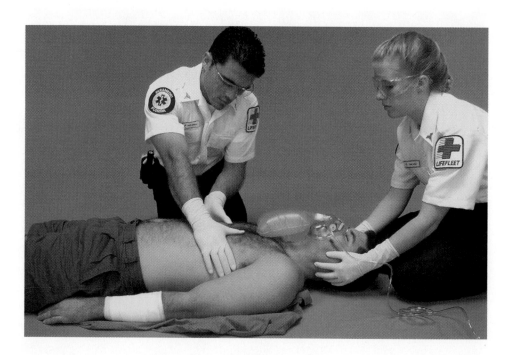

Table 2-1	Percussion Sounds				
Sound	**Description**	**Intensity**	**Pitch**	**Duration**	**Location**
Tympany	Drumlike	Loud	High	Medium	Stomach
Hyperresonance	Booming	Loud	Low	Long	Hyperinflated lung
Resonance	Hollow	Loud	Low	Long	Normal lung
Dull	Thud	Medium	Medium	Medium	Solid organs—liver
Flat	Extremely dull	Soft	High	Short	Muscle, atelectasis

To assess visceral organs such as those in the abdomen, use deep palpation. Apply pressure by placing the fingers of the opposite hand over the sensing fingers and gently pressing in about 4 centimeters. This will increase your sensitivity to any masses, guarding, or other abdominal pathology. Feel for areas of warmth that might reflect injury before significant edema or discoloration occur. Observe how your patient responds with facial expressions while you palpate tender areas. Even if he is unconscious, he may respond to pain with facial expressions or purposeful or purposeless motion.

Palpation begins your physical assessment of your patient. Three commonsense tips will help make it therapeutic and respectful. Keep your hands warm, keep your fingernails short, and be gentle to avoid discomfort or injury to your patient.

To make palpation therapeutic and respectful, keep your hands warm, keep your fingernails short, and be gentle.

Percussion

Percussion is the production of sound waves by striking one object against another. In this technique, you strike a knuckle on one hand with the tip of a finger on the opposite hand. The impact causes vibrations that produce sound waves from 4 to 6 centimeters deep in the underlying body tissue. We hear these sound waves as percussion tones. The density of the tissue through which the sound must travel determines the degree of percussion. The denser the medium, the quieter the tone. The tone's resonance or lack of resonance indicates whether the underlying region is filled with air, air under pressure, fluid, or normal tissue. Listen to each sound and evaluate its meaning (Table 2–1).

percussion
the production of sound waves by striking one object against another.

Move across the area that you are percussing and compare sounds with what you know to be normal there. For example, in the chest you expect to hear the resonant sound of a healthy lung filled with air and tissue. In a pneumothorax or emphysema, however, you may hear the hyperresonant sound of air trapped in the chest. In a hemothorax, you may hear the dull sound of blood in the same area.

Percussion is simple. Place one hand on the area of the body you wish to percuss. Use a finger of that hand (usually the middle finger) as the striking surface. Sharply tap the distal knuckle of that finger with the tip of your other middle finger (Figure 2-3 ▶).

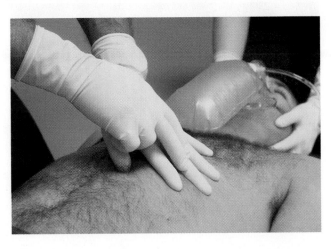

▶ **Figure 2-3** Percuss your patient to evaluate vibrations and sounds.

The tap should come from snapping the wrist, not the forearm or shoulder. Snap the finger back quickly to avoid dampening the sound. When percussing the chest, make sure the finger lies between the ribs and parallel to them. In this way you will percuss the tissue underneath the ribs, not the ribs themselves.

A wall in your home is a good place to practice your percussion skills. As you percuss the air-filled area between studs, you will hear a hollow, resonant sound. Wall spaces filled with insulation will sound less resonant. When you percuss over a wall stud, you will notice a flatter, dull sound. You can apply this principle to the percussion of body cavities. Compare the sounds on the affected side with those on the unaffected side. The key is knowing what is normal, so above all you must practice percussion on healthy people in order to recognize abnormalities in sick or injured patients.

Unfortunately at most emergency scenes, especially those in the street, noise prevents percussing your patient effectively. Your clinical experience and common sense will tell you when to use this valuable assessment technique.

Auscultation

Auscultation involves listening for sounds produced by the body, primarily the lungs, the heart, the intestines, and major blood vessels. It is difficult to master. You may hear some sounds clearly, such as stridor, the high-pitched squeal of a partially obstructed upper airway. Most, however, require a stethoscope. You should perform auscultation in a quiet environment. Unfortunately, this is not always practical in emergency services. Hearing the low-amplitude heart and lung sounds against on-scene noise or in-transit background noise may be especially difficult.

For your patient's comfort, warm the end piece of your stethoscope with your hands before auscultating. To auscultate, hold the end piece of your stethoscope between your second and third fingers and press the diaphragm firmly against your patient's skin (Figure 2-4 ▶). If you are using the bell side, place it evenly and lightly on the skin. Avoid touching the tubing with your hands or allowing it to rub any surfaces. Make sure the earpieces point anteriorly before you put them in your ears.

Listen for the presence of sound and its intensity, pitch, duration, and quality. When reporting and recording lung sounds, always note abnormal sounds (crackles, wheezes), their locations (bilateral, right lower lobe, bases), and their timing during the respiratory cycle (inspiratory, end-expiratory). Sometimes, closing your eyes helps you concentrate on the sounds by eliminating visual stimuli. Try to isolate and concentrate on one sound at a time. Generally, auscultate after you have used other assessment techniques. The only exception is the abdomen, which you should auscultate before palpation and percussion. A paramedic should be proficient in auscultating

You must practice percussion on healthy people in order to recognize abnormalities in sick or injured patients.

auscultation
listening with a stethoscope for sounds produced by the body.

▶ **Figure 2-4** Auscultate body sounds with the stethoscope.

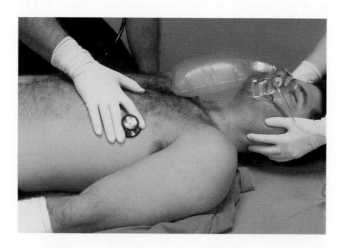

blood pressure, lung sounds, heart sounds, bowel sounds, and arterial bruits. As with any other physical assessment tool, you cannot detect abnormalities unless you know what is normal. Take every opportunity to auscultate lung, heart, and bowel sounds regularly.

Equipment

To conduct a comprehensive physical examination you will need a stethoscope, a sphygmomanometer, an ophthalmoscope, an otoscope, a scale, and other equipment. The ophthalmoscope, otoscope, and scale are not considered prehospital assessment tools.

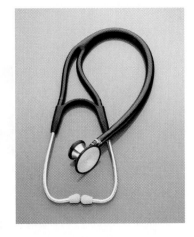

Figure 2-5 Use a stethoscope to auscultate most sounds.

Stethoscope The **stethoscope** is a basic paramedic tool used to auscultate most sounds (Figure 2-5 ▶). It transmits sound waves from the source through an end piece and along rubber tubes to the ear. One side of the end piece is a rigid diaphragm that best transmits high-pitched sounds such as heart sounds and blood pressure sounds. The diaphragm also screens out low-pitched sounds such as lung sounds and bowel sounds. The other side of the end piece is a bell that uses the skin as a diaphragm. The sounds that the bell transmits vary with the amount of pressure exerted. For example, with light pressure the bell picks up low-pitched sounds; with firm pressure it acts like the diaphragm and transmits high-pitched sounds. Whether you use the bell or the diaphragm depends on which sounds you are auscultating. To hear blood pressure or heart sounds, for instance, use the diaphragm; to hear lung or bowel sounds, use the bell side.

Accurate auscultation depends in part on the quality of your instrument. Your stethoscope should have the following important characteristics:

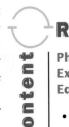

Review

Physical Examination Equipment

- Stethoscope
- Sphygmomanometer
- Ophthalmoscope
- Otoscope
- Scale
- Tongue blades
- Penlight
- Visual acuity chart/card
- Reflex hammer
- Thermometer

stethoscope
tool used to auscultate most sounds.

- ▶ A rigid diaphragm cover
- ▶ Thick, heavy tubing that conducts sound better than thin, flexible tubing
- ▶ Short tubing (30 to 40 cm) to minimize distortion
- ▶ Earpieces that fit snugly—large enough to occlude the ear canal—and are angled toward the nose to project sound toward the eardrum
- ▶ A bell with a rubber-ring edge to ensure good contact with the skin

Sphygmomanometer The circumstances and the patient care setting determine what type of equipment you use to measure blood pressure (Figure 2-6 ▶). Intensive care unit staff commonly use intra-arterial pressure devices for critically ill patients who

Assessment Pearls

Taking an Accurate Blood Pressure in the Morbidly Obese It's important to accurately measure your patient's blood pressure. In order to obtain an accurate reading, the blood pressure (BP) cuff must fit the patient's arm. Ambulances should have an assortment of various sizes of blood pressure cuffs. However, some morbidly obese patients are so large that even your largest cuff isn't big enough. In these cases, take an appropriate-size cuff and apply it to the patient's forearm where there is not as much adipose tissue to interfere with the reading. Place the diaphragm of your stethoscope over the radial artery and measure the blood pressure. Such forearm readings are often more accurate than standard readings in the morbidly obese patient.

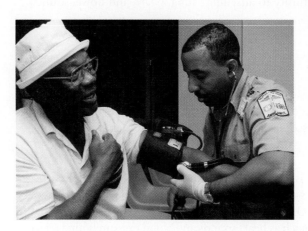

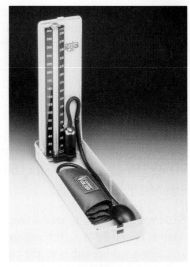

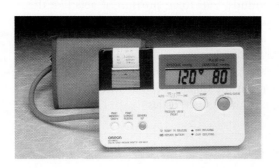

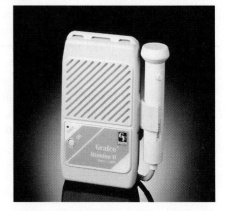

▶ **Figure 2-6** Use a blood pressure device suited to the circumstances. Clockwise from upper left: aneroid sphygmomanometer, mercury sphygmomanometer, digital electronic, and Doppler device.

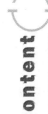

Review

The Upper Airway

- Nasal cavity
- Pharynx
- Larynx

Because your patient's blood pressure is important in evaluating his condition, you must be able to measure it accurately.

sphygmomanometer

blood pressure measuring device comprising a bulb, a cuff, and a manometer.

manometer

pressure gauge with a scale calibrated in millimeters of mercury (mmHg).

need continuous monitoring. When a noisy environment makes auscultation difficult or when the sounds are especially weak, a Doppler device that amplifies the sounds is useful. You will see these devices in the emergency department, newborn nursery, emergency vehicles, and labor and delivery suites. The most familiar blood pressure measuring device is the aneroid **sphygmomanometer.** You will use it with your stethoscope to auscultate the sounds of the blood moving through an artery, usually the brachial artery. Because your patient's blood pressure is important in evaluating his condition, you must be able to measure it accurately.

A sphygmomanometer includes a bulb, a cuff, and a manometer. The cuff has an airtight, flat, rubber bladder enclosed within a fabric cover. Cuffs are available in various sizes and designs. Flexible tubing attaches the rubber bulb to the cuff. Squeezing the bulb pumps air into the cuff's bladder. A control valve allows you to inflate and deflate the cuff. To inflate the cuff, close the valve by turning it clockwise; to deflate the cuff, open the valve by turning it counterclockwise.

The **manometer** is a pressure gauge with a scale calibrated in millimeters of mercury (mmHg). Each line represents 2 mmHg. The heavy lines are 10 mmHg of mercury apart. The aneroid manometer displays the scale on a circular dial. As the pressure in the bladder changes, the needle moves and indicates the pressure reading at

Assessment Pearls

Getting a Closer Look   A comprehensive physical examination is essential in prehospital care. However, it's often difficult to examine the posterior body surface without significantly moving the patient (which usually requires assistance). One trick to help with this is to carry a small hand mirror with you for assessing areas that are hard to view if the patient is seated or immobilized. Thus, you won't have to get on your knees to see the posterior aspect of your patient's body. A small flashlight used in conjunction with the hand mirror will help improve the illumination. A small hand mirror in every ambulance is a cheap investment that will pay off many times over.

On many occasions you'll find yourself in need of magnification. This may be to examine an injury, a skin lesion, a splinter, or something similar. Ambulances should carry at least one ophthalmoscope and an otoscope. Both are excellent for providing magnification and excellent lighting. For larger areas or for injuries for which you're trying to perform a procedure (such as removing a splinter), the otoscope is the better choice. For smaller and more detailed work, the ophthalmoscope can be used. You may need to adjust the diopter of the ophthalmoscope to compensate for your own vision, and then dial up or down until the object you're examining comes into view.

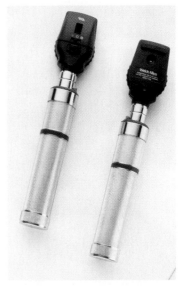

▶ **Figure 2-7**   Visualize the interior of your patient's eyes with an ophthalmoscope.

a given moment. When you use an aneroid sphygmomanometer, keep the dial in plain sight. The aneroid types lose their calibration, so you will need to calibrate them periodically against a mercury-type device.

The mercury sphygmomanometer displays the scale along a glass tube connected to a reservoir of mercury. As pressure in the cuff increases, the mercury in the tube rises. When using a mercury sphygmomanometer, keep the scale at eye level and vertical. Available as portable, wall-mounted, or floor units, mercury sphygmomanometers are more accurate than aneroid, but they are impractical for prehospital use.

Ophthalmoscope   An **ophthalmoscope** allows you to examine the interior of your patient's eyes. It is a handheld device comprised of a light source and a series of lenses and mirrors (Figure 2-7 ▶).

Otoscope   To visualize the ear canal and tympanic membrane, you will need an **otoscope.** The otoscope provides illumination for inspecting the ear canal and tympanic membrane (eardrum) and the internal nose. It has a light source, a speculum you insert into the ear canal, and a magnifying glass through which you visualize the inner structures of the ear (Figure 2-8 ▶).

Scale   The standing platform scale measures weight and height (Figure 2-9 ▶). To measure weight, it uses a system of counterbalanced weights that you calibrate before each use. Your patient simply stands on the scale, and you add or subtract weight in small increments until it balances. To measure your patient's height, pull up the height adjustment and position the head piece at his crown. Electronic scales are becoming more popular. They calculate your patient's weight electronically and display it as a digital readout. You also calibrate them before each use.

Additional Equipment   Besides the above items, you will need sterile tongue blades to inspect inside the mouth and to initiate a gag reflex; a penlight to test your patient's

ophthalmoscope
handheld device used to examine interior of eye.

otoscope
handheld device used to examine interior of ears and nose.

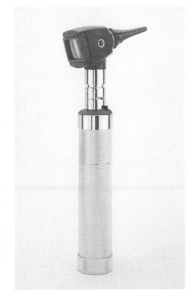

▶ **Figure 2-8**   An otoscope enables you to inspect the ear canal and tympanic membrane.

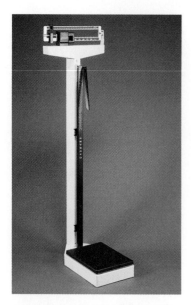

Figure 2-9 Use a platform scale to measure your patient's weight and height.

How you approach your patient, both in the emergency setting and elsewhere, will set the stage for an efficient and effective patient assessment.

pupillary responses; a visual acuity chart or card to measure visual acuity; a reflex hammer to test deep tendon reflexes; and a thermometer to measure body temperature (Figure 2-10 ▶). The danger of breakage limits glass thermometers' usefulness in the prehospital setting, and their inability to record temperatures below 96° F (36° C) prevents them from helping you evaluate the hypothermic patient. Available battery-operated devices measure temperature orally, rectally, and in the ear canal. If your service operates in areas of low environmental temperatures, equip your ambulance with a low-reading thermometer. Some of these items, such as the ophthalmoscope, otoscope, and scale, will be more suited to a medical clinic setting than to a typical prehospital scene.

The General Approach

How you approach your patient, both in the emergency setting and elsewhere, will set the stage for an efficient and effective patient assessment. Most patients are apprehensive about a physical examination. They feel exposed and vulnerable, and they fear painful procedures. This anxiety is multiplied in an emergency. You must recognize your patient's apprehension and take steps to alleviate it. Display confidence and skill while you complete your history and physical exam.

If you systematically assess your patient's complaints and efficiently perform your duties, he should feel safe. Then add the personal touches of active listening, a reassuring voice, and gestures that convey your sincere compassion and interest. Most patients will respond favorably. Let your patient know that you are not just checking off items on a diagnostic list; you are conducting a personal examination of *his* problems.

Proficiency will come only with clinical practice. In time, you will become adept at focusing the exam on your patient's chief complaint and present illness. In the emergency setting, no matter how nervous and apprehensive you may be, never let your patient see anything but a calm, professional, confident demeanor. This will help alleviate his anxiety about disclosing personal information to, and being examined by, a nonphysician. Try to remain objective, even when confronted by alarming or disgusting information. A bad bedsore, a perverted sexual story, or black tarry stools (melena)

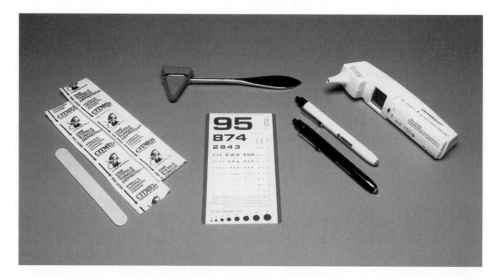

Figure 2-10 Essential assessment tools.

can test even the most experienced clinician's composure. Simply thinking about how embarrassed your patient must be may help you keep your own poise.

OVERVIEW OF A COMPREHENSIVE EXAMINATION

This section gives an overview of the comprehensive physical exam. Later in the chapter we will discuss each component in detail. The key to an effective comprehensive exam is to integrate each individual section into a unified patient assessment. Chapter 3 provides a template for conducting a problem-oriented patient assessment on both medical and trauma patients.

As a paramedic, you will determine which elements of the comprehensive exam to use. You will base your decision on your patient's presenting problem and clinical status. For example, if you are conducting comprehensive physicals for your fire department, you may choose to use the entire examination. If you are assessing a child just struck by an automobile and lying unconscious in the street, you will narrow your focus to the child's injuries. A comprehensive examination should include a general survey and a detailed assessment of anatomical regions.

The General Survey

A general survey is the first part of a comprehensive examination. It begins with noting your patient's appearance and goes on to include vital signs and other assessments.

Appearance

A thorough evaluation of your patient's appearance can provide a great deal of valuable information about his health. Note his level of consciousness, posture, and any obvious signs of distress, such as sitting upright gasping for each breath or slumped to one side. Is his motor activity normal or does he have noticeable tremors or paralysis? Observe his general state of health, his dress, grooming, and personal hygiene. Obvious odors can also provide significant information.

Level of Consciousness   Is your patient awake? Is he alert? Does he speak to you in a normal voice? Are his eyes open, and does he respond to you and others in the environment? If he is not apparently awake, speak to him in a loud voice. If he does not respond to your verbal cues, shake him gently. If he still does not respond, apply a painful stimulus such as pinching a tendon, rubbing his sternum, or rolling a pencil across a nail bed. Note and document his response.

Signs of Distress   Is your patient in distress? For example, does he have a cardiac or respiratory problem, as evidenced by labored breathing, wheezing, or a cough? Is he in pain, as evidenced by wincing, sweating, or protecting the painful area? Is he anxious, as evidenced by his facial expression, cold moist palms, or nervous fidgeting?

Apparent State of Health   Is your patient healthy, robust, and vigorous? Or is he frail, ill looking, or feeble? Does he have an obvious abnormality? Base your evaluation of his general state of health on your observations throughout the interview and physical examination.

Vital Statistics   **Vital statistics,** weight and height, are used widely in clinical medicine. Accurately measuring your patient's weight and height with a scale, however, is not

Review

General Survey

- Appearance
- Vital signs
- Additional assessments
  Pulse oximetry
  Capnography
  Cardiac monitoring
  Blood glucose
  determination

vital statistics
height and weight.

a practical prehospital assessment procedure. You will occasionally estimate your patient's weight to administer medications for which the dose is weight dependent. You also may use a **Broselow tape** to measure your infant patient's length. The Broselow tape provides information concerning drug dosages, airway management adjuncts, and intravenous calculations based on your patient's height.

Note your patient's general stature. Is he lanky and slender, short and stocky, muscular and symmetrical? Does he have any obvious deformities or disproportionate areas? Is he extremely thin or obese? If obese, is the fat evenly distributed or is it concentrated in his trunk? Has he gained or lost weight recently?

Sexual Development   Is your patient's sexual maturity appropriate for his or her age and gender? Consider such indicators as voice, facial and body hair, and breast size.

Skin Color and Obvious Lesions   Is your patient's skin pale, suggesting decreased blood flow or anemia? Does he have central (lips, oral mucosa) or peripheral (nail beds, hands) cyanosis, the bluish color resulting from decreased oxygenation of the tissues? Does he have the yellow color of jaundice or high carotene levels? Note any rashes, bruises, scars, or discoloration.

Posture, Gait, and Motor Activity   Observe your patient's posture and presentation. Is he sitting straight up and forward, bracing his arms (tripoding)? This suggests a serious breathing problem such as acute pulmonary edema or airway obstruction. Does one side of his body droop and seem immobile, suggesting a stroke? Does he sit quietly or does he seem restless? Does he have tremors or other involuntary movements?

Dress, Grooming, and Personal Hygiene   Does your patient dress appropriately for the climate and situation? Are his clothes clean and properly fastened? Are they conventional for his age and social group? Abnormalities in dress might suggest the cold intolerance of hypothyroidism or the hiding of a skin rash or needle marks, or they might simply reflect personal preference. Look at his shoes. Are they clean? Do they have holes, slits, open laces, or other alterations to accommodate painful foot conditions such as gout, bunions, or edema? Does he wear a slipper, or slippers, instead of shoes? Is he wearing unusual jewelry such as a copper bracelet for arthritis or a medical information tag? Do his grooming and hygiene seem appropriate for his age, lifestyle, occupation, and social status? Does his lack of concern over appearance (overgrown nails and hair, for instance) suggest a long illness or depression?

Odors of Breath or Body   Does your patient have any unusual or striking body or breath odors? The acetone breath of a diabetic, the bitter-almond breath of a cyanide poisoning, the putrid smell of bacterial infection, or the obvious smell of alcohol may give important clues to the underlying problem. Avoid tunnel vision when you smell alcohol, which often masks other serious illnesses such as liver failure or injuries such as a subdural hematoma.

Facial Expression   Watch your patient's facial expressions throughout your interaction. His face should reflect his emotions during the interview and physical exam. The patient with hyperthyroidism may stare intently. The Parkinson's patient's face may appear immobile.

Measurement of Vital Signs

The four basic vital signs in medicine are pulse, respiration, blood pressure, and body temperature. While any complete physical examination should include all four, the first three are most important in prehospital care. They are the primary indicators of your patient's health. Measure them early in the physical examination and, in emergency situations, repeat them often and look for trends. For example, in a serious head injury, watch for your patient's systolic blood pressure to rise, his pulse pressure to widen, and his pulse rate to fall. These trends suggest an increase in intracranial pressure, a serious medical emergency. Conversely, a falling blood pressure with an increasing pulse rate may indicate shock. As a paramedic you should become an expert at taking vital signs on patients of every age.

Pulse   As the heart ejects blood through the arteries, a pulse wave results. Each pulse beat corresponds to a cardiac contraction and results from the ejected blood's impact on the arterial walls. The pulse is a valuable indicator of circulatory function. Your patient's pulse rate, rhythm, and quality indicate his hemodynamic (circulatory) status and the critical nature of his condition. **Pulse rate** refers to the number of pulsations felt in 1 minute. It can be slow (bradycardic), normal, or fast (tachycardic). **Pulse rhythm** refers to the pulse's pattern and the equality of intervals between beats. It can be regular, regularly irregular, irregularly irregular, or grossly chaotic. **Pulse quality** refers to the pulse's strength. Terms such as *bounding* or *thready* are used to describe the pulse's quality.

The normal pulse rate for an adult is 60 to 100 beats per minute. Rates below 60 are bradycardic; rates above 100 are tachycardic. **Bradycardia** may indicate an increase in parasympathetic nervous system stimulation. It might also be the result of a head injury, hypothermia, severe hypoxia, or drug overdose. Bradycardia is sometimes a normal finding in the well-conditioned athlete. Treat bradycardia only if it compromises your patient's cardiac output and general circulatory status. **Tachycardia** usually indicates an increase in sympathetic nervous system stimulation with which the body is compensating for another problem such as blood loss, fear, pain, fever, drug overdose, or hypoxia. It is an early indicator of shock and may indicate ventricular tachycardia, a life-threatening cardiac dysrhythmia.

The pulse's rhythm, when present, may be regular, regularly irregular, irregularly irregular, or grossly chaotic. Irregular pulse rates may be due to extra beats, skipped beats, or pacemaker problems and usually indicate a cardiac abnormality. The rhythm's effect on cardiac output determines if intervention is necessary.

The pulse's quality can be weak, strong, or bounding. Weak, thready pulses indicate a decreased circulatory status such as shock. Strong, bounding pulses may indicate high blood pressure, heat stroke, or increasing intracranial pressure. The pulse location may be another indicator of your patient's clinical status. The presence of a carotid pulse generally means that his systolic blood pressure is at least 60 mmHg. The presence of peripheral pulses indicates a higher blood pressure; their absence suggests circulatory collapse. Practice locating each of the pulse locations (Figure 2-11). As with other vital signs, take your patient's pulse frequently in the emergency setting and note any trends.

To take the pulse of a conscious adult or large child, the most accessible and commonly used location is the radial artery. With the pads of your first two or three fingers, compress the radial artery onto the radius, just below the wrist on the thumb side (Procedure 2–1a). In the unconscious patient, begin by checking his carotid pulse. To locate the carotid pulse, palpate medial to and just below the angle of the jaw. Locate the thyroid cartilage (Adam's apple) and slide your fingers laterally until they are between the thyroid cartilage and the large muscle in the neck (sternocleidomastoid). In infants and small children, use the brachial artery or auscultate for an apical pulse. Remember that auscultating an apical pulse does not provide information about your patient's hemodynamic status. To locate the brachial artery, feel just medial to the biceps tendon. Auscultate the apical pulse just below the left nipple. First, note your

Measure vital signs early in the physical examination and, in emergency situations, repeat them often and look for trends.

pulse rate
number of pulses felt in 1 minute.

pulse rhythm
pattern and equality of intervals between beats.

pulse quality
strength, which can be weak, thready, strong, or bounding.

bradycardia
pulse rate lower than 60.

tachycardia
pulse rate higher than 100.

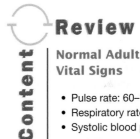

Review

Content

Normal Adult Vital Signs

- Pulse rate: 60–100
- Respiratory rate: 12–20
- Systolic blood pressure ranges:
  Male: 100–135
  Female: 90–125 before menopause, 100–135 after menopause
- Body temperature: 98.6°F (37°C)

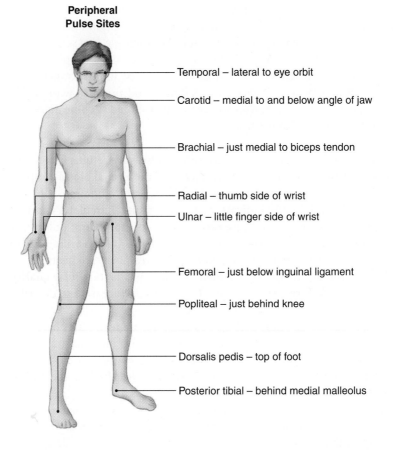

Peripheral Pulse Sites

Temporal – lateral to eye orbit

Carotid – medial to and below angle of jaw

Brachial – just medial to biceps tendon

Radial – thumb side of wrist

Ulnar – little finger side of wrist

Femoral – just below inguinal ligament

Popliteal – just behind knee

Dorsalis pedis – top of foot

Posterior tibial – behind medial malleolus

respiration
exchange of oxygen and carbon dioxide in the lungs and at the cellular level.

Recognizing when your patient's respiration requires rapid intervention often will make the difference between life and death.

respiratory rate
number of times patient breathes in 1 minute.

tachypnea
rapid breathing.

bradypnea
slow breathing.

Very rapid or very slow breathing rates require rapid intervention to ensure that the adequate exchange of gases continues.

respiratory effort
how hard patient works to breathe.

patient's pulse rate by counting the number of beats in 1 minute. If his pulse is regular, you can count the beats in 15 seconds and multiply that number by 4. If his pulse is irregular, you must count it for a full minute to obtain an accurate total. Note also the pulse's rhythm and quality.

Respiration Because oxygen and carbon dioxide exchange is essential to sustain life, **respiration** must occur continuously and must be effective. The lungs supply the arteries with oxygen and maintain the blood's pH by eliminating or retaining carbon dioxide. These two functions occur during respiration. Continuously observe your patient's respiratory rate, effort, and quality. Look for subtle signs of distress. Recognize when your patient requires rapid intervention such as aggressive airway management, positive pressure ventilation, and oxygenation. These interventions often will make the difference between life and death.

Your patient's **respiratory rate** is the number of times he breathes in 1 minute. In general the normal respiratory rate for a healthy adult at rest is 12 to 20 breaths per minute. Rapid breathing (**tachypnea**) can be the result of hypoxia, shock, head injury, or anxiety. Slow breathing (**bradypnea**) can be caused by drug overdose, severe hypoxia, or central nervous system insult. Very rapid or very slow breathing rates require rapid intervention to ensure that the adequate exchange of gases continues.

Your patient's **respiratory effort** is how hard he works to breathe. Normal inhalation involves using the respiratory muscles (diaphragm and intercostals) to increase the chest's inner diameter. It is an active process that requires energy. The increasing space creates negative pressure, like a vacuum, that draws air into the lungs. Exhalation is the passive process of the respiratory muscles' elastic recoil. This normally effortless process can become difficult with some respiratory conditions. For example,

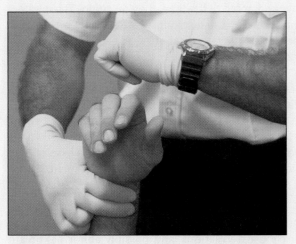

2-1a Assess the pulse as an indicator of circulatory function.

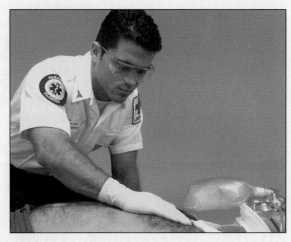

2-1b Count your patient's respirations.

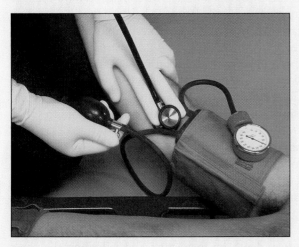

2-1c Assess blood pressure with a sphygmomano-meter and stethoscope.

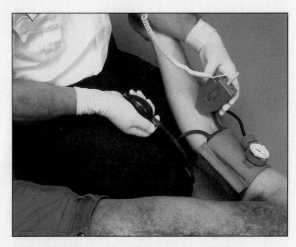

2-1d If you cannot hear blood pressure with a stethoscope, use an ultrasonic Doppler.

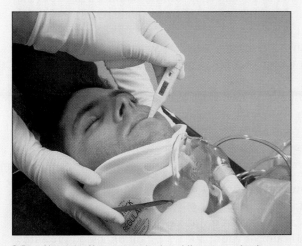

2-1e Use a battery-operated oral thermometer to take your patient's temperature.

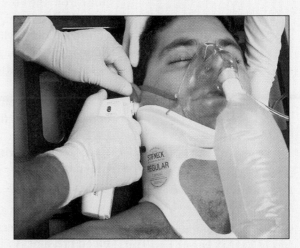

2-1f Use a specially designed, battery-operated thermometer to measure temperature inside the ear.

Assessment Pearls

Obtaining an Accurate Respiratory Rate Often, EMTs and paramedics "guesstimate" the respiratory rate and, most of the time, they're wrong. The importance of accurately obtaining and recording the respiratory rate cannot be overemphasized. A change in respiratory rate is often the first physical exam finding you'll observe with an emergency condition.

People involuntarily change their respiratory rate when they know it's being measured. Thus, if they're aware that you're measuring the respiratory rate, you'll end up with an inaccurate reading. To avoid this, you must distract or mislead the patient. Make the patient think you're still measuring his pulse rate. Place your hand on his wrist and measure the pulse rate for 15–30 seconds. After you've determined the pulse rate, leave your hand in place and then measure the respiratory rate for at least 30 seconds. This should give you an accurate measurement.

an airway obstruction may compromise inhalation. The resultant increased breathing effort is evident in accessory muscle use, retractions, and possibly abnormal breath sounds.

Diseases such as asthma and emphysema, in which the smaller airways collapse and trap air in the distal airways, may obstruct exhalation. Exhalation then becomes an active process that leads to respiratory distress and failure. Some injuries can decrease the respiratory effort. Rib fractures, for example, will cause a decrease in chest wall expansion because it hurts to breathe. A pneumothorax decreases effective gas exchange because the air enters the pleural space instead of the alveoli. Children become tired and decrease their respiratory effort, making their condition even worse. Evaluating your patient's respiratory effort will provide invaluable information about his respiratory status.

quality of respiration
depth and pattern of breathing.

tidal volume
amount of air one breath moves in and out of lungs.

The **quality of respiration** refers to its depth and pattern. The depth, or **tidal volume,** of respiration is the amount of air your patient moves in and out of his lungs in one breath. The normal depth for a healthy adult at rest should be approximately 500 mL, just enough to cause the chest to rise. The tidal volume may increase during exercise or anxiety. It may decrease in the presence of a rib injury when every breath hurts.

Assess your patient's respiratory depth by inspecting and palpating the chest wall for symmetrical chest expansion, by feeling and listening for air movement and noise from the nose and mouth, and by auscultating for lung sounds. The depth may be shallow, normal, or deep. Once again, to recognize inadequate respiratory depth, you must know what is normal. The respiratory pattern should be regular. Variations in respiratory pattern can be associated with specific diseases (Table 2-2). Some irregular patterns such as Cheyne-Stokes may indicate serious brain or brain stem problems.

To measure your patient's respiratory rate, place one hand on your patient's chest and count the breaths he takes in 30 seconds (Procedure 2–1b). Multiply that number by 2. Because your patient may consciously or subconsciously control his breathing, try to evaluate it without his knowing. Also assess his respiratory effort and quality of respiration.

blood pressure
force of blood against arteries' walls as the heart contracts and relaxes.

systolic blood pressure
force of blood against arteries when ventricles contract.

Blood Pressure **Blood pressure** is the force of blood against the arteries' walls as the heart contracts and relaxes. It is equal to cardiac output times the systemic vascular resistance. Any alteration in the cardiac output or the vascular resistance will alter the blood pressure. An important indicator of your patient's condition, blood pressure is measured during both systole and diastole. **Systolic blood pressure** (the higher numeric

Table 2-2	Breathing Patterns	
Condition	Description	Causes
Eupnea	Normal breathing rate and pattern	
Tachypnea	Increased respiratory rate	Fever, anxiety, exercise, shock
Bradypnea	Decreased respiratory rate	Sleep, drugs, metabolic disorder, head injury, stroke
Apnea	Absence of breathing	Deceased patient, head injury, stroke
Hyperpnea	Normal rate, but deep respirations	Emotional stress, diabetic ketoacidosis
Cheyne-Stokes	Gradual increases and decreases in respirations with periods of apnea	Increasing intracranial pressure, brainstem injury
Biot's	Rapid, deep respirations (gasps) with short pauses between sets	Spinal meningitis, many CNS causes, head injury
Kussmaul's	Tachypnea and hyperpnea	Renal failure, metabolic acidosis, diabetic ketoacidosis
Apneustic	Prolonged inspiratory phase with shortened expiratory phase	Lesion in brainstem

value) measures the maximum force of blood against the arteries when the ventricles contract. **Diastolic blood pressure** (the lower numeric value) measures the pressure against the arteries when the ventricles relax and are filling with blood. The diastolic blood pressure is a measure of systemic vascular resistance and correlates well with changes in vessel size. The sounds of the blood hitting the arterial walls are called the **Korotkoff sounds.**

Many factors may influence your patient's blood pressure. Anxiety, for example, may cause it to rise. His position (sitting, lying, standing) also may affect the measurement. If your patient has recently been smoking, exercising, or eating, you must wait at least 5 to 10 minutes to allow his blood pressure to return to a resting level before you measure it. Because of these many intangibles, you should never use blood pressure as the single indicator of your patient's condition. Always correlate it with his other clinical signs of end-organ **perfusion** such as level of response, skin color, temperature, and condition, and peripheral pulses.

The average blood pressure in the healthy adult is 120/80. Females usually will have a lower blood pressure until menopause. **Pulse pressure** is the difference between the systolic and diastolic pressures. For example, a blood pressure of 120/80 represents a pulse pressure of 40 mmHg. A normal pulse pressure is generally 30 to 40 mmHg. In certain conditions, such as pericardial tamponade or tension pneumothorax, the pulse pressure will narrow. In others, such as increasing intracranial pressure or fever, the pulse pressure will widen. Again, take your physiologically unstable patient's blood pressure as often as every 5 minutes to chart trends.

What is normal? This question has no easy answer. Generally, systolic blood pressure in adults ranges from 100 to 135 mmHg, diastolic from 60 to 80 mmHg. **Hypertension** in adults is defined as a pressure higher than 140/90. A blood pressure of 130/70, however, may represent hypertension if a patient's usual pressure is 90/60 or

diastolic blood pressure
force of blood against arteries when ventricles relax.

Korotkoff sounds
sounds of blood hitting arterial walls.

perfusion
passage of blood through an organ or tissue.

Never use blood pressure as the single indicator of your patient's condition; always correlate it with his other clinical signs of end-organ perfusion.

pulse pressure
difference between systolic and diastolic pressures.

hypertension
blood pressure higher than normal.

hypotension

blood pressure lower than normal.

hypotension if his usual pressure is 170/90. The numbers are not as important as detecting trends and assessing end-organ perfusion. Do not define hypotension by numbers but by whether perfusion is adequate to sustain life.

Hypertension can result from cardiovascular disease, kidney disease, stroke, or head injury, where it is a classic sign of increasing intracranial pressure. It may be a predisposing factor to, and preexist in, stroke or cardiovascular disease. Did the hypertension occur before or after the condition? Hypotension usually indicates shock due to cardiac insufficiency (cardiogenic shock), low blood volume (hypovolemic shock), or massive vasodilation (vasogenic shock). Orthostatic hypotension is a decrease in your patient's blood pressure when he stands or sits up.

If you suspect shock due to blood or fluid volume loss and you do not suspect a spinal injury, perform a tilt test. Take your patient's pulse and blood pressure while he is supine. Then have him sit up and dangle his feet, then stand. In 30 to 60 seconds retake his vital signs. The healthy patient's vital signs should not change. The tilt test is positive either if his pulse rate increases 10 to 20 beats per minute or if his systolic blood pressure drops 10 to 20 mmHg. (Research has found that an increase in heart rate is a more sensitive indicator of hypovolemia than a decrease in systolic blood pressure.) This finding is common in patients suspected of having hypovolemia.

To measure your patient's blood pressure, first choose the arm you will use. Remove any clothing that covers the upper arm; do not take the blood pressure over clothing, if possible. Look for a dialysis shunt in patients with renal failure. Do not take a blood pressure in that arm. Place the arm in a slightly flexed position, palm up and fingers relaxed. Support the upper arm at the level of your patient's heart.

Use the correct size cuff to obtain an accurate measurement. Its width should be one half to one third the circumference of your patient's arm. For most adults, unless they are obese or extremely slim, the large size cuff (15 cm wide) will suffice. If your patient has an obese arm, use a larger cuff. If the larger cuff is still too small, use your patient's forearm and place your stethoscope over the radial artery. For all patients,

Assessment Pearls

Pulsus Paradoxus   On most encounters, patients who have chronic obstructive pulmonary disease (COPD) are easy to identify. First, they'll tell you they have emphysema or chronic bronchitis. Often, the physical exam will reveal findings suggestive of the disease (e.g., barrel chest, wheezing, accessory muscle usage). However, the presentation of COPD is not always so clear.

One clinical indicator of emphysema that you can check for during your physical exam is pulsus paradoxus. Normally, the patient's systolic blood pressure will fall during inspiration. Under normal conditions, this fall is less than 10 mmHg. However, patients with COPD (and other conditions) will have an exaggerated fall in systolic blood pressure (greater than 10 mmHg) during inspiration.

To check for pulsus paradoxus, inflate the blood pressure cuff until it is above the patient's systolic pressure. Place your stethoscope over the brachial artery and listen for the Korotkoff sounds (blood pulsing through the vessel) as the cuff is deflated at a rate of approximately 2–3 mmHg per heartbeat. The peak systolic pressure during expiration should be identified and reconfirmed. The cuff is then slowly deflated to determine the pressure at which the Korotkoff sounds are again audible during both inspiration and expiration. When the difference in this reading exceeds 10 mmHg during quiet respiration, a paradoxical pulse is present. In addition to COPD, pulsus paradoxus is associated with asthma, pericardial tamponade, hypovolemia, and pericardial effusions.

use a cuff that covers approximately two thirds of his upper arm or thigh. Using a cuff that is too wide, too narrow, too long, or too short will result in an inaccurate measurement.

Turn the control valve counterclockwise to open it; squeeze all the air out of the bladder before applying the cuff. Locate the brachial artery by palpating on the medial side of the antecubital space until you feel a pulse. Place the lower edge of the cuff 1 inch above the antecubital space. Find the center of the bladder (usually marked on the cuff with an arrow), and place it directly over the artery. Fasten the cuff so it is smooth and fits tightly enough to obtain an accurate reading. If you have difficulty inserting a finger between the cuff and your patient's arm, it is snug enough. Also make sure the rubber tubing is clear of the cuff. Check the placement of the manometer so you can see it easily.

Now palpate the radial artery. With your other hand, turn the control valve completely clockwise and squeeze the bulb rapidly to inflate the cuff to approximately 30 mmHg over the point where the radial pulse disappears. Place your stethoscope directly over the brachial artery and hold it firmly in place without pressing on the artery (Procedure 2–1c). Turn the control valve counterclockwise slowly and steadily to deflate the cuff at a rate of 2 to 3 mmHg per heartbeat. Deflating too slowly or too rapidly will cause an inaccurate reading.

As you slowly deflate the cuff, watch the manometer and listen for the Korotkoff sounds. When you hear the first pulse beat, note the reading on the manometer dial or mercury column. This is the systolic pressure. Continue deflating the cuff until the pulsations diminish or become muffled. This is the diastolic pressure.

If you do not obtain a reading, wait 30 seconds to allow the blood pressure to normalize before inflating the cuff again. Sometimes you can palpate the artery during the deflation. The point at which you feel the pulse return marks the systolic reading. You cannot evaluate the diastolic pressure with the palpation method. To take your patient's blood pressure with a Doppler, follow the same procedure as for the palpation method, but instead of palpating for the return of the pulse, place the Doppler device over the palpated artery and listen for the "whooosh" of flowing blood indicating the systolic measurement (Procedure 2–1d). Record the blood pressure on your patient's chart. Include the systolic and diastolic pressures (for instance, 134/78), the arm used (right/left), and your patient's position (lying, sitting, standing).

Body Temperature   The body works hard to maintain a temperature of approximately 98.6° F (37° C). This temperature reflects the balance between heat production and heat loss through the skin and respiratory system. Even a slight variance can mean that significant events are happening within the body or on the body from environmental factors. Assess your patient's temperature to approximate his internal core temperature.

Even a slight variance in body temperature can mean that significant events are happening within the body.

Assessment Pearls

Crossover Test   Have you ever had a patient tell you that one side of his body was cold? Have you had trouble determining whether one foot was cooler than the other (indicative of peripheral vascular disease)? A simple trick to help with this is the crossover test.

Place one of your hands on the body part to be tested for warmth and your other hand on the opposite (contralateral) body part. After 30 to 60 seconds, cross each hand over to the opposite side. If there's an equal amount of warmth bilaterally, there will be no discernible difference in temperature. You'll find that even subtle temperature differences can be discerned in this manner.

hyperthermia
increase in body's core temperature.

An increase in body temperature (**hyperthermia**) can result from environmental extremes, infections, drugs, or metabolic processes. Ordinarily the body's cooling mechanisms maintain a steady core temperature. In an extremely hot and humid environment or in cases like heat stroke, the cooling mechanisms can fail and the core temperature will rise despite an internal thermostat that wants to maintain a normal temperature. Fever, on the other hand, results when the body tries to make its internal environment inhospitable to invading organisms. It often presents with a history of illness. The skin is somewhat dry until the fever breaks and the body's cooling mechanisms begin to take effect. As the body temperature rises, it begins to threaten body processes, specifically those of the brain. A temperature of up to 102° F (38° C) increases metabolism markedly. As body temperature rises above 103° F (39° C), the neurons of the brain may denature. At temperatures above 105° F (41° C), brain cells die and seizures may occur.

hypothermia
decrease in body's core temperature.

Extreme cold also affects body temperature. When peripheral vasoconstriction and shivering mechanisms can no longer balance heat production and loss, core temperature drops (**hypothermia**). At a body temperature of 93° F (34° C), normal body warming mechanisms begin to fail. As the core temperature drops below 90° F (32° C), shivering stops, heart sounds diminish, and cardiac irritability increases. If the temperature drops much below 70° F (21° C), your patient will present with a deathlike appearance and, possibly, irreversible asystole (absence of heartbeat).

A variety of methods can provide accurate temperature readings. You can use glass thermometers to take oral, rectal, or axillary temperatures. A rectal thermometer is the preferred device for children younger than 6 years old and for patients with an altered level of consciousness. An axillary temperature reading is the least accurate of the three methods.

The type of glass thermometer you use determines how long you must leave it in place to get an accurate reading. To take your patient's temperature orally with a glass thermometer, place the thermometer under his tongue for at least 3 to 4 minutes. It may provide a false reading if your patient has swallowed liquid or smoked within 15 to 30 minutes. To use a rectal thermometer, lubricate it well and then insert it 1.5 inches into the rectum; leave it in place for at least 2 to 3 minutes. If you use an axillary thermometer, it must remain under your patient's armpit at least 10 minutes. If your service uses battery-operated devices, become familiar with them and follow the manufacturer's instructions for their use (Procedure 2–1e). For example, when using the tympanic membrane device, place the speculum into the ear canal, push the button and hold it for 2 to 3 seconds, then remove the device (Procedure 2–1f). The temperature is then displayed on a digital readout.

Additional Assessment Techniques

Additional assessment techniques include pulse oximetry, capnography, cardiac monitoring, and blood glucose determination.

pulse oximeter
noninvasive device that measures the oxygen saturation of blood.

Pulse Oximetry   The **pulse oximeter** is a noninvasive device that measures the oxygen saturation of your patient's blood. It can reliably indicate your patient's cardiorespiratory status because it may tell you how well he is oxygenating the most peripheral vessels of his circulatory system. It also quantifies the effectiveness of your interventions such as oxygen therapy, medications, suctioning, and ventilatory assistance. For example, on room air, your patient's reading is 92 percent; after 2 minutes of high-flow, high-concentration oxygen therapy, it is 99 percent, showing a definite improvement.

The pulse oximeter has a probe sensor and a monitoring unit with digital readouts. Attach the probe-sensor clip to your patient's finger, toe, or earlobe (Figure 2-12 ▶). The probe directs two lights (one red and one infrared) through a small area of tissue. The lights penetrate the tissue and are absorbed. Because saturated and desaturated

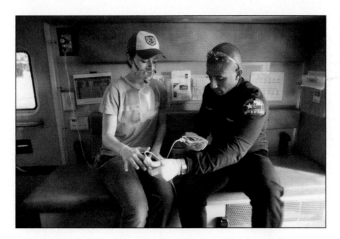

▶ **Figure 2-12** Pulse oximetry allows you to determine quickly and accurately your patient's oxygenation status. (© Scott Metcalfe)

hemoglobin absorb the lights differently, the sensors can determine their individual concentrations. The result is a measurement of your patient's oxygen saturation, or SaO_2.

Normal oxygen saturation at sea level should be between 96 and 100 percent. Generally, if the reading is below 95 percent, suspect shock, hypoxia, or respiratory compromise. Provide your patient with the appropriate airway management and supplemental oxygen and watch him carefully for further changes. Any reading below 90 percent requires aggressive airway management, positive-pressure ventilation, or oxygen administration. The unresponsive patient may require invasive airway management and positive-pressure ventilation.

Several factors affect the accuracy of a pulse oximetry reading. The sensors can accurately measure the oxygen saturation only if blood flow through the tissue is adequate. Most pulse oximeters display a digital readout of the pulse rate; others display a pulsation wave. In either case, if the display does not match your patient's actual pulse, the SaO_2 reading will be erratic. If your patient has decreased blood flow through the tissue, as in hypovolemia or hypothermia, you will obtain a false reading.

In cases of carbon monoxide (CO) poisoning, your saturation readings will be high while your patient's tissues are severely ischemic. This is because the CO molecule saturates the hemoglobin molecule 200 times more easily than does oxygen and the pulse oximetry probe cannot distinguish between hemoglobin that is bound to carbon monoxide and hemoglobin that is bound to oxygen. Your patient's hemoglobin is, in fact, saturated, but with carbon monoxide, not oxygen. Other than these limitations, the pulse oximeter, when teamed with other patient assessment techniques, can be a useful tool in the prehospital setting.

Capnography **Capnography** is a real-time measurement of exhaled carbon dioxide concentrations. A device that makes such measurements is called an **end-tidal carbon dioxide (ETCO₂) detector.** End-tidal CO_2 detectors are available either as disposable colorimetric devices (Figure 2-13 ▶) or as portable electronic devices (Figure 2-14 ▶) that now combine pulse oximetry, $ETCO_2$ detection, blood pressure, pulse rate, respiratory rate, and temperature monitors in one unit.

Although their use in prehospital care is increasing, end-tidal CO_2 detectors are used most commonly to assess proper placement of an endotracheal tube. Carbon dioxide's absence from the exhaled air strongly indicates that the tube is in the esophagus; its presence indicates proper tracheal placement. These devices are attached either in-line or alongside the endotracheal tube and the ventilation device. A color change in the colorimetric device or a light on the electronic monitor confirms proper tube placement. On the colorimetric device, the low CO_2 content of inspired air makes the device purple, whereas the higher CO_2 content of expired air makes it yellow.

capnography
real-time measurement of exhaled carbon dioxide concentrations.

end-tidal carbon dioxide (ETCO₂) detector
a device used in capnography to measure exhaled carbon dioxide concentrations.

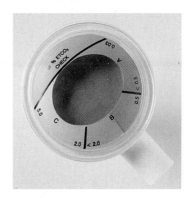

▶ **Figure 2-13** A colorimetric end-tidal CO_2 detector.

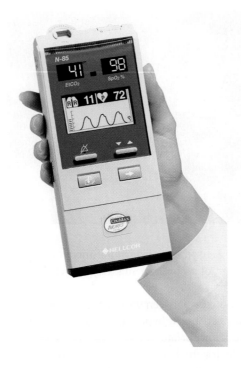

▶ **Figure 2-14** An electronic end-tidal CO₂ detector. *(Reprinted by permission of Nellcor Puritan Bennett LLC, Pleasanton, California)*

Capnography is useful in detecting accidental tracheal extubation, tube obstruction, and disconnection from a ventilation system during transport. In addition, capnography can provide an indirect estimation of cardiac output and pulmonary blood flow and, ultimately, the effectiveness of CPR during cardiac arrest. Unfortunately, although the $ETCO_2$ detector is accurate, the $ETCO_2$ level falls precipitously during cardiac arrest. Therefore, these patients may not cause a color change on the $ETCO_2$ detector despite proper placement of the endotracheal tube.

cardiac monitor

machine that displays and records the electrical activity of the heart.

Cardiac Monitoring The **cardiac monitor** is essential in assessing and managing the patient who requires advanced cardiac life support (ACLS) (Figure 2-15 ▶). The simplest prehospital machines monitor the electrical activity of the heart in three "leads" or positions. These "limb leads" adequately identify life-threatening cardiac rhythms. Also available for prehospital use are 12-lead ECGs. They are essential in gathering data to confirm a myocardial infarction.

▶ **Figure 2-15** The cardiac monitor is essential to managing advanced cardiac life support.

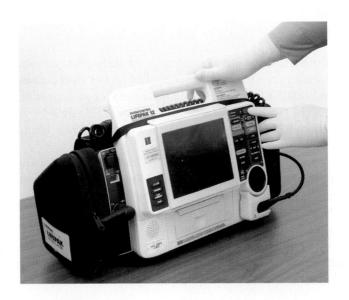

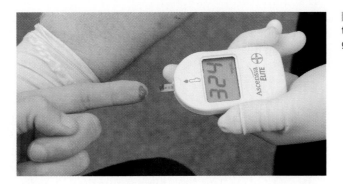

Figure 2-16 Use a glucometer to determine your patient's blood glucose.

Other features of cardiac monitors include pacing capabilities and the "quick-look" paddles and the "hands-off" defibrillation pads used in cardiac arrest. The paddles, which you place on your patient's chest, allow you to check the cardiac rhythm and deliver a rapid electrical countershock. The hands-off defibrillation pads have two large electrodes that you attach to the chest wall. These replace the paddles and allow you to deliver a countershock without fear of injuring yourself.

All monitor-defibrillators can deliver a synchronized countershock in the presence of an unstable tachycardia. Most have a transcutaneous pacemaker that is placed externally on the chest and provides an electrical impulse to stimulate cardiac contraction in cases of bradycardia and heart blocks. This is a temporary measure until a permanent pacemaker can be implanted. Finally, some ECG machines have a "code summary" feature that prints out the electrical record of events and their times. This helps you document your patient's progress while in your care.

The cardiac monitor is a useful tool for measuring electrical activity, but it has one major disadvantage. It cannot tell you if the heart is pumping efficiently, effectively, or at all. The ECG reading does not necessarily correlate with the mechanical function of the heart. Electrical activity can exist with no mechanical contraction. Always assess your patient and compare what you see on the monitor with the rate and quality of the pulse. These are important steps in developing your patient's clinical picture.

Always compare what you see on a cardiac monitor with what you feel for a pulse.

Blood Glucose Determination In cases of altered mental status due to diabetic emergencies, seizures, and strokes, you will want to measure your patient's blood glucose level. The arrival of inexpensive, handheld **glucometers** makes this test easy to perform in the field. Most diabetic patients do it several times each day at home by themselves.

To perform this procedure you will need a glucometer with test strips, a finger-stick device with sterile lancets, an alcohol wipe, and tissue or gauze pads. Simply place a drop of your patient's capillary blood from a finger stick onto a chemical reagent strip (Figure 2-16 ▶). Following the manufacturer's instructions, place the test strip in the glucometer and wait for the reading to appear. This procedure takes less than 1 minute to perform.

Since all glucometers work differently, you must read the manufacturer's instructions carefully. The slightest mistake can alter the measurement's accuracy. For example, make sure the code numbers on the test strips match those on the digital reading. Also make sure you do not allow alcohol to contaminate the blood. Glucometers are moderately accurate when used properly and calibrated daily.

glucometer

tool used to measure blood glucose level.

ANATOMICAL REGIONS

After you complete the general survey, you will examine the body regions and systems in more detail. Again, the specific situation and your experience and common sense

Review

Anatomical Regions

- Skin
- Hair and nails
- Head, eyes, ears, nose, mouth
- Neck
- Chest and lungs
- Abdomen
- Extremities
- Posterior body
- Peripheral vascular
- Neurologic

will determine whether you conduct a thorough examination, as you would when performing physicals for an insurance company, or narrow the focus of your examination, as you might in an emergency setting.

The Skin

The skin is the largest organ in the human body, making up 15 percent of our total body weight. The skin performs many important functions. It protects the body against foreign substance invasion and minor physical trauma. It provides a watertight barrier to keep body fluids in and environmental fluids out. It excretes sweat, urea, and lactic acid and regulates body temperature through radiation, conduction, convection, and evaporation. It provides sensory perception through nerve endings and specialized receptors. It helps regulate blood pressure by constricting skin blood vessels, and it repairs surface wounds by exaggerating the normal process of cell replacement.

The skin consists of two layers that lie atop the subcutaneous fat—the epidermis and the dermis (Figure 2-17 ▶). The thickness of each layer varies with age and body site. The outer layer, the epidermis, is comprised mostly of dying and dead cells that are shed constantly and replaced from beneath by new cells. It is avascular (has no blood vessels), so blood vessels from the underlying dermis must supply its nutrition. The dermis is rich in blood supply and nerve endings. It also contains some hair follicles and sebaceous glands that secrete an oil called sebum. This oil lubricates the epidermis and helps make the watertight seal. The subcutaneous tissue under the dermis contains fat, sweat glands, and hair follicles.

The two types of sweat glands are eccrine glands and apocrine glands. Eccrine glands, also known as merocrine glands, open onto the skin surface and help control body temperature through water excretion. They are widely distributed but are most

▶ **Figure 2-17** The skin.

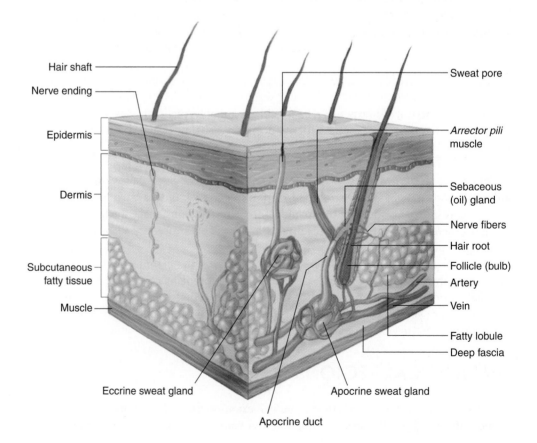

heavily concentrated in the axilla and genital areas. Apocrine glands are found exclusively in the armpits and genital region, and they open into hair follicles. These glands respond to emotional stress. During adolescence, the apocrine glands enlarge and actively increase the axillary sweating that causes adult body odor. Also during this period, the sebaceous glands increase their activity, giving the skin an oily appearance. This predisposes the teenager to acne problems.

As we age, sebaceous and sweat gland activity decreases. As a result, the skin becomes drier and produces less perspiration. The epidermis thins and flattens, and the dermis loses some of its vascularity. The skin wrinkles as it loses turgor. In warmer climates, the skin can become thickened, yellowed, and furrowed and take on a weather-beaten appearance. Elderly people develop a variety of spots on the thin skin of the backs of their hands and forearms. Whitish, depigmented marks are known as pseudoscars. Purple spots (purpura) caused by minor capillary bleeding may appear and fade after a few weeks.

Although you will observe your patient's skin throughout your assessment, a comprehensive physical exam must also include a concentrated inspection of all areas of the skin. The skin provides data on a variety of systemic problems in addition to skin-related disorders. Examining the skin requires good light and a keen eye. The characteristics of normal skin vary with your patients' racial, ethnic, and familial backgrounds. Evaluate its color, moisture, temperature, texture, mobility and turgor, and any lesions. Always wear protective gloves if your patient has any areas of open skin, exudative lesions, or rashes.

Color Normal skin color in light-skinned people is pink, indicating adequate cardiorespiratory function and vascular integrity. This means that the capillaries in the skin are well oxygenated. The bright red oxyhemoglobin in the oxygen-rich blood circulating through the capillary beds gives the epidermis its pink appearance. A pale color suggests decreased blood flow through the skin. This is typical in hypothermia, hypovolemia, and compensatory shock, where blood flow through the distal capillary beds is severely diminished. It also is common in anemia, in which your patient's red blood cell count is low. As the hemoglobin loses its oxygen to the tissues, it changes to the darker, blue deoxyhemoglobin. Increased deoxyhemoglobin causes cyanosis, a bluish skin color. Cyanosis means that less oxygen is available at the tissue level.

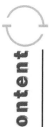

Content ◠**Review**

Skin Characteristics to Assess

- Color
- Moisture
- Temperature
- Texture
- Mobility and turgor
- Lesions

Assessment Pearls

Assessing Skin Abnormalities in Dark-Skinned People To assess skin abnormalities in dark-skinned patients in whom these conditions may not be easily observable, try the following techniques:

Jaundice	Look for a yellow color in the sclera and hard palate.
Pallor	Look for an ashen color in the sclera, conjunctiva, mouth, tongue, lips, nail beds, palms, and soles.
Erythema	Feel for warmth in the affected area.
Petechiae	Look for tiny purplish dots on the abdomen.
Cyanosis	Look for a dull, dark coloring in the mouth, tongue, lips, nail beds, palms, and soles.
Rashes	Feel for abnormal skin texture.
Edema	Look for decreased color and feel for tightness.

Evaluate skin color where the epidermis is thinnest. This includes the fingernails and lips and the mucous membranes of the mouth and conjunctiva. In dark-skinned people, evaluate the sclera, conjunctiva, lips, nail beds, soles, and palms. Note any discoloration caused by vascular changes underneath the skin. Petechiae are small, round, flat, purplish spots caused by capillary bleeding from a variety of etiologies. Ecchymosis is a blue-black bruise resulting from trauma or bleeding disorders. Jaundice first appears in the sclera and then, in the late stages of liver disease, all over the skin. If only your patient's palms, soles, and face are yellow, he may have carotanemia, a harmless nutritional condition caused by eating a diet high in carrots and yellow vegetables or fruits.

Moisture   Inspect and palpate the skin for dryness, increased sweating, and excessive oiliness. Dry skin, common during the cold winter months and in the elderly, may be the result of other conditions. Excessive oiliness, especially where the sebaceous glands are concentrated in the face, neck, back, chest, and buttocks, may suggest acne or hyperthyroidism. Increased sweating may indicate a sympathetic nervous system response to anxiety, fear, or exertion.

Temperature   Use the backs of your fingers to feel the skin temperature in several different locations. Compare symmetrical body areas. Generalized warming or cooling suggests an environmental, infectious, or thyroid problem. Localized warmth may indicate bleeding or swelling.

Texture   Feel your patient's skin. Is it rough or smooth? Are there large patches or small areas of scaling? Observe the skin's thickness. Thin and fragile skin is a sign of debilitating disease in the elderly. Thick skin often occurs with eczema and psoriasis. Inspect the palms and soles for calluses.

turgor
normal tension in the skin.

Mobility and Turgor   Test the skin's **turgor** and elasticity by picking up a fold of skin over a bony prominence and then releasing it. Normal skin immediately returns to its original state. Poor turgor (tenting) results from dehydration. Test the skin's mobility by moving it over the bony prominence. Decreased mobility suggests edema or scleroderma, a progressive skin disease.

lesion
any disruption in normal tissue.

Lesions   A skin **lesion** is any disruption in normal tissue. Skin lesions are classified as vascular, involving a blood vessel (Figure 2-18 ▶); primary, arising from previously normal skin (Figure 2-19 ▶); or secondary, resulting from changes in primary lesions (Figure 2-20 ▶). Skin lesions can take any shape, color, or arrangement. Note their anatomical location and distribution. Are they generalized or localized? Do they involve exposed surfaces or areas that fold over? Do they relate to possible irritants such as wristbands, bracelets, necklaces? Are they linear, clustered, circular, or dermatomal (following a sensory nerve pathway)? What type are they? Inspect and feel all skin lesions carefully. Skin tumors are another variety of skin lesion. These include basal cell and squamous cell carcinomas, malignant melanomas, Kaposi sarcoma in AIDS, actinic keratosis, and seborrheic keratosis.

When you detect a skin lesion, use anatomical landmarks to describe its exact location on the skin's surface. Describe its shape in terms such as *oval, spherical, irregular,* or *tubular.* Sometimes sketching an outline of the lesion is helpful. Record the size of the mass in centimeters, carefully measuring its length, width, and depth. Describe the consistency of the mass exactly as it feels to you (for instance, soft, firm, edematous, cystic, or nodular). Of particular concern is its mobility. If the mass is affixed to a specific structure, suspect a malignancy. Note any pain or tenderness surrounding the mass upon palpation. Pulsation in the mass is another significant finding. For example, a mass that pulsates in all directions suggests an aneurysm.

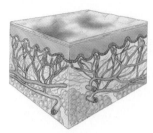

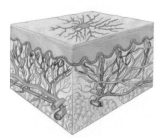

Purpura – Reddish-purple blotches, diameter more than 0.5 cm

Spider angioma – Reddish legs radiate from red spot

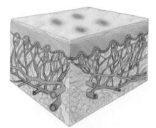

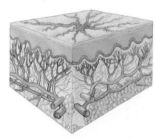

Petechiae – Reddish-purple spots, diameter less than 0.5 cm

Venous star – Bluish legs radiate from blue center

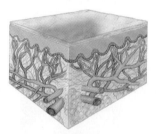

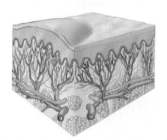

Ecchymoses – Reddish-purple blotch, size varies

Capillary hemangioma – Irregular red spots

The Hair

Hair is a tactile sensory organ, while also playing a role in sexual stimulation and attraction. It covers the entire body except the palms, soles, and parts of the sex organs. Hair develops from the base of the hair follicle, where it is nourished by the papilla, a vast capillary network. An involuntary arrector pili muscle fiber attaches to the base of the hair shaft. When these arrectores pilorum contract, the hair stands erect and goose bumps appear on the skin.

The two types of hair are vellus and terminal. Vellus hair is short, fine, and lacking pigment (similar to "peach fuzz"). Terminal hair is coarser, thicker, and pigmented. It appears on the eyebrows and scalp, in the armpits and groin of both sexes, and on the faces and bodies of males.

With aging the hair turns gray from a decrease in pigmentation and its growth declines. A transition from terminal to vellus hair on the scalp causes baldness in both men and women. The opposite occurs in the nares and ears of men, where terminal hair replaces vellus hair. Both genders generally experience a decrease in body hair as they age. Loss of the lateral third of the eyebrow is also normal in the elderly.

Inspect and palpate the hair, noting its color, quality, distribution, quantity, and texture. Is there hair loss? Is there a pattern to the loss? Patients undergoing chemotherapy for cancer may experience generalized hair loss. Failure to develop normal hair growth during puberty may indicate a pituitary or hormonal problem.

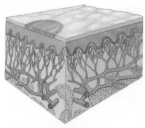

Macule – Flat spot, color varies from white to brown or from red to purple, diameter less than 1 cm

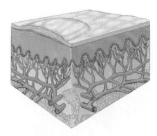

Plaque – Superficial papule, diameter more than 1 cm, rough texture

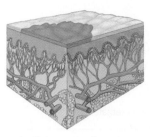

Patch – Irregular flat macule, diameter greater than 1 cm

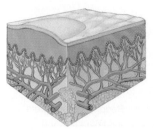

Wheal – Pink, irregular spot varying in size and shape

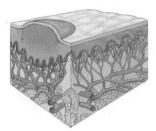

Papule – Elevated firm spot, color varies from brown to red or from pink to purplish red, diameter less than 1 cm

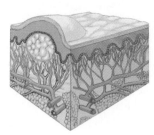

Nodule – Elevated firm spot, diameter 1–2 cm

▶ **Figure 2-19a** Primary skin lesions.

Abnormal facial hair growth in women (hirsutism) also may indicate a hormonal imbalance. Part the hair in several places and palpate the scalp (Figure 2-21 ▶). A normal scalp is clean with no scaling, lesions, redness, lumps, or tenderness. Dandruff is characterized by mild flaking, psoriasis by heavy scaling, and seborrheic dermatitis by a greasy scaling. Try to differentiate the flaking of dandruff from the nits (eggs) of lice. Dandruff flakes off the hair easily, while nits firmly attach themselves to the hair shaft.

Feel the hair texture. In white people a soft hair texture is normal; in black people a coarser texture is normal. Very dry, brittle, or fragile hair is abnormal. Inspect and palpate the eyebrows. Note the quality and distribution of the hair and any scaling of the underlying skin. When assessing hair remember that the normal quantity and distribution of hair is related to gender and racial group. For instance, men have more trunk and body hair than women. Native American men have less facial and body hair than male Caucasians. In addition, Caucasians have more abundant and coarser body hair than Asians.

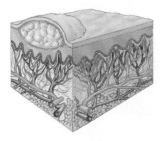

Tumor – Elevated solid, diameter more than 2 cm, may be same color as skin

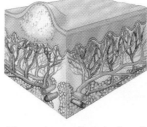

Pustule – Elevated area, diameter less than 1 cm, contains purulent fluid

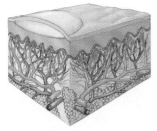

Vesicle – Elevated area, diameter less than 1 cm, contains serous fluid

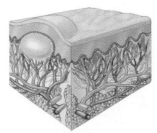

Cyst – Elevated, palpable area containing liquid or viscous matter

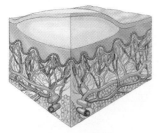

Bulla – Vesicle with diameter more than 1 cm

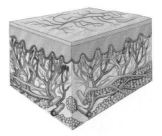

Telangiectasia – Red, threadlike line

▶ **Figure 2-19b** Primary skin lesions, continued.

Assessment Pearls

Always Examine the Fingernails Many EMS providers fail to examine a patient's fingernails. Granted, in the multiple-trauma patient, the appearance of fingernails is of little consequence. But in a medical patient, the nails can provide a great deal of information. Nails grow approximately 1 mm a day. Thus, looking at an intact nail will provide information about the past 3 months or so of the patient's life.

Transverse lines across the nail are referred to as Beau's lines. The presence of these lines on more than one nail often indicates that, sometime during the past 2 to 3 months, the patient had a serious systemic illness. During severe illness, the nails grow slowly, thus forming the lines.

Likewise, clubbing of the nails might indicate that the patient has heart disease. Normally, the angle made by the proximal nail fold and nail plate (Lovibond angle) is less than or equal to 160°. In clubbing, the angle flattens and increases as the severity of the clubbing increases. If the angle is greater than 180°, definitive clubbing exists.

Finally, the cleanliness of the nails can tell you a lot about the patient's hygiene, possible occupation, or what he was doing prior to collapsing.

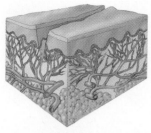

Fissure – Linear red crack ranging into dermis

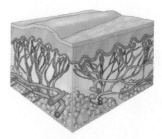

Scar – Fibrous, depth varies, color ranges from white to red

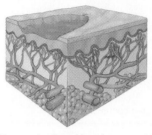

Erosion – Depression in epidermis, caused by tissue loss

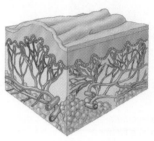

Keloid – Elevated scar, irregular shape, larger than original wound

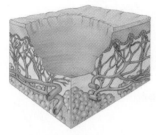

Ulcer – Red or purplish depression ranging into dermis, caused by tissue loss

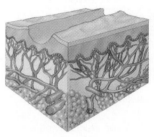

Excoriation – Linear, may be hollow or crusted, caused by loss of epidermis leaving dermis exposed

▶ **Figure 2-20a** Secondary skin lesions.

The Nails

Nails are found at the most distal ends of fingers and toes and are primarily for protection. Nails are strong yet flexible and provide a sharp edge for scratching, scraping, and clawing. They are made up of the nail plate, the nail bed, the proximal nail fold, and the nail root (Figure 2-22 ▶). The angle between the proximal nail fold and the nail plate should be less than 180 degrees. Fingernails grow approximately 0.1 mm daily, slightly faster in the summertime. The nail plate lies on a highly vascular nail bed that gives the nail a pink appearance. Nail edges should be smooth and rounded. The nail plates should be smooth, flat, or slightly curved and should feel hard and uniformly thick. As we age, nail growth diminishes because of decreased peripheral circulation. The nails, especially the toenails, become hard, thick, brittle, and yellowish.

Inspect and palpate the fingernails and toenails. Observe the color beneath the transparent nail. Normally it is pink in Caucasians and black or brown in blacks. Note if the nails appear blue-black or purple, brown, or yellow-gray. Look for lesions,

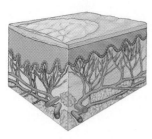

Scale – Elevated area of excessive exfoliation, varies in thickness, shape, and dryness, and ranges in color from white to silver or tan

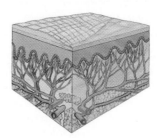

Lichenification – Thickening and hardening of epidermis with emphasized lines in skin, resembles lichen

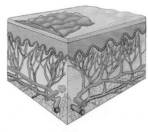

Crust – Reddish, brown, black, tan, or yellowish dried blood, serum, or pus

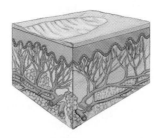

Atrophy – Skin surface thins and markings disappear, semitransparent parchment-like appearance

▶ **Figure 2-20b** Secondary skin lesions, continued.

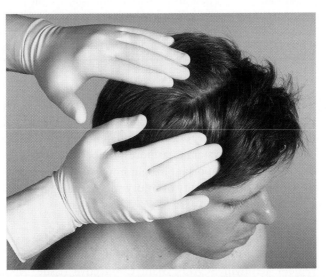

▶ **Figure 2-21** Inspect and palpate your patient's hair and scalp.

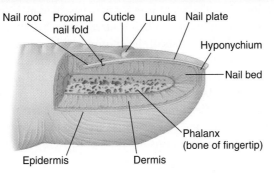

Nail root   Proximal nail fold   Cuticle   Lunula   Nail plate
Hyponychium
Nail bed
Phalanx (bone of fingertip)
Epidermis   Dermis

▶ **Figure 2-22** The nail.

Table 2-3	Abnormal Nail Findings
Condition	**Description**
Clubbing	Clubbing occurs when normal connective tissue and capillaries increase the angle between the plate and proximal nail to greater than 180 degrees. The distal phalanx of each finger is rounded and bulbous. The proximal nail feels spongy. This is caused by the chronic hypoxia found in cardiopulmonary diseases and lung cancer.
Paronychia	This is an inflammation of the proximal and lateral nail folds. It may be acute or chronic. The folds appear red and swollen and tender. The cuticle may not be visible. People who frequently immerse their hands in water are susceptible.
Onycholysis	The nail bed separates from the nail plate. It begins distally and enlarges the free edge of the nail. There are many causes, including hyperthyroidism.
Terry's nails	These appear as a mostly whitish nail with a band of reddish-brown at the distal nail tip. This may be seen in aging and with people suffering from liver cirrhosis, congestive heart failure, and diabetes.
White spots	Trauma to the nail often results in white spots that grow out with the nail. They often follow the curvature of the cuticle and can be the result of overzealous manicuring.
Transverse white lines	These are lines that parallel the lunula, rather than the cuticle. They may appear following a severe illness. They appear from under the proximal nail folds and grow out with the nail.
Psoriasis	These appear as small pits in the nails and may be an early sign of psoriasis.
Beau's lines	These are transverse depressions in the nails and are associated with severe illness. As with the transverse white lines, they form under the nail fold and grow out with the nail. You may be able to estimate the timing or length of an illness by the location of the line.

ridging, grooves, depressions, and pitting (Table 2–3). Depressions that appear in all nails are usually caused by a systemic disease. Gently squeeze the nail between your thumb and forefinger to test for adherence to the nail bed. A boggy nail suggests the clubbing seen in systemic cardiorespiratory diseases. The condition of the fingernails also can provide important insight into your patient's self-care and hygiene. Check the toenails for any deformity or injury such as being ingrown.

The Head

The scalp consists of five layers of tissue. You can remember their names with the convenient acronym SCALP: Skin, Connective tissue, Aponeurosis, Loose tissue, and Periosteum. The scalp is extremely vascular, as it protects and insulates the skull and sensitive brain tissue. When injured, it can bleed profusely.

The skull consists of the cranium and the face. The cranium comprises the frontal, parietal, temporal, occipital, ethmoid, and sphenoid bones and is covered by the scalp (Figure 2-23 ▶). The bones of the skull fuse at their sutures. The face includes the nasal bones, maxillary bones, lacrimal bones, zygomatic bones, the palate, the inferior nasal concha, and the vomer (Figure 2-24 ▶). The facial bones have air-filled compartments called sinuses and have cavities for the eyes, mouth, and nose (Figure 2-25 ▶). The movable mandible joins the skull at the temporomandibular joint (TMJ). The TMJ is

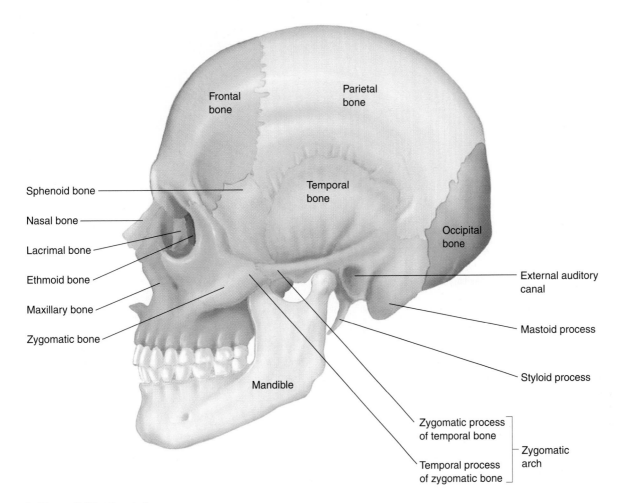

Frontal bone

Parietal bone

Temporal bone

Occipital bone

Sphenoid bone

Nasal bone

Lacrimal bone

Ethmoid bone

Maxillary bone

Zygomatic bone

Mandible

External auditory canal

Mastoid process

Styloid process

Zygomatic process of temporal bone

Temporal process of zygomatic bone

Zygomatic arch

▶ **Figure 2-23** The skull.

in the depression just in front of the ear. It allows you to open and close your mouth and to jut your jaw forward. A variety of muscles gives the face its contour and general shape. Although facial characteristics vary according to race, gender, and body build, the skull and face should appear symmetrical.

You can also examine the skull when you inspect and palpate the scalp and hair. Look for any wounds or active bleeding. Observe the general size and contour of the skull. Palpate the cranium from front to back (Procedure 2–2a). It should be symmetrical and smooth. Note any tenderness or deformities (depressions or protrusions). An indentation in the skull may suggest a depressed skull fracture. Note any areas of unusual warmth.

Inspect the face. Is it symmetrical? Are there any involuntary movements? Note any masses or edema. Observe the bony orbits of the eye for periorbital ecchymosis, a bluish discoloration also known as "raccoon eyes." Also check the mastoid process for discoloration (Procedure 2–2b). These are classic signs of a basilar skull fracture. Discoloration normally will not appear on the scene but will present hours after the injury occurs. Palpate the facial bones for stability and note any crepitus or loose fragments (Procedure 2–2c). Note whether your patient's facial expressions change appropriately with her mood.

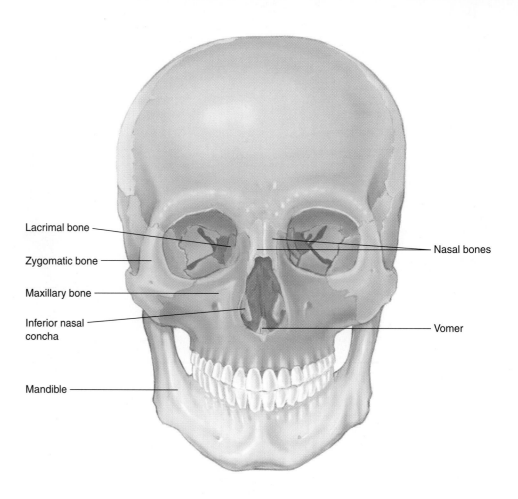

Lacrimal bone

Zygomatic bone

Maxillary bone

Inferior nasal concha

Mandible

Nasal bones

Vomer

Evaluate the TMJ. Place the tip of your index finger into the depression in front of the tragus (the cartilaginous projection just in front of the ear's outer opening) and ask your patient to open her mouth (Procedure 2–2d). The tips of your fingers should drop into the joint space. Palpate the joint for tenderness, swelling, and range of motion. Sometimes, you may hear a clicking or snapping. This is neither unusual nor problematic unless it is accompanied by pain, swelling, and crepitus. Test for range of motion by asking your patient to open and close her mouth, jut and retract her jaw, and move it from side to side. Finally, assess the skin of the face for color, pigmentation, texture, thickness, hair distribution, and lesions.

The Eyes

The eyes comprise external and internal parts. The external eye consists of the eyelid, conjunctiva, lacrimal gland, ocular muscles, and the bony skull orbit (Figure 2-26 ▶). The lacrimal glands, in the temporal region of the superior eyelid, produce tears that moisten the eye. The eyelids distribute the tears over the eye's surface. They also regulate the amount of light entering the eye and protect it from foreign bodies. The eyelashes extend from the eyelid's border. The conjunctiva is a thin membrane that covers the anterior surface of the eye and the inside of the eyelid. It protects the eye from foreign bodies. The ocular muscles (Figure 2-27 ▶) control eye movement and are innervated by three cranial nerves (CNs): the oculomotor (CN-III), trochlear (CN-IV), and abducens (CN-VI).

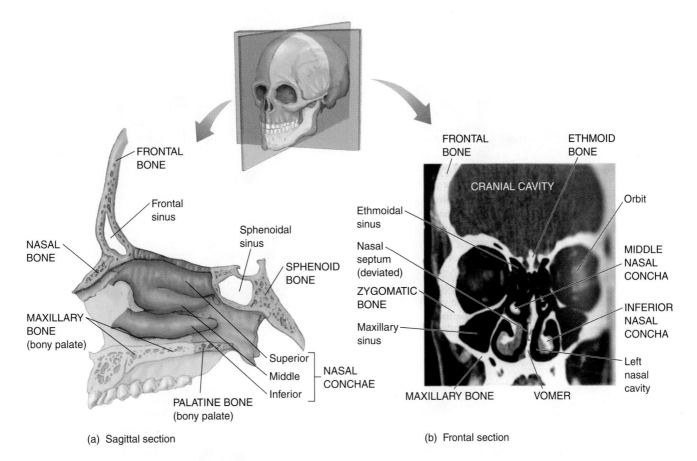

(a) Sagittal section

(b) Frontal section

Figure 2-25 The sinuses and cavities of the skull.

The internal eye consists of the sclera, cornea, iris, lens, and retina (Figure 2-28). The sclera, the white of the eye, is a dense, avascular structure that gives physical shape to the eyeball. The cornea separates the watery fluid in the anterior chamber from the external environment. It also permits light to enter the lens and reach the retina. The iris is a circular, contractile muscle; its pigment produces the color of the eye. The opening in the center of the iris is the pupil. The iris controls the amount of light reaching the retina by constricting and dilating. It is innervated by the optic nerve (CN-II), which senses light, and by the oculomotor nerve (CN-III), which constricts the pupil. The lens is a cellular structure immediately behind the iris. It is convex and transparent, allowing images to focus onto the retina. The retina is the sensory network of the eye. It transforms light rays into electrical impulses that the optic nerve transmits to the brain. Besides the optic nerve, the ophthalmic artery and vein provide necessary circulation to and from the eye. Accurate vision depends on these components functioning effectively.

The ideal environment for an eye exam is a quiet room, free from distractions, in which you can control the lighting and make your patient comfortable. First, test for visual acuity. Place your patient 20 feet from a **visual acuity wall chart** or have her hold a **visual acuity card** 14 inches from her face. Ask her to cover one eye with a card and begin reading the lines (Procedure 2–3a). Record the visual acuity grade next to the smallest line in which she can read at least one half of the letters. The result is written as a fraction. The first number represents the distance away from the chart. The second number is the distance from which a normal eye could read the line. Normal is 20/20. A result of 20/70 means that a normal eye could read the line from 70 feet away but

visual acuity wall chart/card
wall chart or handheld card with lines of letters used to test vision.

Examining the Head

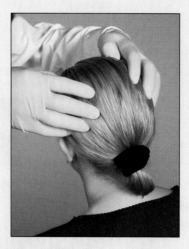

2-1a Palpate the cranium from front to back.

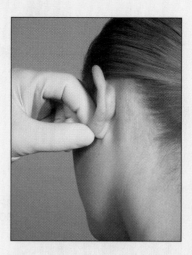

2-1b Inspect the mastoid process.

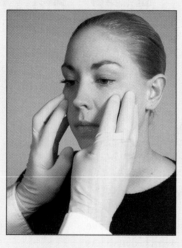

2-1c Palpate the facial bones.

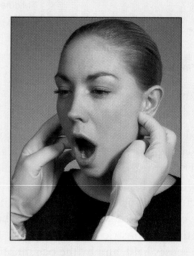

2-1d Palpate the TMJ.

your patient could only read it from 20 feet. If no chart is available, you can have your patient count your raised fingers, read from a distance something you have printed, or distinguish light from dark. This type of exam is routinely conducted as part of a comprehensive physical exam in a clinic setting.

Test the visual fields by confrontation. Sit directly in front of your patient. Have her cover her left eye while you cover your right eye. Ask her to look at your nose. Extend your left arm to the side and slowly bring it toward you. Ask your patient to say when she first sees your finger. Use your own peripheral vision as a guide. If she sees your finger when you do, her visual field is grossly normal in that direction. Do this test in all four quadrants (left and right, up and down). Then perform the same test with the other eye (Procedure 2–3b). Any abnormalities suggest a defect in peripheral

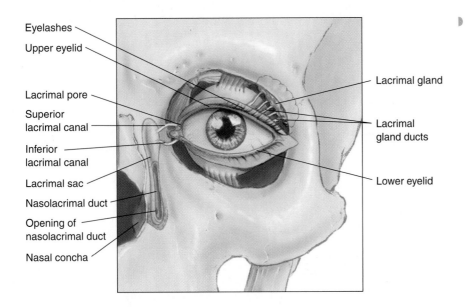

Figure 2-26 The external eye.

Eyelashes
Upper eyelid
Lacrimal pore
Superior lacrimal canal
Inferior lacrimal canal
Lacrimal sac
Nasolacrimal duct
Opening of nasolacrimal duct
Nasal concha

Lacrimal gland
Lacrimal gland ducts
Lower eyelid

vision. Some common abnormalities include a horizontal defect (loss of vision in the upper or lower half of an eye), a blind eye, bitemporal hemianopsia (loss of vision in the outside half of each eye), left or right homonymous hemianopsia (loss of vision in the right half of both eyes or the left half of both eyes), or homonymous quadrantic

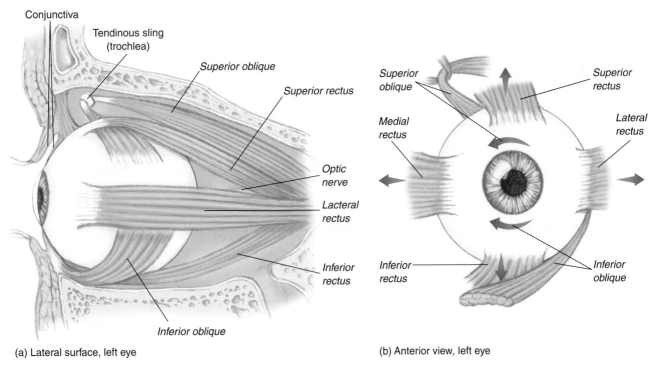

Conjunctiva
Tendinous sling (trochlea)
Superior oblique
Superior rectus
Optic nerve
Lacteral rectus
Inferior rectus
Inferior oblique

Superior oblique
Medial rectus
Inferior rectus

Superior rectus
Lateral rectus
Inferior oblique

(a) Lateral surface, left eye

(b) Anterior view, left eye

Figure 2-27 The extraocular muscles.

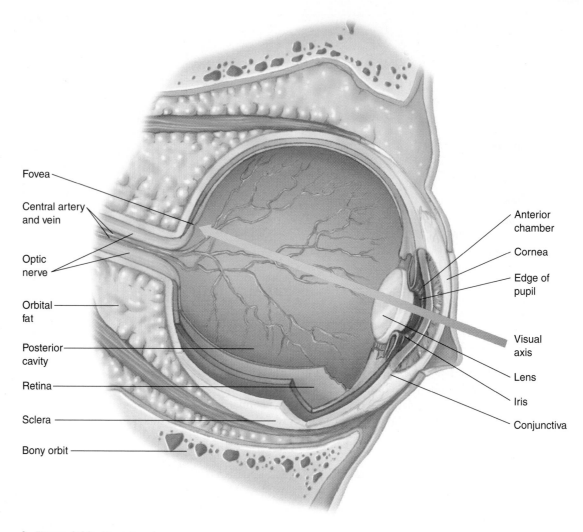

Fovea

Central artery
and vein

Optic
nerve

Orbital
fat

Posterior
cavity

Retina

Sclera

Bony orbit

Anterior
chamber

Cornea

Edge of
pupil

Visual
axis

Lens

Iris

Conjunctiva

▶ **Figure 2-28** The internal eye.

defect (loss of vision in the same quadrant of both eyes). Record the area of defect as illustrated in Figure 2-29 ▶.

Now examine the external eyes. Place yourself directly in front of your patient. Inspect her eyes for symmetry in size, shape, and contour. Do they look alike? Do they protrude (proptosis)? Are they properly aligned? Note the eyelids' position relative to the eyeballs. They should cover the upper quarter of the iris. Are the eyes totally exposed or do the eyelids droop (ptosis)? Have your patient close her eyes. Do they close completely? Do you see any edema, inflammation, or mass? Note the eyelid's color. It should be pink, indicating good central oxygenation. If the lid is pale, your patient could be in shock or anemic. If cyanotic, she could have central hypoxemia. Are there any lesions?

Carefully observe the lids' shape and inspect their contours for any growths. If you see any drainage, note its color and consistency. Do the eyelashes turn inward to scrape against the eyeball or outward to prevent the complete closure of the eye?

Examining the Eyes

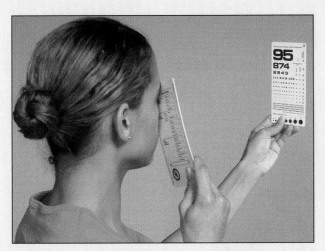

2-3a Use a visual acuity chart to test visual acuity.

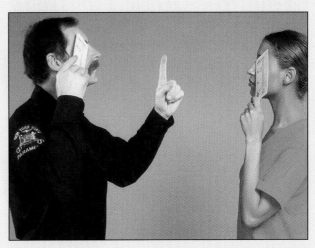

2-3b Test peripheral vision.

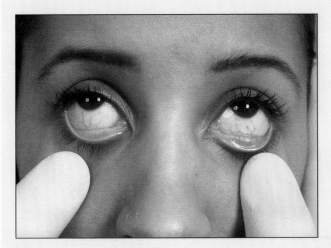

2-3c Inspect the external eye.

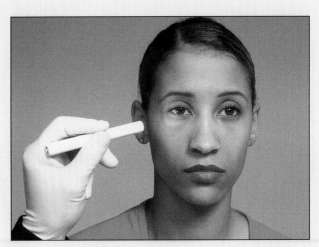

2-3d Test the pupil's reaction to light.

(continued)

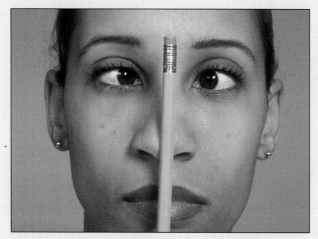

2-3e Test for accommodation.

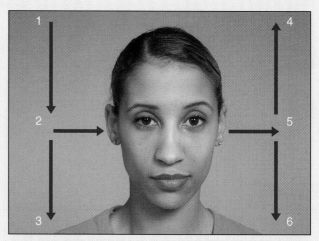

2-3f Move your finger in an *H* pattern to test your patient's extraocular muscles.

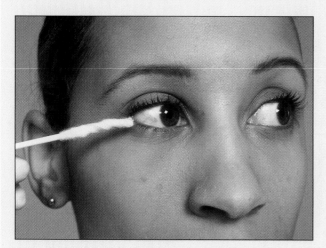

2-3g Check the corneal reflex.

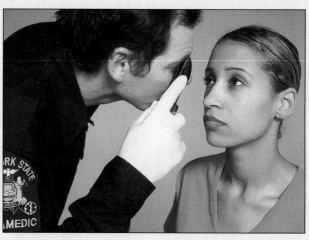

2-3h Visualize the interior eye with an ophthalmoscope.

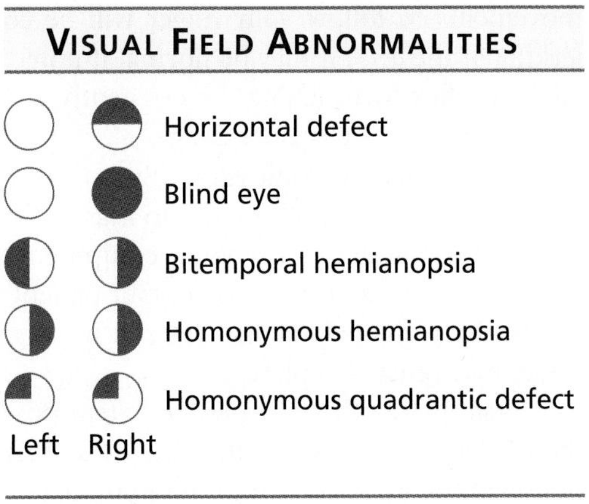

VISUAL FIELD ABNORMALITIES

○ ◑ Horizontal defect

○ ● Blind eye

◐ ◑ Bitemporal hemianopsia

◐ ◑ Homonymous hemianopsia

◔ ◔ Homonymous quadrantic defect

Left Right

Figure 2-29 Visual field abnormalities.

Are they clean and free from debris? Is there a stye (reddened swelling of the inner eyelid)? Quickly assess the regions of the lacrimal sacs and glands for swelling, excessive tearing, or dryness of the eyes.

Now ask your patient to look up while you pull down both lower eyelids to inspect the sclera and conjunctiva (Procedure 2–3c). Be careful not to put pressure on the eyeball. Ask your patient to look left and right, up and down. The conjunctiva should be clear and transparent, with no redness or cloudiness. Redness or a cobblestone appearance suggests an allergic or infectious conjunctivitis. Bright red blood in a sharply defined area surrounded by normal tissue, not extending into the iris, indicates a hemorrhage under the conjunctiva. Look for any nodules, swelling, or discharge. The normal sclera is white. A yellow sclera suggests the jaundice of liver disease.

With an oblique light source, inspect each cornea for opacities. Also check the lens for opacities that you may see through the pupil. Inspect the iris when you inspect the cornea. Shine the light directly from the lateral side and look for a crescent-shaped shadow on the medial side of the iris. Since the iris is flat, the light should cast no shadow. A shadow could suggest glaucoma, caused by a blockage that restricts aqueous humor from leaving the anterior chamber. This increases intraocular pressure and threatens your patient's eyesight.

Inspect the size, shape, and symmetry of the pupils. Are they unusually large (excessive dilation) or unusually small (excessive constriction)? Are they equal? Some patients (20 percent) have unequal pupils, a condition known as anisocoria; if the difference in the pupil's size is less than 2 millimeters and they react normally to light, anisocoria is benign. To test the pupils, first shine a light into one eye and observe that eye's reaction (Procedure 2–3d). This tests the eye's direct response. The pupil should constrict. Repeat this test for the other eye. Now shine a light into one eye and observe the other eye's reaction. This tests the eye's consensual response. Both eyes should react simultaneously to the light. Repeat this test for the other eye.

Normal pupils react to light briskly. A sluggish pupil suggests pressure on the oculomotor nerve (CN-III) from increased intracranial pressure. Bilateral sluggishness may indicate global hypoxia to the brain tissue or an adverse drug reaction. Constricted pupils suggest an opiate overdose, whereas fixed and dilated pupils usually mean brain death.

Now have your patient focus on an object in the distance. Then, ask her to focus on an object right in front of her. As she focuses on the near object, her pupils should constrict (near response). Now have your patient follow your finger or a pen, pencil, or similar object as you move it from a distance to the bridge of her nose (Procedure 2–3e). Her eyes should converge on the object as the pupils constrict (accommodation). Finally, have your patient follow your finger as you move it in an *H* pattern in front of her (Procedure 2–3f). This tests the integrity of the extraocular muscles. Normal eye movements to follow your finger will be conjugate (together). Nystagmus is a fine jerking of the eyes; it may be normal if noted at the far extremes of the test. Check the corneal reflex by touching the eye gently with a strand of cotton and watch for your patient to blink (Procedure 2–3g).

The ophthalmoscopic exam (Procedure 2–3h) may be quite challenging. It requires a significant amount of practice to master this physical exam skill. First, it is necessary to become familiar with your equipment. Locate the aperture, the indicator of diopters, and lens disk. If you or your patient wears glasses, you may remove them unless you or your patient has marked nearsightedness or severe astigmatism. Contact lenses may remain in place.

First, darken the room to the extent possible. Since you will not likely be dilating the patient's pupils, select the narrowest beam of light possible. Dim the light of the ophthalmoscope so as to minimize pupillary constriction. Begin the exam with the lens disk at zero diopters. Keep your index finger on the lens disk so that you can adjust the disk as necessary to focus on the various structures during the exam (Figure 2-30a ▶). Use the same eye as the eye you are examining (i.e., use your right eye to examine the patient's right eye and use your left eye to examine the patient's left eye). Ask your patient to focus on a stationary object straight ahead and slightly above his neutral plane of vision.

Standing laterally and slightly above your patient, look at the eye from about 6 to 15 inches away and aim your light about 15 to 25 degrees nasally. At this distance you should note a red "reflex" while looking through the pupil. The red reflex is simply a reflection of the retina back through the pupil. Absence of the red reflex is commonly secondary to cataracts. Less commonly it may indicate a detached retina (Figure 2-30b ▶), an artificial eye, or, in children, a retinoblastoma.

Place your nonexamining hand on the patient's shoulder or on the patient's forehead in order to gain a sense of proprioception so that you can tell how far away you are from the patient. If your hand is on the patient's forehead, you may assist the patient in keeping his eyelid open by holding the lid up with your thumb

> Examining the eye's interior with an ophthalmoscope is a detailed process that is very difficult to master and requires skill and practice.

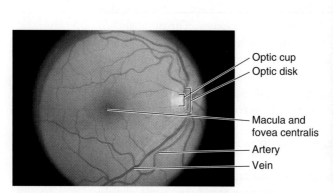

▶ **Figure 2-30a** Normal retina. The fovea is the area of most acute vision and is located within the darker macula. The optic nerve is contiguous with the retina at the optic disk. The paler optic cup is normally less than half of the diameter of the optic disk. Arteries supplying the retina are generally brighter and somewhat smaller than the veins. *(© James P. Gillman/Phototake)*

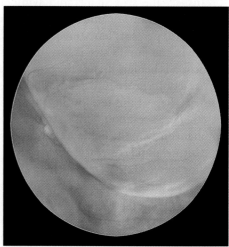

▶ **Figure 2-30b** Retinal detachment. Note the folds on the retina. When performing fundoscopy, each layer of the folds will appear in focus at a different aperture, indicating that the layers are not on the same plane. *(© Chris Barry/Phototake)*

near the eyelashes. While keeping the red reflex in view, slowly move toward your patient's eye while the patient continues to fix his gaze on an object in the distance. Adjust the lens disk as needed to focus on the retina. Farsighted patients will require more "plus" diopters (black or green numbers), whereas nearsighted patients will require more "minus" diopters (red numbers) in order to keep the retina in focus. Try to keep both of your eyes open and relaxed. The optic disk should come into view when you are about 1.5 to 2 inches from the eye while you are still aiming your light 15 to 25 degrees nasally. If you are having difficulty finding the disk, look for a branching (bifurcation) in a retinal blood vessel. Usually the bifurcation will point toward the disk. Follow the vessel in the direction of the bifurcation and you should arrive at the optic disk. The disk should appear as a yellowish orange to pink round structure. Within the center of the disk there should be a central physiological cup, which normally appears as a smaller, paler circle. The cup should be less than half the diameter of the disk. An enlarged cup may indicate chronic open-angle glaucoma. Indistinct borders or elevation of the optic disk may indicate papilledema (Figure 2-30c), which is a marker of increased intracranial pressure. Next, look at the arteries and veins of the retina. The arteries are usually brighter and smaller than the veins. Spontaneous venous pulsations are normal. Abnormalities of the retina such as hemorrhages, arteriovenous (A-V) nicking, and cotton wool spots may indicate local or systemic disease such as retinal vein occlusion (Figure 2-30d), hypertension, or many other conditions.

Finally, look at the fovea and surrounding macula. This area is where vision is most acute. It is located about two disk diameters temporal to the optic disk. You may also find the macula by asking the patient to look directly into the light of your opthalmoscope. Prepare for a fleeting glimpse as this area is very sensitive to light and may be uncomfortable for your patient to maintain. A "cherry red" macula with surrounding pallor of tissue in the setting of acute painless monocular visual loss indicates a central retinal artery occlusion (Figure 2-30e). Irreversible damage occurs within 90 minutes of complete occlusion. Unfortunately, these patients rarely respond to therapy.

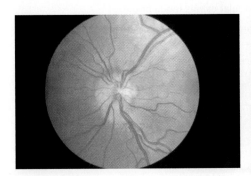

▶ **Figure 2-30c** Papilledema. Bilateral elevation of the optic disks produces the appearance of indistinct disk borders. Flame hemorrhages may be present and microvascular congestion of the disk may also be apparent. Papilledema signifies increased intracranial pressure. *(© Margaret Cubberly/Phototake)*

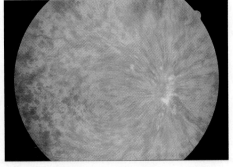

▶ **Figure 2-30d** Central retinal vein occlusion. Note the diffuse "flame hemorrhages" and "cotton wool spots" (white patches) characteristic of central retinal vein occlusion. These findings are so dramatic that the appearance of this condition is often described as "blood and thunder." Unlike central retinal artery occlusion, central retinal vein occlusion is usually subacute and, thus, not a true ophthalmologic emergency. *(© Chris Barry/Phototake)*

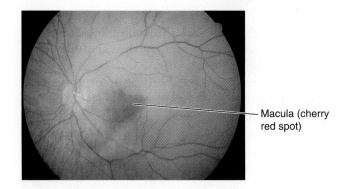

Figure 2-30e Central retinal artery occlusion. Note the "cherry red spot" in the center of the photo. This spot represents the macula, which is thinner than the rest of the retina and, thus, allows the normal color of the choroidal layer to show through. The rest of the retina is thicker and loses its normal transparency when perfusion is blocked. Thus, the macula looks more prominent ("cherry red"), because the rest of the retina becomes less transparent when devoid of blood and prevents the normal color of the underlying choroid from showing through. (© Chris Barry/Phototake)

Macula (cherry red spot)

The Ears

The ear has three components: the outer ear, the middle ear, and the inner ear (Figure 2-31). The outer ear consists of the auricle, the ear canal (external acoustic meatus), and the lateral surface of the tympanic membrane (eardrum). The auricle is the visible, skin-covered cartilage that extends outward from the skull. It comprises the helix (the prominent outer rim), the antihelix (the inner rim), the lobe (which contains no cartilage), the concha (the deep cavity containing the opening to the ear canal), and the tragus (the protuberance that lies just in front of the concha).

Behind the ear lies the mastoid process of the temporal bone. It functions as an attachment for the sternocleidomastoid muscle and is palpable just behind the earlobe. The mastoid bone contains air-filled cells that are continuous with the middle ear. This is why an inner ear infection (otitis) often presents with tenderness in the mastoid area. The ear canal opens behind the tragus and is approximately 2 to 3

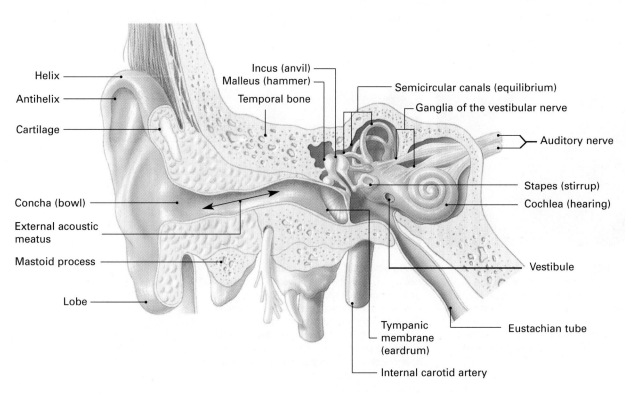

Helix
Antihelix
Cartilage
Concha (bowl)
External acoustic meatus
Mastoid process
Lobe

Incus (anvil)
Malleus (hammer)
Temporal bone
Semicircular canals (equilibrium)
Ganglia of the vestibular nerve
Auditory nerve
Stapes (stirrup)
Cochlea (hearing)
Vestibule
Tympanic membrane (eardrum)
Internal carotid artery
Eustachian tube

Figure 2-31 The ear.

centimeters long in adults. Hair and sebaceous glands that produce wax (cerumen) line the distal third of the canal. At the end of the ear canal, the translucent tympanic membrane separates the ear canal from the middle ear.

The middle ear, an air-filled cavity in the temporal bone, begins with the medial surface of the tympanic membrane. It contains three small bones known as ossicles (the malleus, the incus, and the stapes) that transmit and amplify sound from the tympanic membrane to the inner ear. The irregularly shaped malleus connects directly to the medial surface of the tympanic membrane at the umbo. It pulls the eardrum inward, making it concave. A "cone of light" is visible here during otoscopy. A light shined on the translucent eardrum makes the middle ear somewhat visible. The eustachian tubes help move mucus from the middle ear to the nasopharynx. They also help equalize the pressure between the outside air and the middle ear during swallowing, sneezing, and yawning.

The inner ear cavity contains the vestibule, the semicircular canals, and the cochlea. The cochlea is a coiled structure that transmits sound to the acoustic nerve (CN-VIII). Hearing involves air conduction of vibrations from the environment to the tympanic membrane. These vibrations are transmitted through the eardrum to the ossicles and to the cochlea, which translates them into nerve impulses. The acoustic nerve transmits these nerve impulses to the brain. The labyrinth within the inner ear helps us maintain our balance by sensing the position and movement of our head. It also is innervated by the acoustic nerve.

Begin the examination by simply observing the ears from in front of your patient. Something that just "doesn't look right" warrants further investigation. In particular, look for symmetry. Then examine each ear separately. Inspect each auricle for size, shape, symmetry, landmarks, color, and position on the head. Observe the surrounding area for deformities, lumps, skin lesions, tenderness, and erythema (redness). Lumps on or near the ear may indicate a benign process, such as cutaneous cysts or keloids, a malignant process such as squamous cell or basal cell carcinoma, or a local sign of a systemic process such as gout or rheumatoid arthritis. Pull the helix upward and outward and note any tenderness or discomfort (Procedure 2–4a). Press on the tragus and on the mastoid process (Procedure 2–4b). Pain or tenderness in any of these areas suggests infection such as otitis or mastoiditis. Discoloration in this area is known as Battle's sign, a common, but late, finding in a basilar skull fracture. An earache may arise from the ear itself or be referred from another place through adjoining and shared sensory nerve pathways. Sources of referred pain may include sinus problems, a bad tooth, temporomandibular joint pain, the common cold, a sore throat, and the cervical spine.

Inspect for discharge (otorrhea) from the ear canal (Procedure 2–4c). The discharge may contain mucus, pus, blood, or cerebrospinal fluid that may have leaked from the skull through a fracture in its base. Injuries to the ear itself can result from blunt trauma to the side of the head, causing temporary or permanent damage to the outer or middle ear. A ruptured eardrum can result from sticking a sharp object into the ear canal or from a pressure wave caused by an explosion.

Evaluate your patient's hearing by occluding one canal. Whisper very softly into the other ear (Procedure 2–4d). Begin by exhaling completely before you speak so as to minimize the intensity of your whisper. Use words such as "baseball" that have equally accented syllables. Gradually increase the intensity of your voice until the patient is able to hear you. Do the same for the other ear and evaluate symmetry.

To test for conductive and sensorineural hearing loss you can use a tuning fork (typically 512 Hz) to perform the Rinne and Weber tests. The Rinne test will differentiate a conductive from a sensorineural hearing loss. First place the base of the slightly vibrating tuning fork behind the patient's ear. When the patient can no longer hear the vibration, put the tuning fork up to her ear with the tip of the fork closest to the ear

Examining the Ears

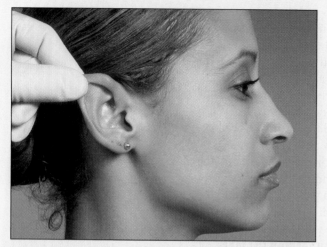

2-4a Examine the external ear.

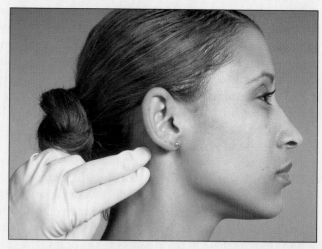

2-4b Press on the mastoid process.

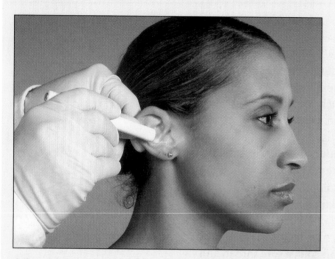

2-4c Inspect the ear canal for drainage.

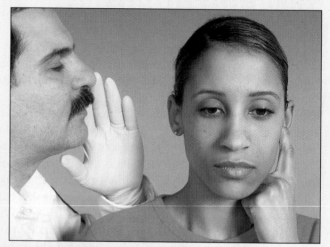

2-4d Whisper into your patient's ear.

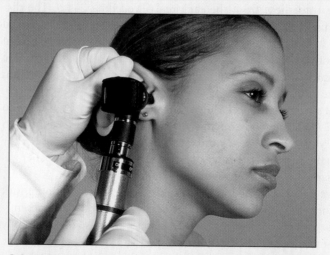

2-4e Visualize the inner ear canal and tympanic membrane.

Procedure 2–6   Examining the Mouth

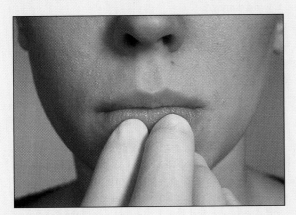

2-6a   Palpate the lips.

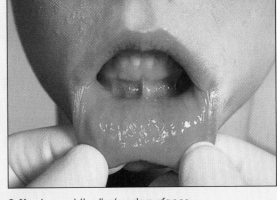

2-6b   Inspect the lips' undersurfaces.

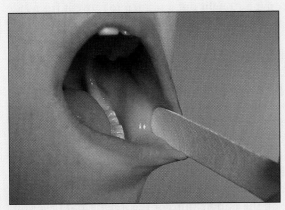

2-6c   Examine the buccal mucosa.

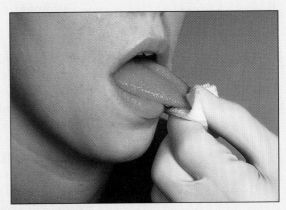

2-6d   Inspect the tongue using a gauze pad and a gloved hand.

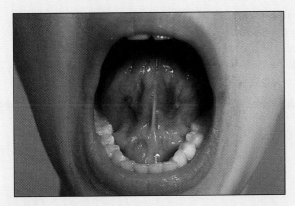

2-6e   Inspect under the tongue.

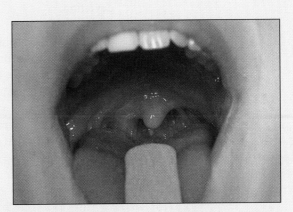

2-6f   Have your patient say "aaahhh" while you examine the soft palate and uvula.

Table 2-4	Lip Abnormalities
Lips	**Cause**
Dry, cracked lips	Dehydration, wind damage
Swelling/edema	Infection, allergic reaction, burns
Lesions	Infection, irritation, skin cancer
Pallor	Anemia, shock
Cyanosis	Respiratory or cardiac insufficiency

oral mucosa for color, ulcers, white patches, and nodules. The oral mucosa should appear pinkish-red, smooth, and moist. Note the color of the gums and teeth. The gums should be pink with a clearly defined margin surrounding each tooth. Inspect the teeth for color, shape, and position. Are any missing or loose? Suspect periodontal disease if the gums are swollen, bleed easily, and are separated from the teeth by large crevices that trap food. Use a tongue blade to move the lateral lip to one side while you examine the buccal mucosa and parotid glands (Procedure 2–6c). Note the buccal mucosa's color and texture.

Ask your patient to stick her tongue straight out and then to move it from side to side. Coating of the tongue indicates dehydration. Note its color and normally velvety surface. Hold the tongue with a 2-inch × 2-inch gauze pad and a gloved hand to manipulate it for inspection (Procedure 2–6d). Make sure to inspect the sides and bottom of the tongue because malignancies are more likely to develop there, especially in patients over age 50 who smoke, chew tobacco, or drink alcohol (Procedure 2–6e). The undersurface should be smooth and pink; often you can see the bluish discoloration of dilated veins or the yellowish tint of early jaundice. Inspect the floor of the mouth, the submandibular ducts, and the fold over the sublingual gland.

Now examine the normally white hard palate and the normally pink soft palate (Procedure 2–6f). Check them for texture and lesions. Observe the posterior pharyngeal wall. Press the blade down on the middle third of the tongue and have your patient say "aaahhh." Examine the posterior pharynx, the palatine tonsils, and the movement of the uvula. Inspect the tonsils for color and symmetry. Look for exudate (pus), swelling, ulcers, or drainage. The uvula should move straight up with no deviation.

Note any odors from your patient's mouth. The smell of alcohol, feces (bowel obstruction), acetone (diabetic ketoacidosis), gastric contents, or the bitter-almond smell of cyanide poisoning may all provide important clues to your patient's problem. Also look for any fluids or unusual matter in your patient's mouth. For example, coffee-grounds-like material suggests an upper gastrointestinal (GI) bleed. Pink-tinged sputum indicates acute pulmonary edema, whereas a green or yellow phlegm suggests a respiratory infection. Pay special attention to anything in your patient's mouth that can eventually obstruct his upper airway, including dentures or missing teeth.

Pay special attention to anything in your patient's mouth that can eventually obstruct his upper airway.

The Neck

The neck houses many life-sustaining structures. It contains the spinal cord, blood vessels delivering blood to (carotid arteries) and from (jugular veins) the brain, and the conduits for air passage (larynx/trachea) into the lungs and food passage (esophagus) into the stomach. Any major disruption of these vital structures can cause

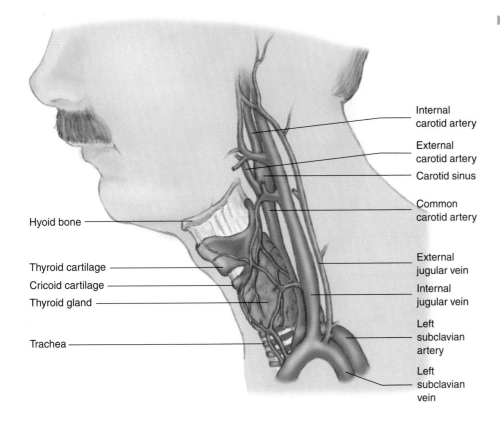

Internal
carotid artery

External
carotid artery

Carotid sinus

Common
carotid artery

External
jugular vein

Internal
jugular vein

Left
subclavian
artery

Left
subclavian
vein

Hyoid bone

Thyroid cartilage

Cricoid cartilage

Thyroid gland

Trachea

rapid deterioration or immediate death. Especially during an emergency, examining the neck can be a critical part of your patient assessment.

From anterior to posterior, the thyroid gland, larynx and trachea, esophagus, and spinal column lie in the midline. The thyroid cartilage is the visible and palpable Adam's apple in the anterior neck midline (Figure 2-37 ▶). Just below it lie the cricoid cartilage and the rings of the trachea. The thyroid gland sits on both sides of the trachea, with its isthmus crossing the trachea. Between the thyroid cartilage and the large sternocleidomastoid muscles, the common carotid arteries extend toward the brain. The internal jugular veins are next to the carotids and are not visible. The external jugular veins extend diagonally across the surface of the sternocleidomastoid muscles and are clearly visible when they are distended or the patient is lying down. The lymph system helps drain fluid from the head and face and assists in fighting infection. A long chain of lymph nodes runs along the side of the neck, behind the ears, and under the chin (Figure 2-38 ▶). The nodes are palpable only when inflamed.

Briefly inspect your patient's neck for general symmetry and visible masses. Note any obvious deformity, deviation, tugging, masses, surgical scars, gland enlargement, or visible lymph nodes. Examine any penetrating injuries to the neck closely for damage to the trachea or major blood vessels; handle gently to avoid dislodging a clot that has halted bleeding. Immediately cover any open wounds with an occlusive dressing to prevent air from entering a lacerated jugular vein during inspiration. Look for jugular vein distention while your patient is sitting upright and at a 45-degree incline.

Palpate the trachea for midline position (Procedure 2–7a). Then gently palpate the carotid arteries, one at a time, and note the rate and quality of their pulses (Procedure 2–7b). Now palpate the butterfly-shaped thyroid gland from behind your patient. Rest

Especially during an emergency, examining the neck can be a critical part of your patient assessment.

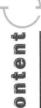

Review

Vital Structures in the Neck

- Spinal cord
- Carotid arteries
- Jugular veins
- Larynx/trachea
- Esophagus

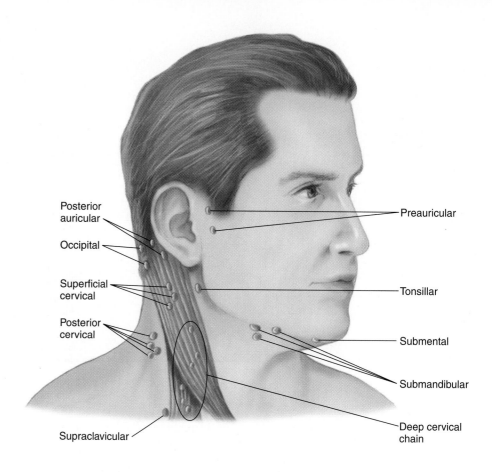

▶ **Figure 2-38** Lymph nodes of the head and neck.

Posterior auricular

Occipital

Superficial cervical

Posterior cervical

Supraclavicular

Preauricular

Tonsillar

Submental

Submandibular

Deep cervical chain

your thumbs on her trapezius muscles and place two fingers of each hand on the sides of the trachea just beneath the cricoid cartilage (Procedure 2–7c). Have your patient swallow and feel for the movement of the gland. If you can feel it, it should be small, smooth, and free of nodules. Examining the lymph nodes requires a systematic approach (Table 2–5). Using the pads of your fingers palpate the nodes by moving the skin over the underlying tissues in each area (Procedure 2–7d). When swollen, the nodes are palpable, sometimes even visible. Note their size, shape, mobility, consistency, and tenderness. Tender, swollen, and mobile nodes suggest inflammation, usually from infection. Hard or fixed nodes suggest a malignancy. Inspect and palpate for subcutaneous emphysema, the presence of air just below the skin. This generally suggests a tear in the tracheobronchial tree or a pneumothorax.

The Chest and Lungs

The chest is a protective cage of bones, muscles, and cartilage (Figure 2-39▶). The bony cage comprises the three bones of the sternum (manubrium, body, and xiphoid process), the 12 pairs of ribs and their cartilaginous attachments, and the spinal column. In most adults, the transverse (side-to-side) diameter exceeds the anterior-posterior (front-to-back) diameter. The chest is divided into three cavities: the mediastinum, the right pleural cavity, and the left pleural cavity. The right chest contains three lung lobes (upper, middle, lower), while the left contains only two (upper, lower), to make room for the heart. The mediastinum contains the heart, the great vessels (vena cava, aorta, and pulmonary arteries and veins), the trachea, and the esophagus.

Examining the Neck

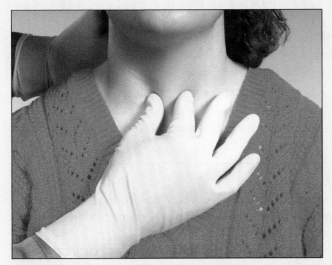

2-7a Assess the trachea for midline position.

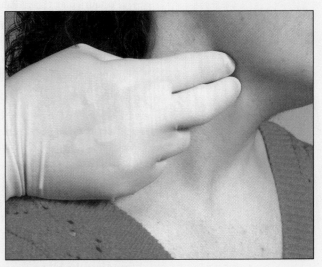

2-7b Palpate the carotid arteries, one at a time.

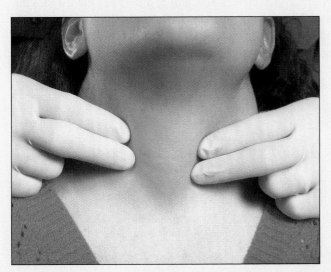

2-7c Palpate the thyroid gland.

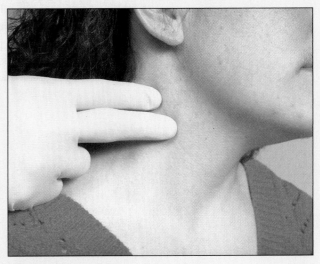

2-7d Palpate the lymph nodes.

The chest wall can expand to create a vacuum that draws air into the lungs and helps return blood to the heart. The primary muscles of respiration are the diaphragm and external intercostals. During inhalation, the diaphragm contracts and moves downward while the external intercostals pull the chest wall upward and outward. The lungs, attached to the inner chest wall by a membrane called the pleura, expand also. The pleura consists of a parietal layer (lining the inner chest wall) and a visceral layer (covering the lungs) that glide over each other during breathing. A small amount of liquid between the layers helps create the vacuum for inhaling and acts as a lubricant. In cases of airway obstruction, a variety of accessory muscles in the neck and chest help

Table 2-5	Lymph Node Exam
Node	**Exam**
Preauricular	Press on the tragus and "milk" anteriorly.
Postauricular	Palpate on or under the mastoid process.
Occipital	Palpate at the base of the skull lateral to the thick bands of muscle.
Submental	Palpate at the base of the mandible under the chin.
Submaxillary	Palpate along the underside of the jawline.
Anterior cervical	Palpate anterior to the sternocleidomastoid muscle.
Posterior cervical	Palpate posterior to the sternocleidomastoid muscle.
Deep cervical	Encircle and palpate the sternocleidomastoid muscle.
Supraclavicular	Palpate just above the clavicle in the deep groove.

lift the chest wall. Exhalation is primarily a passive process of muscle relaxation unless disease or injury forces the use of accessory muscles in the chest and abdomen to help expel air from the lungs.

A neurochemical process controls normal breathing. Specialized chemoreceptors monitor the blood for increases in carbon dioxide, decreases in oxygen, and changes in pH. The brain sends signals to the primary respiratory muscles to begin inspiration. The phrenic nerve, arising from cervical nerves 3, 4, and 5, innervates the diaphragm, while the thoracic spinal nerves innervate their respective intercostal muscles.

To assess the chest and thorax, you will need a stethoscope with a bell and diaphragm, a marking pen, and a centimeter ruler. Have your patient sit upright, if possible, and expose his entire chest. At the same time, try to maintain your female patient's dignity when assessing her thorax and lungs by keeping her breasts covered.

▶ **Figure 2-39** The thorax.

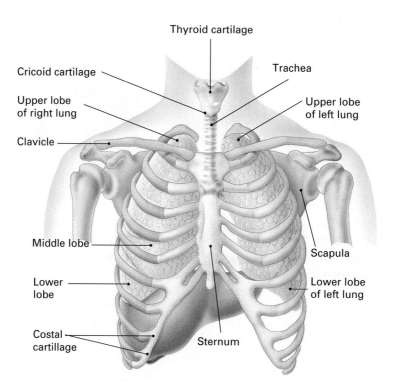

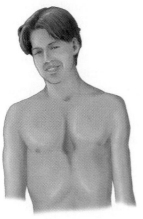
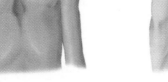

Funnel chest   Pigeon chest   Barrel chest

Perform your exam in the standard sequence—inspect, palpate, percuss, auscultate—and compare the findings from side to side. Always try to visualize the underlying lobes of the lungs during your exam.

Observe your patient's breathing. Look for signs of acute respiratory distress. Now count the respiratory rate and note his breathing pattern. Obviously prolonged inhalation or exhalation indicates difficulty moving air in or out of the lungs. Do you hear sounds of an upper airway obstruction (inspiratory stridor) or a lower airway obstruction (expiratory wheezing, rhonchi)? Any gross abnormalities in the respiratory rate or pattern require rapid emergency intervention.

Inspect the anterior chest wall and assess its symmetry. Funnel chest (pectus excavatum) is a condition in which the lower portion of the sternum is depressed (Figure 2-40 ▶). With a pigeon chest (pectus carinatum), the sternum curves outward. Do both sides of your patient's chest wall rise in unison? Note whether he is using neck muscles during inhalation or abdominal muscles during exhalation. If his skin retracts in the area above his clavicles (supraclavicular), at the notch above his sternum (suprasternal), and between his ribs (intercostal), suspect a ventilation problem. If multiple ribs are fractured, creating a "floating segment" or "traumatic flail chest," you may find paradoxical (opposite) movement of that part of the chest wall during breathing.

Now look at his chest from the side. Normally an adult's thorax is twice as wide as it is deep. That is, the transverse diameter of the chest wall is usually twice the anteroposterior diameter. In infants, the elderly, or patients with chronic pulmonary disease, however, the anteroposterior diameter is increased, giving them a barrel chest appearance.

Posterior Chest Examination

Next examine the posterior chest. Ask your patient to fold his arms across his chest and breathe normally during the exam. This moves his scapulae out of the way and allows you more access to his posterior lung fields. Inspect his posterior chest for deformities and symmetrical movement as he breathes. Some patients may exhibit thoracic kyphoscoliosis, an abnormal spinal curvature that deforms the chest and makes your lung exam more challenging. Inspect the intercostal spaces for retractions or bulging; both are abnormal. Retractions may appear when airflow is impeded during inspiration. Bulging may appear when airflow is impeded during exhalation. Respiratory movement should be smooth and effortless. When it is not, suspect underlying respiratory disease or structural impairment.

Palpate the rib cage for rigidity. Feel for tenderness, deformities, depressions, loose segments, asymmetry, and crepitus. Then evaluate for equal expansion. First, locate

Any gross abnormalities in the respiratory rate or pattern require rapid emergency intervention.

the level of the posterior 10th rib. To do this, find the lowest rib and simply move up two more ribs. An alternate method for locating the posterior 10th rib is to palpate the spinous processes. Ask your patient to touch his chin to his chest. The most prominent spinous process is the 7th cervical vertebra. Locate it and count down to T-10 in the midline. Now place your hands parallel to the 10th rib on your patient's back with your fingers spread. Lightly grasp his lateral rib cage with your spread hands (Procedure 2–8a). Ask him to inhale deeply. Normally the distance between your thumbs will increase symmetrically by 3 to 5 centimeters during deep inspiration. If you detect decreased thoracic expansion or feel unilateral delay, suspect a disorder of the underlying lung, pleura, or diaphragm.

When your patient speaks, you can feel vibrations on his chest wall. This is known as tactile fremitus. Place the palm of your hand on your patient's chest wall and have him say "ninety-nine or one-on-one." As he does, palpate the posterior chest; feel the vibrations in different areas of the chest wall and compare symmetrical areas of the lungs (Procedure 2–8b). Identify and note any areas of increased, decreased, or absent vibrations. You will feel increased fremitus when sound transmission is enhanced through areas of consolidated lung tissue such as in a tumor, pneumonia, or pulmonary fibrosis. You will feel decreased or absent fremitus when sound transmission is diminished in a certain area, as may occur with a pleural effusion, emphysema, or pneumothorax.

Percuss your patient's posterior chest to determine whether the underlying tissues are air filled, fluid filled, or solid. Also percuss to determine the position and boundaries of the diaphragm and underlying organs. Percuss both sides of the chest symmetrically from the apex to the base at 5-centimeter intervals, avoiding bony areas such as the scapulae (Procedure 2–8c). Percuss at least twice in each area and compare both sides of the thorax. Identify and note any area of abnormal percussion. For example, a hyperresonant sound in the right chest may indicate a pneumothorax, whereas a dull sound in the same area may indicate a hemothorax. Assess the percussion sounds according to their quality, intensity, pitch, and duration. Practice percussing the chest so that you will become familiar with the normal resonance of the lungs and be able to identify abnormal sounds.

Next assess for diaphragmatic excursion. Identify the level of the diaphragm during quiet breathing by percussing for dullness as the diaphragm moves during the respiratory cycle. Percuss at the lower rib margin on one side and note when dullness (muscle) replaces resonance (air). With a pen mark the location of the diaphragm at the end of inhalation and at the end of exhalation. The distance between the marks is the diaphragmatic excursion. In the normal healthy adult at rest, the diaphragmatic excursion should be approximately 6 centimeters. Now measure diaphragmatic excursion on the opposite side and compare the marks. If you find asymmetrical diaphragmatic levels, a paralyzed phrenic nerve may be the problem. Here, reevaluate your patient's respiratory depth for adequacy and provide the appropriate intervention as needed.

Auscultate your patient's chest for normal breath sounds, adventitious breath sounds, and voice sounds. Auscultate all lung fields and compare side to side. Evaluate the normal breath sounds produced by airflow through the upper and lower airways. These include tracheal, bronchial, bronchovesicular, and vesicular breath sounds (Table 2–6).

Besides the normal breath sounds already mentioned, you also may hear adventitious sounds. These include crackles, wheezes, rhonchi, stridor, and pleural rubs.

Also known as *rales*, **crackles** are light crackling, popping, nonmusical sounds heard usually during inspiration. They are produced by air passing through moisture in the bronchoalveolar system or from the abrupt opening of closed alveoli. Early inspiratory crackles, associated with chronic bronchitis and heart failure, begin shortly after inspiration starts, and they stop soon thereafter. These are coarse crackles—loud, low pitched, and long, similar to the sound of water boiling. They are often audible at the mouth.

Review

Adventitious Breath Sounds

- Crackles
- Wheezes
- Rhonchi
- Stridor
- Pleural rubs

crackles

light crackling, popping, nonmusical sounds heard usually during inspiration, also called rales.

Examining the Chest

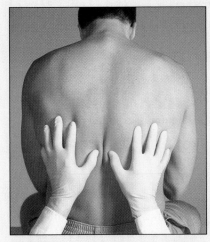

2-8a Palpate the posterior chest for excursion.

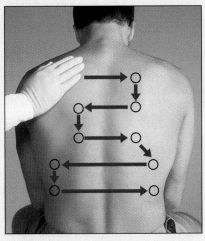

2-8b Palpate the posterior chest for tactile fremitus.

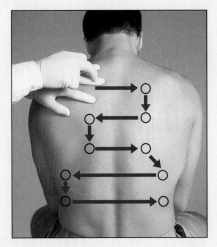

2-8c Percuss the posterior chest.

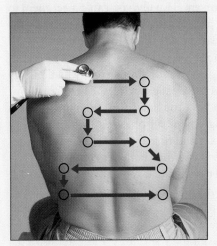

2-8d Auscultate the posterior chest.

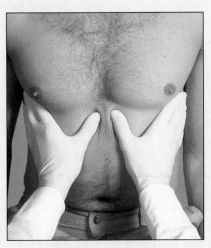

2-8e Palpate the anterior chest for excursion.

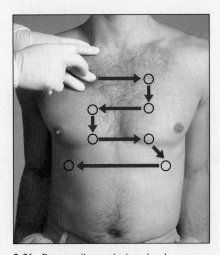

2-8f Percuss the anterior chest.

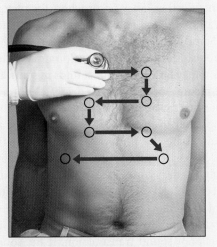

2-8g Auscultate the anterior chest.

Table 2-6	Normal Breath Sounds		
Sound	Description	Location	Duration
Tracheal	Very loud, harsh	Over the trachea	Nearly equal inspiratory and expiratory phases
Bronchial	Loud, high pitch, hollow	Over the manubrium	Prolonged expiratory phase
Broncho-vesicular	Soft, breezy, lower pitch	Between the scapulae/2nd–3rd ICS lateral to the sternum	Approximately equal inspiratory and expiratory phases
Vesicular	Soft, swishy, lowest pitch	Lung periphery	Prolonged inspiratory phase

Late inspiratory crackles, associated with congestive heart failure and interstitial lung diseases, begin in the first half of the inspiratory phase and continue into late inspiration. They are fine crackles—soft, high pitched, and very brief, similar to the sound of Rice Krispies crackling. They commonly appear first at the base of the lungs and move upward as your patient's condition worsens. Usually, you can expect them to shift to dependent regions with changes in your patient's position. For example, if your heart failure patient is sitting up, expect to hear crackles first in the bases. If he is bedridden, expect to hear crackles first in the back.

wheezes
continuous, high-pitched musical sounds similar to a whistle.

Wheezes are continuous, high-pitched musical sounds similar to a whistle. They result when air moves through partially obstructed smaller airways. Their causes include asthma, bronchospasm, and foreign bodies. You may hear them without a stethoscope or by auscultating the chest during any or all phases of the respiratory cycle. They often originate in the small bronchioles and first appear at the end of exhalation. The closer to inspiration they appear, the worse your patient's condition.

rhonchi
continuous sounds with a lower pitch and a snoring quality.

Rhonchi are continuous sounds with a lower pitch and a snoring quality. They are caused by secretions in the larger airways, a common finding in bronchitis (diffuse) and pneumonia (localized). Rhonchi usually appear in early exhalation but may occur in early inspiration as well.

stridor
predominantly inspiratory wheeze associated with laryngeal obstruction.

Stridor is a predominantly high-pitched inspiratory sound. It indicates a partial obstruction of the larynx or trachea.

pleural friction rub
the squeaking or grating sound of the pleural linings rubbing together.

Pleural friction rubs are the squeaking or grating sounds of the pleural linings rubbing together. They occur where the pleural layers are inflamed and have lost their lubrication. Pleural rubs are common in pneumonia and pleurisy (inflammation of the pleura). Because these sounds occur whenever your patient's chest wall moves, they appear during the entire respiratory cycle.

You may hear no breath sounds in some areas. This may result from effusion (fluid in the pleural space causing a decrease in functional lung tissue) or consolidation (infectious pus causing collapsed alveoli). In either case, note the area's size and intervene appropriately to ensure adequate ventilation and oxygenation of your patient.

Auscultate the posterior chest systematically. Have your patient fold his arms across his chest and breathe through his mouth more deeply and slowly than usual. Auscultate the same areas you percussed and compare the bilateral findings (Procedure 2–8d). Listen for at least one full breath at each location. Be alert for patient discomfort or hyperventilation. Note the pitch, intensity, and duration of each inspiratory and expiratory sound. If the sounds are decreased, suspect impaired airflow or poor sound transmission. If the sounds are absent, suspect no airflow. Note whether you hear sounds where you normally should. For example, when you auscultate over the peripheral lung fields, you should not hear tracheal, bronchial, or bronchovesicular breath sounds. Listen carefully and note what you hear, where you hear it, and when you hear it during the respiratory cycle. Also note whether the sounds change when your patient coughs or changes position.

If you hear abnormally located tracheal, bronchial, or bronchovesicular breath sounds, assess your patient's transmitted voice sounds. Ask him to repeat the words "ninety-nine" as you auscultate his chest wall. Normally you should hear muffled, indistinct sounds. Hearing the words clearly is an abnormal finding known as **bronchophony.** Bronchophony occurs when fluid (water, blood) or consolidated tissue (pus, tumor) replaces the normally air-filled lung. After you check your patient for bronchophony, assess him for **whispered pectoriloquy** and **egophony.** For pectoriloquy, ask your patient to whisper "ninety-nine" while you auscultate. As with bronchophony, the words will be clear and distinct if sound transmission through an area is abnormally enhanced. For egophony, ask him to repeat the long *e* sound while you auscultate. You should hear a muffled, long *e*. If vocal resonance is abnormally increased, you will hear an *a* sound instead. This is known as "*e* to *a* egophony."

Anterior Chest Examination

Your examination of the anterior chest will be similar to your examination of the posterior chest. Begin by having your patient lie supine with his arms relaxed but slightly abducted at his sides. Look for any gross deformities or asymmetrical movements. Does the chest wall rise symmetrically? Is there accessory muscle use? Look for abnormal retractions in the suprasternal, supraclavicular, and intercostal areas. Also check for callused elbows from tripodding (leaning with elbows on a table or chair arms), and finger clubbing—both common signs of chronic lung disease. Is the trachea midline or deviated; does it tug during inhalation? In cases of tension pneumothorax, the trachea will deviate away from the affected side. In cases of pulmonary fibrosis and atelectasis, it will tug toward the affected side during inhalation.

Palpate the anterior chest for deformities and areas of tenderness. Check for chest expansion by placing your thumbs along the costal margins on both sides and gently grasping the lateral rib cage (Procedure 2–8e). Ask your patient to inhale deeply. Normally your thumbs will separate symmetrically and the distance between them will increase from 3 to 5 centimeters. If you detect decreased thoracic expansion or feel unilateral delay, suspect a disorder of the underlying lung, pleura, or diaphragm.

As with the posterior chest, test for tactile fremitus, bronchophony, whispered pectoriloquy, and egophony if you detect abnormal breath sounds.

Percuss your patient's anterior chest to help determine whether the underlying tissues are air filled, fluid filled, or solid and to determine the position and boundaries of the diaphragm and underlying organs. Percuss each side of your patient's anterior chest from its apex to its base at 5-centimeter intervals at the midclavicular lines (Procedure 2–8f). Percuss at least twice in each area and compare both sides of the thorax. Identify and note any area of abnormal percussion. Remember that when percussing the right chest, you will hear dullness at the upper border of the liver. On the left side, you will hear the normal resonance of the lung change to tympany when you reach the stomach. You also will percuss an area of cardiac dullness from the 3rd to the 5th intercostal spaces.

Finally, auscultate the anterior and lateral thorax systematically. Have your patient breathe through his mouth more deeply and slowly than usual. Auscultate the same areas you percussed and compare symmetrical areas (Procedure 2–8g). Listen for at least one full breath at each location. Be alert for patient discomfort or hyperventilation. As with posterior chest auscultation, note the pitch, intensity, and duration of each inspiratory and expiratory sound and whether you heard sounds where you should normally expect them. Listen for adventitious sounds. If you hear abnormally

bronchophony
abnormal clarity of patient's transmitted voice sounds.

whispered pectoriloquy
abnormal clarity of patient's transmitted whispers.

egophony
abnormal change in tone of patient's transmitted voice sounds.

Assessment Pearls

Examining for Congestive Heart Failure One physical examination finding in the setting of congestive heart failure (CHF) is jugular venous distension (JVD). JVD results from elevated right atrial pressure, although it can occur with elevated left atrial pressures as well. JVD is best measured with the patient in the supine position and with the upper torso elevated to approximately 45° (20–60° range).

Adjust the head angle so that the top of the jugular vein is generally in the middle of the neck. Measure the height of the venous column from the angle of Louis (i.e., second intercostal space, midsternum). Add 5 cm to this measurement, which determines the measurement from the chest wall to the right atrium.

To determine whether JVD is due to CHF or fluid overload, place your right hand on the patient's midabdomen and apply steady pressure to indent the abdomen about 4–5 cm. When you do this, the blood column in the neck veins will immediately rise. The initial rise usually results when the patient performs a Valsalva maneuver (a forced exhalation against a closed glottis). If the veins remain elevated after the patient has resumed normal breathing (within 10–15 seconds), this finding (referred to as the abdomino-jugular reflex) is indicative of congestive heart failure.

located tracheal, bronchial, or bronchovesicular breath sounds, assess for bronchophony, whispered pectoriloquy, and egophony.

The Cardiovascular System

Mentally picture the heart and great vessels as you inspect the chest (Figure 2-41 ▶). The heart sits just behind the sternum between the 3rd and 6th costal cartilages and rotated to the left. Its most anterior surface, therefore, is the right ventricle. The pulmonary artery, which carries deoxygenated blood to the lungs, leaves the right ventricle at the 3rd costal cartilage, close to the sternum. The left ventricle sits behind

▶ **Figure 2-41** The heart and great vessels.

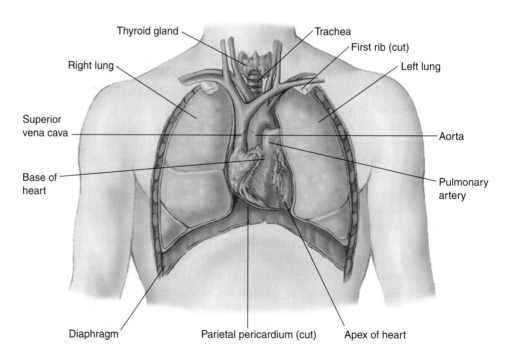

the right ventricle and a little to its left. It forms the left border of the heart and produces the apical impulse at the 5th intercostal space, near the midclavicular line. This is the point of maximal impulse (PMI), usually the same as the apical impulse, which occurs at the apex of the heart. The aorta curves upward from the left ventricle to the level of the sternal angle (2nd costal cartilage), arches backward, and then turns back downward. To the right of the aorta, the superior vena cava returns blood to the right atrium.

To assess cardiac function, you must understand the cardiac cycle (Figure 2-42 ▶). During **diastole,** the heart's resting period, the ventricles relax. The pressure in the atria is greater than the pressure in the ventricles. This opens the tricuspid valve on the right side and the mitral valve on the left, allowing blood from the atria to fill the ventricles. During **systole** the ventricles contract and the tricuspid and mitral valves close, preventing backflow into the atria. The vibrations of these valves' closings generate the

diastole
phase of cardiac cycle when ventricles relax.

systole
phase of cardiac cycle when the ventricles contract.

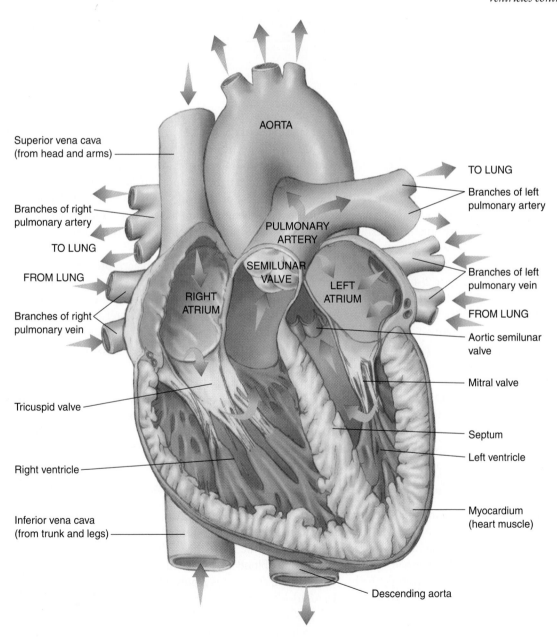

▶ **Figure 2-42** Anatomy of the heart and blood flow.

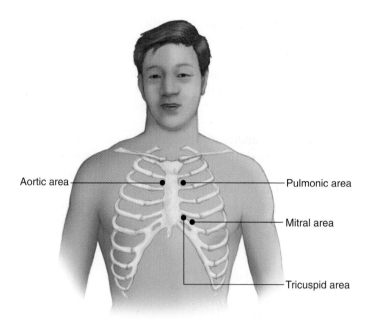

Figure 2-43 Sites for cardiac auscultation.

Aortic area — Pulmonic area

— Mitral area

— Tricuspid area

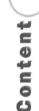

Review

Heart Sounds

- S_1—"lub"
- S_2—"dub"
- Split S_1—"la-lub"
- Split S_2—"da-dub"
- S_3—"lub-dub-dee" (Kentucky)
- S_4—"dee-lub-dub" (Tennessee)
- Click
- Snap
- Pericardial friction rub
- Murmur

cardiac output

the amount of blood the heart ejects each minute, measured in milliliters.

stroke volume

the amount of blood the heart ejects in one beat.

first heart sound—S_1, or the "lub." The increased pressure in the right ventricle opens the pulmonic semilunar valve, sending deoxygenated blood to the lungs. The increased pressure in the left ventricle opens the aortic semilunar valve, sending freshly oxygenated blood to the body. At the end of systole, as pressure in the ventricles falls, the pulmonic and aortic semilunar valves close tightly to prevent backflow. These vibrations generate the second heart sound—S_2, or the "dub." This cycle repeats approximately 60 to 100 times per minute in the healthy adult at rest. Extra sounds known as heart murmurs result when valves do not fully open or close, causing turbulent flow that an experienced clinician can detect.

You must auscultate for heart sounds at the proper places on the chest wall (Figure 2-43 ▶). Always listen downstream. For example, since the tricuspid and mitral valves direct blood flow to the ventricles, which are toward your patient's feet, listen for S_1 at the apex of the heart. This is found near the lower left sternal border. Since the aortic and pulmonic valves direct blood flow to the lungs and aorta, which are toward your patient's head, listen for S_2 at the base of the heart. This is found at the 2nd intercostal space near the sternum.

The heart is an electrical-mechanical pump. Its job is to begin the movement of blood through the circulatory system. Its effectiveness is measured by **cardiac output.** Cardiac output is the amount of blood the heart ejects each minute, measured in milliliters per minute. It is the product of the heart rate and the stroke volume. **Stroke volume** is the amount of blood the heart ejects in one beat. Changes in any of these components may severely affect cardiac output. For example, if your patient's heart rate falls to 30 beats per minute, or if a massive heart attack destroys 30 to 40 percent of his left ventricle, the cardiac output will greatly decrease.

Three factors determine stroke volume: preload, contractile force, and afterload. Preload, also known as end-diastolic pressure, is the amount of blood returned to the heart from the body. The greater the preload, the more the cardiac muscles will stretch, the harder they will contract, and the more blood the heart will eject. Contractile force refers to how forcefully the heart muscle contracts. It is regulated by the autonomic nervous system and the body's needs. Afterload refers to the resistance in the vessels that the heart must overcome to eject blood. It is determined mostly in the medium-sized arterioles.

With each contraction of your patient's heart, you should feel an arterial pulse. Blood pressure is a measurable estimate of the pressure in the circulatory system during systole and diastole. Arterial blood pressure is affected by the stroke volume (left ventricular effectiveness), the condition of the aorta and large arteries, the peripheral vascular resistance (condition of the arterioles), and the circulating blood volume. Changes in any of these components can severely affect your patient's blood pressure. For example, if your patient loses 30 to 40 percent of his blood volume or experiences massive vasodilation, his blood pressure will drop drastically.

Venous pressure, on the other hand, is much lower than arterial pressure. It will remain so unless something restricts blood flow through the heart. For example, in congestive heart failure, a weakened heart cannot effectively move all the blood it receives from the body or the lungs. The resulting backup eventually raises venous pressure. Cardiac tamponade and tension pneumothorax inhibit venous return, causing a dramatic rise in venous pressure. You can easily observe and measure increases in venous pressure in the external jugular veins.

Several changes occur with aging. Since most patients with cardiac complaints are older, an understanding of these changes is essential. Changes in chest wall diameter make it more difficult to find the apical pulse. Extra heart sounds are more common. Many older patients will have heart murmurs, especially affecting the aortic valve, which becomes stenotic over time. The aorta and large arteries stiffen from atherosclerosis, raising blood pressure. Older patients often develop mitral valve murmurs and regurgitation (backflow leakage into the left atrium during ventricular systole).

Begin your cardiovascular assessment by inspecting for signs of arterial insufficiency or occlusion in your patient's trunk and extremities. Look for skin pallor and other signs of decreased perfusion. Now assess the arterial pulses. Inspect the carotid arteries for visible pulsations just medial to the sternocleidomastoid muscles. Palpate the carotid arteries at the level of the cricoid cartilage to avoid pressing on the carotid sinus (Procedure 2–9a). Never palpate both carotids simultaneously; doing so may decrease cerebral blood flow. Assess the carotid pulse for rate, rhythm, and quality. Does its quality vary? Do the variations correspond to respiration? For example, in pulsus paradoxus, the amplitude of the pulse diminishes with inspiration and increases with exhalation. Do you feel a vibration or humming (**thrills**) when you palpate the carotid artery? If so, auscultate the area with your stethoscope for **bruits,** the sounds of turbulent blood flow around a partial obstruction (Procedure 2–9b).

thrill
vibration or humming felt when palpating the pulse.

bruit
sound of turbulent blood flow around a partial obstruction.

If you have not already taken your patient's blood pressure, do so now. Also check for jugular venous pressure, which approximates your patient's right atrial pressure. Position your patient supine, with his head elevated to about 30 degrees. Turning your patient's head away from the side you are assessing, identify the external jugular veins on both sides and locate the pulsations of the internal jugular veins. Look for the pulsation in the area around the suprasternal notch and where the sternocleidomastoid muscle inserts on the clavicle and manubrium.

Now identify the internal jugular vein's highest point of pulsation (the point where the pulse diminishes) and measure its vertical distance from the sternal angle (midline at the 2nd costal cartilage). To do this, place a ruler perpendicular to the chest at the sternal angle and position a straightedge at a right angle to the ruler (Procedure 2–9c). Lower the straightedge until it rests atop the jugular vein pulsation. The corresponding ruler mark is your measurement. Normal venous pressure is 1 to 2 cm. If you cannot visualize the pulsations, observe the point where the external jugular veins collapse and use the same measuring parameters.

Examine the external jugular veins for equality of distention. Abnormal bilateral distention indicates fluid volume overload or that something such as congestive heart failure or cardiac tamponade is blocking venous return to the heart. Unilateral distention suggests a localized problem.

With your patient's head still raised to about 30 degrees, inspect and palpate the chest for the point of maximal impulse (PMI), or apical impulse (Procedure 2–9d).

Assessing the Cardiovascular System

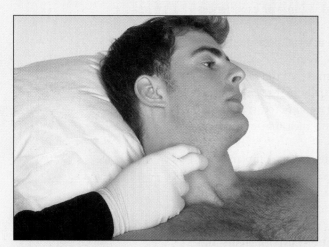

2-9a Assess the carotid pulse.

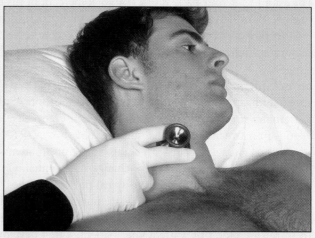

2-9b Auscultate for bruits.

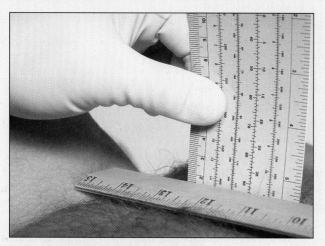

2-9c Measure jugular venous pressure.

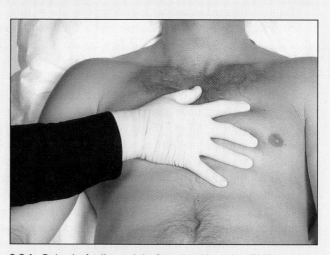

2-9d Palpate for the point of maximal impulse (PMI).

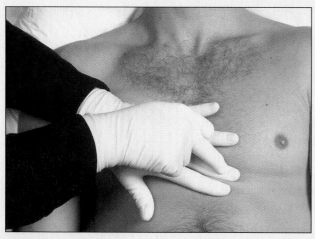

2-9e Percuss for the PMI.

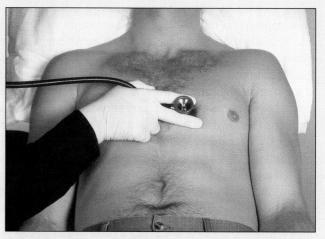

2-9f Auscultate for heart sounds.

When examining a woman with large breasts, gently displace the left breast upward and laterally, if needed, or ask her to do this for you. First, look for a pulsation at the cardiac apex, normally at the 5th intercostal space just medial to the midclavicular line. This pulsation represents the PMI. It helps you locate the left ventricle's apex.

If you cannot see the pulsation, ask your patient to exhale and stop breathing for a few seconds. Lateral displacement of the PMI indicates an enlarged right ventricle. The PMI may be displaced upward and to the left in pregnant women. If your patient is obese or has a very muscular chest wall or a barrel chest you may not detect the PMI. Percussion may help if you have difficulty palpating the PMI. Start lateral and work your way toward the midline (Procedure 2–9e). When you hear a change from resonance (lung) to dull (heart), you have located the PMI.

Using the diaphragm of your stethoscope, auscultate your patient's anterior chest for normal heart sounds and for abnormal or extra heart sounds (Procedure 2–9f). Listen for the high-pitched sounds of S_1 at the 5th intercostal space at the left sternal border (tricuspid valve) and at the PMI (mitral valve) using the diaphragm of your stethoscope. Listen for the high-pitched sounds of S_2 at the 2nd intercostal space at the right sternal border (aortic valve) and 2nd intercostal space at the left sternal border (pulmonic valve). For a comprehensive auscultation of heart sounds, you should also listen at the 3rd and 4th intercostal spaces. Although nothing is specifically behind those spaces, you may hear something there that you will not hear in the other places if the heart is not anatomically perfect.

Because the mitral and aortic valves (left side) close slightly before the tricuspid and pulmonic valves (right side), you may hear two sets of sounds instead of one. This is known as splitting. A split S_1 sounds like "la-lub," a split S_2 like "da-dub." Instead of "lub-dub" you will hear "la-lub—da-dub." Splitting of S_2 during inspiration is normal in healthy children and young adults. Expiratory or persistent splitting suggests an abnormality.

You also may hear extra or abnormal heart sounds, depending on your patient's age and condition. A third heart sound, S_3, is sometimes called the ventricular gallop. It is the "dee" of "lub-dub-dee" and has the same cadence as the word *Kentucky*. This extra heart sound develops from vibrations that result when blood fills a dilated ventricle. Commonly heard in children and young adults, an S_3 is usually considered pathological in patients over age 30. It generally develops with ventricular failure and ventricular volume overload and disappears when the problem is resolved. S_3 is a low-pitched sound heard in early to middiastole. Listen for S_3 at the apex using the bell of your stethoscope with your patient lying on his left side.

Atrial gallop is the fourth heart sound, S_4. It is the "dee" of "dee-lub-dub" and has the same cadence as the word *Tennessee*. An S_4 develops from vibrations produced in late diastole when atrial contraction forces blood into a ventricle that has decreased compliance or that resists filling and causes volume overload. It usually disappears when the problem is resolved. Listen for the low-pitched S_4 at the apex using the bell of your stethoscope with your patient lying on his left side.

Experienced cardiologists can also detect clicks, snaps, friction rubs, and murmurs. An ejection click results from a stiff or stuck valve. An opening snap results when a stenotic mitral or tricuspid valve's leaflets recoil abruptly after ventricular diastole. A pericardial friction rub occurs when inflammation causes the heart's visceral and parietal surfaces to rub together at each heartbeat. A murmur is a rumbling or vibrating noise that results from turbulent blood flow through the heart valves, a large artery, or a septal defect.

The Abdomen

The key to evaluating the abdomen is visualizing the organs in the region you are examining. The abdominal cavity is divided into four quadrants: the right upper (RUQ),

Figure 2-44 The abdominal quadrants.

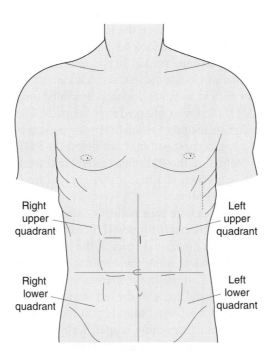

Right upper quadrant

Left upper quadrant

Right lower quadrant

Left lower quadrant

The key to evaluating the abdomen is visualizing the organs in the region you are examining.

right lower (RLQ), left upper (LUQ), and left lower (LLQ). Their dividing lines intersect at the umbilicus (Figure 2-44). Age changes in the abdomen include increased fat storage around the midsection and hips and weakened abdominal musculature. The result is the "beer belly" appearance. Decreased sensation may diminish the normal signs and symptoms of serious disease. The classic signs and symptoms of abdominal diseases are often missing in the elderly.

Abdominal Organs

Major organs of the digestive, urinary, reproductive, cardiovascular, and lymphatic systems lie in the abdomen. The peritoneum, a protective membrane, covers most of them.

Digestive   Food travels down the esophagus to the stomach (in the LUQ) (Figure 2-45). It then passes into the first section of the small intestine, the duodenum, where digestive enzymes from the pancreas (just behind the stomach) and gallbladder (just behind the liver in the RUQ) help digestion. Food then begins its journey through the remainder of the long small intestine (the jejunum and ileum), where the mesentery veins absorb nutrients from the food. Blood travels from the mesentery veins to the liver (RUQ) for processing and detoxification before it returns to the right heart. At the point where the small intestine turns into the large intestine lies the appendix (RLQ). The large intestine, or colon, has three distinct sections: the ascending colon (RLQ to RUQ), the transverse colon (RUQ to LUQ), and the descending colon (LUQ to LLQ). The large intestine is responsible for absorbing water from the feces and returning it to the general circulation. The remaining waste continues through the sigmoid colon (LLQ), rectum (midline), and anus.

Urinary   The kidneys are pear-shaped solid organs imbedded in fat in the retroperitoneal space (RUQ, LUQ) (Figure 2-46). They receive blood from the renal arteries, which branch off the abdominal aorta. The kidneys filter blood and excrete impurities, acids, and electrolytes from the blood before returning it to the general circulation. The waste product is called urine. Ureters bring the urine to the bladder, just behind the pubic bone in the midline. The urethra connects the urinary bladder to the outside.

Female Reproductive   The ovaries (RLQ, LLQ) are walnut-sized organs that manufacture and produce the ova for fertilization (Figure 2-47). The fallopian tubes transport the ova toward the uterus (midline just above the urinary bladder). Fertilization

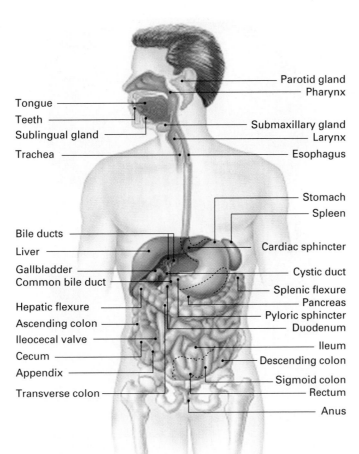

Tongue — Teeth — Sublingual gland — Trachea —

Parotid gland
Pharynx
Submaxillary gland
Larynx
Esophagus

Bile ducts —
Liver —
Gallbladder —
Common bile duct —
Hepatic flexure —
Ascending colon —
Ileocecal valve —
Cecum —
Appendix —
Transverse colon —

Stomach
Spleen
Cardiac sphincter
Cystic duct
Splenic flexure
Pancreas
Pyloric sphincter
Duodenum
Ileum
Descending colon
Sigmoid colon
Rectum
Anus

occurs in the tubes. The fertilized ovum travels and implants in the uterus. The cervix is the opening to the uterus. The vagina is the birth canal.

Male Reproductive The testes are located in the scrotal sac and produce reproductive sperm (Figure 2-48 ◗). The sperm collects in a small reservoir called the epididymis, which can become inflamed. During sex, the sperm travels via the vas deferens (RLQ, LLQ) through an opening in the inguinal ligament known as the inguinal canal. The testicular blood supply also runs through this opening, an anatomical weak point that is the site of male hernias. The vas deferens moves the sperm toward the prostate gland, where it mixes with seminal fluid and is ejected via the penile urethra.

Cardiovascular The large abdominal aorta delivers blood from the heart to all organs of the abdominal cavity (Figure 2-49 ◗). Palpate the aorta just to the left of the umbilicus. The inferior vena cava delivers blood that is deoxygenated and high in carbon dioxide from the abdominal organs and lower extremities to the heart. The mesentery arteries and veins and portal circulation systems deliver blood to and from the intestines and back to the heart for general distribution.

Lymphatic The spleen (LUQ) is the major organ of the lymph system. The vast network of lymph vessels helps drain excessive fluid and return it to the heart and aids the immune and infection control systems.

Abdominal Examination

To examine the abdomen, you need good lighting, a relaxed patient, and exposure from above the xiphoid process to the symphysis pubis. Make sure your patient does

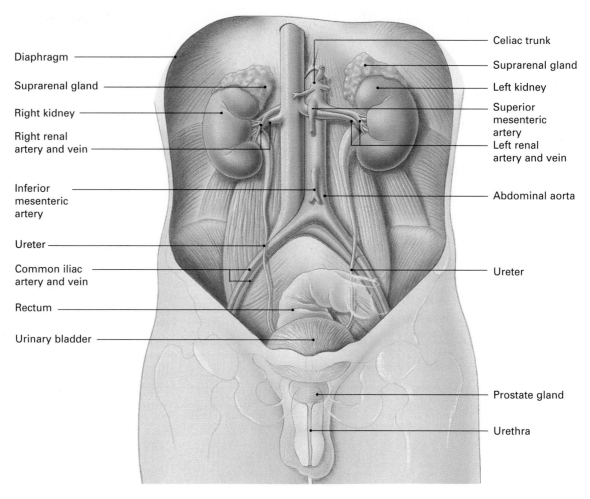

Diaphragm

Suprarenal gland

Right kidney

Right renal
artery and vein

Inferior
mesenteric
artery

Ureter

Common iliac
artery and vein

Rectum

Urinary bladder

Celiac trunk

Suprarenal gland

Left kidney

Superior
mesenteric
artery

Left renal
artery and vein

Abdominal aorta

Ureter

Prostate gland

Urethra

▶ **Figure 2-46** The urinary system.

not have a full bladder. Make him comfortable in the supine position with one pillow under the head and another under the knees. Have him place his hands at his sides. This helps relax his abdominal muscles, making the examination easier for you and more comfortable for him.

▶ **Figure 2-47** The female reproductive system.

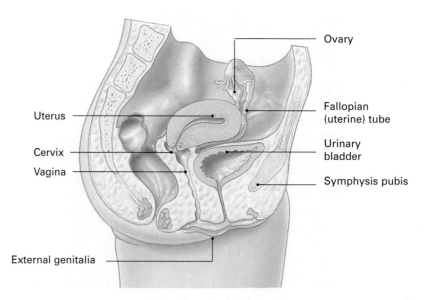

Ovary

Fallopian
(uterine) tube

Urinary
bladder

Symphysis pubis

Uterus

Cervix

Vagina

External genitalia

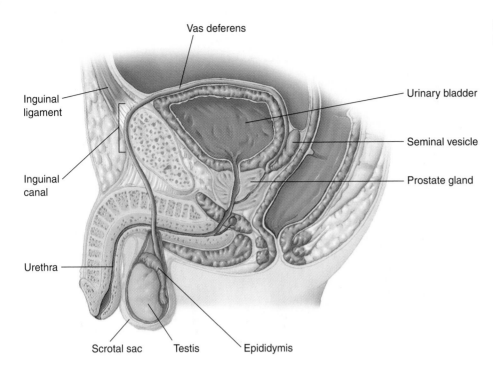

Vas deferens

Inguinal ligament

Inguinal canal

Urethra

Scrotal sac   Testis   Epididymis

Urinary bladder

Seminal vesicle

Prostate gland

Ask your patient to point out any areas of pain or tenderness. Examine these areas last. Use warm hands and a warm stethoscope and keep your fingernails short. If your hands are cold, palpate your patient through his clothes until your hands warm up. Begin your exam slowly and avoid any quick, unexpected movements. Monitor your patient's facial expressions for pain and discomfort. During the exam, distract him with conversation or questions. Use inspection, auscultation, percussion, and palpation to perform the exam. Always auscultate before percussing or palpating, because these manipulations may alter your patient's bowel motility and resulting bowel sounds.

When you examine the abdomen, you will assess the gastrointestinal organs and other nearby organs and structures. Inspect the skin of the abdomen and flanks for scars, dilated veins, stretch marks, rashes, lesions, and pigmentation changes. Look for discoloration over the umbilicus (**Cullen's sign**) or over the flanks (**Grey Turner's sign**); these are late signs suggesting intra-abdominal bleeding. Assess the size and shape of your patient's abdomen to determine whether it is scaphoid (concave), flat, round, or distended. Ask the patient if it is its usual size and shape. Note its symmetry. Check for bulges, hernias, or distended flanks. **Ascites** appears as bulges in the flanks and across the abdomen and indicates edema caused by congestive heart failure. A distended bladder or pregnant uterus can cause a suprapubic bulge. Bulges in the inguinal or femoral areas suggest a hernia.

Now look at your patient's umbilicus. Note its location and contour and observe for any signs of herniation or inflammation. Check for any visible pulsation, peristalsis (the wavelike motion of organs moving their contents through the digestive tract), or masses. You may see the normal pulsation of the aorta just lateral to the umbilicus. If you notice a bounding or exaggerated pulsation, suspect an aortic aneurysm. Visible peristalsis may indicate a bowel obstruction.

Next auscultate for bowel sounds and other sounds such as bruits throughout the abdomen. To auscultate for bowel sounds, first warm your stethoscope's diaphragm in your hand, because a cold diaphragm might cause abdominal tension. Gently place the diaphragm on your patient's abdomen and proceed systematically,

Cullen's sign
discoloration around the umbilicus (occasionally the flanks) suggestive of intra-abdominal hemorrhage.

Grey Turner's sign
discoloration over the flanks suggesting intra-abdominal bleeding.

ascites
bulges in the flanks and across the abdomen, indicating edema caused by congestive heart failure.

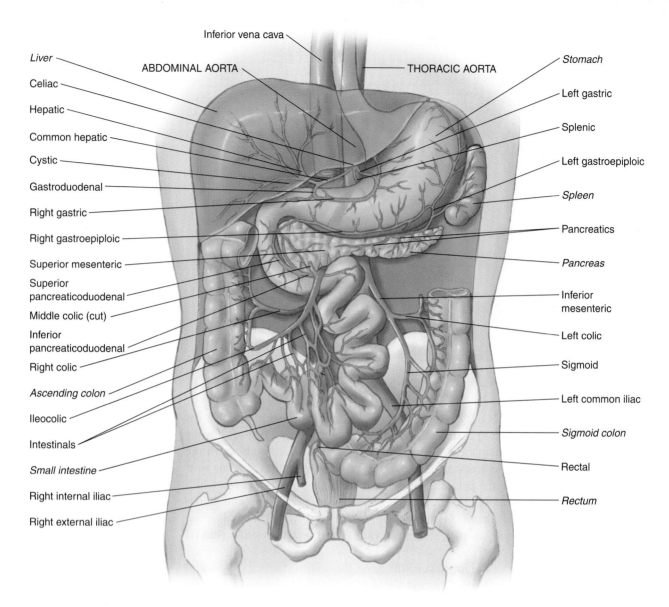

Inferior vena cava

Liver

ABDOMINAL AORTA

THORACIC AORTA

Stomach

Celiac

Left gastric

Hepatic

Splenic

Common hepatic

Left gastroepiploic

Cystic

Spleen

Gastroduodenal

Right gastric

Pancreatics

Right gastroepiploic

Pancreas

Superior mesenteric

Superior pancreaticoduodenal

Inferior mesenteric

Middle colic (cut)

Left colic

Inferior pancreaticoduodenal

Sigmoid

Right colic

Left common iliac

Ascending colon

Sigmoid colon

Ileocolic

Intestinals

Rectal

Small intestine

Right internal iliac

Rectum

Right external iliac

▶ **Figure 2-49** The abdominal arteries.

Assessment Pearls

Examining the Ticklish Patient   Some of your patients will be, frankly, ticklish. Tickling is a tingling, tactile sensation, considered both pleasant and unpleasant, which results in laughter, smiling, and involuntary twitching movements of the head, limbs, and torso. This reaction is probably a remnant of the mammalian scratch-touch reflex. (Ever scratched a dog's stomach and watched as it rhythmically moved a leg?)

Most patients are ticklish when it comes to their abdomen. To help in the assessment of a ticklish patient, have him put his hand on his abdomen and place your hand on top of his. (A person can't tickle himself.) Continue your physical exam, as best you can, using the patient's hand as a buffer. Eventually, the patient will relax and allow you to use your own hand for the exam without a ticklish response. You can then complete a comprehensive examination.

listening for bowel sounds in each quadrant. Note their location, frequency, and character.

Normal bowel sounds consist of a variety of high-pitched gurgles and clicks that occur every 5 to 15 seconds. More frequent sounds indicate increased bowel motility in conditions such as diarrhea or an early intestinal obstruction. Occasionally you may hear loud, prolonged, gurgling sounds known as **borborygmi.** These indicate hyperperistalsis. Decreased or absent sounds suggest a paralytic ileus or peritonitis. Listen at least 2 minutes for bowel sounds if the abdomen is silent. Bruits are swishing sounds that indicate turbulent blood flow. To confirm bruits, use the bell of your stethoscope and listen in areas over abdominal blood vessels such as the aorta and renal arteries (Procedure 2–10a). If you hear a bruit, suspect an arterial disorder such as an abdominal aortic aneurysm or renal artery stenosis.

borborygmi
loud, prolonged, gurgling bowel sounds indicating hyperperistalsis.

Percussing the abdomen produces different sounds based on the underlying tissues. These sounds help you detect excessive gas and solid or fluid-filled masses. They also help you determine the size and position of solid organs such as the liver and spleen. Percuss the abdomen in the same sequence you used for auscultation. Note the distribution of tympany and dullness. Expect to hear tympany in most of the abdomen; expect dullness over the solid abdominal organs such as the liver and spleen.

Palpate the abdomen last to detect tenderness, muscular rigidity, and superficial organs and masses. Before you begin palpation, ask your patient if he has any pain or tenderness. If he does, ask him to point to the area with one finger. Palpate that area last, using gentle pressure with a single finger. Ask him to cough and tell you if and where he experiences any pain. If coughing causes pain, suspect peritoneal inflammation.

Now ask your patient to take slow, deep breaths with his mouth open, and have him flex his knees to relax his abdominal muscles. Perform light palpation by moving your hand slowly and just lifting it off the skin (Procedure 2–10b). Palpate all areas in the same sequence you used for auscultation and percussion. Watch your patient's face for signs of discomfort. Identify any masses and note their size, location, contour, tenderness, pulsations, and mobility. Abdominal pain upon light palpation suggests peritoneal irritation or inflammation. If you feel rigidity or guarding while palpating, determine whether it is voluntary (patient anticipates the pain or is not relaxed) or involuntary (peritoneal inflammation).

Next palpate the abdomen deeply to detect large masses or tenderness. Use one hand on top of another and push down slowly (Procedure 2–10c). Assess for rebound tenderness by pushing down slowly and then releasing your hand quickly off the tender area. If the peritoneum is inflamed, your patient will experience pain when you let go. Alternatively, hold your hand 1 centimeter above your patient's abdomen at rest. Then ask him to push his abdomen out to touch your hand. Limitation by pain suggests peritoneal irritation.

If you note a protruding abdomen with bulging flanks and dull percussion sounds in dependent areas, you might perform two tests for ascites. First assess for areas of tympany and dullness while your patient is supine. Then ask him to lie on one side. Percuss again, noting once more any areas of tympany and dullness. If your patient has ascites, the area of dullness will shift down to the dependent side and the area of tympany will shift up. To test for fluid wave, ask an assistant to press the edge of his hand firmly down the midline of your patient's abdomen (Procedure 2–10d). With your fingertips, tap one flank and feel for the impulse's transmission to the other flank through excess fluid. If you detect the impulse easily, suspect ascites.

The Female Genitalia

The external female genitalia consist of highly vascular tissues that protect the entrance to the birth canal (Figure 2-50). The mons pubis is the hair-covered fat pad

Examining the Abdomen

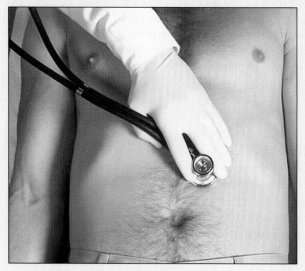

2-10a Auscultate for renal bruits.

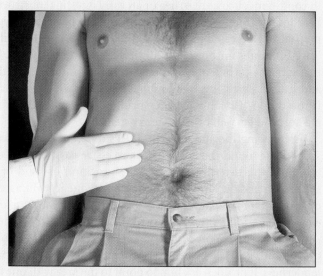

2-10b Light abdominal palpation.

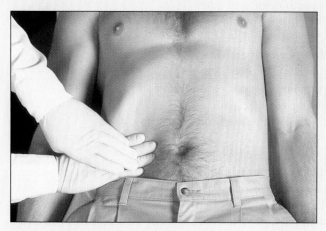

2-10c Deep abdominal palpation.

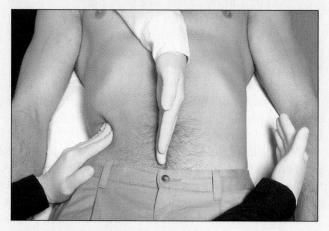

2-10d Test for ascites.

that covers the pubic symphysis. The labia majora and labia minora are rounded folds of tissue that protect the opening to the vagina. Extensions of the labia form the prepuce and clitoris. The vagina is the receptacle for the penis during sexual intercourse. The urethral opening lies between the clitoris and the vagina. The perineum refers to the tissue between the vagina and the anus.

The external genital organs begin to mature and take adult proportions during adolescence. Puberty also marks the appearance of breast buds, pubic hair, and the first period (menarche). The age in which sexual development occurs varies among individuals. As women grow older, ovarian function diminishes, menstrual periods cease, and pubic hair becomes gray and sparse. The labia and clitoris become smaller; the vagina narrows and shortens and its lining (the mucosa) becomes thin, pale, and dry. The ovaries and uterus decrease in size.

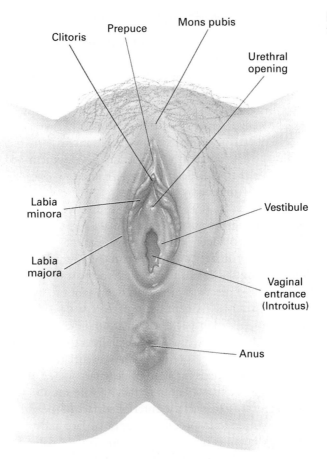

Figure 2-50 The external female genitalia.

Clitoris

Prepuce

Mons pubis

Urethral opening

Labia minora

Labia majora

Vestibule

Vaginal entrance (Introitus)

Anus

Except in cases of trauma or abuse, you rarely would be expected to examine the female genitalia. Before examining the external female genitalia, make sure that the room is warm and quiet and that your patient's bladder is empty. Be sure to maintain privacy during this examination. To reduce any anxiety or embarrassment your patient may feel, explain what you are doing during the exam. Expose her body areas only as necessary, be sensitive to her feelings, and project a professional demeanor. Place a pillow under her head and shoulders to help relax her abdominal muscles.

Begin your assessment by inspecting your patient's external genitalia. Look at the mons pubis, labia, and perineum for abnormalities such as inflammation, swelling, or lesions. These abnormalities may signal a sebaceous cyst or a sexually transmitted disease such as syphilis or herpes simplex virus infection. Check the bases of the pubic hair for signs of lice such as excoriation, or small, itchy, red maculopapules.

Now retract the outer labia and inspect the inner labia and urethral meatus (opening). Assess for vaginal discharge. The normal discharge is clear or cloudy and has little or no odor. A white, curd-like discharge with no odor or a yeasty, sweet odor may suggest a fungal infection (candidiasis). A yellow, green, or gray discharge with a foul or fishy odor may suggest a bacterial infection (gonorrhea or *Gardnerella*). Examining the external female genitalia can be an embarrassing, uncomfortable experience, especially for male clinicians. Remember it is probably twice as awkward for your patient. It is customary for male clinicians to have a female partner present during the examination.

The Male Genitalia

The external male genitalia consist of the penis and scrotum. The penis is the male organ for copulation. It houses the urethra and specialized erectile tissue (Figure 2-51 ▶). The scrotum contains the testes. The glans, a conical structure at the end of the penis, is covered by a fold of skin called the foreskin, or prepuce. The foreskin may have been surgically removed by circumcision.

The genital organs begin to mature and take adult proportions during adolescence. Puberty also marks a noticeable increase in the size of the testes. As in the female, the actual age in which sexual development occurs will vary widely. As men grow older, the penis decreases in size and the testes hang lower in the scrotum. The pubic hair becomes gray and sparse.

Except for trauma, you rarely would be expected to inspect the male genitalia. Before examining the male genitalia, make sure that the room is warm and quiet and that your patient's bladder is empty. Be sure to maintain privacy during this examination. To reduce any anxiety or embarrassment your patient may feel, explain what you are doing during the exam. Expose his body areas only as necessary, be sensitive to his feelings, and project a professional demeanor.

Begin your assessment by inspecting your patient's penis and scrotum. Note any inflammation, and inspect the skin around the base of the penis for abnormalities such as lesions that may be caused by sexually transmitted diseases. Also check the bases of the pubic hair for signs of lice such as excoriation or small, itchy, red maculopapules. Next inspect the glans for signs of degeneration or other abnormalities. If the foreskin is present, ask your patient to retract it. Note any abnormalities and the location of the urethral meatus. Inspect the anterior surface of the scrotum and note its contour. Then lift the scrotum to inspect its posterior surface and note any swelling or lumps. Expect acute epididymitis or testicular torsion if your patient has scrotal swelling and lower abdominal pain. Testicular torsion requires immediate intervention.

priapism

a painful and prolonged erection of the penis.

Priapism is a painful and prolonged erection of the penis. In the trauma patient it may indicate cervical spine injury with autonomic nervous system dysfunction. Nontraumatic causes are many and include sickle cell disease and other blood disorders

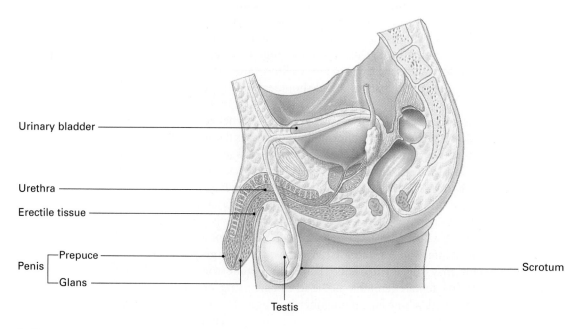

Urinary bladder

Urethra

Erectile tissue

Penis — Prepuce

Glans

Testis

Scrotum

▶ **Figure 2-51** Male reproductive anatomy.

Assessment Pearls

Always Check the Testicles in Males with Abdominal Pain Many cases of male abdominal pain are actually due to problems in the testicles—especially in children. During development, the testicles are in the abdomen and (usually) descend into the scrotum before birth. Thus, pain from the testicles can often be interpreted as abdominal pain because of the innervation of the testicles.

Testicular torsion (twisting of the testicle on the spermatic cord) is the most common pediatric genitourinary emergency. The testicles hang freely in the scrotum and, in certain situations, can twist. (The right testicle usually twists counterclockwise and the left usually twists clockwise.) When this occurs, blood flow to the testicle is cut off, causing pain. The torsed testicle is usually swollen, very tender to touch, and rides higher in the scrotum. Often, associated vomiting is present. If surgery is not provided to relieve the torsion within 6 hours, the testicle may be lost.

---

as well as drug overdose including erectile dysfunction medications such as vardenafil (Levitra). Priapism is a medical emergency requiring prompt intervention by a urologist.

Assess any discharge from the urethral meatus. Normally no discharge is present. A profuse, yellow discharge may be a sign of gonorrhea. A scant, clear or white discharge may suggest a nongonococcal urethritis. Examining the male genitalia can be an embarrassing, uncomfortable experience, especially for female clinicians. Remember it is probably twice as awkward for your patient. It is customary for female clinicians to have a male partner present during the examination.

The Anus

The rectum and anus mark the most distal end of the gastrointestinal system (Figure 2-52 ▶). The anal canal is approximately 2.5 to 4.0 cm long and is kept closed by the internal and external anorectal sphincters. The internal ring has smooth muscle that the autonomic nervous system controls. When the rectum fills with feces the internal sphincter relaxes, resulting in the urge to defecate. Because the external sphincter has striated muscle, defecation is under voluntary control. The lower half of the anal canal contains sensory fibers, whereas the upper half is somewhat insensitive.

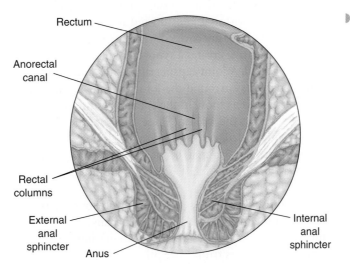

▶ **Figure 2-52** The anus.

Labels: Rectum, Anorectal canal, Rectal columns, External anal sphincter, Anus, Internal anal sphincter

Hence, many problems of the lower anus cause pain, while those in the upper region do not. The lower anus is also rich in venous circulation, promoting internal and external hemorrhoids.

Examining the anus is normally not a prehospital assessment practice. Unless your patient presents with rectal bleeding, there will be no reason for you to examine this area. Because routine internal rectal and prostate examinations are beyond the scope of this course, this section will focus on the external anal exam. As always, your aim is gentleness, a calm demeanor, and talking to your patient about what you are doing.

Before examining the anus, make sure the room is warm and quiet. Be sure to maintain privacy during this examination. To reduce any anxiety or embarrassment your patient may feel, explain what you are doing during the exam. Drape your patient appropriately and expose his body areas only as necessary; be sensitive to his feelings and project a professional demeanor. Place your patient on his left side with his legs flexed and his buttocks near the edge of the examination table. Glove your hands and spread the buttocks apart. Inspect the sacrococcygeal and perianal areas for lumps, ulcers, inflammations, rashes, or excoriation. Palpate any abnormal areas carefully and note any tenderness or inflammation. If appropriate, obtain a fecal sample and test it for occult blood. Simply smear a small sample onto a special test slide and add a couple of drops of developer onto the sample. If it turns blue, there is blood in the stool.

The Musculoskeletal System

The musculoskeletal system consists of at least 206 bones and their associated muscles, tendons, ligaments, and cartilage. Its main functions are to give form to the body and to allow for movement. Skeletal muscle is attached to bone by a tendon (Figure 2-53 ▶). The proximal attachment is the origin, while the distal attachment is the insertion. When a muscle contracts, the distal attachment usually moves toward the origin. Movement of one bone upon another occurs at a joint. In an elaborate system, the muscles and tendons act like ropes, the bones like levers, and the joints like fulcrums to make movement possible.

Each joint's structure, along with the number and size of the surrounding ligaments, determines its range of motion. Hinge joints such as the fingers and elbows allow only flexion and extension (Figure 2-54 ▶). Ball-and-socket joints such as the shoulder and hip allow rotation and a wide range of motion. Saddle joints like those in the thumbs permit movement in several planes. Condyloid joints such as the wrist are similar to ball-and-socket joints but do not allow rotation. Gliding joints such as those in the hands and feet permit a movement in which one bone slides across another. Pivot joints, as in the first two cervical vertebrae, allow a turning motion.

The bones within a joint do not touch each other (Figure 2-55 ▶). Instead, their articulating surfaces are covered with cartilage. A synovial membrane at the outer margins of the cartilage creates a synovial cavity into which it secretes synovium, a viscous lubricating fluid. A joint capsule surrounds and protects the synovial capsule. In turn, strong ligaments surround the joint capsule and extend to the articulating bones. In some joints such as those in the spinal column, cartilaginous disks instead of synovial cavities separate the bones. These disks cushion the vertebrae and absorb shocks. Bursae—fluid-filled, disk-shaped sacs—lie between the skin and the convex surface of a bone where friction may occur. They appear where tendons or muscles might rub against a bone or ligament or another muscle or tendon, such as in the knee and shoulder.

The musculoskeletal system's most obvious physical change with age is the gradual shortening in height. This occurs because the intervertebral disks become thinner and even collapse. As a result, your patient's limbs may appear longer than they should in proportion to his trunk. The other visible change is in posture. The anteroposterior

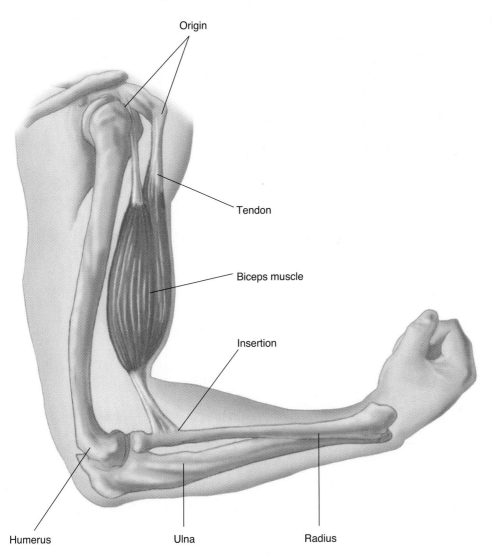

Figure 2-53 Interaction of bone, muscle, and tendon.

Origin

Tendon

Biceps muscle

Insertion

Humerus

Ulna

Radius

diameter of the chest increases due to kyphosis (abnormal curvature of the spine), particularly in women. Also, skeletal muscles decrease in size and strength, and the ligaments lose some of their pliability. As a result, the range of motion decreases. Osteoporosis also contributes to this loss of mobility.

An examination of the musculoskeletal system must include a detailed assessment of function and structure. Inspect and palpate your patient's joints, their structure, their range of motion, and the surrounding tissues. Begin your assessment with a general observation of posture, build, and muscular development. Watch how your patient's body parts move, and observe their resting positions. Begin the exam with your patient sitting to evaluate his head, neck, shoulders, and upper extremities. Then have him stand to assess his chest, back, and ilium; ask him to walk so that you can assess his gait. Finally, ask him to lie down so you can examine his hips, knees, ankles, and feet.

Inspect for swelling in or around joints, changes in the surrounding tissue, redness of the overlying skin, deformities, and symmetry of impairment. Swelling may be caused by trauma to the area or by excess synovial fluid in the joint space or tissues surrounding the joint. Tissue changes may include muscle atrophy, skin changes, and subcutaneous nodules resulting from rheumatoid arthritis or rheumatic fever. Skin redness may suggest inflammation or arthritis. Deformities may be produced by

An examination of the musculoskeletal system must include a detailed assessment of function and structure.

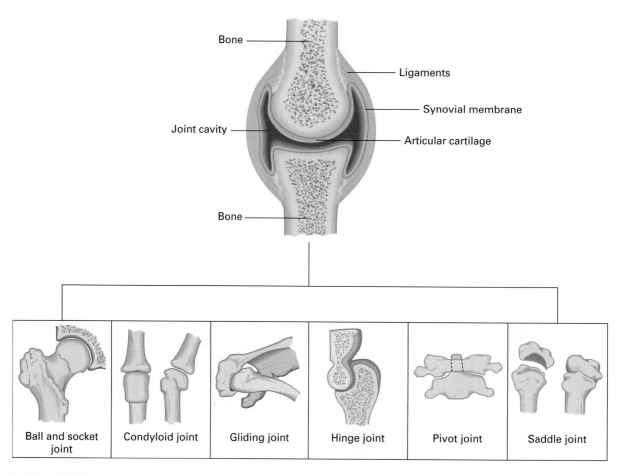

Figure 2-54 Types of joints.

Ball and socket joint | Condyloid joint | Gliding joint | Hinge joint | Pivot joint | Saddle joint

Figure 2-55 A synovial joint.

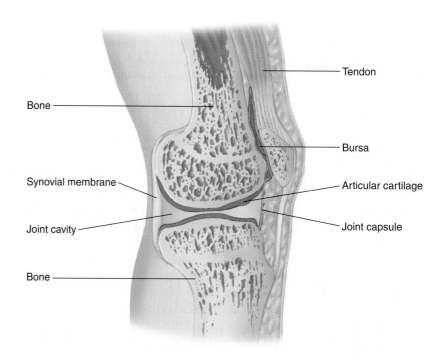

restricted range of motion, misalignment of the articulating bones, dislocation (complete separation of bone ends), or subluxation (partial dislocation). Symmetrical impairment is usually associated with a disorder such as rheumatoid arthritis.

Inspect and palpate each body part, then test its range of motion and muscle strength as explained in the Motor System section later in this chapter. Examine each joint and compare joints on opposite sides for equal size, shape, color, and strength. Swelling in a joint usually involves the synovial membrane or a bursa, which will feel spongy on deep palpation within the joint space. It also may involve the surrounding structures such as ligaments, cartilage, tendons, or the bones themselves. Redness of the overlying skin suggests a nontraumatic joint inflammation such as arthritis, gout, or rheumatic fever. Palpate for tenderness in and around the joint. Try to identify the specific structure that is tender, such as a ligament or tendon. Some common causes of a tender joint include arthritis, tendonitis, bursitis, or osteomyelitis. With the back of your hand, feel over the tender area for increased temperature, which suggests arthritis.

After you have inspected and palpated each body part with your patient at rest, assess range of motion. Test each joint for passive range of motion, range of motion against gravity, and range of motion against resistance. First test the joint's passive range of motion by moving it in the directions that it normally allows. For example, test the elbow, a hinge joint, for flexion and extension. Note any resistance and whether the range of motion is within normal limits. Now test range of motion against gravity by asking your patient to perform the same movements by himself. Again, note the range of motion and any difficulties. Finally, test range of motion against resistance. Have your patient perform the same movements while you apply resistance.

Passive and active range should be equal. A discrepancy indicates either a muscle weakness or a joint problem. If your patient has difficulty with passive and active tests, suspect a joint problem. If he has difficulty only with active tests, suspect a weakened muscle or nerve disorder. A decreased range of motion could indicate arthritis or injury, whereas an increased range of motion suggests a loosening of the structures that support the joint.

Listen for **crepitus,** the crunching sounds of unlubricated parts rubbing against each other, while you manipulate the joint. Crepitus may indicate an inflamed joint or osteoarthritis. An obvious traumatic deformity could indicate a sprained ligament, a bone fracture, or a dislocation. In these cases, modify your manipulation and range-of-motion exam accordingly. Nontraumatic deformities are caused by arthritis or the misalignment of bones. Avoid manipulating a painful joint.

The Extremities

The extremities are the arms and legs. A complete examination of your patient's extremities will include wrists and hands, elbows, shoulders, ankles and feet, knees, and hips.

Wrists and Hands   The radius and ulna articulate with the carpal bones at the wrist, or radiocarpal joint (Figure 2-56). The carpals articulate with the metacarpals. The metacarpals articulate with the proximal phalanges at the metacarpophalangeal (MCP) joint. The proximal phalanges articulate with the middle phalanges at the proximal interphalangeal (PIP) joint. The middle phalanges articulate with the distal phalanges at the distal interphalangeal (DIP) joint. Movement at the wrist includes flexion, extension, radial deviation, and ulnar deviation. Movement at the MCP, PIP, and DIP joints includes flexion and extension. The MCP joints also allow abduction (spreading the fingers out) and adduction (bringing them back together). The major flexor muscles are the flexor carpi radialis and flexor carpi ulnaris (Figure 2-57). The major extensor muscles are the extensor carpi radialis longus, extensor carpi radialis brevis, and extensor carpi ulnaris.

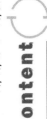

Review

Steps in Evaluating Joints

1. Inspection
2. Palpation
3. Passive range of motion
4. Range of motion against gravity
5. Range of motion against resistance

crepitus
crunching sounds of unlubricated parts in joints rubbing against each other.

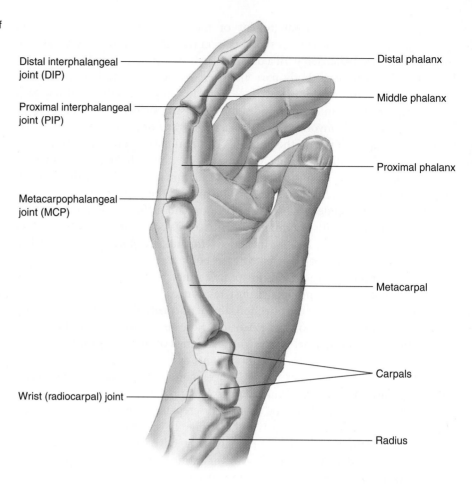

Figure 2-56 Bones and joints of the hand and wrist.

Distal interphalangeal joint (DIP)

Proximal interphalangeal joint (PIP)

Metacarpophalangeal joint (MCP)

Wrist (radiocarpal) joint

Distal phalanx

Middle phalanx

Proximal phalanx

Metacarpal

Carpals

Radius

Begin by inspecting your patient's hands and wrists. Next palpate them by feeling the medial and lateral aspects of the DIP joints and then the PIP joints with your thumb and forefinger (Procedure 2–11a). Note any swelling, sponginess, bony enlargement, or tenderness. Then palpate the tops and bottoms of these joints in the same manner. Now ask your patient to flex his hand slightly so you can examine each MCP. Compress the MCP joints by squeezing the hand from side to side between your thumbs and fingers and note any swelling, tenderness, or sponginess (Procedure 2–11b). Finally, palpate each wrist joint with your thumbs and note any swelling, sponginess, or tenderness (Procedure 2–11c). If your patient has had swelling of both his wrists or finger joints for several weeks, suspect an inflammatory condition such as rheumatoid arthritis.

To assess range of motion, ask your patient to make a fist with each hand and then open his fist and extend and spread his fingers. He should be able to make a tight fist and spread his fingers smoothly and easily. Next ask him to flex and then extend his wrist. Normal flexion is 90°, extension 70° (Procedure 2–11d). Check for radial and ulnar deviation by asking your patient to flex his wrist and move his hands medially and laterally. Normal radial movement is 20°, ulnar movement 45° (Procedure 2–11e).

If your patient complains of hand pain and numbness, especially at night, suspect carpal tunnel syndrome, the painful inflammation of the median nerve. To detect additional signs of this disorder, hold your patient's wrists in acute flexion for 60 seconds (Procedure 2–11f). In carpal tunnel syndrome, he will develop numbness or tingling in the areas innervated by the median nerve—the palmar surface of his thumb, index,

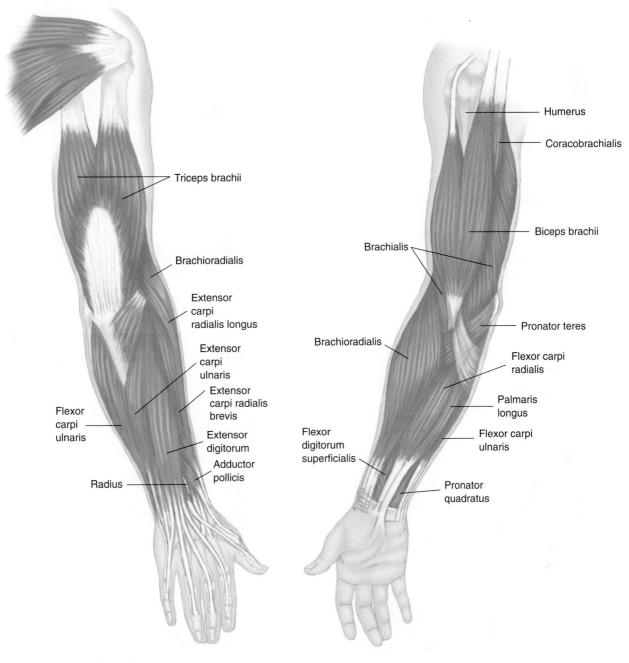

Labels on figure:

Triceps brachii

Brachioradialis

Extensor carpi radialis longus

Extensor carpi ulnaris

Extensor carpi radialis brevis

Flexor carpi ulnaris

Extensor digitorum

Adductor pollicis

Radius

Humerus

Coracobrachialis

Biceps brachii

Brachialis

Pronator teres

Brachioradialis

Flexor carpi radialis

Palmaris longus

Flexor carpi ulnaris

Flexor digitorum superficialis

Pronator quadratus

▶ **Figure 2-57** Muscles of the arm.

and middle fingers, and part of his ring finger. Throughout these maneuvers watch for deformities, redness, swelling, nodules, or muscular atrophy.

Elbows The lateral and medial epicondyles (large rounded edges) of the distal humerus, the olecranon process of the proximal ulna, and the proximal radius comprise the elbow joint (Figure 2-58 ▶). Between the olecranon process and skin lies a bursa. The ulnar nerve (funny bone) extends through the groove between the olecranon process and the medial epicondyle. The elbow is a hinge joint, allowing flexion and extension. The major flexor muscles are the biceps (Figure 2-59 ▶). The major extensor

Procedure 2-11   Examining the Wrist and Hand

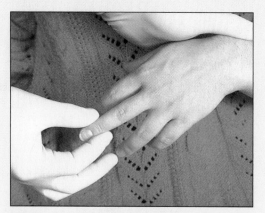

2-11a Palpate the DIP and PIP joints.

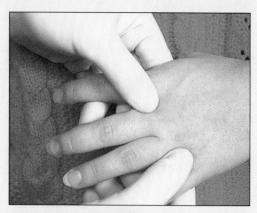

2-11b Palpate the MCP joints.

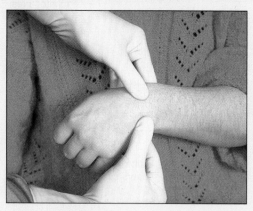

2-11c Palpate the wrist.

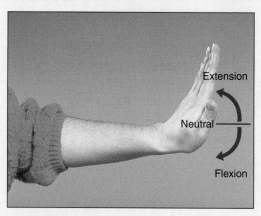

2-11d Assess wrist flexion and extension.

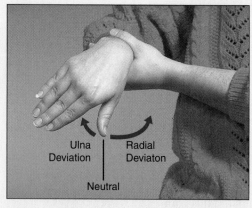

2-11e Assess radial and ulnar deviation.

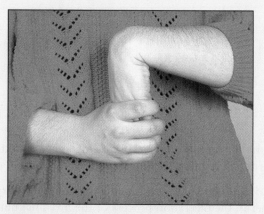

2-11f Test for carpal tunnel syndrome.

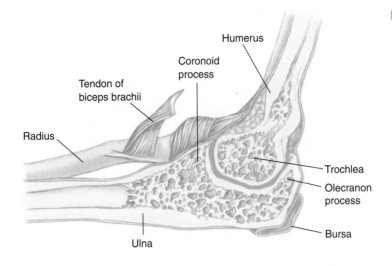

Humerus

Coronoid process

Tendon of biceps brachii

Radius

Trochlea

Olecranon process

Bursa

Ulna

▶ **Figure 2-59** Elbow flexors.

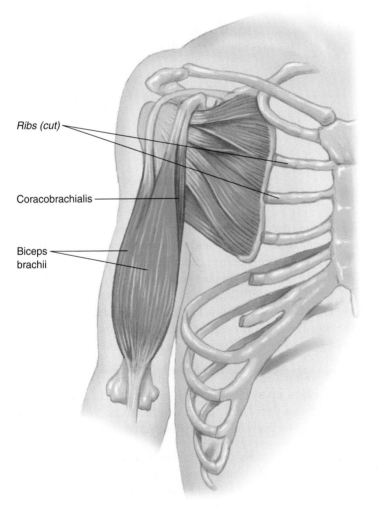

Ribs (cut)

Coracobrachialis

Biceps brachii

Anterior

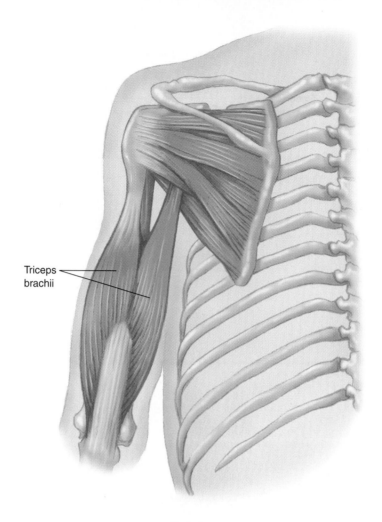

Triceps brachii

Posterior

muscles are the triceps (Figure 2-60 ▶). Just below the elbow, the relationship of the radius and ulna to the pronator and supinator muscles allows the forearm to supinate (turn palm up) and pronate (turn palm down) (Figure 2-61 ▶).

To examine the elbow, support your patient's forearm with your hand so that her elbow is flexed about 70° (Procedure 2–12a). Inspect the elbow joint and note any deformities, swelling, or nodules. Palpate the joint structures for tenderness, swelling, or thickening. Press on the medial and lateral epicondyles (Procedure 2–12b). Inflammation of either the medial epicondyle (tennis elbow) or of the lateral epicondyle (golfer's elbow) suggests tendonitis at those muscle insertion sites. To assess range of motion, ask your patient to flex and extend her elbow (Procedure 2–12c). Normally she will flex her elbow up to 160° and return it back to the neutral position. Then ask her to keep her elbows flexed and her arms at her sides. Now have her turn her palms up and then down. Normally both supination and pronation are 90° (Procedure 2–12d).

Shoulders   The shoulder girdle consists of articulations between the clavicle and the scapula and between the scapula and the head of the humerus (Figure 2-62 ▶). The sternoclavicular joint, which joins the clavicle and the manubrium, is the only bony link between the upper extremity and the axial skeleton. Movement at this joint is largely passive and occurs as a result of active movements of the scapula. The distal clavicle

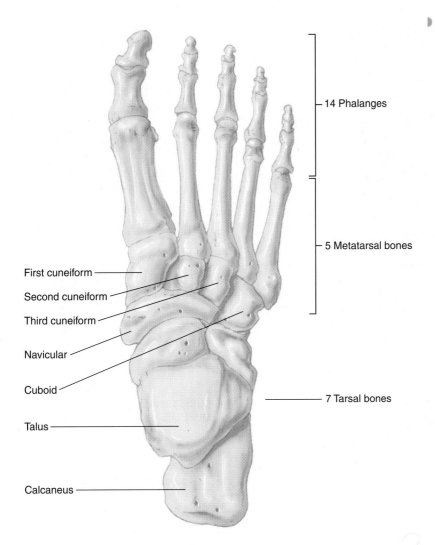

14 Phalanges

5 Metatarsal bones

First cuneiform

Second cuneiform

Third cuneiform

Navicular

Cuboid

7 Tarsal bones

Talus

Calcaneus

causing severe pain upon inversion and plantar flexion. In arthritis, pain and tenderness will accompany movement in any direction. Finally, flex and extend the toes (Procedure 2–14e). Expect a great range of motion in these joints, especially the big toes.

▶ **Figure 2-66** The foot and ankle.

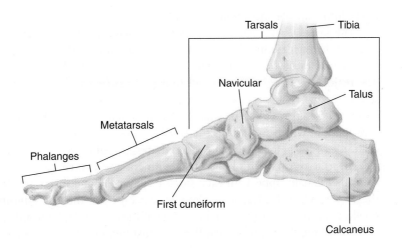

Tarsals

Tibia

Navicular

Talus

Metatarsals

Phalanges

First cuneiform

Calcaneus

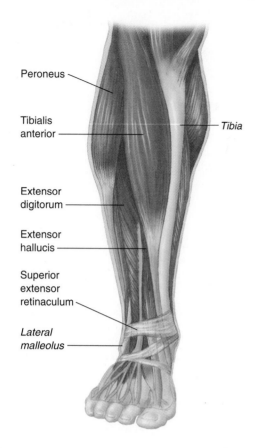

Peroneus

Tibialis
anterior

Tibia

Extensor
digitorum

Extensor
hallucis

Superior
extensor
retinaculum

*Lateral
malleolus*

▶ **Figure 2-67** The dorsiflexors.

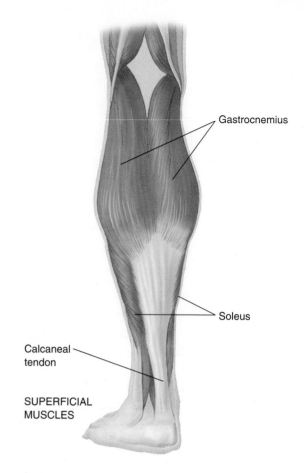

Gastrocnemius

Soleus

Calcaneal
tendon

SUPERFICIAL
MUSCLES

▶ **Figure 2-68** The plantar flexors.

Knees The knee joint involves the distal femur, the proximal tibia, and the patella (Figure 2-69 ▶). The distal femur and the proximal tibia meet at this joint and are cushioned by the lateral meniscus and the medial meniscus, which form a cartilaginous surface for pain-free movement. The joint capsule contains synovial fluid. Several ligaments surround the knee joint and help maintain its integrity. The medial and lateral collateral ligaments provide side-to-side stability and are easily palpable. The anterior and posterior cruciate ligaments, which give the knee front-to-back stability, lie deep within the joint capsule and are not palpable.

The knee is a modified hinge joint, allowing flexion and extension, with some rotation during flexion. The major flexors are a group of three muscles (biceps femoris, semimembranosus, and semitendinosus) known as the hamstrings (Figure 2-70 ▶). The major extensors are a group of four muscles (vastus lateralis, vastus intermedius, vastus medialis, and rectus femoris) known as the quadriceps (Figure 2-71 ▶). The femur can rotate on the tibia slightly. The patella lies deep in the middle of the quadriceps tendon, which inserts on the tibial tuberosity below the knee. Concave areas at each side of the patella and below it contain synovial fluid.

Inspect your patient's knees for alignment and deformities. Look for the concave areas that usually appear on each side of the patella and just above it. The absence of these concavities indicates swelling in the knee or the surrounding structures. If swelling is present, milk the medial aspect of the knee firmly upward two or three times to displace the fluid. Then press the knee just behind the lateral margin of the patella

Examining the Ankle and Foot

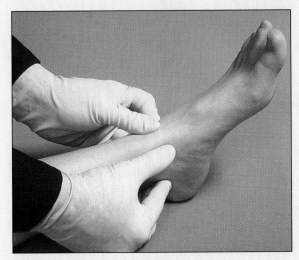

2-14a Palpate the ankle and foot.

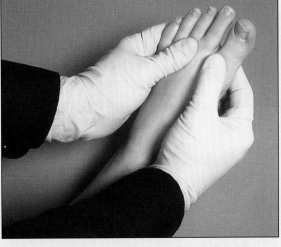

2-14b Palpate the metatarsal-phalangeal joints.

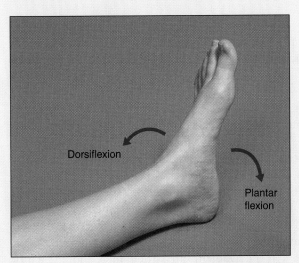

2-14c Assess dorsiflexion and plantar flexion.

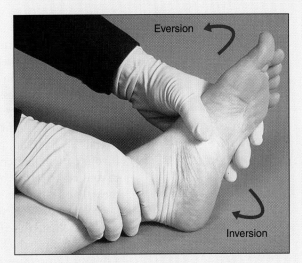

2-14d Assess inversion and eversion of the foot.

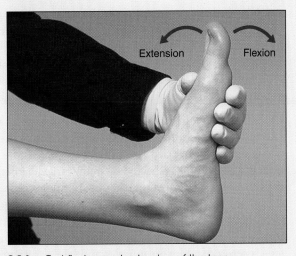

2-14e Test flexion and extension of the toes.

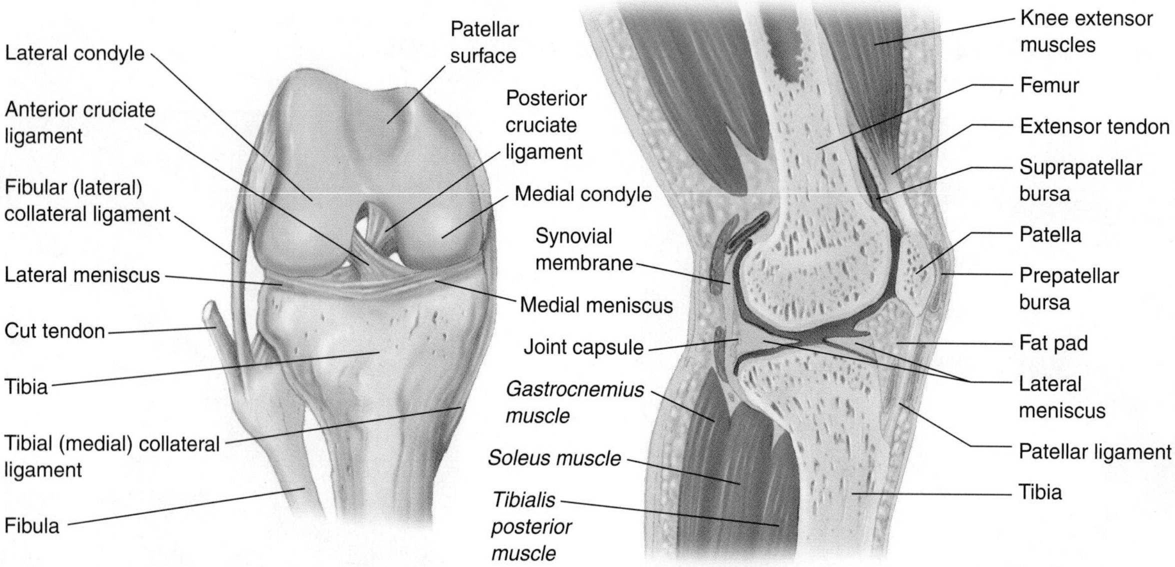

Lateral condyle
Anterior cruciate ligament
Fibular (lateral) collateral ligament
Lateral meniscus
Cut tendon
Tibia
Tibial (medial) collateral ligament
Fibula
Patellar surface
Posterior cruciate ligament
Medial condyle
Medial meniscus
Synovial membrane
Joint capsule
Gastrocnemius muscle
Soleus muscle
Tibialis posterior muscle
Knee extensor muscles
Femur
Extensor tendon
Suprapatellar bursa
Patella
Prepatellar bursa
Fat pad
Lateral meniscus
Patellar ligament
Tibia

Figure 2-69 The knee.

and watch for a return of fluid (a positive sign for effusion) (Procedure 2–15a). Feel for any thickening or swelling around the patella; these suggest synovial thickening or effusion. Compress the patella and move it against the femur (Procedure 2–15b). Note any pain or tenderness.

To test for range of motion, have your patient flex his knee to 90°. Press your thumbs into the joint and palpate along the tibial margins from the patellar tendon laterally. Palpate along the course of each ligament and note any points of tenderness. If your patient has tenderness, expect damage to the meniscus or to lateral ligaments. If you feel irregular bony ridges, suspect osteoarthritis. Now test for stability of the medial and collateral ligaments by moving the knee joint from side to side with the knee flexed to 30° (Procedure 2–15c). There should be little movement if the joint is stable. Evaluate the anterior and posterior cruciate ligaments by using the "drawer" test. Try to move the knee joint anterior and posterior, much like opening and closing a drawer (Procedure 2–15d). Again, if the ligaments are strong, there should be little movement.

Now have your patient sit at the edge of the exam table with his lower legs dangling. Ask him to extend his leg. Normal extension is 90° (Procedure 2–15e). Ask him to lie down on his stomach and try to touch his foot to his back. Normal flexion is 135°. With your patient standing, inspect the posterior surface of his legs, especially the popliteal region behind his knees. Note any deformity or abnormalities such as bowlegs, knock-knee, or flexion contracture, the inability to fully extend the knee.

Hips The hip joint involves the head of the proximal femur (ball) and the acetabulum (socket) of the ischium (Figure 2-72). Although the hip is a ball-and-socket joint like the shoulder, the two are very different. Whereas the shoulder has a wide range of motion, the hip joint is restricted by many large ligaments, a bony ridge in the pelvis, and capsular fibers. Hip flexion, the most important movement, occurs via the iliopsoas muscle group (Figure 2-73). Other movements, though much more limited in range than the shoulder, include extension, abduction, adduction, and internal and external rotation. A number of muscle groups control these movements. One of these is the gluteus, a series of adductor muscles and lateral rotators (Figure 2-74). Three bursae in

Figure 2-70 The knee flexors.

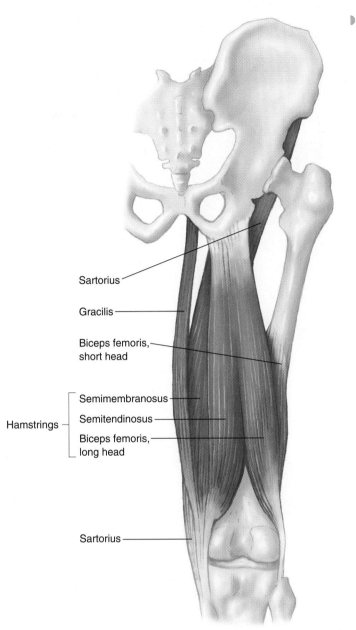

Sartorius

Gracilis

Biceps femoris,
short head

Hamstrings

Semimembranosus

Semitendinosus

Biceps femoris,
long head

Sartorius

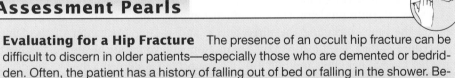

Assessment Pearls

Evaluating for a Hip Fracture   The presence of an occult hip fracture can be difficult to discern in older patients—especially those who are demented or bedridden. Often, the patient has a history of falling out of bed or falling in the shower. Because the patient is nonambulatory, it's difficult to determine whether a fracture exists. One trick is to auscultate for the fracture.

This test is performed by percussing the patella and simultaneously auscultating with the bell of a stethoscope over the symphysis pubis. The percussion note is then compared with the opposite (contralateral) side in a similar fashion. A positive test is one that results in diminished percussion note on the side where pain is felt. A negative test is defined as one in which no difference in percussion note is obtained. This test was first described in 1846 and remains valid. Diagnostic X-rays, of course, will still be needed.

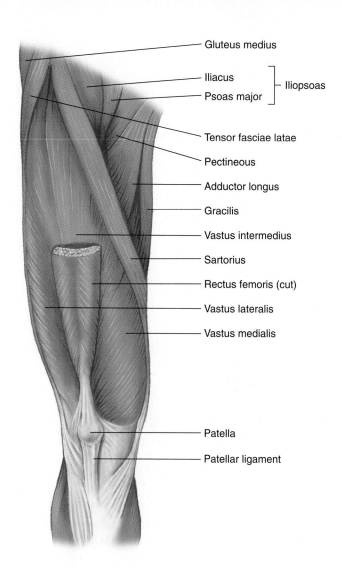

Figure 2-71 The knee extensors. (The vastus intermedius is behind the rectus femoris.)

Gluteus medius

Iliacus

Psoas major

Iliopsoas

Tensor fasciae latae

Pectineous

Adductor longus

Gracilis

Vastus intermedius

Sartorius

Rectus femoris (cut)

Vastus lateralis

Vastus medialis

Patella

Patellar ligament

the hip play an important role in pain-free movement. The iliopectineal bursa sits just anterior to the hip joint. The trochanteric bursa lies just to the side and behind the greater trochanter. The ischiogluteal bursa resides under the ischial tuberosity.

Inspect the hips for deformities, symmetry, and swelling. Palpate for tenderness all around the joint, including the three bursae and greater trochanter of the femur (Procedure 2–16a). Test the hip's range of motion with your patient supine. Ask her to raise her knee to her chest and pull it firmly against her abdomen. Observe the degree of flexion at the knee and hip (normally 120°) (Procedure 2–16b). Now flex the hip at 90° and stabilize the thigh with one hand while you grasp the ankle with the other. Swing the lower leg medially to evaluate external rotation and laterally to evaluate internal rotation (Procedure 2–16c). Normal external rotation is 40°, normal internal rotation 45°. Arthritis restricts internal rotation. To test for hip abduction, have your patient extend her legs. Then while you stabilize the anterior superior iliac spine with one hand, abduct the other leg until you feel the iliac spine move. This marks the degree of hip abduction, which is normally 45° (Procedure 2–16d). If your patient complains of hip pain or if range of motion is limited, palpate the three bursae for swelling (bursitis) and tenderness.

Examining the Knee

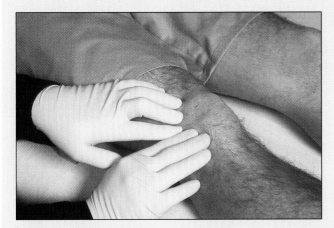

2-15a Palpate the knee.

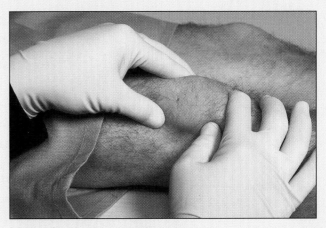

2-15b Palpate the patella.

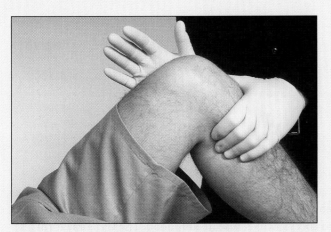

2-15c Test the collateral ligaments of the knee.

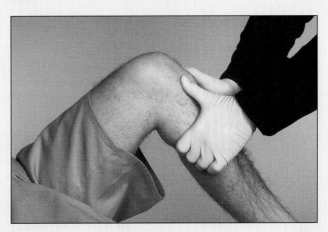

2-15d Test the cruciate ligaments of the knee.

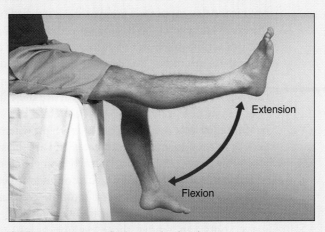

Extension

Flexion

2-15e Assess knee flexion and extension.

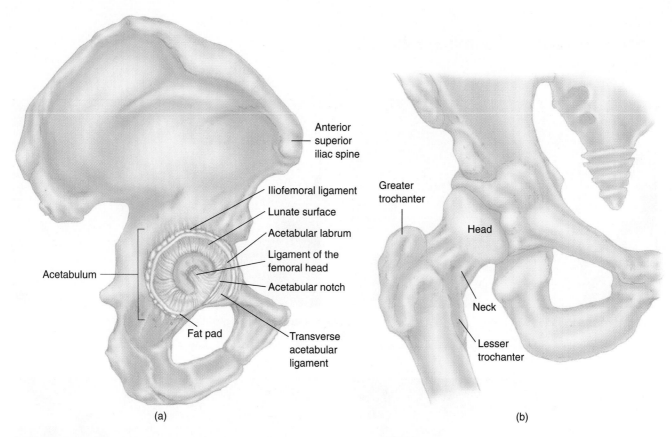

Figure 2-72 The hip joint: (a) lateral view (b) anterior view.

Review

Content

Vertebrae from Head to Tail

- Cervical (C1–C7)
- Thoracic (T1–T12)
- Lumbar (L1–L5)
- Sacral (S1–S5, fused in adulthood)
- Coccygeal

The Spine

The spine comprises the cervical, thoracic, lumbar, sacral, and coccygeal vertebrae (Figure 2-75 ▶). Cartilaginous disks separate the vertebrae from one another, except for those in the sacrum and coccyx, which fuse in adulthood. The vertebrae form a series of gliding joints that permit a variety of movements.

The cervical vertebrae are the most mobile. C1 and C2 share a special structural relationship. C1, also known as the atlas because it supports the head much as the mythical Atlas supported the world, allows flexion and extension between itself and the skull. This enables us to look up and down. C2, also known as the axis, has a finger-like projection called the odontoid process. The atlas sits atop the odontoid process and rotates around it. The cervical spine (C2 through C7) permits flexion, extension, lateral bending, and rotation in a fairly wide range of motion in all directions. The thoracic vertebrae (T1 through T12) articulate with the 12 sets of ribs that protect the vital organs of the chest. The lumbar vertebrae (L1 through L5) are the most massive because they bear most of the body's weight when it is standing erect. Like the cervical vertebrae, they are not well protected and are the site of frequent back problems. They, too, allow flexion, extension, lateral bending, and rotation.

The spinal cord runs through a foramen (opening) in the center of each vertebra. Nerve roots for both sensory and motor nerves leave the spinal cord bilaterally at each level and innervate the various body regions (Figure 2-76 ▶). Damage to the cord or nerve roots can render those regions numb and immobile. Ligaments, tendons, muscles, and various other connective tissues hold the vertebrae in place. When these

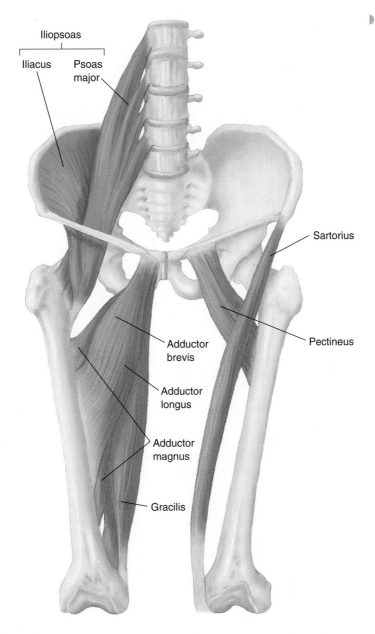

Iliopsoas

Iliacus   Psoas major

Sartorius

Adductor brevis

Pectineus

Adductor longus

Adductor magnus

Gracilis

supporting structures are injured, the risk of damage to the spinal column, and ultimately to the spinal cord, becomes a priority concern.

To assess your patient's spine, first inspect his head and neck for deformities, abnormal posture, and asymmetrical skin folds. The head should be erect and the spine straight. Ask your patient to bend forward slightly while you visually identify the spinous processes, the paravertebral muscles, the scapulae, the iliac crests, and the posterior iliac spines (usually marked by dimples). Draw imaginary horizontal lines across the shoulders and iliac crests. Now draw an imaginary vertical line from T1 to the space between the buttocks (gluteal cleft). Any deviations suggest a variety of pathologies.

Next observe your patient from the side. Evaluate the curves of the cervical, thoracic, and lumbar spine and note any irregularities. Common abnormalities of the spine include lordosis, scoliosis, and kyphosis (Table 2–7). Using the pads of your fingers, palpate the spinous processes for tenderness (Procedure 2–17a). Feel the supporting structures for muscle tone, symmetry, size, and tenderness or spasms. If your

> When the vertebrae's supporting structures are injured, the risk of damage to the spinal column, and ultimately to the spinal cord, becomes a priority concern.

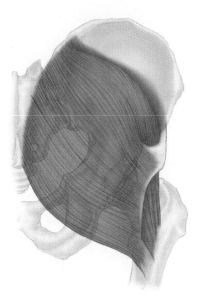

Gluteus maximus

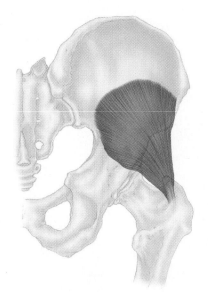

Gluteus minimus

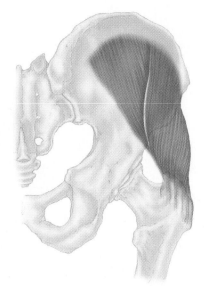

Gluteus medius

▶ **Figure 2-74** The gluteus muscles.

Assessment Pearls

Evaluating for Spinal Disk Disease   Lower back or neck pain are common reasons people summon EMS or go to the emergency department. Most back pain is musculoskeletal in origin and resolves with conservative treatment. However, herniation of a spinal disk can be quite painful and refractory to treatment. How can you differentiate musculoskeletal back pain from diskogenic back pain? It's not always easy, but here are a few pointers.

When you're obtaining the history from the patient, listen for indications that the pain is worse on one side compared with the other. Diskogenic pain tends to be worse in one leg compared with the other.

Other clues to diskogenic pain include worsening of the pain when the patient coughs or bears down while having a bowel movement. Both of these cause an increase in the intrathecal pressure (i.e., the pressure within the spinal canal) and thus push on the herniated disk, which then pushes on the spinal nerve root, exacerbating the pain.

Numbness in one leg, especially along a spinal nerve dermatome, is usually due to diskogenic disease. Bilateral numbness is usually not. The exception would be bilateral numbness on the inside of the thighs (i.e., saddle anesthesia), which is indicative of a cauda equina syndrome and a neurosurgical emergency. (Cauda equina syndrome is compression of the nerve roots in the lower spinal cord, which causes paralysis, and loss of bowel and bladder control. Patients have altered sensation between the legs, over the buttocks, the inner thighs and back of legs [saddle area], and the feet.)

On your physical exam, loss of muscle strength or loss of a deep tendon reflex on one side is indicative of diskogenic disease. Have a patient without recent trauma lie supine and raise both of his feet off the stretcher for about 30 seconds. If he can do this, diskogenic disease is unlikely. If he can't, the weak side is the side where the spinal nerve root is compressed.

Another test is the straight-leg lifting test. With the patient supine, pick up a leg, keeping it straight. If this causes pain before the leg can be completely raised, suspect diskogenic disease.

Examining the Hip

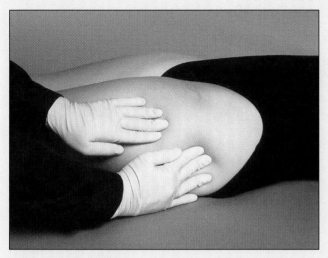

2-16a   Palpate the hip.

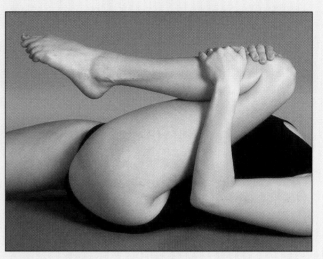

2-16b   Assess hip flexion with the knee flexed.

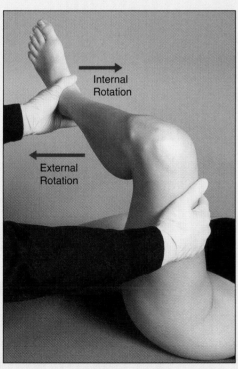

2-16c   Assess external and internal rotation of the hip.

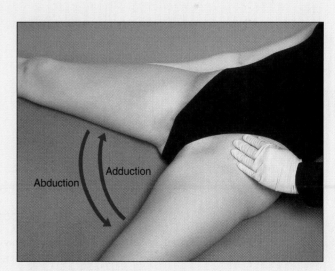

2-16d   Assess hip abduction and adduction.

Figure 2-75 The spinal column.

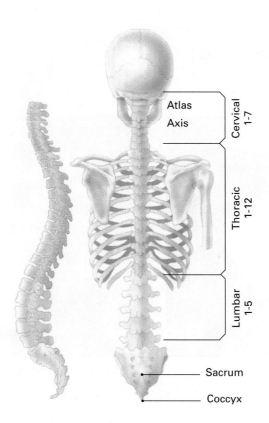

Atlas
Axis

Cervical 1-7

Thoracic 1-12

Lumbar 1-5

Sacrum

Coccyx

Figure 2-76 The vertebrae.

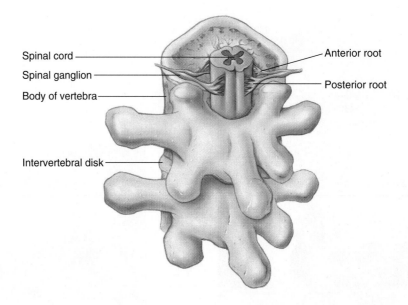

Spinal cord

Spinal ganglion

Body of vertebra

Intervertebral disk

Anterior root

Posterior root

Table 2-7	Spinal Curvatures
Condition	**Description**
Normal	Concave in cervical and lumbar regions, convex in thorax
Lordosis	Exaggerated lumbar concavity (swayback)
Kyphosis	Exaggerated thoracic convexity (hunchback)
Scoliosis	Lateral curvature

Assessing the Spine

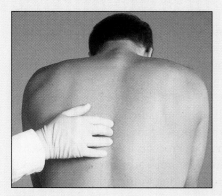

2-17a   Palpate the spine.

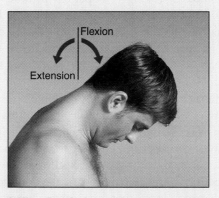

2-17b   Test flexion and extension of the head and neck.

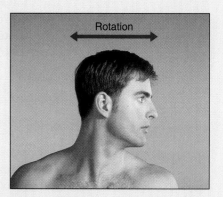

2-17c   Test rotation of the head and neck.

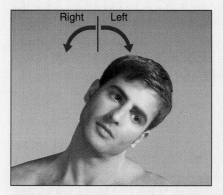

2-17d   Assess lateral bending of the head and neck.

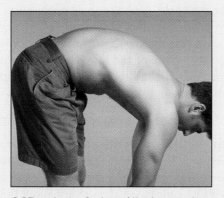

2-17e   Assess flexion of the lower spine.

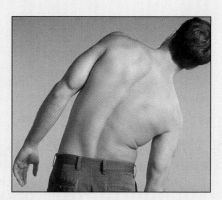

2-17f   Assess lateral bending of the lower spine.

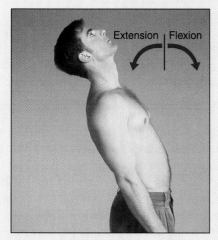

2-17g   Assess spinal extension.

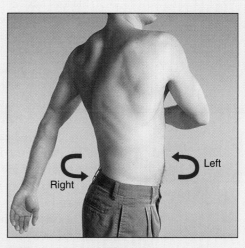

2-17h   Assess spinal rotation.

patient exhibits tenderness of the spinous processes and paravertebral muscles, suspect a herniated intervertebral disk, most commonly found between L4 and S1.

Now test range of motion. First test for flexion by asking your patient to touch his chin to his chest (Procedure 2–17b). Flexion is normally 45°. Next, ask him to bend his head backward. This tests extension, which normally is up to 55°. Now test for rotation by asking your patient to touch his chin to each shoulder (Procedure 2-17c). Normal rotation is 70° on each side. Finally ask him to touch his ears to his shoulders without raising his shoulders. This assesses lateral bending, which normally is 40° on each side (Procedure 2–17d). Now test for flexion of the lower spine with your patient standing. Ask him to bend and touch his toes (Procedure 2–17e). Note the smoothness and symmetry of movement, the range of motion, and the curves in the lumbar region. Normal flexion ranges from 75° to 90°. If the lumbar area remains concave or appears asymmetrical during this exam, your patient may have a muscle spasm. Next stabilize your patient's pelvis with your hands and have him bend sideways; normal lateral bending is 35° on each side (Procedure 2–17f). To assess hyperextension, ask him to bend backward toward you; normal hyperextension is 30° (Procedure 2–17g). Finally test spinal rotation by asking your patient to twist his shoulders one way, then the other. Normally they will rotate 30° to each side (Procedure 2–17h).

If your patient complains of lower back pain radiating down the back of one leg, assess it by having him lie supine on the table. Ask him to raise his straightened leg until he feels pain. Note the angle of elevation at which the pain occurs, as well as the quality and distribution of the pain. Now dorsiflex your patient's foot. If this causes a sharp pain that radiates from your patient's back down his leg, suspect compression of the nerve roots of the lower lumbar region. Repeat this test with the other leg. Increased pain in the affected leg when the opposite leg is raised confirms the finding.

The Peripheral Vascular System

The peripheral arterial system delivers oxygenated blood to the tissues of the extremities (Figure 2-77 ▶). Where the arteries lie close to the skin, the pulse is palpable. The brachial artery runs along the medial humerus and delivers blood to the arm and hands. Palpate the brachial pulse just above the elbow and medial to the biceps tendon and muscle. The brachial artery splits into the radial and ulnar arteries that deliver blood to the forearm and hands. Palpate the radial artery just above the wrist on the thumb side; palpate the ulnar artery just above the wrist on the other side.

In the lower extremities, the femoral artery delivers blood to the legs and feet. Palpate the femoral artery just below the inguinal ligament midway between the anterior-superior iliac spine and the symphysis pubis. The femoral artery then branches into the popliteal artery, which passes behind the knee and is easily palpated there. Below the knee the popliteal artery branches into the posterior tibial artery, which travels behind the tibia and can be felt just below the medial malleolus. The anterior branch can be felt as the dorsalis pedis pulse on top of the foot just lateral to the extensor tendon of the big toe.

The venous system comprises deep, superficial, and communicating veins that return blood to the heart. In the upper extremities, superficial veins are visible in the back of the hand, the inside of the arms, and in the antecubital fossa (crook of the elbow). These veins are used for venous access in the emergency setting. They eventually deliver their blood into the superior vena cava en route to the right atrium. In the legs, the vast majority of venous return happens via deep veins. The superficial veins, however, also play an important role. The great saphenous vein originates in the foot and joins the deep vein system near the inguinal ligament. The small saphenous vein, which also begins in the foot, joins the deep system in the popliteal space behind the knee. The two saphenous systems and the deep system are connected in other places

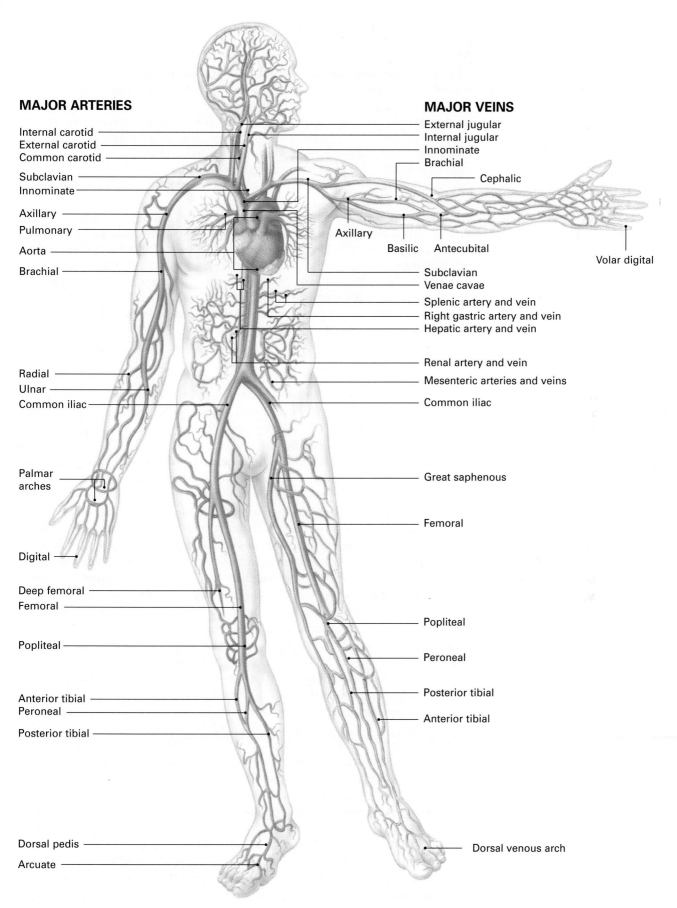

MAJOR ARTERIES

Internal carotid
External carotid
Common carotid

Subclavian
Innominate

Axillary
Pulmonary

Aorta

Brachial

Radial
Ulnar
Common iliac

Palmar
arches

Digital

Deep femoral
Femoral

Popliteal

Anterior tibial
Peroneal

Posterior tibial

Dorsal pedis

Arcuate

MAJOR VEINS

External jugular
Internal jugular
Innominate
Brachial
Cephalic

Axillary

Basilic   Antecubital

Volar digital

Subclavian
Venae cavae
Splenic artery and vein
Right gastric artery and vein
Hepatic artery and vein

Renal artery and vein
Mesenteric arteries and veins
Common iliac

Great saphenous

Femoral

Popliteal

Peroneal

Posterior tibial

Anterior tibial

Dorsal venous arch

▶ **Figure 2-77** The circulatory system.

Assessment Pearls

Checking for Impaired Peripheral Perfusion When you encounter a patient with a penetrating injury to an extremity, such as a gunshot or knife wound, you should always be concerned about the presence of a vascular injury. Ideally, you want to be able to palpate pulses distal to the injury. However, in certain situations, this can be difficult (e.g., cold weather, entrapment). In patients with suspected peripheral vascular disease, the oximeter probe can be placed distally to detect any perfusion. Placing the oximeter probe distal to the injury will help determine the presence and quality of perfusion and can also allow you to monitor perfusion during treatment and transport.

To accomplish this, take the probe from your pulse oximeter and apply it to the toes or fingers of the extremity in question. If peripheral perfusion is present, you should get a reading. Move the probe from toe to toe (or finger to finger) and note any difference. For example, if your patient's pulse ox readings drop off when you move the probe from the third to the fourth and fifth fingers, your index of suspicion about an ulnar artery injury should be raised.

Likewise, when you encounter a patient with a knee or elbow dislocation, you should always worry about vascular compromise.

by communicating veins and anastomotic vessels. The veins of the lower extremities deliver their blood into the inferior vena cava en route to the heart. Venous flow occurs via muscular contractions that push the blood against gravity toward the heart and one-way valves that prohibit backflow.

The lymphatic system (Figure 2-78 ▶) is a network of vessels that drains fluid, called lymph, from the body tissues and delivers it to the subclavian vein. Lymph nodes in the neck, the axilla, and the groin help filter impurities en route to the heart. They are palpable when congested with infectious products.

The lymphatic system plays an important role in the body's immune system. It also plays an important role in our circulatory system. When arterial blood flows into a capillary bed, hydrostatic pressure pushes fluid across the capillary membrane into the tissues. As the blood flows through the capillary bed, this pressure diminishes. Plasma proteins in the capillaries create an oncotic pressure gradient that draws fluid back into the bloodstream. On the venous side of the capillary bed, the oncotic pressure drawing fluid in is greater than the hydrostatic pressure pushing fluid out. The net effect is that fluid returns to the capillary for its return to the heart. In a perfect system, whatever fluid enters the tissues should exit at the other end. In reality, some fluid usually remains. The lymph system acts as an auxiliary drainage system, collecting the remaining fluid from the tissues and returning it to the heart. Tissue edema can occur because of an increase in hydrostatic pressure, a decrease in plasma proteins, or a lymph system blockage.

As we age, the arteries lengthen, stiffen, and develop atherosclerosis. A complete evaluation of your patient's circulatory system is an essential component of any physical exam. Many diseases result from poor circulation, either localized (specific artery occlusion) or generalized (cardiovascular collapse). Carefully assess your elderly patient's end-organ perfusion.

To assess your patient's peripheral vascular system, inspect both arms from the fingertips to the shoulders. Note their size and symmetry. Observe swelling, venous congestion, the color of the skin and nail beds, and the skin texture. Yellow or brittle nails or poor color in the fingertips indicates chronic arterial insufficiency. Palpate the peripheral arteries to evaluate pulsation and capillary refill and to assess skin temperature (Procedures 2-18a and 2-18b). To palpate a peripheral pulse, lightly place your

A complete evaluation of your patient's circulatory system is an essential component of any physical exam.

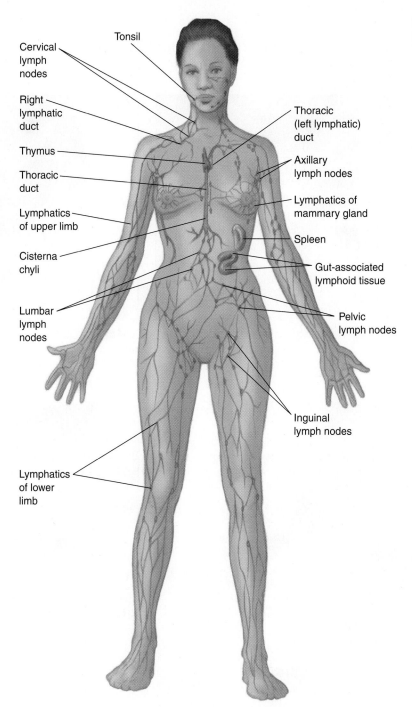

Tonsil

Cervical lymph nodes

Right lymphatic duct

Thymus

Thoracic duct

Lymphatics of upper limb

Cisterna chyli

Lumbar lymph nodes

Lymphatics of lower limb

Thoracic (left lymphatic) duct

Axillary lymph nodes

Lymphatics of mammary gland

Spleen

Gut-associated lymphoid tissue

Pelvic lymph nodes

Inguinal lymph nodes

finger pads over the artery's pulse point. Slowly increase the pressure until you feel a maximum pulsation. Note the rate, regularity, equality, and quality of the pulses. Count the number of beats in 1 minute. Then determine whether the pulse is regular, regularly irregular, or irregularly irregular. Finally, assess the quality of the pulse by noting its amplitude and contour; rate its quality from 0 to 3+ as shown in Table 2–8. Determine if it is absent, normal, weak, or bounding, and note any thrills, humming vibrations that feel similar to the throat of a purring cat. Thrills suggest a cardiac murmur or vascular narrowing. Expect the pulse of a normal adult to range between 60 and 100 beats per minute with a regular rhythm and normal amplitude.

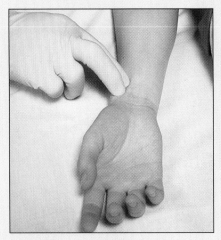

2-18a Palpate the radial artery.

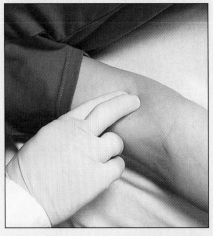

2-18b Palpate the brachial artery.

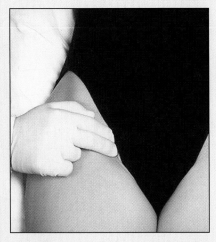

2-18c Palpate and compare the femoral arteries.

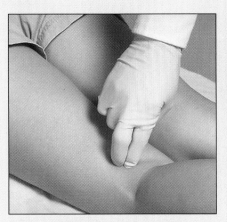

2-18d Palpate the popliteal pulse.

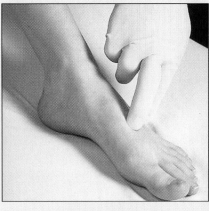

2-18e Palpate the dorsalis pedis pulse.

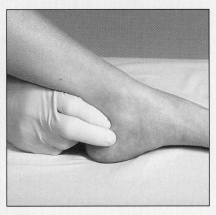

2-18f Palpate the posterior tibial pulse.

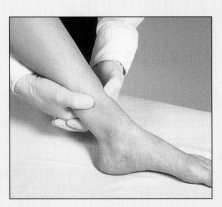

2-18g Palpate for edema.

Table 2-8	Assessing a Peripheral Pulse
Score	**Description**
0	Absent pulse
1+	Weak or thready
2+	Normal
3+	Bounding

Compare peripheral pulses bilaterally. If you detect a weak or absent pulse in one extremity, suspect an arterial occlusion proximal to the pulse point. Also compare distal and proximal pulses for equality. If you cannot palpate a distal artery, move proximally to another artery. For example, if you cannot palpate the radial artery, move to the brachial artery in the antecubital area. While you are at the elbow, you can also assess the epitrochlear lymph nodes; they will be palpable only if inflamed.

Next assess the feet and legs. Have your patient lie down and ask him to remove his socks. Inspect the legs from the feet to the groin. Note their size and symmetry. Evaluate the presence of swelling, venous congestion, the color of the skin and nail beds, and the skin texture. Note any venous enlargement. Evaluate scars, pigmentation, rashes, and ulcers. Palpate and compare the femoral pulses (Procedure 2–18c). Note the rate, regularity, equality, and quality of the pulses. Palpate the popliteal pulse behind the knee, the dorsalis pedis pulse on top of the foot, and the posterior tibial pulse just behind the medial malleolus (Procedures 2-18d through 2-18f). Feel the temperature of the legs, feet, and toes with the back of your fingers and compare both sides. Unilateral coldness indicates an arterial occlusion. Bilateral coldness is due to an environmental problem, bilateral occlusion (saddle embolus), or a general circulatory problem (shock). Palpate the superficial inguinal lymph nodes for enlargement and tenderness.

Observe the legs for edema, the presence of an abnormal amount of fluid in the tissues. Compare one leg and foot with the other. Note their relative size and symmetry. Are veins, tendons, and bones easily visible under the skin? Edema will usually obscure these structures. Palpate for pitting edema by pressing firmly with your thumb for 5 seconds over the top of the foot, behind each medial ankle, and over the shins (Procedure 2–18g). **Pitting** is a depression left by the pressure of your thumb. Normally there should be no depression. If edema is present, evaluate the degree of pitting, which can range from slight to marked (Figure 2-79 ▶). You can grade the depth of the pitting according to the appropriate scale in Table 2–9. Expect the pit to disappear within 10 seconds after you release the pressure. Bilateral edema suggests a central circulatory problem such as congestive heart failure or renal failure; unilateral edema suggests a lower extremity circulation abnormality such as deep venous

pitting
depression that results from pressure against skin when pitting edema is present.

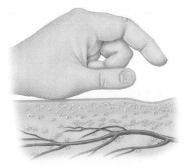 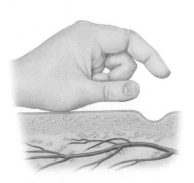

+1 Slight pitting edema   +4 Deep pitting edema

▶ **Figure 2-79** Assessing for edema.

Table 2-9	Pitting Edema Scale
Score	**Description**
1+	One quarter inch or less
2+	One quarter to one half inch
3+	One half to one inch
4+	One inch or more

thrombosis (DVT) or venous occlusion. Note the extent of the edema. How far up the leg does it spread? The higher the edema, the more severe the problem.

During your assessment, look for visible venous distention. An associated swollen, painful leg suggests a DVT. Palpate the femoral vein just medial to the femoral artery. If you detect a tender femoral vein, flex the knee and palpate the calf for tenderness, another classic sign of DVT. Is there a local redness or warmth? Feel for a cordlike vessel. Evaluate the skin for discoloration, ulcers, and unusual thickness. Finally, ask your patient to stand. Evaluate his legs for varicose veins and, if present, palpate them for signs of thrombophlebitis (redness, swelling, pain, and tenderness).

The Nervous System

A comprehensive physical exam includes a thorough evaluation of your patient's mental status and thought processes. On the scene of an emergency, you would limit your mental exam to level of consciousness and basic orientation questions such as "What is your name?" "Where are you right now?" "What day is it today?" If you are conducting a full physical exam or evaluating someone with altered mentation, some or all of the following techniques will be useful.

When you conduct a neurologic exam, you are attempting to answer two vital questions. First, are the findings symmetrical or unilateral? Second, if the signs are unilateral, is the site of origin in the central nervous system (brain and spinal cord) or in the peripheral nervous system (everything else)? You will conduct many parts of the neuro exam while you assess other anatomical areas and systems. For example, you can examine the cranial nerves while evaluating the head and face. You can note any weaknesses or abnormal neurologic findings while evaluating the arms and legs during the musculoskeletal exam.

A nervous system exam covers five areas: mental status and speech, the cranial nerves, the motor system, the sensory system, and the reflexes. This section presents the complete neuro exam. The chief complaint, the clinical condition of your patient, and time constraints will determine which parts you actually use.

Mental Status and Speech

The central nervous system consists of the brain and spinal cord. The brain is the nerve center for the human body. It has three major regions: the brainstem; the cerebrum, or cerebral cortex; and the cerebellum. The brainstem consists of the midbrain, pons, and medulla (Figure 2-80 ▶). The cerebrum and the cerebellum are each divided into left and right hemispheres. Each cerebral hemisphere comprises four lobes—frontal, parietal, temporal, and occipital—which serve diverse functions (Figure 2-81 ▶). Myelin-coated axons (white matter) allow areas of the brain to communicate with one another and transmit their messages to the rest of the body via the spinal cord and peripheral nerves.

The cerebral cortex (gray matter) is the center for conscious thought, sensory awareness, movement, emotions, rational thought and behavior, foresight and

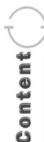

Review

Five Areas of Neurologic Exam

- Mental status and speech
- Cranial nerves
- Motor system
- Sensory system
- Reflexes

Figure 2-80 The brain.

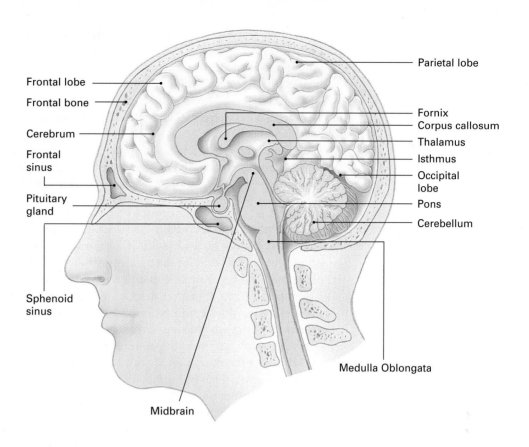

Frontal lobe

Frontal bone

Cerebrum

Frontal sinus

Pituitary gland

Sphenoid sinus

Midbrain

Parietal lobe

Fornix

Corpus callosum

Thalamus

Isthmus

Occipital lobe

Pons

Cerebellum

Medulla Oblongata

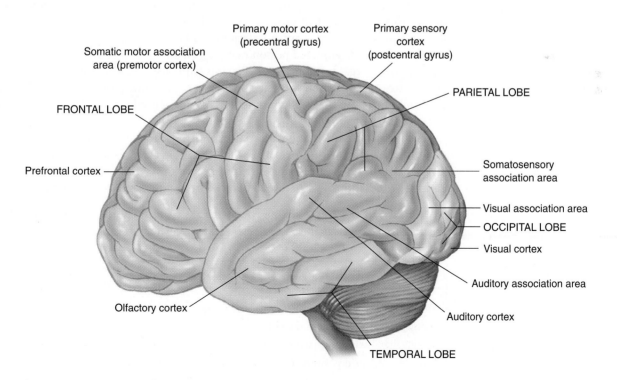

Somatic motor association area (premotor cortex)

Primary motor cortex (precentral gyrus)

Primary sensory cortex (postcentral gyrus)

FRONTAL LOBE

PARIETAL LOBE

Prefrontal cortex

Somatosensory association area

Visual association area

OCCIPITAL LOBE

Visual cortex

Auditory association area

Olfactory cortex

Auditory cortex

TEMPORAL LOBE

Figure 2-81 The cerebrum.

planning, memory, speech, and language and interpretation. The frontal lobe contains a special speech area and the motor strip that controls voluntary skeletal muscle movement. It is also the area associated with personality and behavior. The parietal lobe is responsible for processing sensory data from the peripheral nerves. The occipital lobe houses the primary vision center and interprets visual data. The temporal lobe perceives and interprets sounds and integrates the senses of taste, smell, and balance.

Generally you will evaluate your patient's mental status and speech when you begin your interview. During this time you will assess his level of response, general appearance and behavior, and speech. If you detect abnormalities, continue your assessment with more specific questioning or testing as presented here.

Appearance and Behavior   First, assess your patient's level of response. Is he alert and awake? Does he understand your questions? Are his responses appropriate and timely, or does he drift off the topic easily or lose interest? If you detect an abnormality, continue with more specific questions. Is he lethargic (drowsy, but answers questions appropriately before falling asleep again)? Is he obtunded (opens his eyes and looks at you but gives slow, confused responses)? Sometimes you must arouse your patient repeatedly by gently shaking him or shouting his name. If he does not respond to your verbal cues, assess him with painful stimuli for coma or stupor. The stuporous patient is arousable for short periods but is not aware of his surroundings. The comatose patient is in a state of profound unconsciousness and is totally unarousable.

If your patient is awake and alert, observe his posture and motor behavior. Does he lie in bed or prefer to walk around? His posture should be erect and he should look at you. A slumped posture and a lack of facial expression may indicate depression. Excessive energetic movements or constantly watchful eyes suggest tension, anxiety, or a metabolic disorder. Watch the pace, range, and character of his movements. Are they voluntary? Are any parts immobile? Do his posture and motor activity change with the environment? Some possible findings are listed in Table 2–10.

Observe your patient's grooming and personal hygiene. How is he dressed? Are his clothes clean, pressed, and properly fastened? Is his appearance appropriate for the season, climate, and occasion? A deterioration in grooming and personal hygiene in the previously well-groomed person may suggest an emotional problem, a psychiatric disorder, or an organic brain disease. Patients with obsessive-compulsive behavior may exhibit excessive attention to their appearance. Note your patient's hair, teeth, nails, skin, and beard. Are they well groomed? Compare one side to another. One-sided neglect may suggest a brain lesion.

Also observe your patient's facial expressions. Are they appropriate? Do they vary when he talks with others and when the topic changes or is his face immobile throughout the interaction? Can he express happiness, sadness, anger, or depression? Patients with Parkinson's disease have facial immobility, a mask-like appearance.

Speech and Language   Note your patient's speech pattern. Normally a person's speech is inflected, clear and strong, fluent and articulate, and varies in volume. It should

Table 2-10	Posture and Behavior	
Motor Activity	**Meaning**
Tense posture, restlessness, fidgeting	Anxiety
Crying, hand-wringing, pacing	Agitation, depression
Hopeless, slumped posture, slowed movements	Depression
Singing, dancing, expansive movements	Manic

express thoughts clearly. Is your patient excessively talkative or silent? Does he speak spontaneously or only when you ask him a direct question? Is his speech slow and quiet, as in depression? Is it fast and loud, as in a manic episode? Does he speak clearly and distinctly? Does he have dysarthria (defective speech caused by motor deficits), dysphonia (voice changes caused by vocal cord problems), or aphasia (defective language caused by neurologic damage to the brain)? With expressive aphasia his words will be garbled; with receptive aphasia, his words will be clear but unrelated to your questions. Your patient with aphasia may have such difficulty talking that you mistakenly suspect a psychotic disorder.

Mood   Observe your patient's verbal and nonverbal behavior for clues to his mood. Note any mood swings or behaviors that suggest anxiety or depression. Is he sad, elated, angry, enraged, anxious, worried, detached, or indifferent? Assess the intensity of your patient's mood. How long has he been this way? Is his behavior normal for the circumstances? For example, anxiety is normal for someone having a heart attack; if your heart attack patient did not act frightened and concerned, that would be abnormal. If your patient is depressed, is he suicidal? If you suspect the possibility of suicide, ask him directly, "Have you ever thought of committing suicide? Are you currently thinking of committing suicide?"

Thought and Perceptions   Assess how well your patient organizes his thoughts when he speaks. Is he logical and coherent? Does he shift from one topic to an unrelated topic without realizing that the thoughts are not connected? These "loose associations" are typical in schizophrenia, manic episodes, and other psychiatric disorders. Does he speak constantly in related areas with no real conclusion or end point? Such "flight of ideas" is most often associated with mania. Does he ramble with unrelated, illogical thoughts and disordered grammar? You may see this "incoherence" in severe psychosis. Does he make up facts or events in response to questions? You may see this "confabulation" in amnesia. Does he suddenly lose his train of thought and stop in midsentence before completing an idea? Such blocking occurs in normal people but is pronounced in schizophrenia.

Assess the thought content of your patient's responses as they occur during the interview; for example, "You said you thought you were allergic to your mother. Can you tell me why you think that way?" In this way you can ask about your patient's unpleasant or unusual comments. Allow him the freedom to explore these thoughts with you. Is your patient driven to try to prevent some unrealistic future result (compulsion)? Does he have a recurrent, uncontrollable feeling of dread and doom (obsession)? Does he sense that things in the environment are strange or unreal (feelings of unreality)? Does he have false personal beliefs that other members of his group don't share (delusions)? Compulsions and obsessions are neurotic disorders, while delusions and feelings of unreality are psychotic disorders.

Determine whether your patient perceives imaginary things. Does he see visions, hear voices, smell odors, or feel things that aren't there? Ask him about these false perceptions just as you would ask about anything else. For example, ask "When you see the pink elephants, what are they doing?" Decide whether your patient is misinterpreting what is real (illusions) or seeing things that are not real (hallucinations). Both illusions and hallucinations may occur in schizophrenia, post-traumatic stress disorders, and organic brain syndrome. Auditory and visual hallucinations are common in psychedelic drug ingestion, while tactile hallucinations suggest alcohol withdrawal.

Insight and Judgment   During the interview you will most likely evaluate your patient's insight and judgment. Does he understand what is happening to him? Does he realize that what he thinks and how he feels is part of the illness? Patients with psychotic disorders may not have insight into their illness. Judgment refers to your patient's ability to reason appropriately. Does your mature patient respond appropriately to questions concerning his family and personal life? Ask him what he would do if he cut himself shaving. Proper judgment means that your patient can evaluate the data and provide an adequate response. Impaired judgment is common in emotional problems, mental retardation, and organic brain syndrome.

Your patient should be oriented to person, time, and place and respond appropriately to your questions.

Memory and Attention   Assess your patient's orientation. Does he know his name? Person disorientation suggests trauma, seizures, or amnesia. Does he know the time of day, day of the week, month, season, and year? Time disorientation may suggest anxiety, depression, or organic brain syndrome. Does he know where he is, where he lives, the name of the city and state? Place disorientation suggests a psychiatric disorder or organic brain syndrome. Your patient should be oriented to person, time, and place and respond appropriately to your questions.

To assess your patient's ability to concentrate, use the following three exercises. First, have him repeat a series of numbers back to you (digit span). Normally, a person can repeat at least five numbers forward and backward. Then, ask him to start from 100 and subtract seven each time (serial sevens). A normal person can complete this in 90 seconds with fewer than four errors. Finally, ask your patient to spell a common five-letter word backward (spelling backward). Poor performance in these tests may suggest delirium, dementia, mental retardation, loss of calculating ability, anxiety, multiple sclerosis, fibromyalgia, fetal alcohol syndrome, previous brain injury, medication toxicity, or depression.

Memory can be divided into three grades: immediate, recent, and remote. First, test your patient's immediate memory. Ask him to repeat three or four words that have no correlation such as *desk, toothbrush, six,* and *blue.* This tests immediate recall and is similar to digit span. Next, test your patient's recent memory by asking him what he had for lunch or to repeat something he told you earlier in the interview. Make sure the information you ask for is verifiable. Finally, test for remote memory by asking about facts such as his wife's name, son's birthday, or his social security number. Ask him to describe the house in which he grew up or the schools he attended. Long-term and short-term memory problems may be due to amnesia, anxiety, or organic causes. Finally, test your patient's ability to learn new things. Give him the names of three or four items such as *man, chair, grass,* and *hot dog.* Ask him to repeat them. This tests registration and immediate recall. About 5 minutes later ask him to repeat them again. Normally, he will be able to name all four. Note his accuracy, his awareness of whether he is correct, or if he tries to confabulate by making up new words.

The Cranial Nerves

The 12 pairs of cranial nerves originate from the base of the brain and provide sensory and motor innervation, mostly to the head and face (Figure 2-82 ▶). Each pair bears the name of its function and carries either sensory fibers or motor fibers, or both (Figures 2-83 ▶ through 2-91 ▶). Table 2–11 lists the cranial nerves' names, their specific functions, and the areas they innervate.

Most likely you will conduct parts of the cranial nerve exam when you assess other areas such as the eyes, ears, throat, and musculoskeletal system. The following is the cranial nerve exam in its entirety.

CN-I   Test your patient's olfactory nerve by having her close her eyes and compress one nostril while you present her with a variety of common, nonirritating odors (Procedure 2–19a). Repeat the test with each nostril. Ask her to identify the odor. Most people will do so easily. If your patient cannot, several causes are possible. Bilateral loss of smell suggests head trauma, nasal stuffiness, smoking, cocaine use, or a congenital defect. A unilateral loss of smell without nasal disease suggests a frontal lobe lesion.

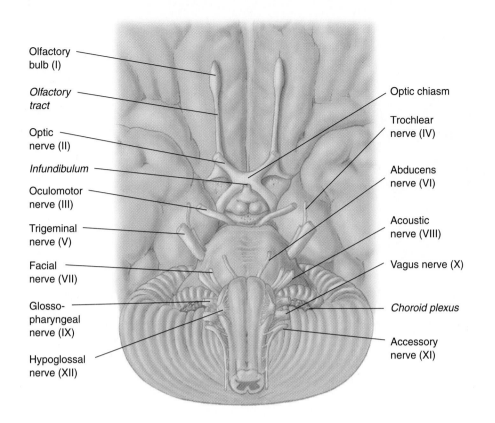

Figure 2-82 The cranial nerves.

Olfactory bulb (I)

Olfactory tract

Optic nerve (II)

Infundibulum

Oculomotor nerve (III)

Trigeminal nerve (V)

Facial nerve (VII)

Glosso-pharyngeal nerve (IX)

Hypoglossal nerve (XII)

Optic chiasm

Trochlear nerve (IV)

Abducens nerve (VI)

Acoustic nerve (VIII)

Vagus nerve (X)

Choroid plexus

Accessory nerve (XI)

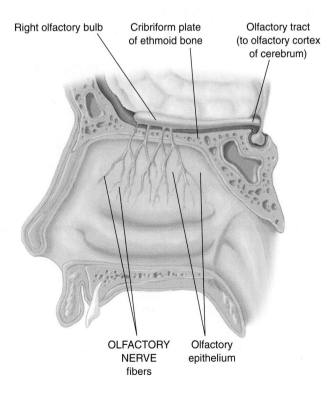

Right olfactory bulb

Cribriform plate of ethmoid bone

Olfactory tract (to olfactory cortex of cerebrum)

Figure 2-83 The olfactory nerve.

OLFACTORY NERVE fibers

Olfactory epithelium

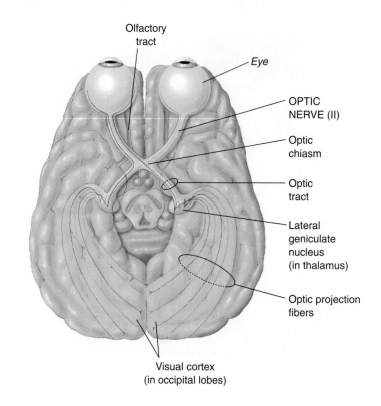

Figure 2-84 The optic nerve.

Olfactory tract

Eye

OPTIC NERVE (II)

Optic chiasm

Optic tract

Lateral geniculate nucleus (in thalamus)

Optic projection fibers

Visual cortex (in occipital lobes)

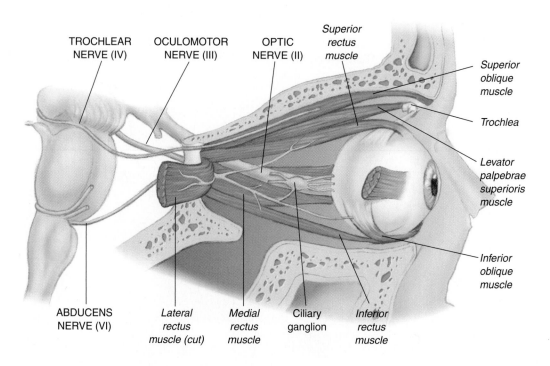

TROCHLEAR NERVE (IV)

OCULOMOTOR NERVE (III)

OPTIC NERVE (II)

Superior rectus muscle

Superior oblique muscle

Trochlea

Levator palpebrae superioris muscle

Inferior oblique muscle

ABDUCENS NERVE (VI)

Lateral rectus muscle (cut)

Medial rectus muscle

Ciliary ganglion

Inferior rectus muscle

Figure 2-85 The oculomotor, abducens, and trochlear nerves.

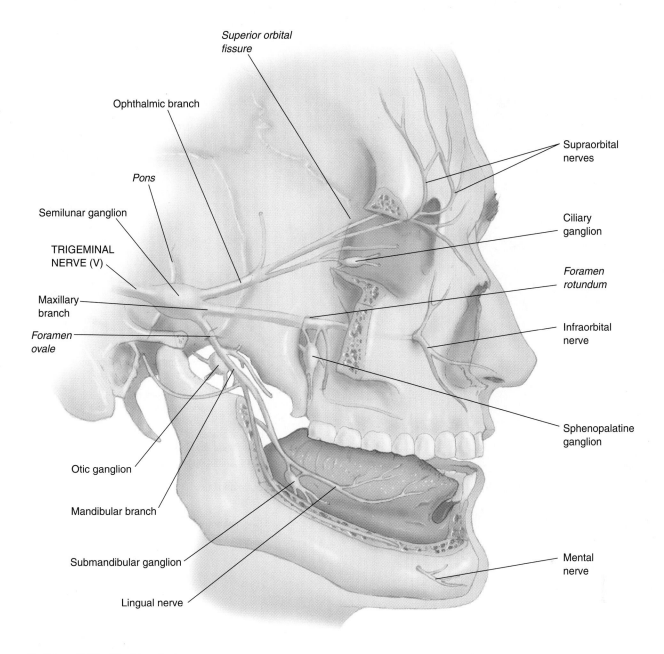

Superior orbital
fissure

Ophthalmic branch

Pons

Semilunar ganglion

TRIGEMINAL
NERVE (V)

Maxillary
branch

Foramen
ovale

Otic ganglion

Mandibular branch

Submandibular ganglion

Lingual nerve

Supraorbital
nerves

Ciliary
ganglion

Foramen
rotundum

Infraorbital
nerve

Sphenopalatine
ganglion

Mental
nerve

▶ **Figure 2-86** The trigeminal nerve.

CN-II   Test the optic nerve with the visual acuity and visual field tests described earlier in this chapter in the Anatomical Regions section on the eyes.

CN-III   Test the oculomotor nerve with the optic nerve when you perform pupil reaction tests. Inspect the size and shape of your patient's pupils and compare one side to the other. A slight inequality may be normal. Usually the pupil is midpoint. Constricted or dilated pupils may result from medications, drug abuse, glaucoma, and neurologic disease. Darken the room, if possible, to test for pupillary reaction. Ask your patient to look straight ahead. Shine a bright light obliquely into one of his pupils. Watch for direct reaction (pupillary constriction in the same eye) and for consensual reaction (pupillary constriction in the opposite eye). Repeat this test on the other side. Now assess for the near-response, asking your patient to follow your finger as you move

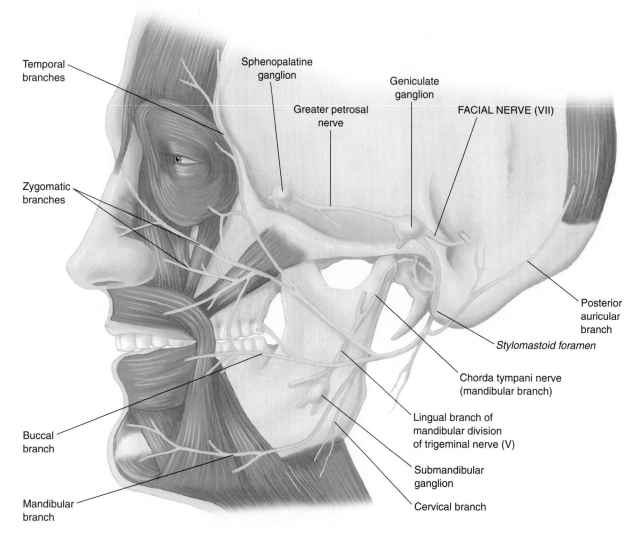

Temporal branches

Zygomatic branches

Buccal branch

Mandibular branch

Sphenopalatine ganglion

Greater petrosal nerve

Geniculate ganglion

FACIAL NERVE (VII)

Posterior auricular branch

Stylomastoid foramen

Chorda tympani nerve (mandibular branch)

Lingual branch of mandibular division of trigeminal nerve (V)

Submandibular ganglion

Cervical branch

▶ **Figure 2-87** The facial nerve.

it in toward the bridge of his nose. Watch for his pupils to constrict and his eyes to converge.

CN-III, IV, VI Test the oculomotor, trochlear, and abducens nerves by evaluating your patient's extraocular movements (EOM). Ask her to follow your finger with only her eyes as you move it through the six cardinal positions of gaze (Procedure 2–19b). Make a wide "H" in the air with your finger. Observe for conjugate (together) movements of your patient's eyes in each direction. Normally your patient can follow your finger with no strabismus (deviation) or nystagmus (involuntary movements). Inability to move in any direction can be the result of a problem with a cranial nerve, an ocular muscle, or an eye orbit that may be fractured and impinging on the muscle or nerve. Finally, look for ptosis (a droopy eyelid) that may be the result of CN-III palsy or myasthenia gravis.

CN-V Test function of the trigeminal nerve by asking your patient to clench her teeth while you palpate the temporal and masseter muscles (Procedure 2–19c). Note the

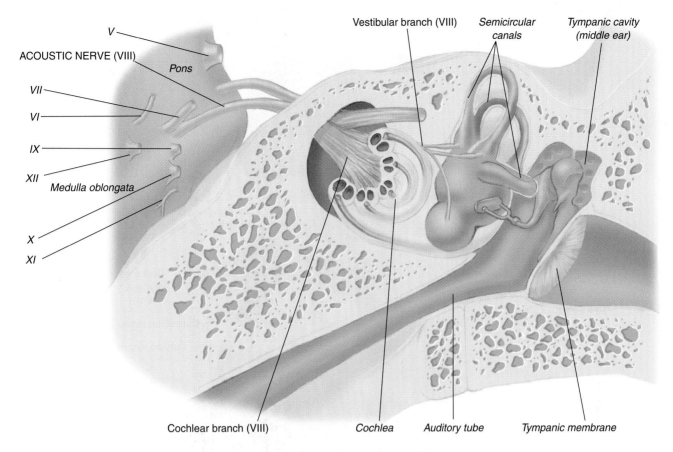

V

ACOUSTIC NERVE (VIII)

Pons

VII

VI

IX

XII

Medulla oblongata

X

XI

Vestibular branch (VIII)

Semicircular canals

Tympanic cavity (middle ear)

Cochlear branch (VIII)

Cochlea

Auditory tube

Tympanic membrane

▶ **Figure 2-88**   The acoustic nerve.

▶ **Figure 2-89**   The glossopharyngeal nerve.

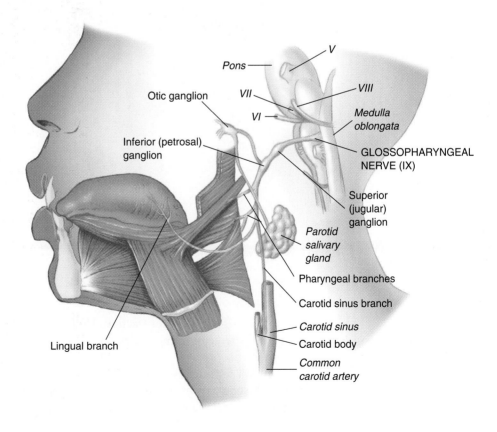

Otic ganglion

Inferior (petrosal) ganglion

Pons

VII

VI

V

VIII

Medulla oblongata

GLOSSOPHARYNGEAL NERVE (IX)

Superior (jugular) ganglion

Parotid salivary gland

Pharyngeal branches

Carotid sinus branch

Carotid sinus

Carotid body

Common carotid artery

Lingual branch

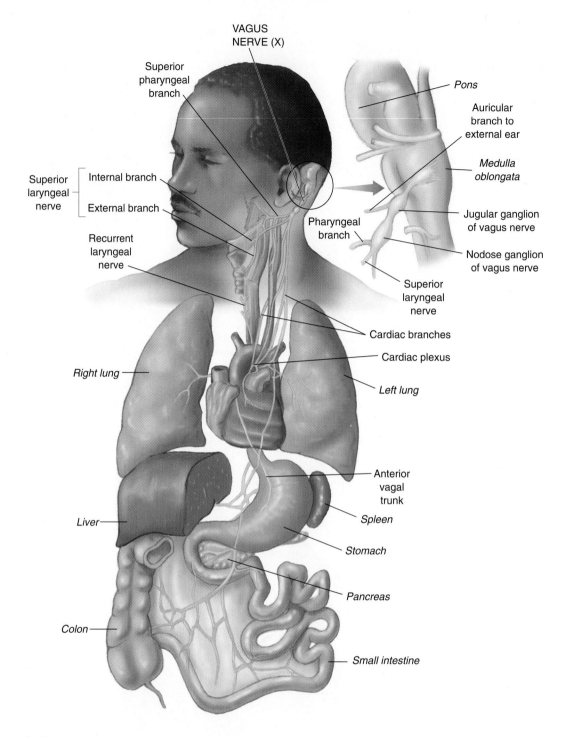

VAGUS
NERVE (X)

Superior
pharyngeal
branch

Pons

Auricular
branch to
external ear

*Medulla
oblongata*

Superior
laryngeal
nerve

Internal branch

External branch

Jugular ganglion
of vagus nerve

Recurrent
laryngeal
nerve

Pharyngeal
branch

Nodose ganglion
of vagus nerve

Superior
laryngeal
nerve

Cardiac branches

Cardiac plexus

Right lung

Left lung

Anterior
vagal
trunk

Spleen

Liver

Stomach

Pancreas

Colon

Small intestine

▶ **Figure 2-90** The vagus nerve.

strength of the muscle contraction. Unilateral weakness or the inability to contract suggests a trigeminal nerve lesion. Bilateral dysfunction suggests motor neuron involvement.

To test for sensory function in the three main divisions of the trigeminal nerve, first ask your patient to close her eyes. Using something sharp and something dull, lightly scrape the objects across the forehead, cheek, and chin on both sides and ask

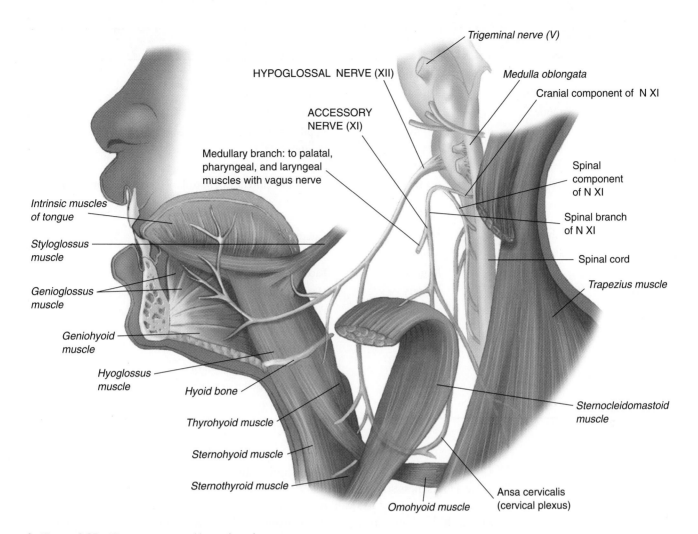

Trigeminal nerve (V)

HYPOGLOSSAL NERVE (XII)

Medulla oblongata

Cranial component of N XI

ACCESSORY
NERVE (XI)

Medullary branch: to palatal,
pharyngeal, and laryngeal
muscles with vagus nerve

Spinal
component
of N XI

Intrinsic muscles
of tongue

Spinal branch
of N XI

Styloglossus
muscle

Spinal cord

Trapezius muscle

Genioglossus
muscle

Geniohyoid
muscle

Hyoglossus
muscle

Hyoid bone

Sternocleidomastoid
muscle

Thyrohyoid muscle

Sternohyoid muscle

Sternothyroid muscle

Ansa cervicalis
(cervical plexus)

Omohyoid muscle

▶ **Figure 2-91** The accessory and hypoglossal nerves.

your patient to distinguish the sensations (Procedure 2–19d). The two ends of a paper clip work well for this procedure; straighten one end and use its tip as the sharp object. Unilateral loss of sensation suggests a trigeminal nerve lesion. Finally, test the corneal reflex. Ask your patient to look up and away as you touch her cornea lightly with some fine cotton fibers. She should blink. Repeat this test on the other eye.

CN-VII First assess your patient's face at rest and during conversation. Note any asymmetry, eyelid drooping, or abnormal movements such as tics. Test the facial nerve by having your patient assume a variety of facial expressions. Ask him to raise his eyebrows, frown, show his upper and lower teeth or smile, and puff out his cheeks. Also ask him to close his eyes tightly so that you cannot open them; then to test muscle strength, try to open them. Bell's palsy is an inflammation of CN-VII. Your patient will present with unilateral facial drooping from paralysis of this nerve.

CN-VIII Ask your patient to occlude one ear with a finger. Then whisper something softly into the other ear. Ask him to repeat what you said. Any loss of hearing warrants further testing to detect air and bone conduction problems. Test the acoustic nerve for the senses of hearing and balance. Ask your patient to stand erect and close his eyes. Now evaluate his balance and then ask him to open his eyes. If he doesn't become dizzy and opens his eyes to your command, the eighth nerve is functioning appropriately.

Table 2–11	Cranial Nerves		
CN	Name	Function	Innervation
I	Olfactory	Sensory	Smell
II	Optic	Sensory	Sight
III	Oculomotor	Motor	Pupil constriction; superior rectus, inferior rectus, inferior oblique muscles
IV	Trochlear	Motor	Superior oblique muscles
V	Trigeminal	Sensory	Opthalmic (forehead), maxillary (cheek), and mandibular (chin) regions
		Motor	Chewing muscles
VI	Abducens	Motor	Lateral rectus muscle
VII	Facial	Sensory	Tongue
		Motor	Face muscles
VIII	Acoustic	Sensory	Hearing balance
IX	Glossopharyngeal	Sensory	Posterior pharynx, taste to anterior tongue
		Motor	Posterior pharynx
X	Vagus	Sensory	Taste to posterior tongue
		Motor	Posterior palate and pharynx
XI	Accessory	Motor	Trapezius muscles; sternocleidomastoid muscles
XII	Hypoglossal	Motor	Tongue

CN-IX, X Test the glossopharyngeal and vagus nerves together. Listen to your patient's voice. Hoarseness suggests a vocal cord problem; a nasal quality suggests a palate problem. Ask your patient to swallow; note any difficulties. Ask him to open his mouth and say "aaahhh"; watch for the soft palate and uvula to rise symmetrically. The posterior pharynx should move medially. If the vagus nerve is paralyzed, the soft palate and uvula will deviate toward the side of the lesion. Test the gag reflex with a tongue blade on the posterior tongue (Procedure 2–19e). Absence of a gag reflex suggests a lesion in one of these nerves.

CN-XI Inspect the upper portions of your patient's trapezius muscles and sternocleidomastoid muscles for symmetry at rest. To test her trapezius muscles, place your hands on her shoulders and ask her to raise her shoulders against resistance (Procedure 2–19f). Now test her sternocleidomastoid muscles. Place your hands along her face and ask her to turn her head to each side as you apply resistance. Note any bilateral or unilateral weaknesses. A supine patient with bilateral weakness of the sternocleidomastoids will have trouble lifting her head.

CN-XII First evaluate your patient's speech articulation. Then ask him to stick out his tongue; watch for a midline projection. A CN-XII lesion will make the tongue deviate away from the affected side. Have your patient move his tongue from side to side as you watch for symmetry.

You may conduct a cranial nerve exam according to this sequence. More likely, you will develop your own efficient system of testing these nerves.

The Motor System

Thirty-one pairs of nerves arise from the spinal foramina on both sides of the spinal column (Figure 2-92). The anterior root of the peripheral nerves carries the motor,

Procedure 2-19   Assessing the Cranial Nerves

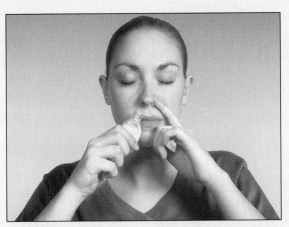

2-19a Test the olfactory nerve by having your patient identify common odors.

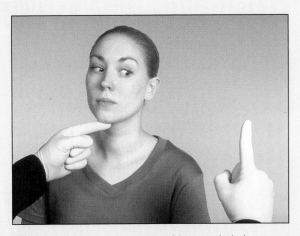

2-19b Test the oculomotor, trochlear, and abducens nerves by evaluating your patient's extraocular movements.

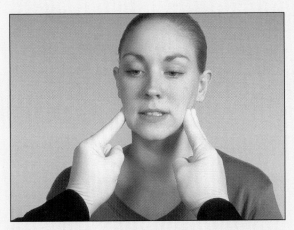

2-19c Test motor function of the trigeminal nerve by palpating the temporal and masseter muscles.

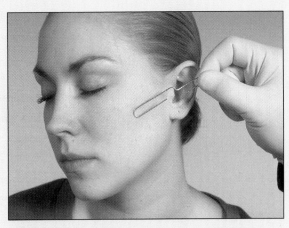

2-19d Test sensory function of the trigeminal nerve with sharp and dull objects.

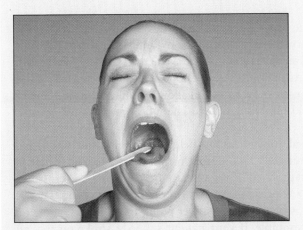

2-19e Test the glossopharyngeal and vagus nerves with a tongue blade.

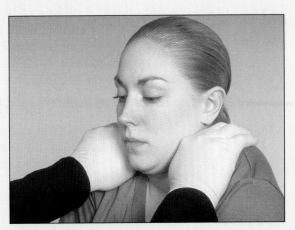

2-19f Test the spinal accessory nerve by having your patient shrug her shoulders against resistance.

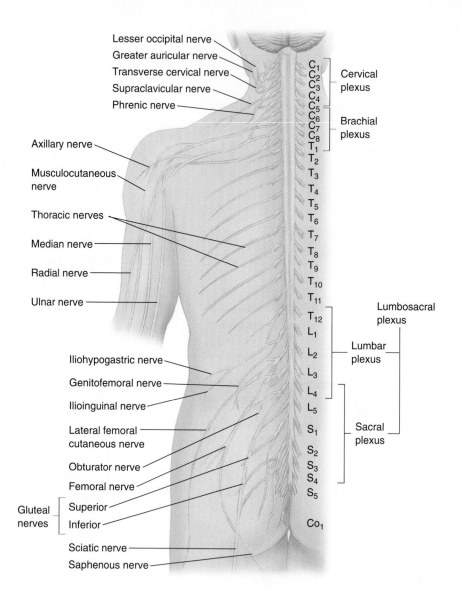

Figure 2-92 The peripheral nerves.

Lesser occipital nerve
Greater auricular nerve
Transverse cervical nerve
Supraclavicular nerve
Phrenic nerve

Axillary nerve
Musculocutaneous nerve

Thoracic nerves
Median nerve
Radial nerve
Ulnar nerve

Iliohypogastric nerve
Genitofemoral nerve
Ilioinguinal nerve
Lateral femoral cutaneous nerve
Obturator nerve
Femoral nerve

Gluteal nerves
Superior
Inferior
Sciatic nerve
Saphenous nerve

C_1 C_2 C_3 C_4 — Cervical plexus
C_5 C_6 C_7 C_8 T_1 — Brachial plexus
T_2 T_3 T_4 T_5 T_6 T_7 T_8 T_9 T_{10} T_{11} T_{12}
L_1 L_2 L_3 L_4 L_5 — Lumbar plexus / Lumbosacral plexus
S_1 S_2 S_3 S_4 S_5 — Sacral plexus
Co_1

or efferent, nerve fibers from the brain and spinal cord through three pathways: the pyramidal, extrapyramidal, and cerebellar systems. The pyramidal tract, which begins in the motor cortex of the brain, mediates voluntary movements. Its fibers travel down the brainstem, where they crisscross to innervate the opposite sides of the body. These tracts guide voluntary skeletal muscle movement and allow for fine motor movements by stimulating some muscles and inhibiting others. The motor system's net effect is coordinated, skilled movements.

When this system is damaged, function is lost below the level of the injury, and movements become weak or paralyzed. Inhibition is lost, so muscle tone is increased and deep tendon reflexes are exaggerated. If the damage occurs above the crossover point in the brainstem, then the effects will be seen on the opposite (contralateral) side of the body. If the damage is below the crossover point, the damage will be on the same (ipsilateral) side. For example, if your patient suffers a stroke on the left motor strip controlling the hands, then the motor deficiencies will appear in the right hand. If your patient has swelling of the spinal cord from an injury that impinges on the left motor nucleus, the motor deficiencies will appear on the left side of his body.

The extrapyramidal tract controls body movements and maintains muscle tone through motor fibers and pathways outside the pyramidal system. Since the extrapyramidal tract is mostly inhibitory, damage to this system causes increased muscle tone, abnormal gait and posture, and involuntary movements. This is commonly seen in patients who have adverse reactions to drugs in the phenothiazine class. They appear flushed and stiff, with motor control problems. The cerebellar system coordinates muscular activity and helps to maintain equilibrium and posture through its motor fibers. Cerebellar damage causes abnormal changes in gait, coordination, and equilibrium.

Inspect your patient's general body structure, muscle development, positioning, and coordination. What is his position at rest? Is he erect or does he slump to one side, suggesting unilateral paralysis or weakness? Note any obvious asymmetries, deformities, or involuntary movements. Are there tremors, tics, or fasciculations (twitches)? If so, note their location, rate, quality, rhythm, amplitude, and relation to your patient's posture, activity, fatigue, emotion, and other factors. For example, if your patient's hand begins to shake only when you ask him to perform a task with it such as writing his name or lifting a spoon, this suggests a postural tremor. Conversely, a tremor at rest that may disappear with voluntary movement suggests Parkinson's disease. To assess involuntary movement, observe your patient throughout the exam.

To determine your patient's muscle bulk, observe the size and contour of his muscles. Look for atrophy, a decrease in bulk and strength; hypertrophy, an increase in bulk and strength; or pseudohypertrophy, an increase in bulk and decrease in strength, as in muscular dystrophy. Flattened or concave contours, especially with fasciculations, may result from lower motor neuron disease. Some degree of muscle atrophy may be a normal part of the aging process or may result from the effects of diabetes on the peripheral nervous system. Look for signs of general muscle atrophy by checking for flattening of the thenar (thumb) muscle and for furrowing between the metacarpals. Unilateral muscle atrophy in the hands suggests median or ulnar nerve paralysis.

To assess muscle tone, feel the muscle's resistance to passive stretching in the extremities. Ask your patient to relax one of her arms. Then put the arm, wrists, hands, and elbows through a moderate range-of-motion exam (Procedure 2–20a). Repeat the exam in the lower extremities. If you detect decreased resistance, shake the hand loosely back and forth. It should move freely, but it should not be floppy (flaccid). Increased resistance may be caused by tension. Does the resistance persist throughout the motion (lead-pipe rigidity) or does it vary? If the resistance increases at the extreme limits of the movement, it is called spasticity. A ratchet-like jerkiness in the resistance is known as "cog-wheel rigidity," a common finding in a patient faking her symptoms or trying to resist your examination. Table 2–12 describes some common muscle tone findings.

Now focus on your patient's muscle strength. First, assess the strength of her grip. Test both grips simultaneously and compare them. Cross your middle finger over the top of your index finger to prevent your fingers from being hurt, then ask your patient to squeeze them as hard as possible (Procedure 2–20b). Normally you will have difficulty removing your fingers from your patient's grip. Continue testing all of the muscle groups listed in Table 2–13. While assessing muscle strength remember that each patient's age, gender, size, and muscular training will affect your exam results. When comparing sides, your patient's dominant side will be stronger. Test for muscle strength by having your patient move actively against your resistance (Procedure 2–20c). If the muscle is too weak to perform against resistance, have her try the movement against gravity or with gravity eliminated (you support the limb). Grade muscle strength on a scale from 0 to 5 (Table 2–14).

Assessing the Motor System

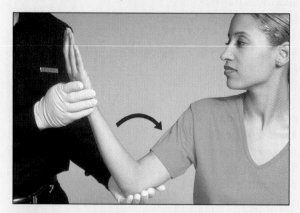

2-20a Assess the elbow's range of motion.

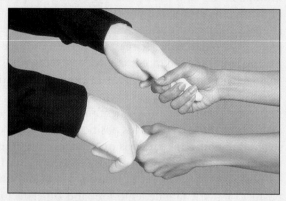

2-20b Test your patient's grip.

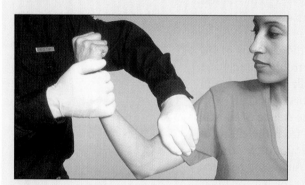

2-20c Test arm strength.

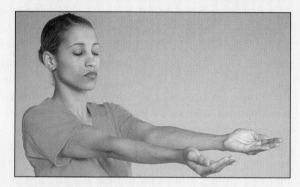

2-20d Test for pronator drift.

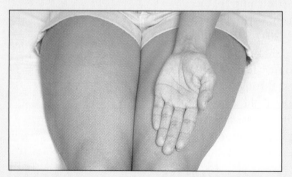

2-20e Test for coordination with rapid alternating movements.

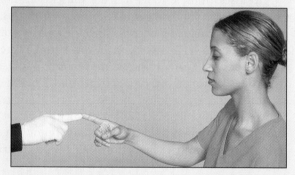

2-20f Test coordination with point-to-point testing.

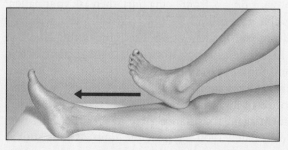

2-20g Assess coordination with heel-to-shin testing.

Table 2-12	Muscle Tone
Finding	Description
Spasticity	Increased tone when passive movement applied, especially at the end of range. Common in stroke.
Rigidity	Increased rigidity throughout movement (lead-pipe). Common in Parkinson's disease and extrapyramidal reactions. Cog-wheel motion is a patient-applied resistance.
Flaccidity	Loss of muscle tone causing limb to be loose. Common in stroke, spinal cord lesion, and Guillain-Barré syndrome.
Paratonia	Sudden changes in tone with passive movement. Can be increased or decreased resistance. Common in dementia.

Table 2-13	Muscle Strength Tests	
Muscles	Nerves	Test
Biceps	C5, C6	Flexion of the elbow
Triceps	C6, C7, C8	Extension of the elbow
Wrist extensors	C6, C7, C8, radial nerve	Extension of the wrist
Fingers	C8, T1, ulnar nerve	Finger abduction
Thumb	C8, T1, median nerve	Thumb opposition
Iliopsoas	L2, L3, L4	Hip flexion
Hip extensor	S1	Hip extension
Hip abductors	L4, L5, S1	Hip abduction
Hip adductors	L2, L3, L4	Hip adduction
Quadriceps	L2, L3, L4	Knee extension
Hamstrings	L4, L5, S1, S2	Knee flexion
Feet	L4, L5	Dorsiflexion
Calf muscles	S1	Plantar flexion

Table 2-14	Muscle Strength Scale
Score	Description
5	Active movement against full resistance with no fatigue
4	Active movement against some resistance and gravity
3	Active movement against gravity
2	Active movement with gravity eliminated
1	Barely palpable muscle contraction with no movement
0	No visible or palpable muscle contraction

To assess your patient's position sense and coordination, first observe his gait. Ask him to walk across the room, turn, and come back. Normally he will be able to maintain his balance, swing his arms at his side, and turn easily. If his gait is ataxic—uncoordinated, reeling, or unstable—suspect cerebellar disease, loss of position sense, or intoxication. Next ask him to walk heel-to-toe in a straight line. This "tandem walking" may reveal an ataxia not previously seen. Now ask your patient to walk first on his toes, then on his heels. This will assess plantar flexion and dorsiflexion of the ankle as well as balance. Next, ask him to hop in place on each foot in turn. Difficulty hopping may result from leg muscle weakness, lack of position sense, or cerebellar dysfunction. Now ask him to do a shallow knee bend on each leg in turn. Difficulty doing this suggests muscle weakness in the pelvic girdle and legs. If your patient is old and unable to hop or do knee bends, have him rise from a sitting position without arm support, or step up onto a stool.

Next perform the Romberg test. Ask her to stand with her feet together and eyes open. Now have her close her eyes for 20 to 30 seconds. Observe her ability to remain upright with minimal swaying and no support. Losing her balance indicates a positive Romberg test caused by ataxia from a loss of position sense. An inability to maintain her balance with her eyes open and feet together represents a cerebellar ataxia. Now check your patient for pronator drift. Ask her to stand with her arms straight out in front of her with her palms up and her eyes closed (Procedure 2–20d). Ask her to maintain this position for 20 to 30 seconds. Normally your patient can do this easily. If one forearm pronates, suspect a mild hemiparesis. If it drifts sideways or upward, suspect a loss of position sense.

To assess your patient's coordination, test for rapid alternating movements. These maneuvers can be difficult to describe, so you should always demonstrate them to your patient. Ask him to repeat them as rapidly as possible while you observe for speed, rhythm, and smoothness. He should repeat all movements with both sides of the body. Keep in mind that his dominant hand usually will perform better than his nondominant hand. If his movements are slow, irregular, and clumsy, suspect cerebellar or extrapyramidal tract disease or upper motor neuron weakness.

First, have your patient tap the distal joint of her thumb with the tip of her index finger as rapidly as possible. Then ask her to place her hand, palm up, on her thigh, quickly turn it over palm down, and return it palm up (Procedure 2–20e). Have her repeat this movement as quickly as possible for 15 seconds; evaluate both hands. Next have her perform point-to-point testing. Ask her to alternate touching your index finger and her nose several times while you observe for accuracy and smoothness (Procedure 2–20f). Note any tremors or difficulty performing this task, indicating cerebellar disease; evaluate both hands. Now assess for point-to-point testing in her legs. Ask her to touch her heel to the opposite knee, then run it down her shin to her big toe (Procedure 2–20g). Note the smoothness and accuracy of her actions. Repeat the test with the other leg. To test your patient's position sense, have her close her eyes and repeat this test for both legs. Abnormalities suggest cerebellar disease.

Assessment Pearls

Two-Point Sensory Discrimination Assessing peripheral sensory function is important for the trauma patient with possible spinal cord injury (or for the back-pain patient with reported sensory loss). Formerly, it was common practice to use a sharp object, such as the pin out of a reflex hammer or a sterile needle, to test for sensory function. However, testing with a sterile needle will often result in bleeding, thus potentially exposing EMS personnel to bloodborne diseases. Instead, pick up a bunch of individually wrapped toothpicks (available at restaurant supply stores). When needed, open the wrapper, take out the toothpick and break it in half. You can use the sharp end to test for sharp sensation and the dull end to test for dull sensation. Take both parts of the broken toothpick, separate them, and test for two-point discrimination. When through, drop the toothpick into the trash.

The Sensory System

The posterior root of the peripheral nerves carries the sensory, or afferent, nerve fibers to the spinal cord and brain along two pathways. The spinothalamic tracts conduct the sensations of pain, temperature, and crude touch. The posterior column of the spinal cord conducts the sensations of position, vibration, and fine touch. Areas of the skin innervated by these afferent fibers are known as dermatomes. A dermatome chart is a road map depicting bands of skin innervated by sensory nerve fibers at each particular spinal level (Figure 2-93 ▶). By learning some basic landmarks, you can begin to identify approximate areas of spinal cord lesions according to the absence of skin sensation.

To assess the sensory system, test for pain, light touch, temperature, position, vibration, and discriminative sensations. Remember to compare distal areas to proximal areas, to compare symmetrical areas bilaterally, and to scatter the stimuli to assess most of the dermatomes. Ask your patient to close his eyes for each of these tests. To test for pain sensation, touch your patient's skin with a sharp object and ask him to tell you whether it is sharp or dull. Compare areas as you move along the different regions, intermittently substituting a dull object for the sharp one. To test for light touch, softly touch him with a fine piece of cotton. Ask him to tell you whenever he feels the cotton. An abnormality suggests a peripheral neuropathy. Test for temperature sensation by touching his skin with a vial filled with either hot or cold liquid. Then test for position

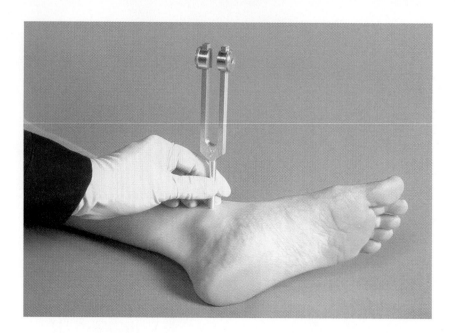

Figure 2-94 Test vibration sense with a tuning fork.

sense by pulling one of his toes upward and asking him to tell you whether it is up or down. Test for vibration sense by placing the stem of a vibrating tuning fork against a bony prominence (Figure 2-94 ▶). Finally, test for discriminative sensation by putting a familiar object, such as a key, in your patient's hand and asking him to identify it.

Reflexes

The sensory pathways manage conscious sensation and participate in the reflex arc. The reflex arc connects some sensory impulses directly to motor neurons, triggering immediate responses to noxious stimuli such as touching your hand to a flame. Deep tendon reflexes are a similar involuntary response to direct muscular stretch. Striking a slightly flexed tendon with a reflex hammer sends an impulse to the spinal cord, where a reflex arc occurs (Figure 2-95 ▶). This immediately sends a motor response back to the tendon, which begins the muscle contraction.

When you perform a nervous system exam, also test your patient's superficial and deep tendon reflexes. Always compare one side to the other. Grade the reflexes on a scale of 0 to 4+ (Table 2–15) and record your findings on a stick figure (Figure 2-96 ▶). A hyperactive response suggests upper motor neuron disease. A diminished response or no response suggests damage to the lower motor neurons or spinal cord.

Deep tendon reflexes can be tested at several places on the body. Use the pointed end of a reflex hammer for striking small areas, the flat end for striking larger areas. First ask your patient to relax. Then properly position the limb you are testing. Quickly strike the tendon using wrist motion only.

Biceps   Support your patient's arm in the slightly flexed position with your thumb directly over the distal biceps tendon in the antecubital space (Procedure 2–21a). Strike your thumbnail with the point of the reflex hammer and watch for contraction of the biceps muscle and the resulting flexion of the elbow. This tests for spinal nerves C5 and C6.

Triceps   Flex your patient's arm at a right angle. With the point of your reflex hammer, strike the triceps tendon along the posterior aspect of the distal humerus (Procedure 2–21b). Watch for triceps contraction and the resulting elbow extension. This tests spinal nerves C6, C7, and C8.

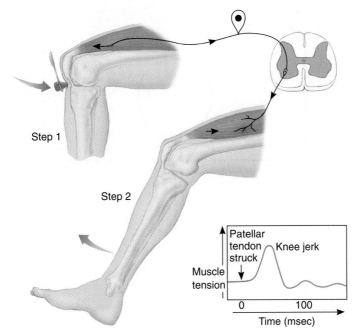

Step 1

Step 2

Patellar tendon struck

Knee jerk

Muscle tension

0   100

Time (msec)

Assessment Pearls

Assessing Deep Tendon Reflexes   For various reasons, it's difficult to test for deep tendon reflexes (DTRs) in some patients. To enhance DTRs, use a technique referred to as augmentation. Have the patient isometrically tense muscles not directly involved in the reflex being tested. For example, if testing patellar DTRs, have the patient grab the fingers of his opposite hand, clench his fists, and try and pull both hands apart with fingers interlocked. When testing upper-extremity DTRs, have the patient clench his jaw or contract his quadriceps. These procedures will augment DTRs and provide a more accurate reading.

Brachioradialis   Support your patient's arm with the forearm slightly pronated (Procedure 2–21c). Now strike his radius about 2 inches above his wrist. Watch for contraction of the brachioradialis and the resulting flexion and supination of the forearm. This tests cervical nerves C5 and C6.

Table 2-15	Reflex Scale
Grade	**Description**
0	No response
+	Diminished, below normal
++	Average, normal
+++	Brisker than normal
++++	Hyperactive, associated with clonus

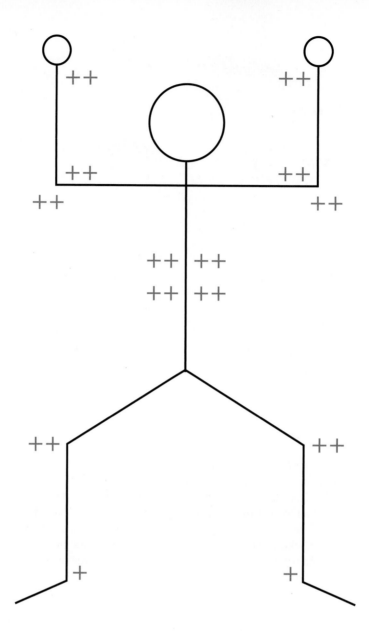

Quadriceps   Have your patient sit with his leg hanging off the end of the exam table. Tap the tendon just below the patella and watch for the quadriceps to contract and extend the knee (Procedure 2–21d). This tests lumbar nerves L2, L3, and L4.

Achilles   With your patient sitting, dorsiflex the foot at the ankle and strike the Achilles tendon (Procedure 2–21e). Watch for the calf muscles to contract and cause plantar flexion of the foot. This tests sacral nerves S1 and S2.

Abdominal/Plantar   Now test the superficial abdominal reflexes and plantar response. These are initiated by stimulating the skin instead of muscle. Assess the plantar reflex by stroking the lateral aspect of the sole from the heel to the ball of your patient's foot, curving medially across the ball (Procedure 2–21f). Begin with the lightest stimulus that will elicit a response. If you detect no response, be more firm. Watch for plantar flexion of the toes. Note if the big toe dorsiflexes while the other toes fan out. Known as a positive **Babinski's response,** this indicates a central nervous system lesion.

Babinski's response

big toe dorsiflexes and the other toes fan out when sole is stimulated.

Test the abdominal reflex by lightly stroking each side of the abdomen above and below the umbilicus with an irregular object such as a reflex hammer, a broken

Testing the Reflexes

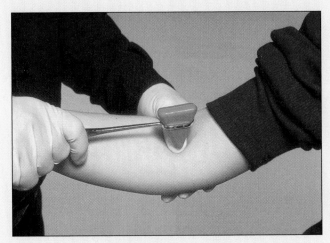

2-21a Test the biceps reflex (cervical nerves C5 and C6).

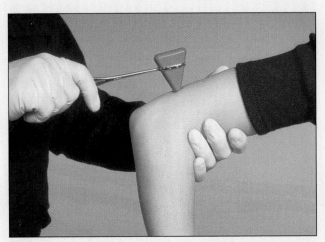

2-21b Test the triceps reflex (cervical nerves C6, C7, and C8).

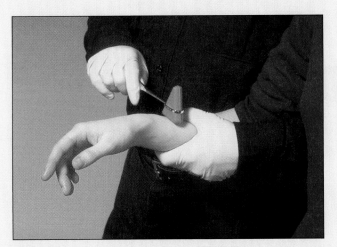

2-21c Test the brachioradialis reflex (cervical nerves C5 and C6).

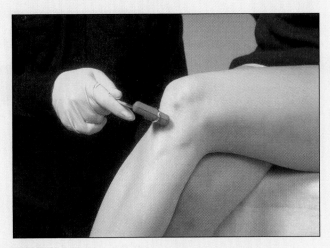

2-21d Test the quadriceps reflex (lumbar nerves L2, L3, and L4).

(continued)

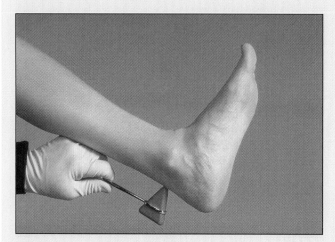

2-21e Test the Achilles reflex (sacral nerves S1 and S2).

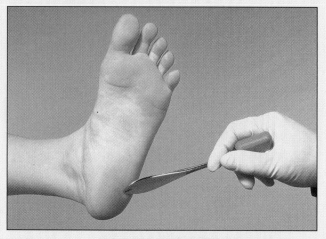

2-21f Test the plantar reflex (central nervous system).

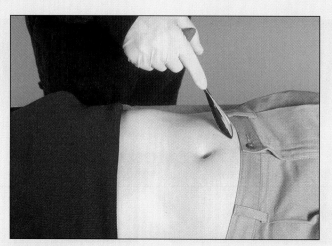

2-21g Test abdominal reflexes (thoracic nerves T8, T9, T10, T11, and T12).

cotton swab, or a split tongue blade (Procedure 2–21g). Note the contraction of the abdominal muscles and how the umbilicus deviates to the stimulus. The area above the umbilicus is innervated by thoracic nerves T8, T9, and T10. The area below the umbilicus is innervated by thoracic nerves T10, T11, and T12. The absence of abdominal reflexes can suggest either a central or peripheral nervous system disorder.

PHYSICAL EXAMINATION OF INFANTS AND CHILDREN

Conducting a physical examination of a sick or injured child can challenge any clinician. Your success will depend on several factors. First, you must be familiar with the anatomical differences between children and adults. Second, you must understand the physical and psychological developmental stages of the different age groups. Most importantly, you must practice these skills daily.

Building Patient and Family Rapport

Children are not just small adults, and you cannot treat them as if they were. Children are naturally apprehensive of strangers and new things. A sick or injured child is a frightened child. He fears pain, separation from his family, and unfamiliar surroundings. Dealing with these fears paves the way for a successful encounter with the child and his parents. You are a stranger. In uniform, you become even more ominous. Gaining your pediatric patient's trust becomes a vital part of your assessment. Unless he requires emergency critical care, take time to establish a rapport with him. This will help to ensure continuous cooperation.

While different age groups have specific fears and characteristics, the following general rules apply to pediatrics as a whole. Remain calm and confident. Be direct and honest about what you are doing, especially if you are performing a painful procedure. If possible, do not separate the child from his parents. Instead, elicit their help in obtaining the history and allow them to help hold the child while you conduct your exam. The more invasive the procedure, the later in the exam you should perform it—unless, of course, your patient is critically ill or injured. (Never delay important procedures or techniques on the critically ill or injured child.) Once your patient begins crying and carrying on, the more difficult the rest of your exam will be, if not impossible. Finally, provide continuous reassurance and feedback to your patient and his family members. This helps reduce everyone's anxiety over what is wrong, what you are doing, and what comes next.

Position yourself at the child's eye level, use a soft voice, and smile a lot. Often a small toy, such as a teddy bear, can distract your patient while you examine him. If you are using diagnostic equipment, allow the child to handle it while you explain how it works. Make sure your movements are slow and deliberate, and explain everything you are doing.

General Appearance and Behavior

Evaluate the child's general appearance and behavior. Ask the parents if his behavior seems normal. Observe his body position and muscle tone, keeping in mind the normal physical and psychological developmental stages of children. Ask yourself two questions: Does your patient look and act like a normal child in the same age group? Do his actions appear normal to you and to his parents? It is best to leave children in a parent's arms while you examine them (Figure 2-97 ▶).

Children are not just small adults, and you cannot treat them as if they were.

The more invasive the procedure, the later in the exam you should perform it.

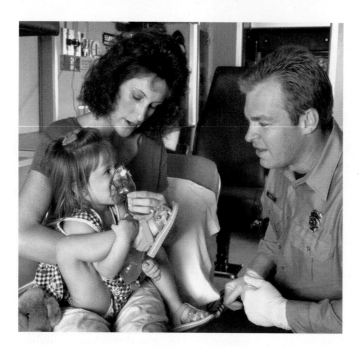

▶ **Figure 2-97** Have parents hold young children while you examine them.

Infants (Newborn–1 Year)   In the newborn or young infant, the arms and legs will flex slightly and move equally (Figure 2-98 ▶). Infants recognize their parents' faces and voices at about 2 months. They are normally alert and like to look around. They also like to be held and kept warm. They are frightened by loud noises and bright lights and may be soothed by having something to suck on. They are somewhat easy to assess because they are not very strong. At 4 to 6 months, they begin to sit up, and they can do so without assistance by 8 months. They are easily distracted by a toy or shiny object. They are very distressed by separation from their parents. Since they will not understand what you are doing or why you are there, they probably will resist being examined. It is best to examine any child under the age of 1 from toe to head.

Toddlers (1–3 Years)   Toddlers should be able to walk by their 18th month (Figure 2-99 ▶). They love to disagree with everyone and everything, and they trust no one but their parents. They are the most difficult age group to examine, even when they are not sick or hurt. They do not want you to touch them, so be prepared to take opportunities to assess areas as they become available. You may want to limit your assessment of the very ill or injured toddler to the most important areas. For example, focus on the chest and lungs of any child in respiratory distress. Do the vital areas first, before the child becomes agitated and makes the rest of your exam nearly impossible. Toddlers do like to be distracted with toys; if possible, make a game of the examination. In addition, because toddlers are beginning to sense their dignity, always respect their modesty.

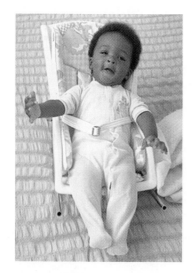

▶ **Figure 2-98** Infant (newborn–1 year).

Preschoolers (3–6 Years)   Preschoolers (Figure 2-100 ▶) are particularly distrusting of strangers. Talk with them, gain their trust, and answer their questions honestly. Always prepare them if something you are going to do may hurt. Tell them it may hurt and that it's all right to cry. They have a great fear of being hurt and of the sight of their own blood. They fear mutilation of their bodies, and the slightest injury may result in a temporarily hysterical child. Always cover a preschooler's wounds quickly, so he won't have to look at them. Often, injured or sick children in this age group feel guilty about their problem, as if it is their fault, regardless of the circumstances. Approach them slowly and offer a calming reassurance that they will be all right.

Assessment Pearls

Estimate a Child's Weight Pediatric drug dosages and other therapies are often based on a child's weight. Because of this, it's important to try to determine a pediatric patient's weight. Often, a parent can provide a fairly reliable weight from a recent doctor's visit or measurement at home, but, sometimes, they're unsure. Fortunately, children tend to grow at approximately the same rate. Therefore, height should correspond to weight.

Before your next pediatric patient, place a starting mark low on a pediatric backboard or immobilization device and mark each centimeter up the board. Thus, when you have a child whose weight is undetermined, lay the child on the board with his feet at 0 cm and measure his height. Once you have the height, look at a pediatric growth chart. If you have a boy who is 18 months old and 32 cm in length, his weight is likely +/– 18 kg (40 lb.).

These charts are commonly used by pediatricians and pediatric units and give the average weight, by percentile, for a given height. Charts are available for children from birth to 26 months of age (one for boys and one for girls) and for older children ages 2 to 19 years (again, separate charts for boys and girls). Most pediatricians will give you these charts, or you can get them from a hospital nursery. Laminate and keep them for reference.

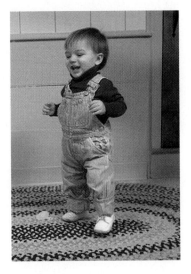

▶ **Figure 2-99** Toddler (1–3 years).

School-Age (6–12 Years)

School-age children (Figure 2-101 ▶) will cooperate with you if you gain their trust. They want to participate and to remain somewhat in control. Allow them to participate in the exam and to make treatment choices whenever possible. They have a basic understanding of their bodies, but they still fear separation, pain, and punishment. Modesty becomes more important, and they will not like being examined. Talk honestly with them about what you are doing and prepare them for what will come next as you proceed.

Adolescents (13–18 Years)

Adolescents (Figure 2-102 ▶) can be treated much the same as adults. Since a teenager's modesty is extremely important, have a person of the same sex examine this patient if possible. Otherwise, conduct the physical exam just as you would for an adult patient.

Always cover a preschooler's wounds quickly, so he won't have to look at them.

Allow school-age children to participate in the exam and to make treatment choices whenever possible.

Hoarseness, suggesting an upper airway obstruction, or moaning, suggesting decreased consciousness, requires intervention and rapid transport.

Anatomy and the Physical Exam

To assess a child properly, you must understand his unique anatomy (Figure 2-103 ▶). The anatomical differences among age groups will alter your interpretation of physical findings. For example, since an infant's skin is thinner and contains less subcutaneous fat, you can expect environmental temperature extremes to affect him more severely.

This section deals with examining infants and children in the clinical situation. The pediatric chapter in Volume 5, *Special Considerations/Operations*, discusses a more detailed pediatric assessment.

General Appearance

Especially in the emergency setting, note whether your patient looks toxic, or sick. A toxic child appears not to recognize or respond to his parents. He may look tired and have a decreased respiratory effort and may have mottled skin or a generalized rash. He may be gray or cyanotic and just look very sick, usually from some type of bacterial process. These children, who present with the signs and symptoms of respiratory

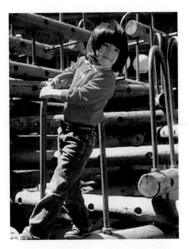

▶ **Figure 2-100** Preschooler (3–6 years).

failure or shock, usually require rapid transport while you provide aggressive resuscitation procedures (advanced airway management, oxygenation and ventilation, intravenous access, and rapid fluid administration).

Head and Neck

The bones of the skull are soft and the fontanelles ("soft spots," spaces between a child's cranial bones) stay open until about 18 months (Figure 2-104 ▶). From this time until about age 5, cartilage connects the sutures. This allows the skull to expand as the brain grows. Check the sutures for bulging (increased intracranial pressure) or sunkenness (dehydration). In infants, a soft bulging spot following a history of trauma suggests a head injury with increasing intracranial pressure. The same finding associated with a fever suggests meningitis.

Because a child's airways are so much smaller than an adult's, a minor obstruction can create an acute respiratory problem. Watch the child's face for signs of distress and increased respiratory effort, such as nasal flaring. Children in acute respiratory distress will appear anxious and not interested in their surroundings. Also watch for retractions and head bobbing. Listen for stridor, wheezing, and grunting as further signs of severe breathing problems. As the child speaks, listen for hoarseness (upper airway obstruction) or moaning (decreasing level of consciousness). These findings always require appropriate intervention and rapid transport. Remember, a crying or screaming child has a patent airway.

Observe the child's face for signs of pain and discomfort as you continue your examination. Inspect his eyes as you would an adult's. Assess the outer ear for position. The top of the ear should be on a horizontal line with the outer corner of the eye. As a child grows, the anatomy of the external ear canal changes. In infancy the canal curves downward, so you should pull down the auricle to see the tympanic membrane at the distal end of the canal. As the child grows, the canal starts to move up and backward, and the ear is relatively higher and farther back on the head. Remember to pull the auricle upward and backward to afford the best view with the otoscope. Brace your hand against the child's skull to prevent injury from sudden movement.

Choose the largest speculum that will fit comfortably into the child's ear. Tilt the child's head away from you. Hold the otoscope firmly in one hand and, with your free hand, pull the ear appropriately to straighten the ear canal. Slowly insert the speculum one fourth to one half inch into the canal. Observe the amount, texture, and color of wax and the presence of foreign bodies. Inspect the tympanic membrane for color, light reflex, and bony landmarks. Repeat the same steps for the other ear.

Inspect the child's mouth much the same as you would for the adult. A young child's mouth is small, while the tongue is relatively large, so examining his oral cavity will be a challenge. Examine the nose using the nasal speculum and penlight or the appropriate attachment to the otoscope. To examine the mucous membrane, tip the child's head back and use the otoscope to inspect for color or swelling.

Evaluate the child's neck for stiffness, which—when associated with a fever—suggests meningitis. Evaluate for lymphadenopathy (enlarged lymph nodes) in the neck by assessing the nodes' size, warmth, tenderness, and mobility. Certain infectious diseases like mononucleosis, rubella, and mumps are associated with lymphadenopathy. Nodes commonly feel enlarged due to recurrent upper respiratory infection.

Chest and Lungs

The rib cage in infants and small children is elastic and flexible. Because it comprises more cartilage than bone at this age, rib fractures are rare. On the other hand, lung contusions are common, because the lung tissue is very fragile. Small children also

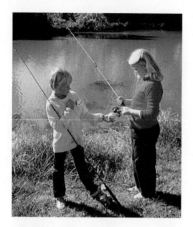

▶ **Figure 2-101** School-age (6–12 years).

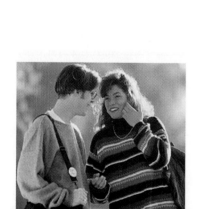

▶ **Figure 2-102** Adolescent (13–18 years). (© Index Stock Imagery, Inc.)

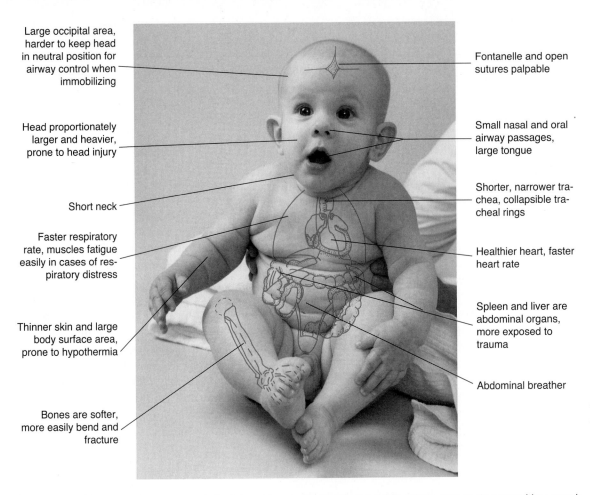

Large occipital area, harder to keep head in neutral position for airway control when immobilizing

Head proportionately larger and heavier, prone to head injury

Short neck

Faster respiratory rate, muscles fatigue easily in cases of respiratory distress

Thinner skin and large body surface area, prone to hypothermia

Bones are softer, more easily bend and fracture

Fontanelle and open sutures palpable

Small nasal and oral airway passages, large tongue

Shorter, narrower trachea, collapsible tracheal rings

Healthier heart, faster heart rate

Spleen and liver are abdominal organs, more exposed to trauma

Abdominal breather

▶ **Figure 2-103** Pediatric anatomy and physiology. You must understand a child's unique anatomy to assess him properly.

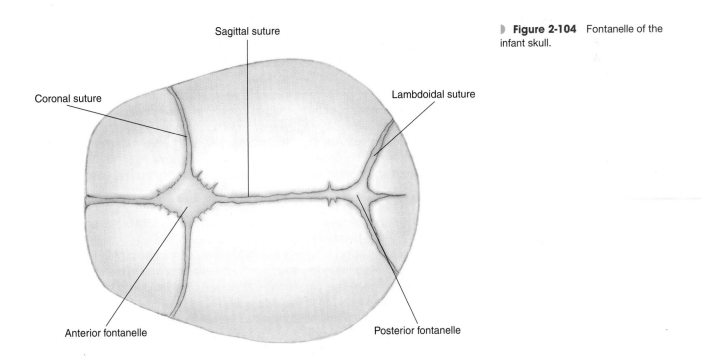

Sagittal suture

Coronal suture

Lambdoidal suture

Anterior fontanelle

Posterior fontanelle

▶ **Figure 2-104** Fontanelle of the infant skull.

Table 2-16	Normal Pediatric Vital Signs		
Age Group	Respiratory Rate	Heart Rate	Systolic BP
Newborn	30–60	100–180	60–90
Infant	30–60	100–160	87–105
Toddler	24–40	80–110	95–105
Preschooler	22–34	70–110	95–110
School-age	18–30	65–110	97–112
Adolescent	12–26	60–90	112–128

have a mobile mediastinum with a greater tendency to develop a tension pneumothorax. The chest muscles are not well developed, so children are mostly diaphragm breathers until about age 7.

The chest muscles are considered accessory muscles in the young child; to evaluate his breathing, observe both the chest and abdomen for movement. A child in severe respiratory distress may exhibit a "see-saw" pattern in which his sternum and abdomen rise and fall in opposition to each other. Count the respiratory rate without touching your patient, if possible. Assess the rate, quality, and depth of his respirations. Normal respiratory rates vary with age, but generally they decrease as the child grows older. Table 2–16 gives normal vital signs for the various pediatric age groups. Auscultate for breath sounds with the bell of your stethoscope at the midaxillary line (Figure 2-105 ▶). Use this location to avoid hearing transmitted breath sounds from the opposite lung fields.

Assessment Pearls

Assessing Pediatric Breath Sounds   Many EMS calls involving children are for respiratory system complaints, and it's critical to adequately assess the child's respiratory system, including breath sounds. This can prove challenging when the child is frightened, as they often are in the presence of strangers—especially when they're ill. Try to obtain their trust; consider having the child sit in his parent's lap.

It's often difficult to get a child to take a deep breath. Either he doesn't understand what you're asking, or he's afraid to comply. In these cases, some visual imagery often proves helpful. Engage the parent's assistance by pretending to hold a candle or birthday cake. Ask the child to blow, just as if he's blowing out a candle. Get the parent to do this once, and the child will often follow.

When the child prepares to "blow out the candle," listen to his chest. He will take a deep breath, and you can usually accurately auscultate the chest. Have him repeat the "candle blowing" until your auscultation is complete. As an alternative, use your fingers as the candles, folding them down as the child blows and repeating as many times as needed for adequate auscultation.

Another visualization technique is to ask the child if he's heard of the story "The Three Little Pigs." If so, have the child imitate the big bad wolf in the story and attempt to blow down the little pigs' house. When the child inhales to blow down the pigs' house, you can hear breath sounds well.

Always follow a standardized approach when assessing the chest: inspection, palpation, percussion (if indicated), and auscultation.

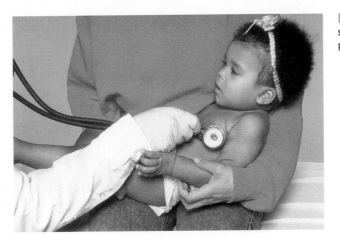

Figure 2-105 Place your stethoscope along your young patient's midaxillary line.

Cardiovascular

Unless the child has a congenital defect, his heart will be strong and healthy. His heart rate will vary with age, but generally it will decrease as he gets older. If the child is alert and uncooperative, measure his pulse rate by listening to the heart. Place your stethoscope between the sternum and nipple on your patient's left side. Children have thin chest walls, so you will usually be able to observe the apical impulse of the heart. Remember that tachycardia or bradycardia can be a response to hypoxia in infants and young children. Bradycardia is the initial response to this condition in the newborn; without aggressive intervention, cardiopulmonary arrest will soon follow. Blood pressure will vary in children, but generally it will rise as they grow older. Children respond to hypovolemia by increasing cardiac function.

Tachycardia or bradycardia can be a response to hypoxia in infants and young children; without aggressive intervention, cardiopulmonary arrest will soon follow.

Abdomen

A child's liver and spleen are proportionally larger and more vascular than an adult's. Thus they extend beyond the rib cage and are more exposed. Likewise, the child's immature abdominal muscles provide less protection than an adult's. Inspect the abdomen first for movement. Normally only respiratory movements should be visible; peristalsis is not normally observable. Next, assess contour. The abdomen normally bulges by the end of inspiration. Note any asymmetry. Inspect the groin area for inguinal hernias, common in male children. Finally, look at the umbilicus for any hernias, common in children under 3 years. Percuss and auscultate the abdomen as in the adult.

Before you begin palpating the abdomen, make sure the child is comfortable. Bend his knees to relax the abdominal muscles and make palpation easier. Your hands should be warm. If the child is ticklish, cover his hands with yours as you palpate. Begin with light palpation and gradually increase the pressure (Figure 2-106 ▶). Palpate all four quadrants. Deep palpation is performed next. You are feeling for masses and tenderness. The child's facial expression is a better guide to pain than his words, since he may interpret your pressure as pain.

Musculoskeletal

Evaluate pulses, sensation, movement, and warmth in all four extremities. Check for capillary refill (Figure 2-107 ▶) and feel for peripheral pulses. Evaluate the skin, which reveals important clues in children. Its color, turgor, moisture, and temperature are key indicators of his cardiovascular system's condition. Unlike the adult's, the child's

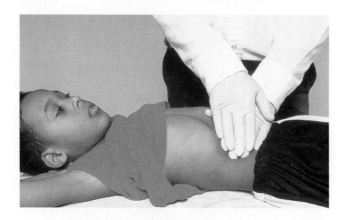

Figure 2-106 Gradually increase the pressure when palpating a young patient's abdomen.

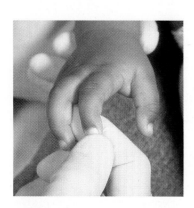

Figure 2-107 Pressing a child's fingernail is one of several ways to assess capillary refill. The child's capillary refill time is a good indicator of the child's peripheral perfusion status.

capillary refill time accurately reflects his peripheral perfusion status. When examining the musculoskeletal system, remember the growth and posture at different stages of the child's development. For example, a toddler walks with a broad base for support and is likely to appear bowlegged. A teenager with poor posture may suffer from a skeletal problem such as scoliosis.

Palpate the upper and lower extremities for swelling, tenderness, and contractions. Next have the child demonstrate the range of motion of his joints while you feel for smoothness of movement. Examine all joints. Check muscle strength in all muscle groups by asking the child to prevent you from moving a part of his body. A child's bones are more likely to break at the ends, where growth takes place. Until the child reaches adolescence, when these areas become as strong as the rest of the bone, injuries that occur near the joints are more likely to damage the bone than the ligaments or tendons. Assess the child's muscle coordination by having him stand and then hop on one foot. Repeat this for the other foot. Children usually enjoy this aspect of the physical examination. You can also have the child skip or jump.

Nervous System

The child's general behavior, level of consciousness, and orientation are signs of cerebral function. You have asked the parents to comment on their child's behavior during the history taking. You have observed the child's behavior throughout the examination and already have learned much about his cerebral function by interacting with him. Now test specific functions such as language and recall. You will have checked most of the 12 cranial nerves during your head and neck exam.

You can test for cerebellar function with several games that children usually enjoy. First, as you move your finger, ask the child to touch his nose and then your finger. Consistent past-pointing should arouse your suspicion. An alternate test is to have the child pat his knees alternately with the palms and backs of his hands. Check for sensation over the child's face, trunk, arms, and leg. Check for hot and cold sensation by alternately touching the skin with warm and cold test tubes. Ask the child to close his eyes and tell you which he feels. Be sure to test for reflexes on both sides of the body, just as with an adult. If the child has difficulty relaxing, test the parent's reflexes to show that it does not hurt.

Remember, the most important characteristic of a physical assessment is thoroughness. Be systematic in your approach and, with practice, you will be able to do a complete and accurate physical assessment.

The most important characteristic of a physical assessment is thoroughness.

RECORDING EXAMINATION FINDINGS

After you perform the history and physical examination, it is time to record the findings on your patient's chart, or permanent medical record. The information you enter enables you and other members of the health care team to identify health problems, make a diagnosis, plan the appropriate care, and monitor your patient's response to treatment. The patient record is only as good as the accuracy, depth, and detail you provide.

All health care clinicians follow a standard format when charting patient information. Using it and appropriate medical terminology will allow everyone to easily read and understand your assessment findings. While your first attempts at writing a complete history and physical exam will be lengthy and possibly disorganized, clinical experience will eventually lead to a more efficient and organized record.

Your patient's chart is a legal document, and any information you enter may be used in court. Proper documentation is vital to your protection. Present the data legibly, accurately, and truthfully. They should represent the findings of your history and physical examination—no more, no less. State your assessment, your analysis of the problem, and your management plan clearly and exactly. No question should ever arise about your assessment or care of your patient if you document it properly.

Be sure to include all data about your assessment. You cannot formulate an impression unless you have clearly spelled out the positive and negative details upon which it was made. Remember that the absence of a sign or symptom (pertinent negative) may be just as important as its presence. Record everything in writing. If you do not document a neuro exam, you will never convince anyone that you performed it, especially not a plaintiff's lawyer or a jury. Be complete but avoid unnecessary words. For example, say "pale," not "pale in color." Also avoid lengthy repetitive phrases such as "patient states." Use accepted abbreviations and symbols whenever possible. Avoid using vague adjectives such as *good, normal,* and *poor,* because they are open to interpretation by other providers. Document what your patient tells you, not what you infer or interpret. Use direct quotes whenever possible.

The universally accepted organization for patient charts follows the SOAP format. SOAP stands for *S*ubjective, *O*bjective, *A*ssessment, and *P*lan. Use this format when writing your patient's chart. Subjective information is what your patient tells you. It comprises the chief complaint, the history of present illness, the past history, the current health status, and the review of systems. Objective information includes the data collected from the general survey, vital signs, head-to-toe anatomical exam, systems-oriented exam, and neurologic exam, including the mental status. These are the data you gathered by inspection, palpation, percussion, auscultation, and other techniques of physical examination. Objective information also includes the results of any laboratory tests. The assessment summarizes the relevant data for each problem identified in the history and physical exam. The plan outlines your management strategy in three categories: diagnostic (how you will assess progress), therapeutic (any treatments), and educational (what you need to teach your patient). Figure 2-108 offers an example of documentation for a comprehensive physical examination. Chapter 6 deals with prehospital documentation in detail.

The patient record is only as good as the accuracy, depth, and detail you provide.

Record everything in writing.

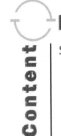

Review

Content

SOAP

- *S*ubjective
- *O*bjective
- *A*ssessment
- *P*lan

Screening Exam Report

Patient: Jane Doe
Location: University Hospital
Date: 11/11/1998
Examiner: David Cywinski, MD
Jane Doe is a healthy appearing 24 yo white female who has come into the office for a physical for entrance into medical school.

Past History

General Health Good	
Childhood illnesses	Measles and chickenpox
Adult illnesses	2 year history of PUD
	Appendectomy 1992 without sequelae
	Last physical exam 1995 for college athletics
Psychiatric illnesses	None
Injuries	None
Operations	None

Current Health Status

Medications	Zantac
Allergies	Sulfa drugs
	Bee stings
Tobacco	5 pack year smoker (no desire to quit, will follow up)
Alcohol/drugs	2-3 drinks/week, CAGE negative
Tests	PAP smear 05/1997 normal, no mammograms
Exercise/leisure	No time

Family History

Single female living alone
Mother   54 yo — healthy
Father   57 yo — MI 1993
Brother   20 yo — healthy
Grandparents both deceased prior to patient's birth, no information available
Patient denies history of genetic diseases

Psychosocial History

Born in Syracuse, NY. Grew up here.
Graduated from University of Rochester (Biology)

Review of Systems

General: Patient reports to be in good health.

HEENT: Denies headaches, diplopia, blurred vision, eye pain or redness, decreased visual acuity. Also denies hearing loss, tinnitus, vertigo. No report of sinusitis, PND, epistaxis, bleeding from gums, oral ulceration or growths, sore throats.

Pulmonary: Denies cough, hemoptysis, dyspnea, pleuritic chest pain, wheezing, asthma, or recurrent infections. No history of occupational exposures. Last TB test done 3 weeks ago by school. Results — negative.

Cardiac: Denies chest pain or pressure, palpitations, orthopnea, PND, SOB, pedal edema, heart murmur, HTN, or MVP.

GU: Denies dysuria, hematuria, polyuria. No history of UTIs or renal calculi. Onset of menses at 13 yoa. States she has a regular 28 day cycle with 4 days of bleeding. No history of abnormal vaginal discharge, STDs. No history of pregnancy. SBE done monthly, instructed by her OB/GYN physician.

GI: Denies weight gain or loss, nausea, vomiting, diarrhea, melena, hemorrhoids. History of PUD that started 2 years ago when she decided to go to medical school and had to "buckle down" and do well in school. Pain becomes worse when her workload increases and when she eats spicy food. She describes the pain as burning and sometimes ascending into esophagus. Medication and relaxation alleviate the symptoms.

Neuro: Denies dizziness, syncope, seizures, paresthesia, weakness, or tremors.

Rheum: Denies arthritic pain, joint stiffness or swelling. No history of Lyme disease, back pain.

Vascular: Denies phlebitis, varicose veins, cramping or Raynauds.

Endocrine: Denies polyuria, polydipsia, polyphagia, cold-heat intolerance, tachycardia, fatigue.

▶ **Figure 2-108**   Patient documentation for a comprehensive physical examination.

(continued)

Heme: Denies easy bruising, bleeding, or anemia. No prior history of transfusion. Patient reports A+ blood group, does donate blood with Red Cross. Denies lymph node enlargement.

Derm: Denies rashes, nevi, dryness, pruritis, or pigmentation change.

Psych: Denies depression, panic-anxiety attacks, memory disturbances, personality changes, or hallucinations.

Physical Exam

General appearance: Jane Doe is an alert, oriented, well developed 24 yo white female in no apparent distress.

VS: BP — 124/78, Pulse — 64 regular both radials, Resp — 16, Temp — not taken, appears afebrile.

HEENT: Head — Normocephalic with scar above OS, pt had sutures above OS from falling off coffee table when she was 2 yoa. Eyes — Visual acuity 20/20 with pocket chart, does not wear glasses. PERLA, EOM intact, sclera white, visual fields intact. Retinal vessels visualized and appeared normal. Ears — Pinnae nontender as well as external ear canal. Gross hearing intact to whispers. Weber test lateralizes to left ear with a normal Rhinne test. Tympanic membrane grey without erythema. Nose — mucosa pink with exudate, no polyps noted. Throat — mucosa, buccal and gingival, pink without exudate, no ulcers or growths noted. Uvula midline.

Neck: Trachea midline, no JVD noted at 45 degrees, thyroid not palpable. Good cartoid pulses. ROM intact. No carotid bruits heard.

Pulmonary: Chest symmetrical, normal respiratory expansion, breath sounds clear bilaterally, no egophony or whispered pectoriloquy. Diaphragmatic excursion equal at 6 cm. Normal resonance to percussion.

Cardiac: PMI not palpated, S_1, S_2 heard at aortic and pulmonic locations. Tricuspid and mitral valves not auscultated. S_1, S_2 at above noted sites sounded clear without murmurs, clicks or snaps.

Abdomen: Small scar 3 cm noted in right lower quadrant, appears to have healed well. Otherwise, abdomen is symmetrical. Bowel sounds heard in all four quadrants. No bruits heard over renals, iliacs, or aorta. Liver not palpable, span 8 cm with percussion and scratch test. Spleen not palpable. No CVA tenderness. No masses noted on palpation. Aorta 2 cm in width.

GU/Rectal: Not done.

Musculoskeletal: General muscle tone appears good, no atrophy noted, gross symmetry apparent. No joint swelling or deformity noted. Range of motion intact for all four extremities. Spinal contour appropriate without scoliosis noted.

Nodes: Submental, submandibular, preauricular, postauricular, occipital, cervical chain, supraclavicular, axillary, epitrochlear, inguinal nodes not palpable.

Breast: Not done.

Vascular/Pulses:

Carotid 2+   2+
Radial 2+   2+
Aorta 2+
Femoral 2+ 2+
Popliteal 1+ (equal bilateral)
Dorsalis 1+   1+

No varicose veins noted, bruits were not heard in carotid, aorta, renal, femoral regions.

Extremities: No clubbing, cyanosis, edema, pigmentation change noted. Capillary refill < 2 seconds, nails nonpitted.

Neuro: Patient is alert and responsive.
Cranial Nerves I — XII
    I — not tested
    II — PERLA
    III — PERLA EOM, intact
    IV — EOM intact
    V — Facial sensation intact, muscles of mastication intact/operable
    VI — EOM intact
    VII — Muscles of facial expression intact, symmetrical
    VIII — Hearing grossly intact to whispers, balance intact

(continued)

IX — Gag reflex intact
X — Gag reflex intact, uvula midline
XI — Sternocleidomastoid, trapezius functioning symmetrically
XII — Tongue protrudes midline

Sensory intact to both sharp and dull stimuli. Rhomberg negative. Joint position and sense intact. Two-point discrimination intact and appropriate. Reflexes as follows:

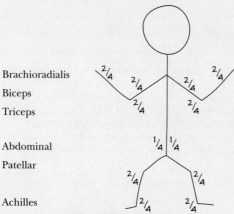

Brachioradialis

Biceps

Triceps

Abdominal

Patellar

Achilles

Babinskis were downgoing bilateral.

Problem list: 1. PUD
2. Abnormal Weber test
3. Smoker

Plan: 1. Continue medications for PUD and instruct patient on stress reduction techniques. If PUD continues, consider biopsy for *H. Pylori*.
2. Refer patient for audiogram
3. At next visit, discuss perils of smoking and advantages of cessation program

David Cywinski, MD
SUNY HSC @ Syracuse

▶ **Figure 2-108** *(continued)*

▶ Summary

This chapter has presented both a regional and a systems approach to physical examination. The setting, chief complaint, and clinical status of your patient will dictate how much of the physical exam you actually use. For example, if you are hired to conduct preemployment physicals, you may decide to conduct a complete examination. If you are at the scene of a critically ill or injured patient, you will assess only those areas relevant to the situation. If your patient presents with a minor, isolated musculoskeletal injury, you may focus your exam on that area and system. As you become more experienced, making these decisions will become easier.

▶ You Make the Call

Your crew from the Barnes Ambulance Service is at a standby at the annual 10K fun run to benefit the St. Joseph's Hospital pediatric clinic. Several hundred runners began the race on this very warm and muggy day. Thirty minutes into the race, when the serious runners begin crossing the finish line, you receive a call to the turnaround point 3 miles away. Approaching the scene, you find a woman in her 30s on the side of the road. She is in moderate distress, clutching her right ankle. You ask the runner what happened. The runner says that she stepped into a small pothole and twisted her ankle. You instruct your partner, EMT-Basic Darlene Harris, to remove the victim's shoes and socks.

1. How would you begin the exam?
2. What is your differential field diagnosis?
3. What elements of the history are appropriate to ask this patient?
4. Outline your physical exam.

See Suggested Responses at the back of this book.

▶ Review Questions

1. In addition to assessing your patient's skin condition and peripheral pulses, you may choose to use this technique as a reassuring gesture.
   a. fremitus
   b. percussion
   c. touch
   d. auscultation

2. Four basic techniques form the foundation of a formal physical examination. These techniques include all of the following EXCEPT:
   a. inspection.
   b. palpitation.
   c. auscultation.
   d. percussion.

3. During a physical examination, primary indicators of your patient's health include pulse, respiration, blood pressure, and body temperature. These indicators are called the:
   a. initial assessment.
   b. preferred devices.
   c. vital signs.
   d. critical evaluators.

4. Terms such as *bounding* or *thready* are used to describe the quality of your patient's:
   a. blood pressure.
   b. respiration.
   c. pulse.
   d. voice.

5. Which of the following is not commonly noted in a patient who presents with bradycardia?
   a. head injury
   b. hypothermia
   c. severe hypoxia
   d. fever

6. The amount of air your patient moves in and out of his lungs in one breath is the:
   a. tidal volume.
   b. minute volume.
   c. PEEP.
   d. CPAP.

7. The sounds of the blood hitting the arterial walls are called:
   a. bruits.
   b. heart sounds.
   c. diastolic murmurs.
   d. Korotkoff sounds.

8. The term _____ refers to blood pressure greater than normal.
   a. hypotension
   b. hypertension
   c. normotension
   d. hypovolemia

9. Hypovolemia may be suggested if, after performing a tilt test, the patient's pulse rate has:
   a. decreased by 10 to 20 beats per minute.
   b. decreased by 6 to 8 beats per minute.
   c. increased by 6 to 8 beats per minute.
   d. increased by 10 to 20 beats per minute.

10. To conduct a comprehensive physical examination, you will need all of the following equipment EXCEPT a/an:
    a. stethoscope.
    b. sphygmomanometer.
    c. modulator.
    d. ophthalmoscope.

11. In reference to the physical exam, your patient's vital statistics include his:
    a. height and weight.
    b. age and height.
    c. weight and sex.
    d. weight and age.

12. As you are conducting the physical examination on your patient, you note a large mass that pulsates. This finding is suggestive of a/an:
    a. malignancy.
    b. aneurysm.
    c. sarcoma.
    d. cyst.

13. The cochlea is a coiled structure that transmits sound to the:
    a. vagus nerve.
    b. optic nerve.
    c. facial nerve.
    d. acoustic nerve.

14. The medical term _____ refers to discharge from the ear canal.
    a. otorrhea
    b. rhinorrhea
    c. mastoiditis
    d. Battle's sign

15. The liver is normally located in which abdominal quadrant?
    a. LLQ
    b. RLQ
    c. RUQ
    d. LUQ

16. The medical term for the crunching sounds of unlubricated parts rubbing against each other is:
    a. arthritis.
    b. crepitus.
    c. bursitis.
    d. tendonitis.

17. The medical term _____ refers to a droopy eyelid.
    a. nystagmus
    b. strabismus
    c. conjugate
    d. ptosis

18. Abnormal nail findings include all of the following EXCEPT:
    a. clubbing.
    b. paronychia.
    c. scoliosis.
    d. onycholysis.

19. You note an increase in your patient's pulse pressure. This change may indicate:
    a. decreasing intracranial pressure.
    b. increasing intracranial pressure.
    c. impending hypertension.
    d. late-stage hypotension.

20. The bell of your stethoscope should be used to auscultate:
    a. blood pressure.
    b. arterial bruits.
    c. heart sounds.
    d. lung sounds.

See Answers to Review Questions at the back of this book.

▶ Further Reading

Bates, Barbara, Lynn S. Bickley, and Robert A. Hoekelman. *A Guide to Physical Examination and History Taking.* 9th ed. Philadelphia: Lippincott, Williams & Wilkins, 2005.

Bledsoe, B. E., and F. Martini. *Anatomy and Physiology for Emergency Care.* 2nd ed. Upper Saddle River, N.J.: Pearson/Prentice Hall, 2008.

Bledsoe, B. E., R. A. Porter, and R. A. Cherry. "Twenty-five Tricks and Pearls of Physical Examination." *Journal of Emergency Medical Services (JEMS)*, March 2005.

Bradford, C. A. *Basic Ophthalmology for Medical Students and Primary Care Residents.* 8th ed. San Francisco: American Academy of Ophthalmology, 2004.

DeLorenzo, Robert. "Sneezes, Wheezes, and Breezes—Listening to the Chest." *Journal of Emergency Medical Services* 20 (October 1995): 58–69.

Eichelberger, Martin R., et al. *Pediatric Emergencies: A Manual for Prehospital Care Providers.* 2nd ed. Upper Saddle River, N.J.: Pearson/Prentice Hall, 1998.

Epstein, Owen, et al. *Clinical Examination.* 3rd ed. St. Louis: Mosby, 2003.

Foltin, George, et al. *Teaching Resource for Instructors in Prehospital Pediatrics for Paramedics.* New York: Center for Pediatric Medicine, 2002.

Netter, F. H. *Netter's Atlas of Human Anatomy.* 4th ed. St. Louis, Mosby, 2006.

Ralston, M., et al., eds. *Pediatric Advanced Life Support Provider Manual.* Dallas: American Heart Association, 2006.

Seidel, Henry M., et al. *Mosby's Guide to Physical Examination.* 6th ed. St. Louis: Mosby, 2006.

Spaite, David W., et al. "A Prospective Evaluation of Prehospital Patient Assessment by Direct In-field Observation: Failure of ALS Personnel to Measure Vital Signs." *Prehospital and Disaster Medicine* 5 (October–December 1990): 325–333.

Willms, Janice L., Henry Schniederman, and Paula S. Algranati. *Physical Diagnosis: Bedside Evaluation of Diagnosis and Function.* Baltimore: Williams & Wilkins, 1994.

Yanoff, M., et al. *Ophthalmology.* 2nd ed. St. Louis: Elsevier Science, 2004.

▶ Media Resources

See the Student CD at the back of this book for quizzes, animations, videos and other features related to this chapter. In particular, take a look at the Virtual Tours of the airway, cardiovascular system, heart, nervous system, and musculoskeletal system. See the animations on flexion, extension, and other movements of the extremities. In addition, look at the interactivities on use of the otoscope and the oral exam as well as videos on various specific aspects of the physical exam. Also, visit the Companion Website for Brady's paramedic series at **www.prenhall.com/bledsoe,** where you will find additional reinforcement and links to other resources.

Patient Assessment in the Field

Objectives

After reading this chapter, you should be able to:

1. Recognize hazards/potential hazards associated with the medical and trauma scene. (pp. 187–194)
2. Identify unsafe scenes and describe methods for making them safe. (pp. 187–194)
3. Discuss common mechanisms of injury/nature of illness. (pp. 196–198)
4. Predict patterns of injury based on mechanism of injury. (pp. 196–197, 211–213)
5. Discuss the reason for identifying the total number of patients at the scene. (pp. 195–196)
6. Organize the management of a scene following size-up. (pp. 195–196)
7. Explain the reasons for identifying the need for additional help or assistance during the scene size-up. (pp. 190–196)
8. Summarize the reasons for forming a general impression of the patient. (pp. 198–199)
9. Discuss methods of assessing mental status/levels of consciousness in the adult, child, and infant patient. (pp. 200–201)
10. Discuss methods of assessing and securing the airway in the adult, child, and infant patient. (pp. 201–206)
11. State reasons for cervical spine management for the trauma patient. (p. 199)
12. Analyze a scene to determine if spinal precautions are required. (pp. 196–197, 211–213)
13. Describe methods for assessing respiration in the adult, child, and infant patient. (pp. 206–207)
14. Describe the methods used to locate and assess a pulse in an adult, child, and infant patient. (pp. 207–210)

15. Discuss the need for assessing the patient for external bleeding. (p. 207)

16. Describe normal and abnormal findings when assessing skin color, temperature, and condition. (p. 207)

17. Explain the reason and process for prioritizing a patient for care and transport. (pp. 210–211)

18. Use the findings of the initial assessment to determine the patient's perfusion status. (pp. 207–210)

19. Describe orthostatic vital signs and evaluate their usefulness in assessing a patient in shock. (p. 228)

20. Describe the medical patient physical examination. (pp. 223–231)

21. Differentiate among the assessment for an unresponsive, altered mental status, and alert medical patient. (pp. 222–231)

22. Discuss the reasons for reconsidering the mechanism of injury. (pp. 211–213)

23. Recite examples and explain why patients should receive a rapid trauma assessment. (p. 213)

24. Describe the trauma patient physical examination. (pp. 213–221)

25. Describe the elements of the rapid trauma assessment and discuss their evaluation. (pp. 213–221)

26. Identify cases when the rapid assessment is suspended to provide patient care. (pp. 213–218)

27. Discuss the reason for performing a focused history and physical exam. (pp. 211, 224, 230)

28. Describe when and why a detailed physical examination is necessary. (pp. 231–232)

29. Discuss the components of the detailed physical examination. (pp. 232–238)

30. Explain what additional care is provided while performing the detailed physical exam. (pp. 232–238)

31. Distinguish between the detailed physical exam that is performed on a trauma patient and that of the medical patient. (pp. 232–238)

32. Differentiate between patients requiring a detailed physical exam and those who do not. (pp. 231–232)

33. Discuss the rationale for repeating the initial assessment as part of the ongoing assessment. (pp. 238–240)

34. Describe the components of the ongoing assessment. (pp. 238–241)

35. Describe trending of assessment components. (pp. 238–241)

36. Discuss medical identification devices/systems. (p. 220)

37. Given several preprogrammed and moulaged medical and trauma patients, provide the appropriate scene survey, initial assessment, focused assessment, detailed assessment, and ongoing assessments. (pp. 186–241)

Key Terms

advanced life support
   (ALS), p. 187
Battle's sign, p. 232
chief complaint,
   p. 222

circulation assessment,
   p. 207
Cullen's sign, p. 218
decerebrate, p. 201
decorticate, p. 201

detailed physical exam,
   p. 231
focused history and
   physical exam, p. 211
general impression, p. 198

Grey Turner's sign, p. 218
index of suspicion, p. 197
initial assessment, p. 198
major trauma patient,
    p. 211
mechanism of injury,
    p. 196
patient assessment,
    p. 186

periorbital ecchymosis,
    p. 232
personal protective
    equipment (PPE), p. 188
rapid trauma assessment,
    p. 213
scene safety, p. 190
semi-Fowler's position,
    p. 214

Standard Precautions,
    p. 188
subcutaneous
    emphysema, p. 215

Case Study

En route to the scene, paramedic Chris Johnson and EMT-Basic Nick Farina prepare for the worst. The initial report from bystanders at the scene says that a woman jumped from a fourth-floor balcony at the downtown shopping mall. She reportedly landed four stories below on the marble floor and lies bleeding with multiple injuries. If this is true, Chris thinks, she and Nick will find a significant mechanism of injury and probable serious injuries.

Upon arrival, Chris's worst fears come true. A woman in her mid-30s lies on the floor in a pool of blood with signs of obvious multiple trauma. Immediately, Chris directs her partner to stabilize the woman's head and neck and manually open her airway with a jaw thrust. Nick, also a part-time respiratory therapist, is well suited for the job.

Chris begins the initial assessment by evaluating their patient's level of response. She quickly notes that their patient is unresponsive to all stimuli. She then assesses the airway, which is noisy with gurgling blood. She immediately suctions the oropharynx and listens for air movement. Their patient has shallow respirations at a rate of 38 per minute. Chris instructs Nick to insert an oropharyngeal airway and begin ventilations with a bag-valve mask and supplemental oxygen at a rate of 12 per minute while she continues her assessment.

Because the patient exhibits signs of severe respiratory distress, Chris decides to assess her neck and chest before proceeding with the initial assessment. Chris quickly exposes their patient's chest and notices deformity to the right side with probable multiple rib fractures. She auscultates the chest and, noticing decreased breath sounds on the right side, suspects a pneumothorax or pulmonary contusion. Chris feels for radial and carotid pulses. She notes the absence of a radial pulse and the cool, pale look of their patient's skin. The carotid pulse is weak at a rate of approximately 130 beats per minute. Nick comments that their patient is in shock. Chris designates her as a priority 1, indicating rapid transport to the appropriate medical facility.

While Nick continues to maintain manual stabilization of their patient's neck, Chris begins a rapid trauma assessment. She starts at the head and quickly palpates a depressed skull fracture. Chris notes that her patient's trachea is midline and jugular veins are flat, temporarily ruling out a tension pneumothorax. She notices a rigid, distended abdomen and suspects an intra-abdominal bleed, which is most likely causing the profound shock. Next Chris palpates the pelvis and notes an unstable pelvic ring, indicating fracture. She also notes severe deformity and angulation to both femurs, suggesting bilateral fractures.

As additional help from the fire department arrives, Chris instructs them to immobilize her patient with the pneumatic antishock garment while she prepares the back of the ambulance for transport.

Once in the ambulance, Chris reassesses her patient's mental status and ABCs during the 4-minute ride to Duethorn Memorial Hospital. At this time, she takes a full set of vital signs and notes the following: heart rate—130 and weak; blood pressure—76/40; respirations—38 and shallow. Chris decides to administer a rapid fluid bolus. Firefighter EMT-Intermediate Joe Armstrong performs the procedure and runs both lines "wide open." Chris contacts the hospital and gives a quick report to Dr. Prasad, the attending physician. Upon arrival, they transfer their patient to the emergency department staff and watch as an experienced team of trauma specialists prepares the patient for a quick ride to surgery.

INTRODUCTION

patient assessment

problem-oriented evaluation of patient and establishment of priorities based on existing and potential threats to human life.

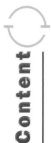

Review

Content

Components of Patient Assessment

- Scene size-up
- Initial assessment
- Focused history and physical exam
- Ongoing assessment
- Detailed physical exam

Patient assessment means conducting a problem-oriented evaluation of your patient and establishing priorities of care based on existing and potential threats to human life. In the previous two chapters you studied the techniques of performing a comprehensive history and physical exam. Such all-inclusive evaluations are best suited for patients without a chief complaint. They also establish a baseline health evaluation for patients admitted to the hospital. As a paramedic, however, you will certainly never perform a comprehensive exam in the acute setting. It is too time consuming and yields too much irrelevant information. Instead you will use your foundation of knowledge, skills, and tools to assess the acutely ill or injured patient. With time and clinical experience, you will learn which components of the comprehensive exam apply to each particular patient.

Now you can use the pertinent components of the comprehensive history and physical exam to perform patient assessments—problem-oriented assessments based on your patient's chief complaint. The basic components of patient assessment include the initial assessment; the focused history and physical exam, including vital signs; an ongoing assessment; and in some cases, a detailed physical exam.

Your patient's condition will determine which components you use and how you use them. For example, for trauma patients with a significant mechanism of injury, you will perform an initial assessment followed by a rapid trauma assessment (a head-to-toe exam aimed at traumatic signs and symptoms) and, if time allows, a detailed physical exam en route to the hospital. For patients with minor, isolated trauma, an initial assessment followed by a focused physical exam is warranted. For the responsive medical patient, you will conduct an initial assessment followed by a focused history and physical exam. Finally, for the unresponsive medical patient, you will perform an initial assessment followed by a rapid medical assessment (a head-to-toe exam aimed at medical signs and symptoms). In all cases, you will perform an ongoing assessment en route to the hospital to detect changes in patient condition.

The initial assessment's goal is to identify and correct immediately life-threatening conditions. These include airway compromise, inadequate ventilation, and major hemorrhage. During this rapid evaluation you use a variety of maneuvers and special equipment to manage any life threats as you find them. Immediately following the initial assessment you will establish the priorities of care. People such as the trauma patient with unstable vital signs and the unresponsive medical patient require a rapid head-to-toe exam and immediate transport to the hospital. Patients with minor, isolated trauma

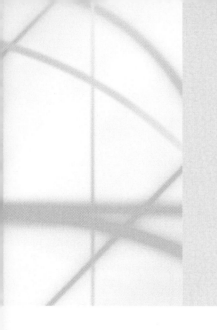

and most medical emergencies allow time to perform further assessments and provide care before transport.

Your proficiency in performing a systematic patient assessment will determine your ability to deliver the highest quality of prehospital **advanced life support (ALS)** to sick and injured people. Paramedic patient assessment is a straightforward skill, similar to the assessment you might have performed as an EMT-Basic. It differs, however, in depth and in the kind of care you will provide as a result. Your assessment must be thorough, because many ALS procedures are potentially dangerous. Safely and appropriately performing advanced procedures such as administration of drugs, defibrillation, synchronized cardioversion, needle decompression of the chest, or endotracheal intubation will depend on your assessment and correct field diagnosis. If your assessment does not reveal your patient's true problem, the consequences can be devastating.

As always, common sense dictates how you proceed in the field. When you assess the responsive medical patient, the history reveals the most important diagnostic information and takes priority over the physical exam. For the trauma patient and the unresponsive medical patient, the reverse is true. Yet trauma may cause a medical emergency, and, conversely, a medical emergency may cause trauma. Only by performing a thorough patient assessment can you discover the true cause of your patient's problems. This chapter provides problem-oriented patient assessment templates based on the information and techniques presented in the previous two chapters. You will need to refer to those chapters for the details of taking a history and conducting a physical exam.

advanced life support (ALS) *life-support activities that go beyond basic procedures to include adjunctive equipment and invasive procedures.*

If your assessment does not reveal your patient's true problem, the consequences can be devastating.

Only by performing a thorough patient assessment can you discover the true cause of your patient's problems.

SCENE SIZE-UP

Scene size-up is the essential first step at any emergency. Before you enter a scene, take the necessary time to judge the situation. Fire officers drive just past a burning house so they can see three of its sides before they make strategic decisions. Follow their lead. Never rush into any situation; first stop and look around (Figure 3-1 ▶).

Upon arrival, determine whether the scene is safe. Does the situation require special body substance isolation precautions? Is the mechanism of injury or the nature of illness obvious? Are there multiple patients? Do you need immediate additional resources? After an initial scene assessment, if necessary, report to your dispatcher what you have, what you need, and what you are doing. This way, you keep everyone informed and your dispatcher can send any necessary additional support.

Although size-up is your initial responsibility, remember that it is also an ongoing process. Emergency scenes are dynamic and can change suddenly. An injury to a child call can erupt into a violent domestic dispute if one parent blames the other. A hazardous

Never rush into any situation; first stop and look around.

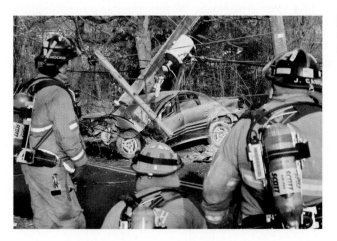

▶ **Figure 3-1** Always stop to size up the scene before going in. *(© On Scene Photography)*

Always be alert for subtle signs of danger.

Sizing up the scene gives you important information that will guide your actions.

Review

Components of Scene Size-Up

- Standard Precautions
- Scene safety
- Location of all patients
- Mechanism of injury
- Nature of the illness

Standard Precautions

a strict form of infection control that is based on the assumption that all blood and other body fluids are infectious.

The best defense against bloodborne, body-fluid-borne, and airborne pathogens is to take standard precautions.

personal protective equipment (PPE)

equipment designed to protect against infection. The minimum recommended personal protective equipment includes protective gloves, masks and protective eyewear, HEPA and N-95 respirators, gowns, and disposable resuscitation equipment.

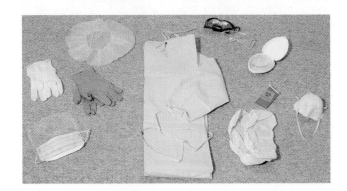

▶ **Figure 3-2** Always wear the appropriate personal protective equipment to prevent exposure to contagious diseases.

material spill can ignite. An improperly stabilized car can shift. Always be alert for subtle signs of danger, and avoid becoming a patient yourself.

Sizing up the scene gives you important information that will guide your actions. In trauma, a brief size-up of the accident scene reveals the mechanism of injury. From this, you can estimate the degree of energy transfer and possible seriousness of injuries. In a medical emergency, you can sometimes determine the nature of your patient's illness from clues at the scene. The smell of a lower gastrointestinal bleed, the sound of a hissing oxygen tank, or the sight of drug paraphernalia provides clues and an initial insight into your patient's situation. Learn to use all your senses when sizing up the scene.

The components of a scene size-up include:

▶ Standard Precautions
▶ Scene safety
▶ Location of all patients
▶ Mechanism of injury
▶ Nature of the illness

Standard Precautions

Standard Precautions is a strategy that includes the major features of *Universal Precautions (UP)*, which are blood and body fluid precautions that are designed to reduce the risk of transmission of bloodborne pathogens, and body substance isolation (BSI), which is designed to reduce the risk of transmission of pathogens from moist body substances. Standard Precautions applies these two concepts to all patients receiving care, regardless of their diagnosis or presumed infection status. Standard Precautions apply to:

▶ Blood
▶ All body fluids, secretions, and excretions except sweat, regardless of whether or not they contain visible blood
▶ Nonintact skin
▶ Mucous membranes

Standard Precautions are designed to reduce the risk of transmission of microorganisms from both recognized and unrecognized sources of infection in hospitals.

Standard Precautions dictate that all EMS personnel take the same (standard) precautions with every patient. To achieve this, appropriate **personal protective equipment (PPE)** should be available in every emergency vehicle (Figure 3-2 ▶). The minimum recommended PPE includes the following:

▶ *Protective gloves.* Wear disposable protective gloves before initiating any emergency care. When an emergency involves more than one patient,

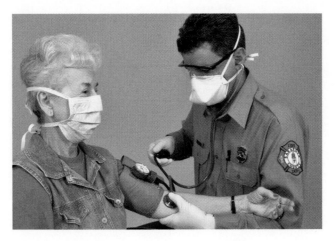

Figure 3-3 With a suspected tuberculosis patient, you may place a surgical-type mask on the patient while you wear a NIOSH-approved respirator. Monitor the patient's airway and breathing carefully.

change gloves between patients. When gloves have been contaminated, remove and dispose of them properly as soon as possible.

▶ *Masks and protective eyewear.* These should be worn together whenever blood spatter is likely to occur, such as with arterial bleeding, childbirth, endotracheal intubation and other invasive procedures, oral suctioning, and clean-up of equipment that requires heavy scrubbing or brushing. Both you and your patient should wear masks whenever the potential for airborne transmission of disease exists.

▶ *HEPA and N-95 respirators* (Figure 3-3 ▶). Due to the resurgence of tuberculosis (TB), you must protect yourself from infection through the use of a high-efficiency particulate air (HEPA) or N-95 respirator. Wear one whenever you care for a patient with confirmed or suspected TB. This is especially true during procedures that involve the airway, such as the administration of nebulized medications, endotracheal intubation, or suctioning.

▶ *Gowns.* Disposable gowns protect your clothing from splashes. If large splashes of blood are expected, such as with childbirth, wear an impervious gown.

▶ *Disposable resuscitation equipment.* Use disposable resuscitation equipment as your primary means of artificial ventilation in emergency care. Such items should be used once then disposed of properly.

The garments and equipment previously described are intended to serve the paramedic by protecting against infection through contact with both potentially contaminated body substances, such as blood, vomit, and urine, as well as other agents, such as airborne droplets. These garments and equipment will assist you in achieving, to the extent possible, the universal precautions recommended by the Centers for Disease Control, which help to protect against bloodborne infection. When you are finished with them, place all contaminated items in the appropriate biohazard bag (Figure 3-4 ▶).

Infectious diseases also are minimized through the use of appropriate work practices and equipment especially engineered to minimize risk. For example, most invasive equipment is now used on a one-time, disposable basis. Of course, it is important to launder reusable clothing with infection control in mind.

General cleanliness and appropriate personal hygiene will do much to prevent infection. Probably the most important infection control practice is hand washing (Figure 3-5 ▶). As soon as possible after every patient contact and decontamination procedure, thoroughly wash your hands. To do so, first remove any rings or jewelry from your hands and arms. Then use soap and water. Lather your hands vigorously

Always use all the equipment recommended for a particular procedure or patient to maximize your protection against communicable diseases.

Washing your hands is the most effective method of preventing disease transmission between you and your patients.

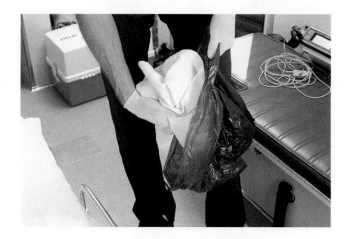

Figure 3-4 Place all contaminated items in the appropriate biohazard bag.

front and back for at least 15 seconds up to 2 or 3 inches above the wrist. Be sure to lather and rub between your fingers and in the creases and cracks of your knuckles. Scrub under and around the fingernails with a brush. Rinse your hands well under running water, holding your hands downward so that the water drains off your fingertips. Dry your hands on a clean towel.

Plain soap works perfectly well for hand washing. At those times when soap is not available, you might use an antimicrobial hand washing solution or an alcohol-based foam or towelette.

Scene Safety

Scene safety simply means doing everything possible to ensure a safe environment for yourself, your crew, other responding personnel, your patient, and any bystanders—in that order. Your personal safety is the top priority at any emergency scene. Make sure you are not injured while providing care. If you become a patient yourself, you will do your own patient little good. You must determine that no hazards may endanger the lives of people on the scene. If your scene is unsafe, either make it safe or wait until someone else does (Figure 3-6).

As the first unit on the scene, you may overestimate your capability to manage a rescue situation. Do not attempt a hazardous rescue unless you are properly clothed, equipped, and trained. Individual acts of courage are sometimes necessary, but modern rescue operations emphasize safety first, not heroics. Foolish heroics often end in tragedy. If in doubt, it is better to err on the side of caution than to risk personal harm.

scene safety
doing everything possible to ensure a safe environment.

Review

Content

Order of Priorities for Scene Safety

1. You
2. Your crew
3. Other responding personnel
4. Your patient
5. Bystanders

Your personal safety is the top priority at any emergency scene.

Figure 3-5 Careful, methodical hand washing helps reduce exposure to contagious disease.

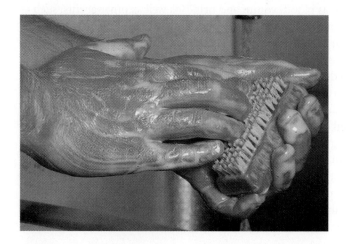

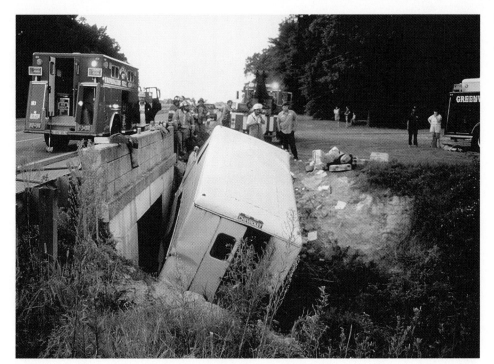

▶ **Figure 3-6** Look for potential hazards during scene size-up. (© Robert J. Bennett)

Many factors can make an emergency scene unsafe. Through experience you will learn to identify them quickly. Do not become complacent. Sometimes even the most nonthreatening, harmless-looking scene can turn into a disaster (Figure 3-7 ▶). If you are not sure the scene is safe, do not enter. As you approach a scene, immediately evaluate the surrounding area. Is it as your dispatcher's information has led you to expect, or does something just not look right? What do the bystanders' faces tell you? Are they angry, scared, or panicked? Be alert for situations that look or feel suspicious. If necessary, wait until law enforcement personnel secure the scene. Use all your senses to evaluate a scene and learn to trust your intuition. If your instincts tell you not to enter or to get out, follow them. They are the subconscious sum of your experiences. Listen to them; they are probably correct.

Carefully look for and identify on-scene hazards before even attempting to reach your patient. To do otherwise places you, other rescuers, and your patient at risk. Remember that you may find such dangers at either medical or trauma scenes. Potential hazards include fire, structural collapse, traffic, unstable surfaces, and broken glass or jagged metal. Other risks involve hazardous materials—chemical spills, radiation, or gas leaks—that might ignite or explode. A simple spark can set off a gas

Listen to your instincts; they are probably correct.

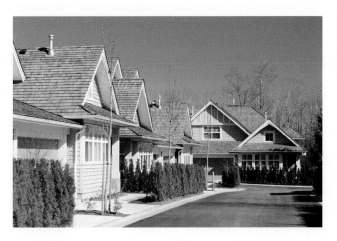

▶ **Figure 3-7** Even the most peaceful-looking scene can pose potential dangers. (© Rob Melnychuk/Getty Images, Inc.—Photodisc)

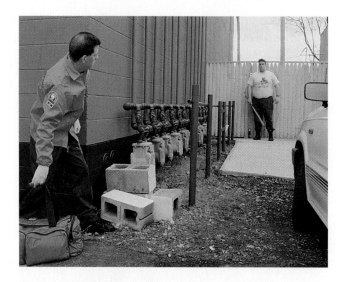

leak or oil spill. Electric wires threaten both fire and electric shock. Look around to determine the possibility of lightning, avalanche, rock slides, cave-ins, or similar dangers. Other potential hazards include poisonous or caustic substances; biological agents; germ-infested materials; confined spaces such as vessels, trenches, mines, silos, or caves; and extreme heights. In every case, let common sense dictate scene management.

Crime scenes pose a special threat. When responding to a call in which the initial dispatch includes words such as *shooting*, *stabbing*, or *domestic dispute*, wait for law enforcement personnel to secure the scene before entering (Figure 3-8). In fact, do not even enter the neighborhood, because sitting in your ambulance on the scene may undermine an already unstable environment. If possible, turn off your lights and siren and stage your vehicle a few blocks away, where it cannot be seen from the scene. Refer to the crime scene awareness chapter in Volume 5, *Special Considerations/Operations,* for more information on this topic.

Crash scenes requiring heavy-duty rescue procedures, scenes where toxic substances are present, crime scenes with a potential for violence, or scenes with unstable surfaces such as slippery slopes, ice, or rushing water all call for specialized crews, additional medical supplies, and sophisticated equipment (Figure 3-9). Do not even consider entering such situations unless you have the proper clothing, equipment, and training to work in them. Because getting backup requires extra time, this phase is critical. A prompt call to your dispatch center can save critical minutes in a life-threatening situation.

Without the appropriate protective gear, you will jeopardize your safety and your patient's. To participate in a rescue operation, you should have at least the following equipment immediately available: four-point suspension helmets, eye goggles or industrial safety glasses, high-quality hearing protection, leather work gloves, high-top steel-toed boots, insulated coveralls, and turnout gear (Figure 3-10). Only personnel thoroughly trained in hazardous material (HAZMAT) suits or self-contained breathing apparatus (SCBA) should use them (Figure 3-11). These items are often supplied on specialty support vehicles such as HAZMAT response units and heavy-rescue trucks (Figure 3-12).

After you ensure that responding personnel have adequate safety equipment to manage the rescue scene, consider patient safety. Many considerations for rescuer safety also apply to patients. Additionally, patient safety equipment should at least include construction-type hard hats, eye goggles, hearing and respiratory protection, protective blankets, and protective shielding. You will need these to protect

In every case, let common sense dictate scene management.

Do not even consider entering hazardous scenes unless you have the proper clothing, equipment, and training to work in them.

A prompt call for backup can save critical minutes in a life-threatening situation.

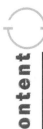

Review

Content

Minimum Rescue Operation Equipment

- Four-point suspension helmets
- Eye goggles or industrial safety glasses
- High-quality hearing protection
- Leather work gloves
- High-top steel-toed boots
- Insulated coveralls
- Turnout gear

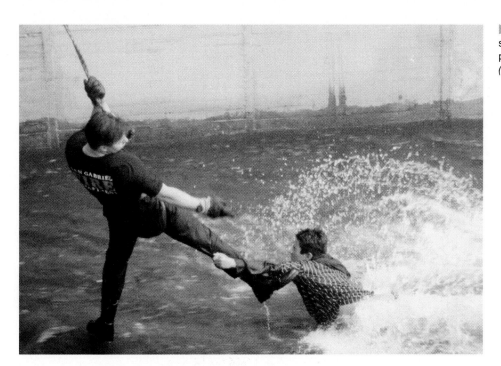

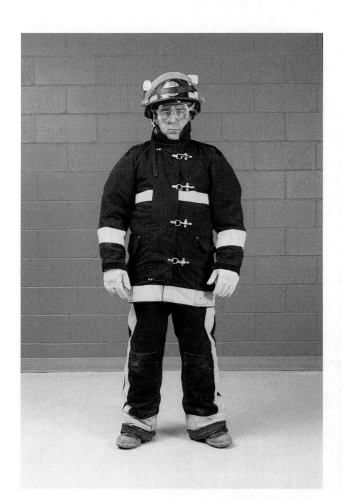

Figure 3-10 Full protective gear, including eye protection, helmet, turnout gear, and gloves.

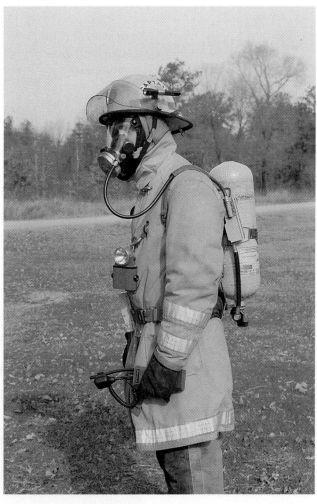

Figure 3-11 Self-contained breathing apparatus (SCBA).

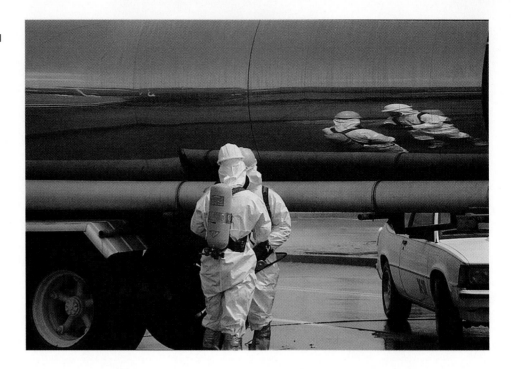

Review

Minimum Patient Safety Equipment

- Construction-type hard hats
- Eye goggles
- Hearing and respiratory protection
- Protective blankets
- Protective shielding

Safe, orderly, and controlled incident management is essential for everyone's safety.

your patient during rescue operations (Figure 3-13 ▶). Patient safety also includes simple measures such as removing them from unstable environments such as temperature extremes, smoky rooms, or hostile crowds. For example, the simplest way to begin managing a patient suffering from hypothermia is to move him into a warm environment.

Safe, orderly, and controlled incident management is essential for everyone's safety. Call for specialty personnel to stabilize wreckage or turn off electrical power. Make sure someone routes traffic safely around a vehicle collision. Control bystanders and spot potential human hazards. Be certain that a hostile crowd or someone who assaulted your patient is not ready to attack you. Scenes involving toxic exposures, environmental hazards, and violent patients are especially worrisome. When possible, have law enforcement personnel establish a tape line to cordon off the hazard zone to protect bystanders who do not realize the potential dangers of watching operations (Figure 3-14 ▶).

Figure 3-13 Protect the patient from hazards at the scene.

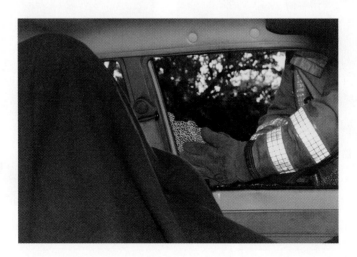

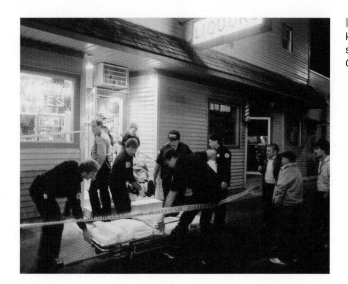

Location of All Patients

Scene size-up also includes a search of the area to locate all of the patients. Ask yourself if other persons could be involved in the crash or affected by the medical problem. Determine where you are most likely to find the most seriously affected patients and how many patients will need transport. The mechanism of injury or the nature of the illness can help you determine the number of patients. For example, a two-car crash must include at least two drivers. Clues such as diaper bags, child auto seats, toys, coloring books, clothing, or twin spider-web impact marks in the windshield should lead you to search for more patients, especially children, than those who may be readily apparent. Some medical situations such as carbon monoxide poisoning can affect an entire household. A hazardous liquid spill in the chemistry lab can affect students and staff in an entire wing of a school.

If you find more patients than you can safely and effectively manage, call for assistance early. If possible, you should do this before you make contact with any patients, because you are less likely to call for help once you become involved with patient care. Often, as you proceed into a scene, more patients become apparent. It is wise to overestimate when asking for help at the scene.

Initiate the incident management system according to local protocols (Figure 3-15). Again, try not to become immediately involved in patient care, because two important functions must occur in the initial stages of any multiple-casualty incident: command

> Search the area to locate all patients.

> Call for assistance early; it is wise to overestimate when asking for help.

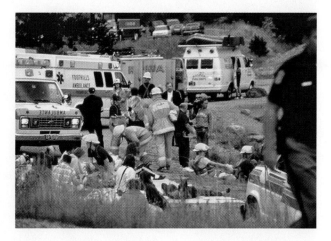

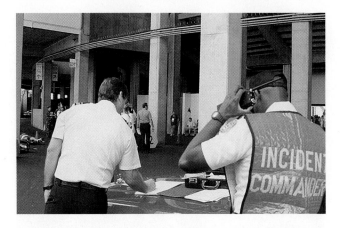

▶ **Figure 3-16** The incident commander directs the response and coordinates resources at a multiple-casualty incident.

and triage. If you and your partner find yourselves in a situation that overwhelms your resources, one of you should establish command while the other begins triaging patients. The command person performs a scene size-up, determines the needs of the incident, makes a radio report requesting the necessary additional help, and directs oncoming crews to their duties (Figure 3-16 ▶). The triage person performs a triage exam on every patient and prioritizes them for immediate or delayed transport (Figure 3-17 ▶). He may perform simple lifesaving procedures such as opening the airway or controlling bleeding, but as a rule he should not stop to provide intensive care for any one patient.

Mechanism of Injury

mechanism of injury
combined strength, direction, and nature of forces that injured your patient.

The **mechanism of injury** is the combined strength, direction, and nature of forces that injured your patient. It is usually apparent through careful evaluation of the trauma scene and can help you anticipate both the location and the seriousness of injuries. Identify the forces involved, the direction from which they came, and the bodily locations potentially affected (Figure 3-18 ▶). For example, in a fall injury, how high was the patient, what did he land on, and what part of his body hit first? If your patient jumped from a height and landed on his feet, expect lower extremity, pelvic, and lumbar spine injuries.

▶ **Figure 3-17** The triage person examines and prioritizes patients.

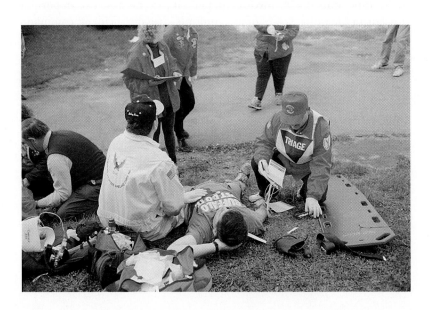

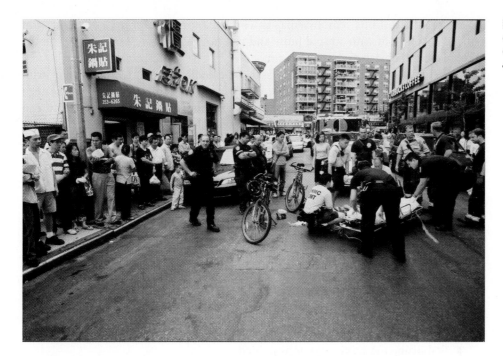

▶ **Figure 3-18** With trauma, try to determine the mechanism of injury during scene size-up. (© *Craig Jackson/In the Dark Photography*)

In an automobile crash, the mechanism of injury is the process by which forces are exchanged between the automobile and what it struck, between your patient and the automobile's interior, and among the various tissues and organs as they collide with one another within the patient. Close inspection of the automobile and the forces, or various collisions, can lead to an **index of suspicion** (a prediction of injuries based on the mechanism of injury) for possible injuries. What does the car look like? If the windshield is cracked, expect head and neck injuries. If the steering wheel is bent, expect chest and abdominal injuries. With a major intrusion into the passenger compartment, expect major trauma.

index of suspicion
your anticipation of possible injuries based on your analysis of the event.

Expect a pedestrian struck by a car to have fractures of the lower extremities. If the auto was moving at 20 miles per hour, expect less severe fractures than if it had been moving at 55 miles per hour. Also, internal injuries are less likely at lower speeds than at higher speeds. By evaluating the strength and nature of impact, you can anticipate which organs are injured and the degree of their damage.

For a gunshot patient, determine the type of gun used, the range of the shot, and if an exit wound exists. This information will enable you to estimate the damage along the bullet's path and to formulate an index of suspicion for your patient's possible injuries. Expect the internal injuries from serious blunt trauma to be more extensive and severe than those you see externally. Often the mechanism of injury is the only clue to the possibility of serious internal injury. The chapters on blunt and penetrating trauma in Volume 4, *Trauma Emergencies*, describe the mechanisms of these injuries in depth.

Often the mechanism of injury is the only clue to the possibility of serious internal injury.

Nature of the Illness

Determine the nature of the illness from bystanders, family members, or your patient himself. If he is alert and oriented, he is usually the best source of information about his problem. If he is unresponsive, disoriented, or otherwise unable to provide information, rely on family members, bystanders, or visual cues for this information.

The scene can give additional clues to your patient's condition. How is he positioned? Does he sit bolt upright gasping to breathe? Are pill bottles or drug paraphernalia nearby? Is medical care equipment such as an oxygen tank, a nebulizer, or a glucometer in the room? For example, if you respond to a "difficulty breathing" call and your patient is using his nebulizer when you arrive, suspect a history of pulmonary disease such as asthma, emphysema, or chronic bronchitis. If your patient is an agitated 17-year-old with a rapid pulse and you notice crack cocaine ampules on the floor, suspect a substance abuse problem.

Sometimes the nature of the illness is not readily apparent. Your patient with severe difficulty breathing, for instance, may be suffering from respiratory disease, a cardiac problem, an allergic reaction, or a toxic exposure. Remember that the nature of your patient's illness may be very different from his chief complaint.

THE INITIAL ASSESSMENT

The **initial assessment** exemplifies the basis of all prehospital emergency medical care. Its goal is to identify and correct immediately life-threatening patient conditions of the *A*irway, *B*reathing, or *C*irculation (*ABC*s). If you find these conditions during this part of your assessment, treat them at once. For example, open a closed airway, provide ventilation, or control hemorrhage before moving on. Immediately following the initial assessment, decide priority regarding immediate transport or further on-scene assessment and care. The initial assessment consists of the following steps:

- Forming a general impression
- Stabilizing the cervical spine as needed
- Assessing a baseline mental status
- Assessing the airway
- Assessing breathing
- Assessing circulation
- Determining priority

The initial assessment should take less than 1 minute, unless you have to intervene with lifesaving measures. Perform the initial assessment as part of your ongoing assessment throughout the patient contact, especially after any major intervention or whenever your patient's condition changes.

Forming a General Impression

The **general impression** is your initial, intuitive evaluation of your patient. It will help you determine his general clinical status (stable vs. unstable) and priority for immediate transport. Base your first impression on the information you gather from the environment, the mechanism of injury, the nature of the illness, the chief complaint, and your instincts.

Your patient's age, gender, and race often influence your index of suspicion. Very old and very young patients are more apt to have severe complications from injury or illness. For example, age is a factor in burn mortality, along with degree and body percentage. A 25-year-old patient with third-degree burns over 50% of his body has a 75% chance of mortality. A 45-year-old patient with the same burns has a 95% chance of mortality. Suspect a female of childbearing age with lower abdominal pain and vaginal bleeding to have a life-threatening gynecological emergency known as ruptured ectopic pregnancy. Black Americans have a higher incidence of hypertension and cardiovascular disease than members of other races.

Determine whether your patient's problem results from trauma or from a medical problem. Sometimes this will not be readily apparent. For example, did your patient slip and fall or get dizzy and fall? Note your patient's face and his posture and decide whether rapid intervention or a more deliberate approach is warranted. With experience you will be able to recognize even the most subtle clues of a patient in critical condition. Generally, the more serious the condition, the quieter your patient will be. Look at, listen to, and smell the environment. Gather as many clues as possible as you enter the scene.

initial assessment
prehospital process designed to identify and correct life-threatening airway, breathing, and circulation problems.

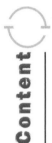

Review

Content

Steps of Initial Assessment

1. Form general impression
2. Stabilize cervical spine as needed
3. Assess baseline level of response
4. Assess airway
5. Assess breathing
6. Assess circulation
7. Assign priority

The initial assessment should take less than 1 minute, unless you have to intervene with lifesaving measures.

general impression
your initial, intuitive evaluation of your patient.

Patho Pearls

Developing Your "Sixth Sense" Patient assessment actually starts as soon as you approach the scene. Clues about the patient's underlying pathophysiology might be evident from such things as positioning of the vehicle, downed power lines, or the appearance and actions of bystanders. However, your safety, and that of your fellow rescuers, is always paramount. Never approach a scene that appears unsafe. With time, you will develop a "sixth sense" about emergency scenes and bystanders.

As you begin the patient encounter, process all that you see into your patient assessment and care. For example, consider this scenario: A car with two 16-year-old girls fails to negotiate a turn on a country road and overturns into a flowing creek adjacent to the road. Although the ambient temperature is in the 60s, you know that the temperature of the water in this area often is in the 40s. Thus, you should immediately suspect the possibility of hypothermia.

As the girls are removed from entrapment, no obvious injuries are noted. Vital signs are normal other than a slight tachycardia. However, peripheral pulses are weak and the skin is pale and cool. Is it shock? Is it hypothermia? Is it both? Your index of suspicion is high for both hypothermia and blunt force trauma. You follow local protocols with regard to immobilization, fluid therapy, and monitoring. Once in the ambulance and wrapped in blankets, both girls start to show signs that blood flow to the skin is improving. By the time you reach the hospital, their skin has a normal color and their pulse rate is normal.

Following a comprehensive assessment in the emergency department, the girls are discharged to their parents with no apparent injuries. Thus, your instincts were right. The potential for shock was a greater risk to the girls than hypothermia, and you had to treat based on this risk. But hypothermia turned out to be the principal problem. Integrating information from the scene size-up, patient history, and patient examination gave you a clear picture of the patients' underlying pathophysiological process.

Take the necessary Standard Precautions with every patient. Then, if your patient is alert, identify yourself and begin to establish a rapport. For example, "Hello, I'm Jen Stevens, a paramedic with ALS Ambulance Service. I'm here to help you." This establishes your level of training, authority, and reason for being at your patient's side. It also allows your patient to refuse care. As discussed in the chapter on medical/legal aspects of advanced prehospital care (Volume 1, *Introduction to Advanced Prehospital Care*), you cannot provide care without either implied or informed consent.

Reassure your patient. Listen to him and do not trivialize his complaints. Frequently we forget how significant an injury or illness, even a minor one, seems to a patient. With your experience, his problem may seem small, but for your patient it is a real concern. The ill or injured patient may worry about the long-term consequences for work, child care, and finances. Understand these fears and support your patient psychologically as well as physiologically.

Listen to your patient and do not trivialize his complaints.

If the mechanism of injury is significant or if your patient is unresponsive, have your partner manually stabilize your patient's head and neck (Figure 3-19a). Do this before establishing his mental status and continue manual stabilization until you fully immobilize him to a long spine board. If your patient is awake, explain what you are doing and ask him not to move his neck. You do not want him to turn his head when you try to assess mental status. Ask your partner to maintain your patient's head in a neutral position as you begin your assessment. If your patient is a small child, place a small towel or pad beneath the shoulders to maintain proper alignment of the cervical spine (Figure 3-19b). This will compensate for the large occiput of the child's head, which normally would flex his neck when he is placed on a flat surface.

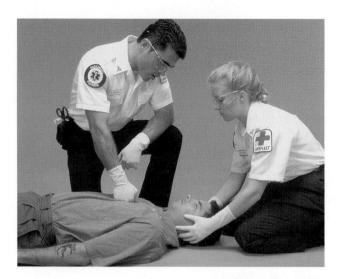

Figure 3-19a Manually stabilize the head and neck on first patient contact.

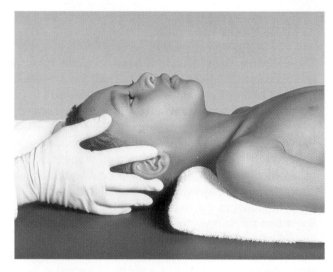

Figure 3-19b Place a folded towel under your young patient's shoulders to keep the airway aligned.

Mental Status

Your assessment of baseline mental status is crucial for all patients. For example, when you deliver your head injury patient to the emergency department, the neurosurgeon will want a chronological report of your patient's mental status from the time you arrived on the scene. This vital information helps the surgical team diagnose a deteriorating brain injury. If the patient was alert and oriented when you arrived, then became sleepy en route, and within 30 minutes was responsive only to deep pain stimuli, the suspicion for epidural hematoma is high. Rapid surgical intervention can save lives in most cases if the diagnosis is made quickly. Your baseline mental status documentation is critical to these patients' emergency care. Establishing a baseline mental status is also crucial in assessing the variety of medical situations that cause altered levels of response. Drug overdoses, poisonings, diabetic emergencies, sepsis, hypoxia, and hypovolemia are just a few of the many conditions that result in altered mentation. For the stroke patient, identifying the time of the symptoms' onset is critical for the emergency physician to consider administering clot-dissolving drugs within the 3-hour window of opportunity. This is possible only with your accurate assessment of your patient's change in mental status.

AVPU Levels

Review

Content

AVPU

- *A*lert
- *V*erbal stimuli
- *P*ainful stimuli
- *U*nresponsive

To record your patient's mental status, use the acronym **AVPU.** Your patient either is *A*lert, responds to *V*erbal stimuli, responds only to *P*ainful stimuli, or is *U*nresponsive. Perform this exam by starting with verbal, then moving to painful stimuli only if he fails to respond to your verbal cues.

Alert An alert patient is awake, as evidenced by open eyes. He may be oriented to person (who he is), place (where he is), and time (day, month, and year) and give organized, coherent answers to your questions. He also may be disoriented and confused. For example, the patient with a suspected concussion will often present as dazed and confused. The hypoxic or hypoglycemic patient may present as combative. The shock patient may be restless and anxious. If his eyes are open and he appears awake, he is categorized as alert. Children's responses to your questions will vary with their age-related physical and emotional development. Infants and young children usually will be curious but cautious when a stranger approaches. Their level of response may not indicate the gravity of their condition. In fact, the quiet child is usually the seriously injured or ill child.

Verbal   If your patient appears to be sleeping but responds when you talk to him, he is responsive to verbal stimuli. He can respond by speaking, opening his eyes, moaning, or just moving. Note the level of his verbal response. Does he speak clearly, mumble inappropriate words, or make incomprehensible sounds? Children may respond to your verbal commands by turning their heads or stopping activity. For infants you may have to shout to elicit a response.

Pain   If your child or adult patient does not respond to verbal stimuli, try to elicit a response with painful stimuli. Pinch his fingernails or rub your knuckles on his sternum and watch for a response. Again, he may respond by waking up, speaking, moaning, opening his eyes, or moving. Note the type of motor response to the painful stimuli. Is his response purposeful or nonpurposeful? If he tries to move your hand away or to move himself away from the pain, it is purposeful. **Decorticate** (arms flexed, legs extended) or **decerebrate** (arms and legs extended) posturing is nonpurposeful and suggests a serious brain injury. For the infant, flick the soles of the feet and expect crying as the appropriate response.

decorticate
arms flexed, legs extended.

decerebrate
arms and legs extended.

Unresponsive   The unresponsive patient is comatose and fails to respond to any noxious stimulus. The AVPU scale describes your patient's general mental status. Avoid using terms such as *semiconscious*, *lethargic*, or *stuporous* because they are broadly interpreted and you have not had a chance to conduct a comprehensive neurologic exam at this point. Your patient's response to stimulation will tell you a great deal about his condition. Any alteration or deterioration in mental status may indicate an emergent or already serious problem. A patient with an impaired mental status may have lost, or be in danger of losing, the ability to protect his airway. Take immediate steps to protect your patient's airway by proper positioning, use of airway adjuncts, or intubation, as appropriate. Provide oxygen to any patient with diminished mental status and seek out its cause.

Any alteration in mental status may indicate an emergent or already serious problem.

Airway Assessment

If your patient is responsive and can speak clearly, you can assume that his airway is patent. If your patient is unconscious, however, his airway may be obstructed. The supine unconscious patient's tongue often obstructs his upper airway. Because the mandible, tongue, and epiglottis are all connected, gravity allows these structures to block your patient's upper airway as his facial muscles relax (Figure 3-20a).

You can open your patient's airway with one of two simple manual maneuvers: the jaw-thrust maneuver or the head-tilt/chin-lift maneuver. For the trauma patient with a suspected cervical spine injury, use the jaw thrust to avoid movement of the cervical spine. Place your thumbs on your patient's cheeks and lift up on the angle of the jaw with your fingers (Figure 3-20b). For all other patients, use the head-tilt/chin-lift maneuver. Place one hand on your patient's forehead and lift up under the chin with the fingers of your other hand (Figure 3-20c). To open the airways of infants and young children, apply a gentle and conservative extension of the head and neck (Figure 3-20d). These patients' upper airway structures are very flexible and are easily kinked when their necks are flexed or hyperextended. You must constantly readjust their airways to maximize patency.

To assess your patient's airway, look for chest rise while you listen and feel for air movement. If the airway is clear, you should hear quiet airflow and feel free air movement. A noisy airway is a partially obstructed airway. Snoring occurs when the tongue partially blocks the upper airway. In this case, reposition the head and neck and reevaluate. Gurgling indicates that fluid such as blood, secretions, or gastric contents is blocking the upper airway. Gently open and examine the mouth for foreign bodies you can

You must constantly adjust infants' and young children's airways to maximize patency.

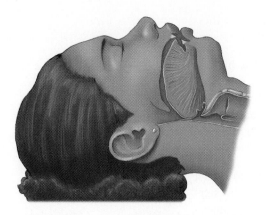

▶ **Figure 3-20a** Your unconscious patient's tongue may fall and close the upper airway.

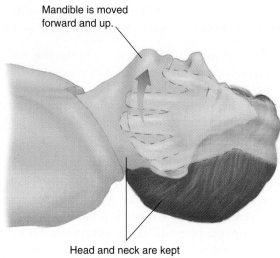

Mandible is moved forward and up.

Head and neck are kept in neutral in-line position.

▶ **Figure 3-20b** Use the jaw-thrust maneuver to open your patient's airway if you suspect a cervical spine injury.

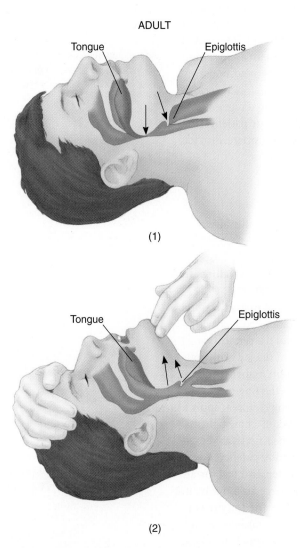

ADULT

Tongue

Epiglottis

(1)

Tongue

Epiglottis

(2)

▶ **Figure 3-20c** The head-tilt/chin-lift maneuver in an adult.

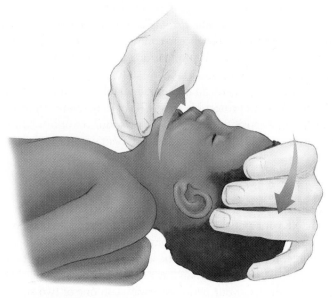

▶ **Figure 3-20d** The head-tilt/chin-lift maneuver in an infant. Do not overextend the head and neck.

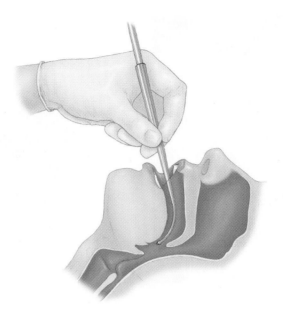

Figure 3-21 Suction fluids from your patient's airway.

remove easily and quickly. Use aggressive suctioning to remove blood, vomitus, secretions, and other fluids (Figure 3-21 ▶).

The high-pitched inspiratory screech of stridor is caused by a life-threatening upper airway obstruction that may be due to a foreign body, severe swelling, allergic reaction, or infection. If you suspect a foreign body obstruction and your patient exhibits poor air movement, a weak cough, or a diminishing mental status, immediately deliver abdominal thrusts to dislodge the object. If your patient is less than 1 year old, use back blows and chest thrusts instead of abdominal thrusts. If these maneuvers are ineffective, remove the object under direct laryngoscopy with Magill forceps.

Other causes of stridor require vastly different approaches. Upper respiratory infections such as croup or epiglottitis call for blow-by oxygen and a quiet ride to the hospital; respiratory burns demand rapid endotracheal intubation; and anaphylaxis necessitates vasoconstrictor medications. Because these vastly different management techniques are potentially life-threatening when applied inappropriately, your correct field diagnosis is critical. If your patient presents with stridor, take time to evaluate the history and clinical signs and symptoms for foreign body obstruction (sudden onset while eating), epiglottitis (fever, illness, drooling, inability to swallow), respiratory burns (history of facial burns, hoarseness), and anaphylaxis (hives, history of allergies).

The softer, expiratory whistle of wheezing is caused by constricted bronchioles, the smaller, lower airways. You will hear it in cases such as asthma, bronchitis, emphysema, or other causes of bronchospasm. Bronchiolitis, a lower respiratory infection, often causes these sounds in infants and young children. Wheezing patients require a bronchodilator medication to dilate the bronchioles and reduce airway resistance.

If your patient is not moving air, he is in respiratory arrest. Immediately provide ventilation with a bag-valve mask (Figure 3-22 ▶). Give 2 rescue breaths, each over 1 second, with enough volume to produce visible chest rise. Be careful not to overventilate (by breathing either too fast or too deeply). Ventilate adult patients at a rate of 10–12 breaths per minute and all children at a rate of 12–20 breaths per minute. If you cannot ventilate the lungs, reposition the head and neck and try again. If there is still no air movement, assume a complete obstruction and begin measures to correct it.

Once you have cleared the airway, keeping it open may require constant attention. In these cases, insert a basic airway adjunct to help keep the tongue from blocking the upper airway. If your patient is unconscious and lacks a gag reflex, insert an oropharyngeal airway (Figure 3-23 ▶). If he has a gag reflex or significant orofacial

Stridor signals a potentially life-threatening airway obstruction.

Once you have cleared the airway, keeping it open may require constant attention.

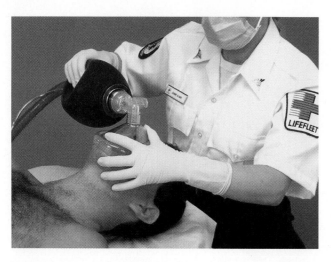

Figure 3-22 Immediately use a bag-valve mask to ventilate patients who are not moving air.

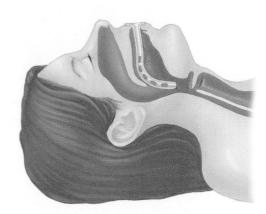

Figure 3-23 Use an oropharyngeal airway for unconscious patients without a gag reflex.

trauma, insert a nasopharyngeal airway (Figure 3-24 ▶). Be cautious when using a nasopharyngeal airway if you suspect a basilar skull fracture. If he has no gag reflex and cannot protect his airway, you will need to use advanced techniques to maintain airway patency. These include endotracheal intubation, multi-lumen airways such as the pharyngotracheal lumen (PL) airway and the Esophageal Tracheal CombiTube® (ETC), and transtracheal techniques such as needle or surgical cricothyroidotomy (Figures 3-25 ▶ through 3-28 ▶). The multi-lumen airways are not appropriate for use in children. All of these devices for maintaining upper airway patency are described in detail in the airway management and ventilation chapter of Volume 1, *Introduction to Advanced Prehospital Care.* If your patient has an airway problem or an altered mental status, administer high-flow, high-concentration oxygen by nonrebreather mask.

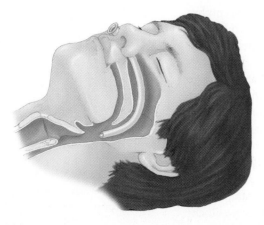

Figure 3-24 The nasopharyngeal airway rests between the tongue and the posterior pharyngeal wall.

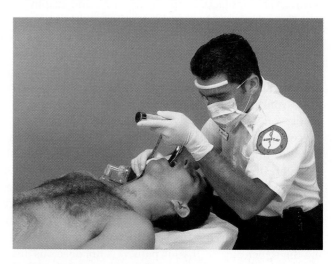

Figure 3-25 Endotracheal intubation.

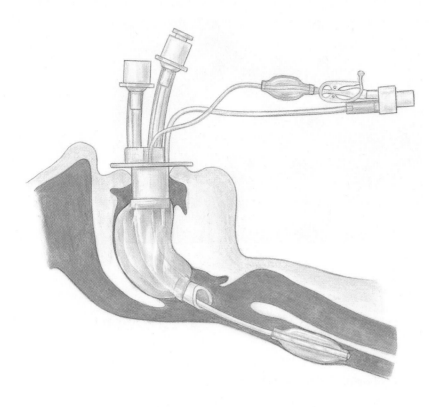

▶ **Figure 3-26** Pharyngotracheal lumen airway.

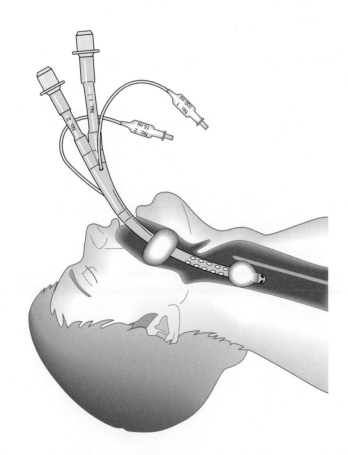

▶ **Figure 3-27** Esophageal Tracheal CombiTube®.

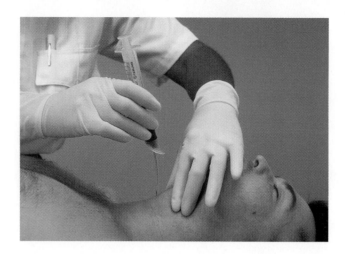

Breathing Assessment

Assess your patient for adequate breathing. Immediately note any signs of inadequate breathing. These include:

Review

Signs of Inadequate Breathing

- Altered mental status
- Shortness of breath
- Retractions
- Asymmetric chest wall movement
- Accessory muscle use
- Cyanosis
- Audible sounds
- Abnormal rate or pattern
- Nasal flaring

▶ Altered mental status, confusion, apprehension, or agitation

▶ Shortness of breath while speaking

▶ Retractions (supraclavicular, suprasternal, intercostal)

▶ Asymmetric chest wall movement

▶ Accessory muscle use (neck, abdominal)

▶ Cyanosis

▶ Audible sounds

▶ Abnormally rapid, slow, or shallow breathing

▶ Nasal flaring

Assess the respiratory rate and quality. Normal respiratory rates vary according to your patient's age. Abnormally fast or slow rates (Table 3–1) actually decrease the amount of air that reaches the alveoli for gas exchange. For patients with abnormally fast or slow respiratory rates and decreased tidal volumes, provide positive-pressure ventilation with, for example, a bag-valve mask and supplemental oxygen, to ensure full lung expansion and maximum oxygenation. Note the respiratory pattern. Rapid (tachypneic), deep (hyperpneic) respirations are a compensatory mechanism and suggest the body is attempting to rid itself of excess acids. They may indicate a diabetic

Table 3–1	Respiratory Rates	
Age	**Low Rate**	**High Rate**
Newborn	30	60
Infant (<1 year)	30	60
Toddler (1–2 years)	24	40
Preschooler (3–5 years)	22	34
School age (6–12 years)	18	30
Adolescent (13–18 years)	12	26
Adult (>18 years)	12	20

problem, severe acidosis, or head injury. They also may result from hyperventilation syndrome or from simple exertion. Kussmaul respirations (deep, rapid breathing) accompanied by a fruity breath odor are a classic sign of a patient in diabetic ketoacidosis. In either case, always ensure an adequate inspiratory volume and administer high-flow, high-concentration oxygen. Cheyne-Stokes respirations, a series of increasing and decreasing breaths followed by a period of apnea, most likely result from a brainstem injury or increasing intracranial pressure. Biot's respirations, identified by short, gasping, irregular breaths, may signify severe brain injury. Again, ensure adequate inspiratory volume and provide ventilation with supplemental oxygen as needed.

If your trauma patient's breathing is inadequate, immediately conduct a rapid trauma assessment of the neck and chest before moving on to circulation. Identify and correct any life-threatening conditions such as a sucking chest wound, a flail chest, or a tension pneumothorax. If your patient exhibits adequate breathing, move directly to circulation.

> If your patient's breathing is inadequate, immediately conduct a rapid trauma assessment of the neck and chest and provide positive-pressure ventilation with supplemental oxygen.

Circulation Assessment

The **circulation assessment** consists of evaluating the pulse and skin and controlling hemorrhage. Go directly to the wrist and feel for a radial pulse (Procedure 3-1a). Its presence suggests a systolic blood pressure of at least 80 mmHg. If the radial pulse is absent, check for a carotid pulse (Procedure 3-1b). The carotid pulse's presence suggests a systolic blood pressure of at least 60 mmHg. In the infant, palpate the brachial pulse (Procedure 3-1c) or, if necessary, auscultate the apical pulse. If the pulse is absent in the adult patient, begin chest compressions immediately, evaluate the cardiac rhythm, and provide prompt defibrillation as needed. In the child, immediately begin cardiopulmonary resuscitation (CPR).

circulation assessment
evaluating the pulse and skin and controlling hemorrhage.

Assess your patient's pulse for rate and quality as detailed in Chapter 2. The normal heart rate varies with your patient's age (Table 3–2). Very fast rates (tachycardia) and very slow rates (bradycardia) may indicate a life-threatening cardiac dysrhythmia. Note the quality of the pulse. The normal pulse should be regular and strong. An irregular pulse may indicate a cardiac dysrhythmia requiring advanced cardiac life support procedures. In head injury, heat stroke, or hypertension, you will often find a strong, bounding pulse. A weak, thready pulse usually indicates poor perfusion due to fluid loss, pump failure, or massive vasodilation.

Stop your patient's bleeding if you haven't already done so (Procedure 3-1d). Major bleeding usually originates with trauma, but it also can result from a medical emergency. For example, vaginal bleeding, rectal bleeding, and even a nosebleed associated with hypertension can result in life-threatening blood loss. For external bleeding, employ any appropriate measures for hemorrhage control, including direct pressure and elevation, pressure dressings, pressure points, and the tourniquet. New hemostatic agents such as HemCon and QuickClot, used by the military to stop uncontrolled hemorrhage, may soon be used by civilian EMS responders. Internal bleeding is not easily controlled in the prehospital setting and demands initiating transport as soon as possible.

> Internal bleeding is not easily controlled in the prehospital setting and demands initiating transport as soon as possible.

Assess the skin for temperature, moisture, and color (Procedure 3-1e). Peripheral vasoconstriction decreases peripheral perfusion to the skin early in shock. The skin may appear mottled (blotchy), cyanotic (bluish), pale, or ashen. It may also feel cool and moist (clammy). This often indicates that warm, circulating blood has been shunted away from the skin to the core of the body to maintain perfusion of vital organs. If you find any of these signs, suspect conditions related to or caused by poor perfusion. In infants and young children capillary refill is a reliable indicator of circulatory function (Procedure 3-1f). In adults, smoking, medications, cold weather, or chronic conditions of the elderly may affect capillary refill, so you should always also consider the other indicators of circulatory function.

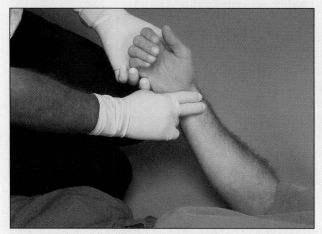

3-1a To assess an adult's circulation, feel for a radial pulse.

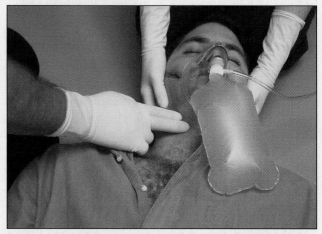

3-1b If you cannot feel a radial pulse, palpate for a carotid pulse.

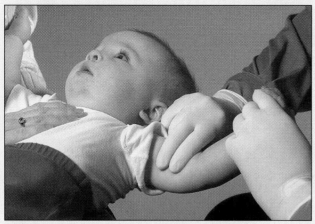

3-1c To assess an infant's circulation, palpate the brachial pulse.

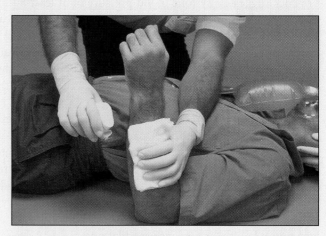

3-1d Control major bleeding.

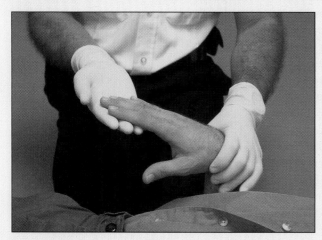

3-1e Assess the skin.

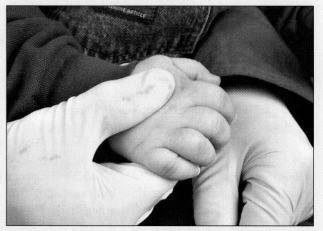

3-1f Capillary refill time provides important information about the circulatory status of infants and young children.

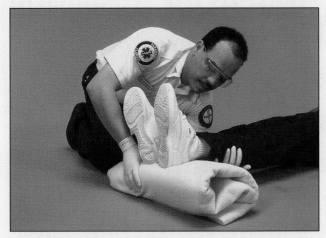

3-1g Elevate your patient's feet if you suspect circulatory compromise.

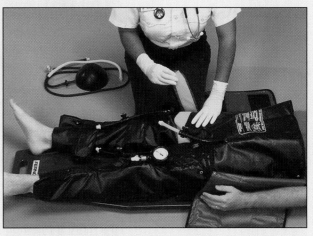

3-1h Apply a pneumatic antishock garment according to your local protocol.

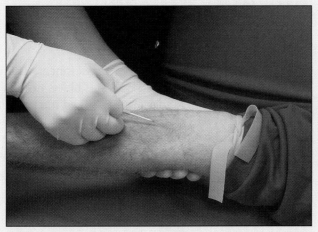

3-1i En route to the hospital, establish an IV.

If your patient shows signs of circulatory compromise, consider elevating his legs to support venous return to the vital organs (Procedure 3-1g). Keep him warm, and on adult patients only, apply and inflate the pneumatic antishock garment as indicated by your local protocol (Procedure 3-1h). The chapter on hemorrhage and shock

Table 3-2	Normal Pulse Rate Ranges	
Age	**Low Rate**	**High Rate**
Newborn	100	180
Infant (<1 year)	100	160
Toddler (1–2 years)	80	110
Preschooler (3–5 years)	70	110
School age (6–12 years)	65	110
Adolescent (13–18 years)	60	90
Adult (<18 years)	60	100

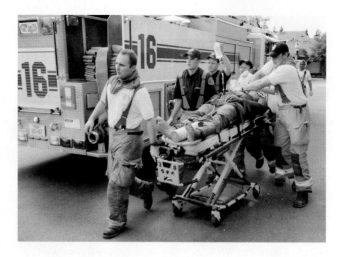

Figure 3-29 Expedite transport for a high-priority patient and continue assessment and care en route. (© Glen E. Ellman)

in Volume 4, *Trauma Emergencies*, explains this procedure fully. Consider starting large-bore intravenous lines en route to the hospital and infusing fluids to augment your patient's circulating blood volume (Procedure 3-1i). New hemoglobin-based oxygen-carrying solutions such as PolyHeme and HemoPure show promise and may soon be available for prehospital use. Also consider using vasoconstricting drugs and antidysrhythmic medications for other specific causes of poor perfusion.

Priority Determination

Once you have conducted an initial assessment, determine your patient's priority. If his initial assessment suggests a serious illness or injury, conduct a rapid head-to-toe assessment to identify other life threats and transport him immediately to the nearest appropriate facility that can deliver definitive care (Figure 3-29 ▶). Do not delay transport for detailed assessments and procedures that you can provide en route to the hospital. Consider top priority and rapid transport for the following patients:

▶ Patients with a poor general impression
- Apnea
- Pulselessness
- Obvious severe distress

▶ Patients with altered mental status

▶ Patients with airway compromise
- Obstructive sounds such as gurgling, snoring, or stridor
- Vomitus, secretions, blood, or foreign bodies obstructing the airway
- Inability to protect the airway (absence of a gag reflex)

▶ Patients with abnormal breathing
- Rates less or greater than normal for age
- Absent or diminished air movement and breath sounds
- Retractions
- Accessory muscle use

▶ Patients with poor circulation
- Weak or absent peripheral pulses
- Pulse rates less or greater than normal for age
- Irregular pulse

Do not delay transport for detailed assessments and procedures that you can provide en route to the hospital.

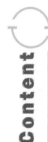

Review

Content

Top Priority Patients

- Poor general impression
- Unresponsive
- Responsive but cannot follow commands
- Airway compromise
- Difficult breathing
- Signs and symptoms of hypoperfusion
- Multiple injuries
- Complicated childbirth
- Chest pain and blood pressure below 100 systolic
- Uncontrolled bleeding
- Severe pain

- Pale, cool, diaphoretic skin
- Uncontrolled bleeding
▶ Obvious serious or multiple injuries
▶ Complicated childbirth

In these cases, decide whether to stabilize your patient on the scene or expedite transport and initiate advanced life support procedures en route. On the way to the hospital you can conduct a detailed history and physical exam and provide additional care as time allows. If your patient is stable, before transport you can conduct a focused history and physical exam—a problem-oriented patient assessment—followed by a detailed physical exam either at the scene or during transport as the situation requires, if time allows.

The initial assessment is the crucial first step in providing lifesaving measures to seriously ill or injured patients. It should take you less than 1 minute to perform, yet it will provide you with enough vital information to confirm your priority determination.

THE FOCUSED HISTORY AND PHYSICAL EXAM

The **focused history and physical exam** is the second stage of patient assessment. It is a problem-oriented process based on your initial assessment and your patient's chief complaint. How you conduct the focused history and physical exam will depend on which of four general categories your patient's initial presentation falls under:

▶ Trauma patient with a significant mechanism of injury or altered mental status

▶ Trauma patient with an isolated injury

▶ Responsive medical patient

▶ Unresponsive medical patient

Each type of patient requires a vastly different approach.

The Major Trauma Patient

The **major trauma patient** is one who has sustained a significant mechanism of injury or has an altered mental status from the incident. For serious trauma patients, you will conduct an initial assessment followed by a rapid trauma assessment, package your patient, provide rapid transport to the emergency department, and perform an ongoing assessment en route, in that order. If time allows, you can also perform a detailed assessment.

Mechanism of Injury

Begin the focused history and physical exam for major trauma patients by reconsidering the mechanism of injury (Figure 3-30 ▶). Although trauma poses a serious threat to life, its appearance often masks your patient's true condition. Extremity injuries, for example, are frequently obvious and grotesque, yet they rarely cause death. Conversely, life-threatening problems such as internal bleeding and rising intracranial pressure often occur with only subtle signs and symptoms. Your assessment of trauma patients must look beyond obvious injuries to the mechanism of injury for evidence that suggests life-threatening situations. Certain mechanisms predictably cause serious internal injury:

▶ Ejection from a vehicle

▶ Fall from higher than 20 feet

▶ Rollover of the vehicle

focused history and physical exam
problem-oriented assessment process based on initial assessment and chief complaint.

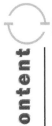
Review
Types of Patients
- Trauma patient with significant mechanism of injury or altered mental status
- Trauma patient with isolated injury
- Responsive medical patient
- Unresponsive medical patient

major trauma patient
person who has suffered significant mechanism of injury.

Review
Order of Focused History and Physical Exam for Major Trauma Patients
- Initial assessment
- Rapid trauma assessment
- Packaging
- Rapid transport and ongoing assessment

Your assessment of trauma patients must look beyond obvious injuries to the mechanism of injury.

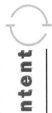
Review
Predictors of Serious Internal Injury
- Ejection from vehicle
- Death in same passenger compartment
- Fall from higher than 20 feet
- Rollover of vehicle
- High-speed vehicle collision
- Vehicle-pedestrian collision
- Motorcycle crash
- Penetration of head, chest, or abdomen

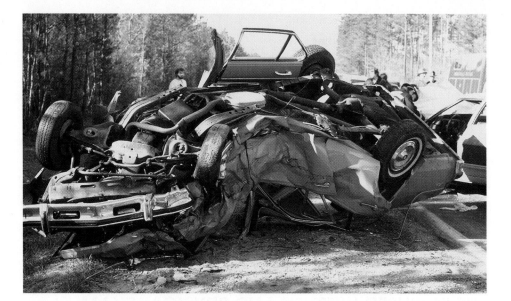

Figure 3-30 Evaluate the trauma scene to determine the mechanism of injury. *(Robert J. Bennett)*

Review

Content

Additional Predictors of Serious Internal Injury for Infants and Children

- Fall from higher than 10 feet
- Bicycle collision
- Medium-speed vehicle collision

Quickly transport patients with a high likelihood of internal injury to an appropriate medical facility.

Do not rule out serious injury just because your patient wore a seat belt.

Always lift a deployed air bag and inspect the steering wheel for deformity.

- High-speed vehicle collision with resulting severe vehicle deformity
- Vehicle-pedestrian collision
- Motorcycle crash
- Penetration of the head, chest, or abdomen

Additional considerations for infants and children include:

- Fall from higher than 10 feet
- Bicycle collision
- Medium-speed vehicle collision with resulting severe vehicle deformity

These mechanisms' presence suggests a high index of suspicion for serious injury. Quickly transport patients to a trauma center when either the mechanism of injury or your patient's clinical presentation indicates a likelihood of internal injury.

Other significant mechanisms of injury can result from seat belts, air bags, and child safety seats. Do not rule out serious injury just because your patient wore a seat belt. Seat belts can actually cause injuries, even when worn properly. Always ask your patient if he wore a seat belt and look for bruises across the chest or around the waist. If present, expect hidden internal injuries.

In general, air bags have been effective devices in preventing serious injury by protecting passengers from hitting the windshield, steering wheel, and dashboard. Originally, they deployed only when the front of the car hit another object. Many automakers currently have installed side air bags that deploy when the car is struck from the side. But they are not without complication. For example, they are designed to cushion the chests of large adults. If the passenger is a child or a short adult, the air bag will hit him in the face, possibly causing injury. Also, air bags are designed to deflate automatically within seconds after inflation, which may allow passengers to be propelled into the steering wheel or dashboard. For this reason, they may not be effective without the seat belt. Always lift the deployed bag and inspect the steering wheel for deformity. If you discover a bent steering wheel, suspect serious internal injury (Figure 3-31 ▶). There is also danger of the bag not deploying in the crash. It may deploy during the rescue operation, putting rescuers in danger of serious injury.

A child safety seat, when used appropriately, also can save a life. But if the safety seat is not securely fastened to the car seat, it can come loose and be thrown when the

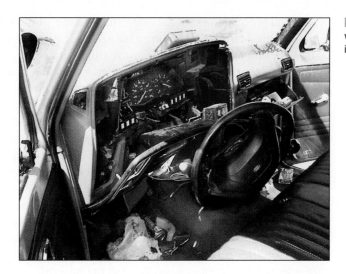

▶ **Figure 3-31** A bent steering wheel signals potentially serious injuries. (*© Michael Grill*)

collision occurs, causing severe head, neck, and body cavity trauma to its occupant. If the harness straps are not tight on the child, the child may come out of the seat during the crash. If the safety seat is used in the car's front seat, the child can suffer a serious injury when the air bag deploys.

If your initial assessment rules out any immediate life threat, examine the suspected area of trauma. Physical signs of trauma such as abrasions or contusions confirm your index of suspicion. If you do not identify any physical evidence, reexamine the mechanism of injury and evaluate your patient's vital signs. You will miss many serious injuries if your index of suspicion is too low.

Usually you will distinguish between those patients who need on-the-scene stabilization and those who need rapid transport after your initial assessment and rapid trauma assessment. Whether to transport your patient immediately or to attempt more extensive on-the-scene assessment and care is among your most difficult decisions, but the care you provide will be more effective if you decide quickly. As a rule, patients who experience the mechanisms of injury listed earlier or who display serious clinical findings should be transported quickly with intravenous access and other procedures attempted en route. Remember, you often arrive at the patient's side only minutes after the crash. He may not yet have lost enough blood internally to demonstrate signs of shock or progressive head injury. If in doubt, transport to an appropriate medical facility without delay. It is always best to err on the side of precaution.

It is always best to err on the side of precaution.

Rapid Trauma Assessment

After you finish your initial assessment, conduct a **rapid trauma assessment** to identify all other life-threatening conditions. Every trauma patient with a significant mechanism of injury, altered mental status, or multiple body-system trauma should receive a rapid trauma assessment. If your patient is responsive, ask him about symptoms as you proceed with your exam. Do not, however, focus totally on the areas your patient identifies as his chief problem. A patient with multiple injuries usually complains about his most painful injury. Sometimes, this may not be his most serious problem. Assess your patient systematically and avoid the tunnel vision invited by dispatch information, first responders' reports, and your patient's chief complaint.

rapid trauma assessment
quick check for signs of serious injury.

Avoid the tunnel vision invited by dispatch information, first responders' reports, and your patient's chief complaint.

Assume that any trauma patient has a spinal injury if he has injuries above the shoulders, has a significant mechanism of injury, or complains of weakness, numbness, or spinal pain. Maintain spinal immobilization throughout your rapid trauma exam.

As you proceed through the exam and discover additional information about your patient, reconsider your decision to transport. Things can change unexpectedly, especially with children. For example, your child patient who appeared stable suddenly deteriorates, requiring you to expedite transport to the closest appropriate facility. The hallmark of an experienced paramedic is the ability to improvise, adapt to new situations, and overcome obstacles that hinder good patient care.

The rapid trauma assessment is not a detailed physical exam but a fast, systematic assessment for other life-threatening injuries. Because you perform it before packaging your patient for transport, you must conduct it quickly. First, reassess your patient's mental status using the AVPU mnemonic and compare your findings with the baseline mental status from your initial assessment. Pay special attention to the head, neck, chest, abdomen, and pelvis. Injuries in these areas can occur with limited signs and symptoms, yet they may rapidly lead to patient deterioration and death. When inspecting an area for injury, keep in mind that the discoloration of contusions will develop over time and may not be apparent at first. Remember, your major concern may not be the injury you see but the internal injuries beneath the superficial wounds. Palpate to identify other signs such as tenderness, deformity, crepitus, symmetry, subcutaneous emphysema, or paradoxical movement. Compare muscle tone and tissue compliance from one side of the body or from one limb to another.

The mnemonic **DCAP-BTLS** may be helpful. The letters represent eight common signs of injury for which you are looking during most of this assessment: *D*eformities, *C*ontusions, *A*brasions, *P*enetrations, *B*urns, *T*enderness, *L*acerations, and *S*welling.

Head Assess the head for DCAP-BTLS and crepitus (Procedure 3-2a). The scalp is extremely vascular and lacks the protective vasospasm mechanism that helps control bleeding. Thus even the most minor lacerations tend to bleed profusely. Inspect the scalp for lacerations that are hidden under hair matted with clotted blood. Look for blood flowing into the hair, and examine your gloved fingers periodically for blood or other body fluids (Procedure 3-2b). If you detect uncontrolled bleeding from the scalp, apply a direct pressure dressing immediately. A simple scalp laceration can cause a life-threatening hemorrhage.

Palpate the skull for open wounds, depressions, protrusions, lack of symmetry, and any unusual warmth. Use cupped hands and do not probe with your fingers. If you feel a depression, stop palpating it, because this risks pushing a broken piece of bone into the brain. If you find an impaled object, stabilize it in place with bulky dressings. If your patient presents with an altered mental status and any abnormality in the structure of the skull, consider this a serious emergency and expedite transport while you continue your assessment and treatment.

Neck Inspect and palpate the neck for DCAP-BTLS and crepitus (Procedure 3-2c). Immediately cover any lacerations that may involve the major blood vessels, such as the carotid arteries and jugular veins, with an occlusive dressing. This is a high-pressure area and your patient can suffer significant blood loss quickly. Because inspiration generates negative pressures in the chest, the jugular veins may draw in air. This can result in a massive air embolus that prevents the heart from pumping blood.

Examine the jugular veins for abnormal distention. In a patient lying supine without circulatory compromise, these veins should distend slightly. If they do not, your patient may be hypovolemic. In the **semi-Fowler's position** (sitting up at 45°), the veins should not distend. Distention beyond 45° is significant because something is inhibiting blood return to the chest. In the trauma patient, this may be the result of cardiac tamponade or tension pneumothorax.

Inspect and palpate the trachea just superior to the sternal notch. It should lie midline and remain fixed during the breathing cycle. Tugging to one side during inspiration

Review

DCAP-BTLS

- Deformities
- Contusions
- Abrasions
- Penetrations
- Burns
- Tenderness
- Lacerations
- Swelling

Immediately cover any neck lacerations that may involve the major blood vessels.

semi-Fowler's position
sitting up at 45°.

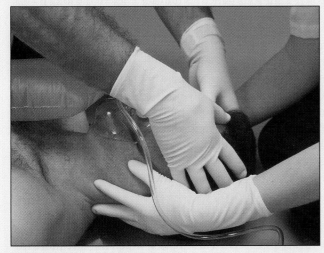

3-2a   The first step in the rapid trauma assessment is to palpate the head.

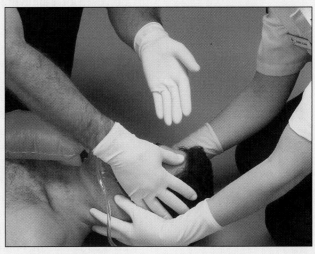

3-2b   Periodically examine your gloves for blood.

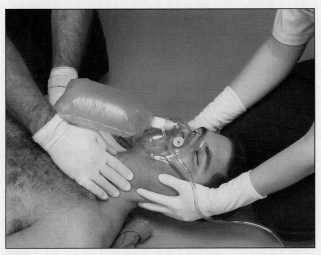

3-2c   Inspect and palpate the anterior neck. Pay particular attention to tracheal deviation and subcutaneous emphysema.

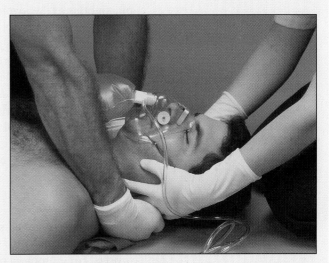

3-2d   Inspect and palpate the posterior neck. Note any tenderness, irregularity, or edema.

suggests a pneumothorax on that side. Displacement to one side may indicate a tension pneumothorax on the opposite side as the entire mediastinum is pushed away from the injury.

Finally, inspect and palpate the neck for **subcutaneous emphysema,** the crackling sensation caused by air just underneath the skin. This condition is the result of air leaking from the respiratory tree into the tissues of the neck. It strongly indicates a serious neck or chest injury.

Now palpate the posterior neck for evidence of spinal trauma (Procedure 3-2d). Gently feel the spinous processes and note any deformities, swelling, and tenderness. If you feel a muscle spasm, consider it a reflex sign following injury somewhere along the

subcutaneous emphysema
crackling sensation caused by air just underneath the skin.

spinal column. When a corroborating mechanism of injury is present, suspect a significant spinal injury requiring immobilization. At this point you can apply a cervical spinal immobilization collar (CSIC). Have someone maintain head and neck stabilization even after applying the collar until your patient is fully fastened to the long board.

Chest Look for signs of acute respiratory distress. If your patient has an upper airway obstruction, he may need to create tremendous negative pressures within his chest just to draw in air. To do so he will use accessory muscles in his neck and chest to help lift the chest wall. These negative pressures may cause suprasternal, supraclavicular, and intercostal retractions. A patient with a lower airway obstruction may have difficulty moving air out. To do so, he may use his abdominal muscles to force the diaphragm upward and inward. He also may purse his lips during exhalation in an attempt to maintain a back pressure to keep the airways open. Infants and small children grunt to maintain this back pressure. Accessory muscle use always indicates a patient in respiratory distress due to a difficulty in moving air. Assist these patients with positive-pressure ventilation and supplemental oxygen as needed.

Quickly inspect and then palpate the chest. Begin palpating at the clavicles and work down and around the rib cage, checking for stability. Palpate the clavicles over their entire length, bilaterally (Procedure 3-3a). These bones, which fracture more frequently than any other bone in the human body, are located directly over the subclavian artery and vein and the superior-most aspect of the lung. Their fracture and displacement may lacerate the vessels or puncture lung tissue, leading to hemothorax, pneumothorax, hypovolemia, or all three.

Be especially careful when palpating the ribs. Beneath each rib lie an artery, a vein, and a nerve that overaggressive palpation can easily damage. Classical soft-tissue injury signs may not be present because the ecchymotic coloration of bruising likely will not have had time to develop. Look for erythema caused by impact to the ribs. The first three ribs are well supported by muscles, ligaments, and tendons. Because of the energy required to fracture them, you should suspect major damage to the underlying organs, especially vascular structures, when they are broken.

If you notice the crackling of subcutaneous emphysema during chest palpation, suspect pneumothorax or a tracheobronchial tear. This condition results when air collects in the soft tissues. Subcutaneous air will normally flow from the upper chest to the neck and head. In some cases, it will drastically change your patient's facial features before your eyes.

Observe for equal, symmetrical, effortless chest rise. The chest should rise with inhalation and fall with exhalation. An abnormality in the chest wall may inhibit this process. For example, a patient with a rib fracture hesitates to expand his chest because it hurts. The fracture of two or more adjacent ribs in two or more places causes an unstable flail (floating) segment, which may be evidenced by paradoxical chest wall movement. Paradoxical movement may not appear early in a flail segment because the muscles surrounding the fractured ribs may contract spasmodically, securing the ribs in place. As the muscles fatigue and relax, the flail segment becomes obvious in the paradoxical movement. A flail chest greatly reduces air movement. The underlying lung contusion and subsequent decreased tidal volume limit the air available for gas exchange. To ensure enough air movement for adequate gas exchange, assist ventilation with a bag-valve mask and supplemental oxygen. If the flail segment is loose, stabilize it to the chest wall with a large pad and tape (Procedure 3-3b).

Inspect your patient's chest front and back for open wounds. The lungs expand because they adhere to the inner chest wall. This adherence is made possible by the presence of two thin membranes: the visceral pleura, which covers the lungs, and the parietal pleura, which covers the inner chest wall. A film of liquid between these two layers creates a negative-pressure bond that forces the lungs to expand with the chest

Rapid Trauma Assessment—The Chest

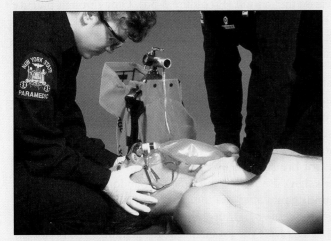

3-3a Palpate the clavicles.

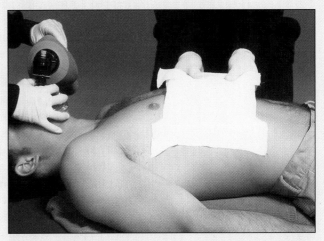

3-3b Stabilize a flail chest.

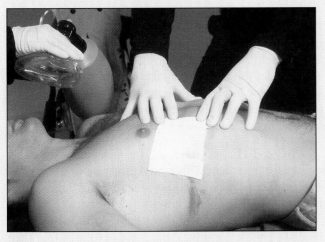

3-3c Seal any sucking chest wound with tape on three sides.

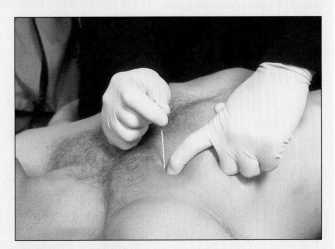

3-3d Perform needle decompression to relieve tension pneumothorax if authorized.

wall. Any opening in this system can disrupt adherence and cause the lung to collapse. Because air follows the path of least resistance, it may enter the chest cavity through the hole instead of through the respiratory tract. Thus, you should seal any open wounds with an occlusive dressing such as Vaseline gauze at the end of exhalation. Tape the dressing on three sides only to create a "one-way valve" effect, allowing air to escape but not be drawn in (Procedure 3-3c). Remember to check carefully under the armpits and back for knife and small-caliber gunshot wounds. You can easily miss these because the elastic skin closes quickly over the wound and limits external bleeding.

Auscultate both lungs quickly at each midaxillary line for equal and adequate air movement. Unequal air movement may indicate the presence of a collapsed lung from a pneumothorax or hemothorax. Absent sounds on one side and diminished sounds on the other may suggest a life-threatening condition known as tension pneumothorax. This condition also presents with severe respiratory distress, accessory muscle use, retractions, tachycardia, hypotension, narrowing pulse pressure, and distended neck veins.

Tracheal deviation may be a late sign of tension pneumothorax. If authorized, perform needle decompression immediately. Insert a large-bore IV catheter into the pleural space at the 2nd intercostal space over the top of the 3rd rib, midclavicular line, allowing the trapped air to escape and release the tension (Procedure 3-3d). Only through practice and repetition will you gain the confidence to recognize the difference between adequate and diminished lung sounds. Again, for patients with inadequate lung sounds, administer 100 percent oxygen and assist ventilation with a bag-valve mask and intubate as needed.

Abdomen   Inspect and palpate the abdomen for DCAP-BTLS and crepitus. Note any areas of bruising and guarding. Exaggerated abdominal wall motion to assist respiration may result from spinal injury, airway obstruction, or respiratory muscle failure. Solid organs such as the kidneys, liver, and spleen can bleed enough blood into the abdominal cavity to cause profound shock.

Two characteristic areas for bruising are over the umbilicus (**Cullen's sign**) and over the flanks (**Grey Turner's sign**). Both signs indicate intra-abdominal hemorrhage but usually will not occur until hours after the injury. Perform deep palpation over each quadrant and note any tenderness, rigidity, and guarding. Be careful, because deep palpation sometimes can aggravate the problem. Avoid spending time needlessly trying to make a specific diagnosis. You need only to recognize the possibility that an intra-abdominal hemorrhage exists and that your patient requires immediate transport to an appropriate medical facility for surgery.

Hollow organs such as the stomach and intestines, when injured, spill their toxic contents into the abdomen, irritating the peritoneum, the inner abdominal lining. Testing for rebound tenderness will help you determine if your patient's peritoneum is irritated. Gently palpate an area and let your hand up quickly. If your patient experiences pain with this release, it is likely due to peritoneal irritation. If you suspect intra-abdominal hemorrhage, provide oxygen and expedite transport. En route to the hospital, provide IV fluid resuscitation as needed.

Pelvis   Examine the pelvis for DCAP-BTLS and crepitus. The importance of a stable pelvic ring cannot be overemphasized. A patient with a pelvic fracture or dislocation risks lacerating the iliac arteries and veins, major blood vessels running through that area. He can easily lose a significant amount of blood into the pelvic cavity.

Evaluate the pelvic ring at the iliac crests and symphysis pubis. With the palms of your hands, direct pressure medially and posteriorly (Procedure 3-4a and 3-4b). Then press posteriorly on the symphysis pubis, being careful not to entrap the penis or cause injury to the urinary bladder. Any pain, instability, or crepitus suggests a pelvic fracture. Always immobilize the pelvis before transport to prevent movement and a possible circulatory catastrophe. Many devices are available to immobilize an unstable pelvic fracture. These include the pneumatic antishock garment, air and vacuum splint devices, even blankets and pillows. Use whichever technique does the job.

Extremities   Inspect and palpate all four extremities for DCAP-BTLS and crepitus (Procedures 3-4c and 3-4d). Splint fractures en route to the hospital if your patient is unstable. Do not spend time splinting fractures on the scene.

Before placing your patient on a backboard and immobilizing his spine, evaluate distal neurovascular function by checking for pulses, sensation, and the ability to move (Procedures 3-4e and 3-4f). If you cannot locate a pulse, determine the adequacy of perfusion by assessing the temperature, color, and condition of the skin of the extremity. Assume vascular compromise if pulse is absent, the extremity is cool, or the skin is ashen or cyanotic. The inability to feel and move both legs indicates complete spinal cord disruption. Diminished sensation, paresthesias, or diminished motor ability may indicate a partial disruption. Weakness or disability on only one side of the body suggests brain injury due to a stroke or head injury. Evaluate these functions again after

Cullen's sign
bruising over the umbilicus.

Grey Turner's sign
bruising over the flanks.

Avoid spending time needlessly trying to make a specific diagnosis during rapid trauma assessment of the abdomen.

Do not spend time splinting an unstable patient's fractures on the scene.

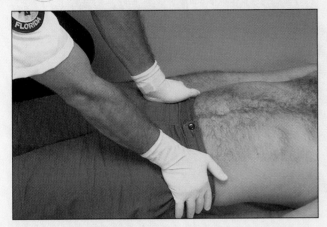

3-4a Assess the integrity of the pelvis by gently pressing medially on the pelvic ring.

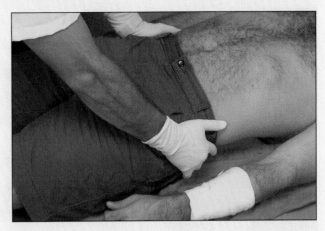

3-4b Compress the pelvis posteriorly.

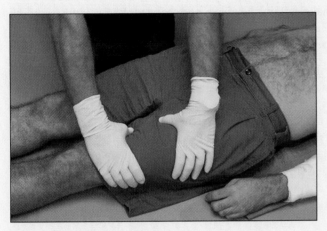

3-4c Palpate the legs.

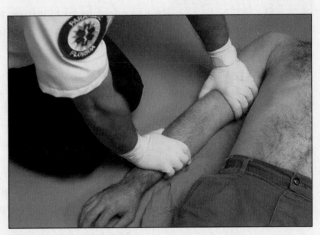

3-4d Palpate the arms.

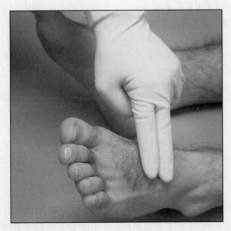

3-4e Palpate the dorsalis pedis pulse to evaluate distal circulation in the leg.

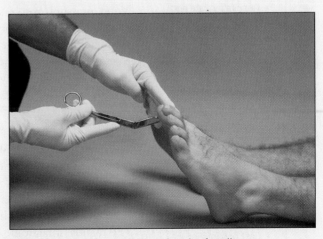

3-4f Assess distal sensation and motor function.

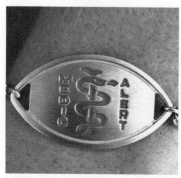

(a)

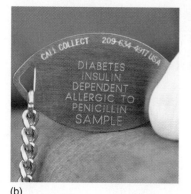

(b)

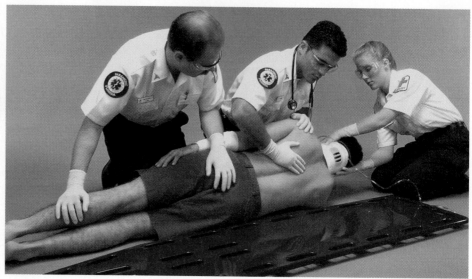

▶ **Figure 3-33** Inspect and palpate the posterior body.

▶ **Figure 3-32** Medic Alert tags can give important information about the patient's condition and medical history.

spinal immobilization to make certain they have not changed. Report and record all extremity function tests. Check for Medic Alert tags, which will identify a medical condition that may complicate the injury (Figure 3-32 ▶).

Posterior Body   Log-roll the patient onto his side to inspect the posterior body. If you suspect a spinal injury, carefully maintain manual stabilization of the head and spine during this procedure. Then inspect and palpate the posterior trunk for DCAP-BTLS and crepitus (Figure 3-33 ▶). Particularly note any tenderness in the spinal area. Palpate the buttocks to rule out hemorrhage, contusion, or other injury. Though predominantly soft tissue, this area is a large mass and can conceal considerable internal blood loss. Next log-roll the patient into a supine position on a long spine board while maintaining manual stabilization of the head and neck. He is now ready to be secured to the spine board and transported.

Vital Signs

Take a baseline set of vital signs, either at the scene or during transport, as your patient's condition and circumstances allow. These vital signs include pulse rate and quality, blood pressure, respiratory rate and quality, and skin temperature and condition. During your EMT-Basic training, you may have learned to include pupils as part of your vital sign check. Including a basic pupil response check (direct response to light) as part of your baseline and serial vital sign assessment is acceptable; however, during the detailed physical exam you may perform an expanded assessment of the pupils (consensual response, near-far response, and accommodation) as outlined in Chapter 2.

History

The history consists of four elements: the chief complaint, the history of present illness, the past history, and the current health status. (Refer to Chapter 1 for a detailed description of taking a history.) For major trauma cases when time is critical, use an abbreviated format that forms the acronym *SAMPLE: Symptoms, Allergies, Medications, Pertinent past medical history, Last oral intake, and Events leading up to the incident. This handy mnemonic is especially useful for eliciting a quick history from your trauma patient. If your patient cannot provide this information, attempt to elicit it from family, friends, and bystanders.

Review

Baseline Vital Signs

- Pulse rate and quality
- Blood pressure
- Respiration rate and quality
- Skin temperature and condition

Review

SAMPLE History

- *Symptoms*
- *Allergies*
- *Medications*
- *Pertinent past medical history*
- *Last oral intake*
- *Events leading up to the incident*

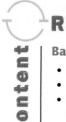

The Isolated-Injury Trauma Patient

Some trauma patients sustain an isolated injury such as a cut finger or sprained ankle. These patients have no significant mechanism of injury and show no signs of systemic involvement such as poor peripheral perfusion, altered mental status, tachycardia, or breathing problems. They do not require an extensive history or comprehensive physical exam. To treat the trauma patient with an isolated injury, first ensure his hemodynamic status via the initial assessment. Then conduct your focused history and physical exam on the specific isolated injury. Use the mnemonic DCAP-BTLS to evaluate the injured area and take a full set of vital signs. Then, if time allows, this is an excellent opportunity to use some of the advanced assessment techniques you learned in Chapter 2. After your exam of the isolated injury, take a SAMPLE history. Remember that some trauma patients may complain of an isolated problem but actually have more significant injuries. Avoid tunnel vision and develop a low threshold for suspecting other injuries based on the mechanism of injury and your patient's story.

Focus your minor trauma assessment on the specific injury and conduct a DCAP-BTLS exam in that area.

In the Field

1. Your patient is a young football player who twisted his knee and lies on the ground, complaining loudly of knee pain. After a quick initial assessment and DCAP-BTLS assessment, you conclude that your patient is in stable condition with no signs or symptoms of systemic involvement and good distal neurovascular function. Before splinting your patient's leg, you decide to elicit more information through a detailed exam of the knee. You inspect the normal concavities for evidence of excessive fluid in the joint by "milking the knee joint" on one side and looking for a fluid wave on the opposite side. Next you palpate the medial and lateral collateral ligaments for tenderness. Then, if doing so does not cause your patient undue pain, you examine the stability of the collateral ligaments with the "side-to-side" test and the cruciate ligaments with the "drawer test." Finally, you assess the knee's passive range of motion (flexion and extension) and note any limitations.

2. Your patient sustains a laceration to the palm of his hand from a bread knife. After you have controlled the bleeding and ensured no systemic involvement or major loss of blood, you decide to examine the hand further before bandaging it. You conduct a DCAP-BTLS exam and note that distal neurovascular function is intact. Knowing that the flexor tendons all run through the palm of the hand, you examine each tendon's function through a full range-of-motion exam. You ask your patient to make a fist, then open his hand and extend all of his fingers. You note any abnormalities, pain, or limitations in the range of motion.

3. Your patient is a teenager who was punched in the eye during a minor altercation with a classmate. After determining that he had no loss of consciousness and that he is alert and oriented with stable vital signs, equal and reactive pupils, and no signs or symptoms of serious head injury, you may conduct a more detailed exam of the injured eye. First, you inspect the external structures for discoloration, deformity, or swelling and find all three. You palpate the orbit of the eye for tenderness and deformity. You look for evidence of hyphema (blood in the anterior chamber), indicating severe blunt trauma. You then examine your patient's visual acuity with a visual acuity card. With a penlight, you check for direct and consensual response to light and for the near-far reflex and accommodation. Finally, you assess the integrity of the extraocular muscles with the H test.

▶ **Figure 3-34** Begin treatment while you assess your responsive medical patient.

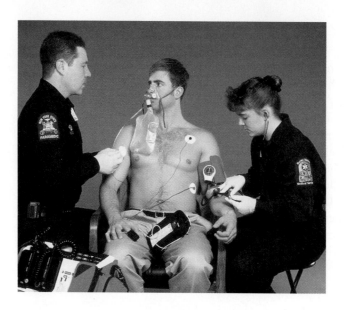

The Responsive Medical Patient

Assessing the responsive patient with a medical emergency is entirely different from assessing the trauma patient for two reasons. First, the history takes precedence over the physical exam. This is because, in the majority of cases, you will formulate your field diagnosis from your patient's story. The physical exam serves mostly to support your diagnostic impression. Second, your physical exam is aimed at identifying signs of medical complications such as inflammation, infection, and edema rather than signs of injury. The focused physical exam evaluates pertinent areas suggested by the history. Remember that you will begin treatment as you conduct your assessment. For example, while interviewing your patient who complains of chest pain, simultaneously take vital signs, administer oxygen, provide cardiac monitoring, and start an IV if appropriate (Figure 3-34 ▶). The following focused history and physical exam pertains to the responsive medical patient. For a more detailed description of the information and techniques outlined here, refer to Chapters 1 and 2.

The History

Listen to your patient; he will tell you what is wrong.

Conscious, alert patients can usually tell you a great deal about their illness. Remember the old medical adage, "Listen to your patient; he will tell you what is wrong." Ask questions and then listen intently to your patient's answers. Because children may not be able to describe their illness and medical history clearly, look to their parents for this information. Elderly patients may pose several obstacles to the clear communication of medical information. They are more likely to be confused, to have poor short-term and long-term memory, and to have hearing, speech, or sight difficulties. Obtaining an accurate history from such patients requires patience, empathy, and outstanding communication skills.

The history consists of four elements: the chief complaint, the history of the present illness, the past history, and the current health status.

chief complaint

the pain, discomfort, or dysfunction that caused your patient to request help.

The Chief Complaint   The **chief complaint** is the pain, discomfort, or dysfunction that caused your patient to request help. Ask your patient, "What seems to be the problem?"

History of the Present Illness   Discover the circumstances surrounding the chief complaint, following the acronym *OPQRST–ASPN*:

Onset	What was your patient doing when the problem/pain began? Did emotional or environmental factors contribute to the problem?
Provocation/**P**alliation	What makes the problem/pain worse or better?
Quality	Can your patient describe the problem/pain?
Region/**R**adiation	Where is the problem/pain and does it radiate anywhere?
Severity	How bad is the problem/pain? Can your patient rate it on a scale of one to ten?
Time	When did the problem/pain begin? How long does the pain last?
Associated **S**ymptoms	Is your patient having any other problems?
Pertinent **N**egatives	Are any likely associated symptoms absent?

Past Medical History   The past medical history may provide significant insights into your patient's chief complaint and your field diagnosis. It includes your patient's general state of health, childhood and adult diseases, psychiatric illnesses, accidents and injuries, and surgeries and hospitalizations. If your history taking reveals significant medical problems, investigate in more detail. Note when your patient first recognized the problem and how it affected him. How frequently did it happen and what medical care did he seek? Was the treatment effective or did the problem recur?

Current Health Status   The current health status assembles all of the factors regarding your patient's medical condition. It tries to gather information that will complete the puzzle surrounding your patient's primary problem. The elements of the current health status include current medications, allergies, tobacco use, alcohol and substance abuse, diet, screening exams, immunizations, sleep patterns, exercise and leisure activities, environmental hazards, the use of safety measures, and any pertinent family or social history. Look for clues and correlations among the various sections of this part of the history. If your patient is critical and your time is limited, use the abbreviated SAMPLE format to elicit the history.

Focused Physical Exam

Once you have obtained the history, begin a focused physical exam based on the information you elicited from your patient. Let the diagnostic impression you formed during the history guide your examination. For example, if you suspect a myocardial infarction, examine areas pertinent to a patient having a heart attack: cardiac and respiratory systems, chest, neck, and peripheral perfusion. It would be pointless and impractical to test deep tendon reflexes, extraocular movements, or the elbow's range of motion. Use those exam techniques presented in Chapter 2 that pertain to your patient's special situation and clinical status.

Three common presentations among your responsive medical patients will be cardiac chest pain/respiratory distress, altered mental status, and acute abdomen. The following sections outline problem-oriented physical exams for those complaints. Note that for each of these cases, the focused physical exam is different. As you gain clinical experience you will be able to quickly assess your patient's pertinent areas according to your suspected field diagnosis. Likewise, clinical judgment and the seriousness of your patient's condition will determine which exam techniques you use on the scene and which you use en route to the hospital.

Review

History for the Responsive Medical Patient

- Chief complaint
- History of present illness
- Past history
- Current health status

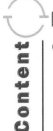

Review

OPQRST–ASPN

- Onset
- Provocation/Palliation
- Quality
- Region, radiation
- Severity
- Time
- Associated Symptoms
- Pertinent Negatives

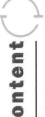

Review

Past Medical History

- General state of health
- Childhood and adult diseases
- Psychiatric illnesses
- Accidents and injuries
- Surgeries and hospitalizations

Review

Current Health Status

- Current medications
- Allergies
- Tobacco use
- Alcohol/substance abuse
- Diet
- Screening exams
- Immunizations
- Sleep patterns
- Exercise/leisure activities
- Environmental hazards
- Use of safety measures
- Family history
- Social history

Chest Pain/Respiratory Distress   For a patient complaining of chest pain or respiratory distress, assess the following:

HEENT (Head, Eyes, Ears, Nose, and Throat)   Note the color of the lips. Lip cyanosis is an ominous sign of central circulatory hypoxia. Examine the oral mucosa for pallor suggesting decreased circulation as in shock. Inspect any fluids in the mouth. Pink, frothy sputum (the result of plasma proteins mixing with air and red blood cells in the alveoli) is a classic sign of acute pulmonary edema. Aggressively suction any fluids from the oropharynx that may compromise the upper airway. Note any swelling, redness, or hives, suggesting an allergic reaction.

Neck   Observe the neck for accessory muscle use and retractions, signs of acute respiratory distress. Retractions in the supraclavicular (above the clavicles) and suprasternal (above the sternum) notches indicate your patient is having difficulty inhaling. Palpate the carotid arteries (one at a time) for rate, quality, and equality; if you detect weak or unequal pulses, auscultate for bruits. Examine the jugular veins for abnormal distention. In a patient lying supine without circulatory compromise, these veins should distend slightly. This is normal. If the jugular veins do not distend in the supine position, your patient may be hypovolemic. In the semi-Fowler's position (sitting up at 45°), the veins should disappear. Distention beyond 45° is significant because something is inhibiting blood return to the chest. This may be the result of cardiac tamponade, tension pneumothorax, or right heart failure. Inspect and palpate the position of the trachea. It should lie midline and remain fixed during the breathing cycle. Tugging to one side during inspiration suggests a pneumothorax on that side. Displacement to one side may indicate a tension pneumothorax on the opposite side as the entire mediastinum is displaced.

Chest   Assess the respiratory rate and pattern again and administer oxygen or ventilation as needed. Note the length of the inspiratory and expiratory phases. A prolonged inspiratory phase suggests an upper airway obstruction. A prolonged expiratory phase suggests a lower airway obstruction such as in asthma and emphysema. Inspect and palpate the chest wall for symmetry of movement and intercostal retractions. A barrel chest suggests a history of emphysema. Look for the classic midline scar from open heart surgery or the typical bulge of an implanted pacemaker or defibrillator.

Auscultate all lung fields (anterior to posterior, apices to bases) and compare side to side. Report and record the sounds you hear (crackles, wheezes), where you hear them (in the bases, apices, diffuse), and when they occur during the respiratory cycle (inspiratory, expiratory). For example, if your patient has bilateral inspiratory crackles, you might suspect congestive heart failure or pulmonary edema. If he has diffuse expiratory wheezing, you might suspect the bronchospasm associated with asthma or chronic obstructive pulmonary disease. The presence of both would suggest acute pulmonary edema. A localized wheeze might indicate a pulmonary embolism, a foreign body aspiration, or an infection. Patients with unilateral (one-sided) decreased breath sounds require further testing such as tactile fremitus, bronchophony, egophony, or whispered pectoriloquy. Percuss the chest and back for hyperresonance (asthma, emphysema, pneumothorax) and dullness (pulmonary edema, pleural effusion, pneumonia).

Cardiovascular   Inspect for signs of arterial insufficiency or occlusion in your patient's trunk and extremities. Look for skin pallor and other signs of decreased perfusion. Inspect and palpate the chest for the point of maximum impulse (PMI) at the 5th intercostal space near the midclavicular line. Assess central and peripheral pulses for equality, rate, regularity, and quality. Auscultate for heart sounds, identifying S_1, S_2, and any additional sounds.

Abdomen   Look for exaggerated abdominal muscle use during exhalation, a sign of lower airway obstruction as seen in asthma and emphysema. Inspect and palpate the abdomen for distention due to air or fluid. Ascites is an accumulation of fluid within the

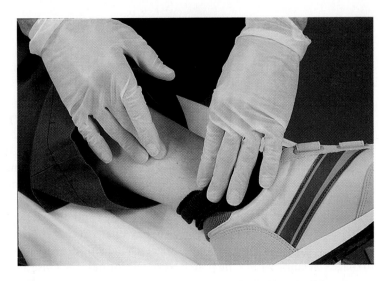

Figure 3-35 Check for peripheral edema.

abdominal cavity caused by increased pressure in the systemic circulation as seen in patients with right heart failure. It is also common in patients with cirrhosis of the liver, where portal circulation (to and from the liver) is increased. This is often seen in patients with right heart failure or cirrhosis of the liver. Inspect and palpate the flanks and pre-sacral area for edema in bedridden patients suspected of having congestive heart failure. Check for unusual pulsation of the descending aorta, just left of the umbilicus. Palpate for liver enlargement or upper quadrant tenderness suggesting ulcer disease, gallbladder disease, or pancreas problems, all of which can be confused as chest pain.

Extremities Perform neurovascular checks on both hands and feet. These consist of checking for pulses, sensation, and the ability to move. Pay special attention to the equality of pulses in all extremities. Unequal pulses in the upper extremities suggest a thoracic aneurysm; unequal pulses in the lower extremities suggest an abdominal aneurysm. Assume vascular compromise if the pulse is absent, the limb is cool, or the skin is cyanotic or ashen. In cardiac and respiratory emergencies, evaluate the lower extremities for pitting edema. Depress the skin on the tibial plateau (Figure 3-35 ▶). If the depression remains after you remove your finger, pitting edema exists. This is a sign of chronic fluid retention as seen in heart and renal failure. Examine the fingernails for pitting. Check the wrists for Medic Alert identification.

Assessment Pearls

Taking a Glucometer Reading for All Patients with Altered Mental Status In a recent case, an unresponsive patient was transported to a community hospital by an ALS ambulance and then later transported by helicopter to a tertiary care facility. Once at the specialty-care hospital, the first thing they did was check the patient's blood sugar. It was 40 mg/dL. The EMS crew and community hospital staff had overlooked this simple diagnostic test. The patient was given lunch and discharged within 1 hour of helicopter arrival.

Granted, this type of case is not a common occurrence; neither is it uncommon. Always, always check the blood glucose level in any patient with altered mental status—or any unexplained physical exam finding—because the condition might be due to hypoglycemia. Many medical conditions, such as hemiparesis, headaches, delirium, abnormal behavior, coma, facial palsies, seizures, and many more, can be attributed to hypoglycemia. The test is easy to administer and the treatment easily provided. When in doubt about a patient's condition, always return first to the basics.

Altered Mental Status   For a patient with an altered mental status, assess the following:

HEENT   Inspect and palpate the head to rule out any evidence of trauma. For example, your stroke patient may have suffered a skull fracture from falling on the floor. Palpate the fontanels of the infant for sunkenness (dehydration) and bulging (increasing intracranial pressure). Examine the face for symmetry. Unilateral facial drooping may indicate a stroke or inflammation of the facial nerve (Bell's palsy). Examine the pupils for direct and consensual response to light. One pupil's getting larger or reacting more slowly to light could indicate a deteriorating brain pathology such as a stroke. A small portion of the population, however, has unequal pupils, a benign condition known as anisocoria. Bilaterally sluggish pupils usually suggest decreased blood flow to the brain and hypoxia. Fixed and dilated pupils indicate severe brain anoxia. Your patient's pupils also may dilate from sympathomimetic or anticholinergic drug use. Pinpoint pupils suggest a narcotic drug overdose or pontine hemorrhage (bleeding within the pons). Next, test for near response and accommodation. Test the integrity of the extraocular muscles with the "H" test. Normally your patient will move his eyes conjugately (together) to follow your finger. He may exhibit a nystagmus, a fine jerking of the eyes. At the far extremes of the test, nystagmus may be normal, but if you observe it during all extraocular movements it suggests a pathology. Examine the conjunctiva for redness (irritation), pallor (hypoperfusion), or cyanosis (hypoxia). Inspect the sclera for jaundice.

Chest   Inspect, palpate, and auscultate the chest for any signs of cardiorespiratory involvement.

Abdomen   Look for evidence of trauma or internal bleeding. Listen for bowel sounds that may be absent in anticholinergic drug ingestions.

Pelvis   Look for evidence of incontinence.

Extremities   Perform neurovascular checks on both hands and feet. These consist of checking for pulses, sensation, and the ability to move. Assume vascular compromise if the pulse is absent, the limb is cool, or the skin is cyanotic or ashen. Because the motor and sensory nerves run along different pathways in the spinal cord, you must check your patient's extremities both for mobility and for sensation of light touch and pain. As with trauma patients, the inability to feel and move both legs indicates complete spinal cord disruption. Diminished sensation or diminished motor ability indicates a partial disruption. Weakness or disability on only one side suggests brain dysfunction such as a stroke. Report and record all extremity function tests.

Posterior Body   Inspect the posterior body for deformities of the spine. Also check for evidence of incontinence or bleeding. In the supine patient, inspect the flanks for presacral edema.

Neuro   Reassess your patient's level of consciousness and compare his response to your earlier findings. Note his speech pattern and any deficits in speech or language. Observe mood swings or behaviors that suggest anxiety or depression. Determine your patient's person, time, and place orientation. Does he know his name, the day of the week, and where he is? Perform the 1-minute cranial nerve exam outlined in Table 3–3. Inspect general body structure, muscle development, positioning, and coordination. Note any obvious asymmetries, deformities, or involuntary movements. Assess muscle tone by feeling the muscle's resistance to passive stretching in the extremities. Note the degree of resistance. Test for muscle strength by applying resistance during the range-of-motion evaluation. Check for pronator drift and watch for any drifting sideways or upward. Assess for coordination and cerebellar function, using rapid alternating movements and

Table 3-3	One-Minute Cranial Nerve Exam
Cranial Nerves	**Test**
I	Normally not done.
II, III	Direct response to light.
III, IV, VI	"H" test for extraocular movements.
V	Clench teeth; palpate masseter and temporal muscles. Test sensory to forehead, cheek, and chin.
VII	Show teeth.
IX, X	Say "aaaahhhh"; watch uvula movement. Test gag reflex.
XII	Stick out tongue.
VIII	Test balance (Romberg test) and hearing.
XI	Shrug shoulders, turn head.

point-to-point testing. Note seizure activity tremors. Ask the primary caregivers whether your patient's presentation is normal for him or if this represents a change.

Acute Abdomen   For a patient complaining of abdominal pain, assess the following:

HEENT   Notice any unusual odors coming from your patient's mouth. The smell of alcohol does not rule out a serious medical condition. The sweet or fruity smell of ketones suggests diabetes. A fecal odor may indicate a lower bowel obstruction. The acidic smell of gastric contents means that your patient has vomited and may again. Inspect any fluids in the mouth. "Coffee-grounds" emesis (vomiting) results from blood mixing with stomach acids and suggests an upper gastrointestinal (GI) bleed. Fresh blood usually means recent hemorrhage from the upper GI tract.

Chest   Listen to breath sounds. Crackles may indicate pneumonia, a cause of upper abdomen pain.

Abdomen   Look for discoloration over the umbilicus (Cullen's sign), or over the flanks (Grey Turner's sign), suggesting intra-abdominal bleeding. Check for any visible pulsation, peristalsis, or masses. If you notice a bounding or an exaggerated pulsation, suspect an aortic aneurysm. Visible peristalsis may indicate a bowel obstruction. Auscultate for bowel sounds and renal bruits. Percussing the abdomen produces different sounds based on the underlying tissues. Percuss the abdomen in the same sequence you used for auscultation. Note the distribution of tympany and dullness. Expect tympany in most of the abdomen; expect dullness over the solid abdominal organs such as the liver and spleen.

Palpate the abdomen last to detect tenderness, muscular rigidity, and superficial organs and masses. The normal abdomen is soft and nontender. Abdominal pain on light palpation suggests peritoneal irritation or inflammation. If you feel rigidity or guarding while palpating, determine whether it is voluntary (patient anticipates the pain or is not relaxed) or involuntary (peritoneal inflammation). Then palpate the abdomen deeply to detect large masses or tenderness. If the peritoneum is inflamed, your patient will experience pain when you let go.

Posterior Body   Inspect the posterior body for evidence of rectal bleeding.

Baseline Vital Signs

Prehospital medicine employs four basic vital signs: blood pressure, pulse, respiration, and temperature. As mentioned earlier, you may add a basic pupil assessment to this list. Your patient's vital signs are your windows to what is happening inside his body. They provide a unique, objective capsule assessment of his clinical status. Vital signs indicate severe illness and the urgency to intervene. Subtle alterations in these vital signs are often the only indication that your patient's condition is changing. They can warn you that your patient is deteriorating, or they can reassure you that he is responding to therapy.

Of the physical assessment techniques, taking accurate sets of vital signs reveals the most important information. As a paramedic you must assess these signs on every patient you evaluate. If your patient is with you for an extended time, measure and record his vital signs at intervals as his clinical condition dictates. Always reevaluate the vital signs after invasive procedures such as endotracheal intubation or fluid resuscitation and after any sudden change in your patient's condition. Accurate records of these numbers are invaluable when documenting your patient assessment.

If you suspect your patient of being hypovolemic, consider performing an orthostatic vital sign exam, commonly known as the tilt test. Take your patient's pulse and blood pressure while he is supine. Then have him sit up and dangle his feet. Finally, tell him to stand. Then in 30 to 60 seconds retake the vital signs. They should not change in the healthy patient. An increase in the pulse rate of 10 to 20 beats per minute or a drop in blood pressure of 10 to 20 mmHg is a positive tilt test. This is a common finding in patients suspected of hypovolemia. Chapter 2 describes vital sign evaluation in detail.

Additional Assessment Techniques

Additional techniques include pulse oximetry, capnography, cardiac monitoring, and blood glucose determination. Refer to Chapter 2 for detailed descriptions of these techniques.

Pulse Oximetry   The pulse oximeter is a noninvasive device that measures the oxygen saturation of your patient's blood. It is usually a good indicator of cardiorespiratory status because it tells you how well your patient is oxygenating the most distal ends of his circulatory system. It also quantifies the effectiveness of your interventions such as oxygen therapy, medications, suctioning, and ventilatory assistance. Normal oxygen saturation at sea level should be between 96 and 100 percent. Generally, if the reading is below 95 percent, suspect shock, hypoxia, or respiratory compromise. Provide your patient with the appropriate airway management, supplemental oxygen, and watch him carefully for further changes. Any reading below 90 percent requires aggressive airway management, positive-pressure ventilation, or oxygen administration.

Capnography   End-tidal CO_2 ($ETCO_2$) detectors are used most commonly to assess proper placement of an endotracheal tube. These devices are attached either in-line or alongside the endotracheal tube and the ventilation device. A color change in the colorimetric CO_2 detector or a light on the electronic monitor indicates the presence of exhaled carbon dioxide, which confirms proper tube placement. Capnography is useful in detecting accidental tracheal extubation, tube obstruction, or disconnection from a ventilation system during transport. In addition, capnography can provide an indirect estimation of cardiac output and pulmonary blood flow and thus, ultimately, the effectiveness of CPR during cardiac arrest. This is the case because, unfortunately, although the $ETCO_2$ detector is accurate, the CO_2 level falls precipitously during cardiac arrest. Therefore, if the patient is in cardiac arrest and CPR is ineffective, there will be no color change or light on the $ETCO_2$ detector, and this will indicate an absence of exhaled carbon dioxide.

Cardiac Monitoring   The cardiac monitor, which measures electrical activity, is essential in assessing and managing the patient who requires advanced cardiac life support (ACLS) measures. You should apply it to any patient you suspect of having a serious illness or injury. Its one major disadvantage, however, is that it cannot tell you if the heart is pumping efficiently, effectively, or at all. Always assess your patient and compare what you see on the monitor with what you feel for a pulse. If available, perform 12-lead ECG monitoring to identify the presence and location of a possible myocardial infarction.

Always reevaluate vital signs after invasive procedures and after any sudden change in your patient's condition.

Review

Content

Additional Assessment Techniques

• Pulse oximetry
• Capnography
• Cardiac monitoring
• Blood glucose determination

Apply the cardiac monitor to any patient you suspect of having a serious illness or injury.

Blood Glucose Determination   In cases of altered mental status, such as diabetic emergencies, seizures, and strokes, measure your patient's blood sugar level. The arrival of inexpensive, handheld glucometers makes this test simple and easy to perform in the field.

Emergency Medical Care

After conducting your physical exam, provide the necessary emergency medical care authorized by your medical director via standing orders. Then contact the on-line medical direction physician to request further orders. For example, you may administer 50 percent dextrose to an adult patient (25 percent dextrose to a pediatric patient) with documented hypoglycemia (Figure 3-36), intubate a patient in severe respiratory distress, or apply external cardiac pacing to a patient with third-degree heart block. Always base your emergency care on your patient's signs and symptoms as obtained through a thorough focused history and physical exam. Finally, en route to the hospital conduct an ongoing assessment as described later in this chapter.

Again, if time allows, in certain situations you may wish to selectively use some of the advanced assessments described in Chapter 2. For example, en route to the hospital you might conduct a complete neurologic exam for your patient who complains of stroke-like symptoms. This would comprise a full mental status assessment including orientation, appearance and behavior, speech and language, mood, thoughts and perceptions, insight and judgment, and memory and attention; a cranial nerve exam; a motor system assessment including muscle bulk, tone, and strength; a sensory exam including sharp and dull identification, temperature discrimination, position and vibration sense, and discriminative sensation; and deep tendon, as well as superficial, reflex tests. For your patient with upper respiratory distress and flu symptoms, you may decide to examine the posterior pharynx and tonsils for redness and exudate; palpate the cervical lymph nodes for presence and tenderness; and thoroughly assess the lungs for tactile fremitus, egophony, bronchophony, and whispered pectoroloquy. For your patient suspected of having acute appendicitis, you may wish to use the psoas test. Ask your patient to bring his right knee to his chest, contracting the iliopsoas muscle group. This motion usually causes pain as the muscles rub against the inflamed appendix. Your clinical experience and judgment will guide these types of decisions. The scope of paramedic practice is changing, not in procedures but in assessment capabilities. You will learn much more than your predecessors about anatomy and physiology, pathophysiology, and patient assessment. In time, you will learn which exam techniques yield the most relevant information and use them in your daily practice.

Always base care of responsive medical patients on your patient's signs and symptoms as obtained through a thorough focused history and physical exam.

Expedite transfer of unresponsive medical patients to the hospital and perform an ongoing assessment every 5 minutes en route.

The Unresponsive Medical Patient

Since he cannot tell you what is wrong, the unresponsive medical patient requires an entirely different approach than the responsive patient. Assess the unresponsive medical patient much as you would a trauma patient. Begin with the initial assessment; then conduct a rapid head-to-toe exam known as the rapid medical assessment; and finally take a brief history from family or friends. This approach to the unresponsive medical patient also will help you to detect whether trauma may be involved.

After conducting the initial assessment, position your patient so that his airway is protected. If the cervical spine is not involved, place your patient in the recovery position—laterally recumbent. This will prevent secretions from obstructing his airway. Now begin the rapid medical assessment. The rapid medical assessment is similar to the rapid trauma assessment, except that you will look for signs of illness, not injury. Assess the head, neck, chest, abdomen, pelvis, extremities, and posterior aspect of the body. Perform the entire exam with the unresponsive patient. Then, assess baseline vital signs: pulse, blood pressure, respiration, and temperature. Finally, obtain a history from bystanders, family members, friends, or medical identification devices or services. If possible this history should include the chief complaint, history of the present illness, past medical history, and current health status.

Evaluate your data and provide emergency medical care while performing additional tests such as cardiac monitoring, blood glucose determination, and pulse oximetry as needed. Consider your unresponsive patient unstable and expedite transport to the hospital, performing an ongoing assessment every 5 minutes en route.

In the Field

The rapid assessment is not a comprehensive history and physical exam, but a practical, systematic assessment aimed at quickly identifying the cause of your patient's unresponsive condition. Your care for a patient with a coma of unknown origin, for example, might go something like this:

You are dispatched to aid an "unresponsive person" in a residential neighborhood. Your patient is an elderly man who presents laterally recumbent on the floor of his bathroom. You conduct an initial assessment while your partner elicits information from the patient's wife:

General:	Your patient appears pale and diaphoretic, moaning unintelligibly. You find no apparent signs of trauma, and he appears to have slumped to the floor from the toilet.
Mental Status:	You establish your patient's mental status with the AVPU mnemonic. He responds to your voice but cannot answer your questions.
Airway:	You open your patient's airway with a head-tilt/chin-lift maneuver and observe his breathing. His airway is clear. His breathing is rapid and shallow but not labored. You ask another rescuer to administer positive-pressure ventilation with supplemental oxygen while you continue with your assessment.
Circulation:	You palpate his radial pulse, and note its absence. His carotid pulse is slow, regular, and weak. His skin is pale, cool, and clammy, indicating poor peripheral perfusion.

You assign this patient a high priority because of his altered mental status; his rapid, shallow breathing; and his poor peripheral perfusion. You suspect shock and begin a rapid medical assessment.

HEENT:	You note lip cyanosis, a sign of central hypoxia. You see no lip pursing, nasal flaring, or other signs of increased breathing effort such as retractions or accessory muscle use. You smell no unusual odors or fluids from the mouth. The face is symmetrical; the pupils are equal and round but react to light sluggishly. The trachea is midline, there is no jugular vein distention (JVD).
Chest:	You note symmetrical chest wall movement and an equal and adequate rise and fall of the chest with each ventilation. You note some crackles in the lung bases. Your patient has no surgical scars.
ABD:	You see no ascites or abdominal distention, no rigidity or guarding, no rebound tenderness, no renal or carotid bruits, no needle marks, no surgical scars or pulsating masses.
Pelvis:	You see no evidence of bladder or bowel incontinence or of rectal bleeding.
Extremities:	No finger clubbing, no medical identification, no needle marks. Peripheral circulation is poor with no radial or pedal pulses. You note no needle marks but some pitting edema in lower extremities.
Posterior:	You note some edema in your patient's flanks.
Vitals:	Heart rate, 46 and regular; blood pressure, 78/38; respirations, 36 and shallow.
Additional:	ECG monitor shows third-degree AV block; pulse oximetry, 92 percent on room air, 99 percent with oxygen; blood glucose, 110.

Your patient's wife reveals his long history of heart disease and a long list of cardiac medications. Your field diagnosis is cardiogenic shock due to the bradycardic rate of the third-degree block. While your partner initiates an IV, you set up for immediate external cardiac pacing.

THE DETAILED PHYSICAL EXAM

The **detailed physical exam** uses many components of the comprehensive evaluation presented in the previous two chapters. It is a careful, thorough process of eliciting the history and conducting a physical exam. The detailed physical exam is a luxury, designed for use en route to the hospital, if time allows, for patients with significant trauma or serious medical illnesses. Ironically, with critical patients you usually will not have time to perform this in-depth exam because you will be preoccupied with performing ongoing assessments and providing emergency care. So you will seldom, if ever, perform a complete exam in the field. In fact, physicians in the emergency department rarely perform a detailed exam on their critical patients. It is too comprehensive and time consuming and yields little relevant information.

In the emergency setting, use a modified approach. You can individualize the exam to your patient's particular situation in many ways. For example, for the multiple-trauma patient, perform a head-to-toe survey that is more detailed and slower than the rapid trauma assessment yet focuses on injury. For the 17-year-old football player who presents with shoulder pain, you may perform the entire portion of the shoulder exam. Palpating the abdomen and auscultating heart sounds would yield little useful

detailed physical exam
careful, thorough process of eliciting the history and conducting a physical exam.

In the emergency setting, individualize the exam to your patient's particular situation.

information. For your stable patient who complains of abdominal pain, you may conduct an extensive history as detailed in Chapter 1, instead of the abbreviated SAMPLE history. Often you will elicit vital information from a seemingly obscure question during the review of systems. Again, clinical experience and your patient's condition will determine how you proceed with the detailed exam.

Components of the Comprehensive Exam

When you conduct the detailed exam you will use components of the comprehensive exam presented in Chapters 1 and 2. Refer to those chapters for a complete description of the components outlined in this section. Interview your patient to ascertain the history, then conduct a systematic head-to-toe physical exam. Place special emphasis on those areas suggested by your patient's chief complaint and current problem. Remember that the physical exam can be an anxiety-provoking experience for both the patient and the examiner. Using a professional, calm demeanor will minimize this anxiety. The following example illustrates how you might conduct a detailed physical exam for a multiple-trauma patient en route to the hospital.

Head Palpate the cranium from front to back for symmetry and smoothness (Procedure 3-5a). Note any tenderness, deformities, and areas of unusual warmth. Inspect and palpate the facial bones for stability and note any crepitus or loose fragments (Procedure 3-5b). Any instability or asymmetry of the eye orbits, nasal bones, maxilla, or mandible suggests a facial bone fracture. In these cases, pay careful attention to the upper airway for obstruction from blood, bone chips, and teeth. Suction these patients aggressively to keep the upper airway clear.

When the base of the skull is fractured, blood and fluid from the brain can seep into the soft tissues around the eyes and ears and can drain from the ears or nose. Observe the bony orbits of the eye and the mastoid process behind the ears for discoloration. **Periorbital ecchymosis** (raccoon's eyes) is a black and blue discoloration surrounding the eye sockets. **Battle's sign** is a similar discoloration over the mastoid process just behind the ears (Procedure 3-5c). They are both late signs and usually are not visible on the scene unless a previous injury exists. Evaluate the temporomandibular joint for tenderness, swelling, and range of motion.

Eyes Examine the external structure of the eyes for symmetry in size, shape, and contour. Inspect the sclera and conjunctiva for discoloration, swelling, and exudate. Inspect the eyes for discoloration, foreign bodies, or blood in the anterior chamber (hyphema). Hyphema suggests that a tremendous blunt trauma to the anterior part of the eye has occurred. Check the pupils for equality in size and reaction to light (Procedure 3-5d). Bilaterally sluggish pupils usually suggest decreased cerebral perfusion and hypoxia. Fixed and dilated pupils indicate severe cerebral anoxia. Unequal pupils may indicate a variety of pathologies, including brain lesions, meningitis, drug poisoning, third-nerve paralysis, and increasing intracranial pressure.

Examine the eyes for conjugate movement, that is, their ability to move together. Muscle or nerve damage to the eyes and use of certain drugs can cause dysconjugate gaze, in which the eyes seem to look in different directions. Check for extraocular movements. Note any inability of the eyes to follow your finger as you draw a large imaginary "H" in front of them; this indicates either nerve damage or an orbital fracture impinging on the extraocular muscles (Procedure 3-5e). Test for visual acuity and peripheral vision, if appropriate.

Ears Examine the external ears and observe the surrounding area for deformities, lumps, skin lesions, tenderness, and erythema. Examine the ear canal for drainage (Procedure 3-5f). A basilar skull fracture can cause blood and clear cerebrospinal fluid

Aggressively suction patients with facial fractures to keep the upper airway clear.

periorbital ecchymosis
black and blue discoloration surrounding the eye sockets.

Battle's sign
black and blue discoloration over the mastoid process.

Detailed Physical Exam—The Head and Neck

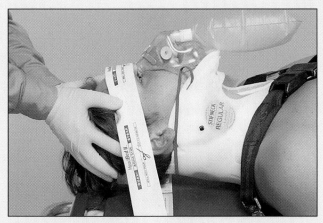

3-5a Inspect and palpate the cranium from front to back.

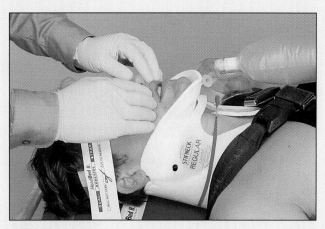

3-5b Inspect and palpate the facial bones.

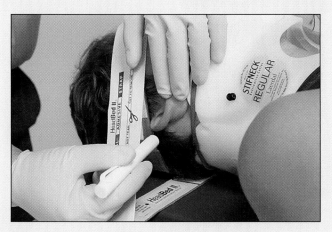

3-5c Inspect the mastoid process for Battle's sign.

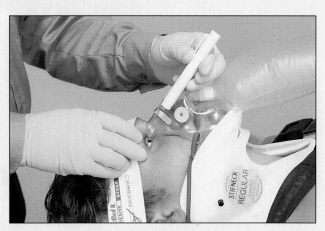

3-5d Check the pupils for reaction to light.

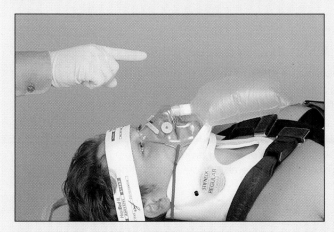

3-5e Check for extraocular movement.

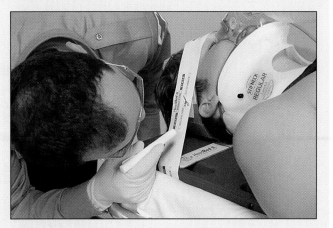

3-5f Inspect the ear canal for drainage.

(continued)

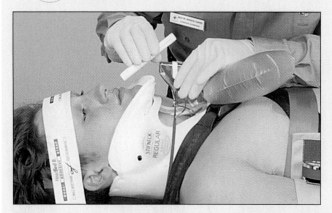

3-5g Examine the nasal mucosa for drainage.

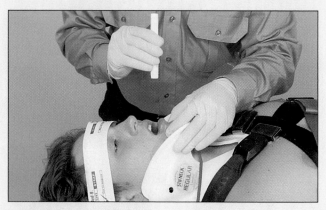

3-5h Examine the oral mucosa for pallor.

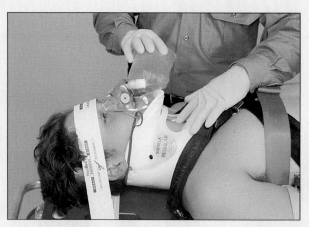

3-5i Palpate the trachea for midline position.

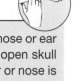

Assessment Pearls

Recognizing Cerebrospinal Fluid   Clear fluid drainage from the nose or ear in the setting of trauma is a worrisome finding that points to a possible open skull fracture. How can you determine whether clear fluid coming from the ear or nose is cerebrospinal fluid (CSF) or another fluid? Most paramedics are familiar with the "halo test," in which a drop of the fluid is placed onto filter paper, a sheet, or a towel. If CSF is present, a ring or "halo" will form (i.e., a dark red circle surrounded by a lighter, yellowish circle). This is due to the erythrocytes migrating only a short distance while the CSF migrates farther.

Although the halo test has proven fairly accurate in detecting CSF, it can be difficult to interpret. If the halo test is suspect, consider the following test.

CSF normally has approximately half the glucose content of blood. So use your glucometer to test the clear fluid and obtain a glucose reading on it. Repeat the glucometer test on the patient's blood. If the glucose reading in the clear fluid is much less than that of the blood, CSF leakage is likely.

(CSF) to leak into the auditory canals and flow to the outside. Do not try to block this flow; just cover it with sterile gauze to prevent an easy route for infection. Check for hearing acuity as appropriate.

Nose and Sinuses   Check your patient's nose from the front and from the side and note any deviation in shape or color. Palpate the external nose for depressions, deformities, and tenderness. Examine the nares for flaring, a sign of respiratory distress, especially in small children. Pay special attention to infants less than 3 months old. They are mainly nose breathers and need a clear, unobstructed nasal cavity for respiration. Examine the nasal mucosa for evidence of drainage and note the color, quantity, and consistency of the discharge (Procedure 3-5g). A clear, runny discharge may indicate leaking CSF from a basilar skull fracture. Test for nasal obstruction.

The nasal cavity has a rich blood supply to warm the inspired air. Unfortunately, this can make bleeding in the nasal cavity severe and very difficult to control. If unconscious, these patients require aggressive suctioning. The patient who swallows this blood may complain later of nausea and vomiting.

Mouth and Pharynx   Note the condition and color of the lips. Lip cyanosis is an ominous sign of central circulatory hypoxia. Examine the oral mucosa for pallor, suggesting poor perfusion as in shock (Procedure 3-5h). Ask your patient to extend his tongue straight out and then move it from side to side. Press a tongue blade down on the middle third of the tongue and have your patient say "aaahhh." Examine the movement of the uvula. Asymmetrical movement of the uvula suggests a cranial nerve lesion. Note any odors or fluids coming from your patient's mouth; they can provide clues to infection, poisoning, and metabolic processes such as diabetic ketoacidosis.

Neck   Briefly inspect the neck for general symmetry. Note any obvious deformity, deviation, tugging, masses, surgical scars, gland enlargement, or visible lymph nodes. Examine any penetrating injuries to the neck closely for injury to the trachea or major blood vessels. Look for jugular vein distention while your patient is sitting up and at a 45° incline. Palpate the trachea for midline position (Procedure 3-5i). Then, palpate the carotid arteries and note their rate and quality.

Chest and Lungs   Observe your patient's breathing. Look for signs of acute respiratory distress. Count his respiratory rate and note his breathing pattern. Inspect the anterior and posterior chest walls for symmetrical movement. Note the use of neck muscles (sternocleidomastoids, scalene muscles) during inhalation or abdominal muscles during exhalation. Accessory muscle use suggests partial airway obstruction and difficulty moving air. Inspect the intercostal spaces for retractions or bulging.

Palpate the rib cage for rigidity (Procedure 3-6a). Feel for tenderness, deformities, depressions, loose segments, asymmetry, and crepitus. Evaluate for equal expansion. Percuss the chest symmetrically from the apices to the bases. Identify and note any area of abnormal percussion. Auscultate all lung fields and compare side to side (Procedure 3-6b).

Percussion can also provide evidence regarding chest pathology. If the region is hyperresonant, the thorax may contain air under pressure (tension pneumothorax). If the region is dull to percussion, it may be filled with blood (hemothorax) or other fluid (pleural effusion). Be sure to compare the sounds left to right and, during examination of the posterior body, front to back to confirm your evaluation.

Cardiovascular System   Look for skin pallor and other signs of decreased perfusion. Inspect and palpate the carotid arteries for rate, rhythm, and quality or amplitude. Inspect and palpate the chest for the PMI. Auscultate for normal, abnormal, and extra heart sounds.

Abdomen   Inspect the skin of the abdomen and flanks for scars, dilated veins, stretch marks, rashes, lesions, and pigmentation changes. Look for Cullen's sign or Grey Turner's

Lip cyanosis is an ominous sign of central circulatory hypoxia.

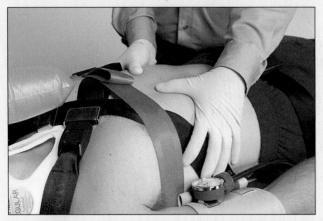

3-6a   Palpate the rib cage.

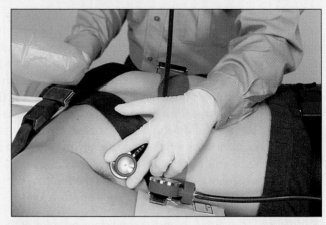

3-6b   Auscultate the lungs.

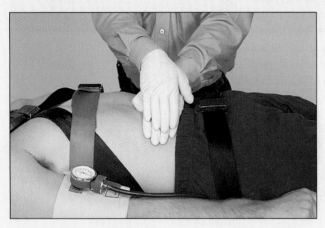

3-6c   Palpate the abdomen.

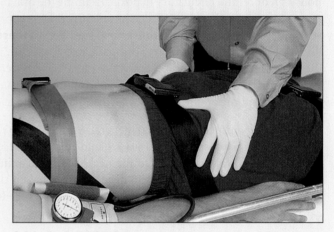

3-6d   Evaluate the pelvis.

sign, suggesting intra-abdominal bleeding. Assess the size and shape of your patient's abdomen and note its symmetry. Palpate the abdomen last to detect tenderness, muscular rigidity, and superficial organs and masses (Procedure 3-6c). Assess for rebound tenderness, a classic sign of peritoneal irritation, by pushing down slowly and then releasing your hand quickly off the tender area.

Pelvis   Reevaluate the pelvic ring at the iliac crests and symphysis pubis (Procedure 3-6d). With the palms of your hands, direct pressure medially and posteriorly. Then press posteriorly on the symphysis pubis, being careful not to entrap the penis or cause injury to the urinary bladder. Any pain, instability, or crepitus suggests a pelvic fracture. Always immobilize the pelvis before transport to prevent movement and a possible circulatory catastrophe. If your patient presents in shock with an unstable pelvis, apply and inflate the pneumatic antishock garment.

Genitalia   The external genitalia are extremely vascular and can bleed profusely when lacerated. Control hemorrhage in this area with direct pressure. Examine the male organ for priapism, a painful, prolonged erection usually caused by spinal cord injury or blood disturbances. Suspect a major spinal cord injury in any patient with a priapism. The female genitalia are somewhat well protected from all but penetrating injury.

If you suspect that your patient may have been raped or sexually abused, limit your assessment and management to only those techniques that are essential to patient stabilization. If possible, have a member of the same sex treat these patients. This may relieve any hostilities and anxiety that might be directed toward a caregiver of the opposite sex. Encourage the patient not to bathe. One of your most important tasks is to provide emotional support and reassurance. (For more on this subject, see the abuse and assault chapter in Volume 5, *Special Considerations/Operations.*)

One of your most important tasks for possible victims of rape or sexual abuse is to provide emotional support and reassurance.

Anus and Rectum   Examining the anus is normally not a prehospital assessment practice. If your patient presents with severe rectal bleeding, apply direct pressure to the area with sterile pads and be prepared to treat him for shock. You will have no other reason to examine this area.

Peripheral Vascular System   Inspect all four extremities, noting their size and symmetry. Palpate the peripheral arteries for pulse rate and quality. Assess the skin for temperature, moisture, color, and capillary refill.

Musculoskeletal System   Reinspect and palpate all four extremities. Inspect and palpate your patient's joints, their structure, their range of motion, and the surrounding tissues. Inspect for swelling in or around joints, changes in the surrounding tissue, redness of the overlying skin, deformities, and symmetry of impairment. Compare both sides for equal size, shape, color, and strength. Palpate for tenderness in and around the joint. Try to identify the specific structure that is tender, such as a ligament or tendon.

Test for range of motion passively and against gravity and resistance. Difficulty during passive range-of-motion tests suggests a joint problem. Difficulty with gravity or against resistance suggests a muscular weakness or nerve problem. Listen for crepitus, the crunching sounds of unlubricated parts rubbing against each other, while you manipulate the joint. Perform distal neurovascular checks.

Nervous System   A nervous system exam covers five areas: mental status and speech, the cranial nerves, the motor system, the reflexes, and the sensory system.

Mental Status and Speech   First, assess your patient's level of consciousness and compare his response to your earlier findings. Observe his posture and motor behavior and his grooming and personal hygiene. Note his speech pattern and use of language. Observe your patient's mood from his verbal and nonverbal behavior. Assess his thought content, perceptions, insight and judgment, memory, attention, and learning ability.

Cranial Nerves   Test any cranial nerves that you have not already checked. (Review Table 3–3 for a quick, reliable, practical, cranial nerve exam that should take no longer than 1 minute to perform.)

Motor System   Inspect your patient's general body structure, muscle development, positioning, and coordination. Note any obvious asymmetries, deformities, or involuntary movements. Assess muscle tone by feeling the muscle's resistance to passive stretching in the extremities. Test for muscle strength by applying resistance during the range-of-motion evaluation. Check for pronator drift and watch for any drifting sideways (laterally) or upward (superiorly). Assess for coordination and cerebellar function, using rapid alternating movements and point-to-point testing.

Reflexes   Test your patient's deep tendon reflexes with a reflex hammer and note any hyperactive or diminished response. Check the biceps, triceps, brachioradialis, quadriceps, and Achilles reflexes. Test the superficial abdominal reflexes and plantar response.

Sensory System   Test for pain, light touch, temperature, position, vibration, and discriminative sensations. Compare distal areas to proximal areas, symmetrical areas

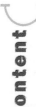

Review

Content

Areas of Nervous System Exam

- Mental status and speech
- Cranial nerves
- Motor system
- Reflexes
- Sensory system

Review

Content

Reflex Tests

- Biceps
- Triceps
- Brachioradialis
- Quadriceps
- Achilles
- Abdominal
- Plantar

Review

**Sensory System
Tests**

- Pain
- Light touch
- Temperature
- Position
- Vibration
- Discriminative

bilaterally, and scatter the stimuli to assess most of the dermatomes. Assess your patient's ability to distinguish sharp from dull sensations.

Vital Signs

Take another set of vital signs and compare them to earlier sets to detect any trends, patterns that indicate either an improvement or deterioration in your patient's condition. These trends include a rising or falling pulse rate and blood pressure; an increasing or decreasing respiratory rate and effort; changing skin temperature, color, and condition; and changing pupillary equality and response to light. Such trends may suggest specific pathologies that you will learn about in Volume 3, *Medical Emergencies*, and Volume 4, *Trauma Emergencies*.

Recording Exam Findings

Record all exam findings on the appropriate run sheet or chart. Remain objective and nonjudgmental when recording the data. Chapter 6, "Documentation," gives detailed instructions on writing patient care reports.

ONGOING ASSESSMENT

Review

**Ongoing
Assessment**

- Detects trends
- Determines changes
- Assesses interventions'
  effects

En route to the hospital, conduct an ongoing series of assessments to detect trends, determine changes in your patient's condition, and assess the effectiveness of your interventions. Patient condition can change suddenly. You must steadfastly reassess mental status, airway patency, breathing adequacy, circulation, and any deterioration in areas already compromised (Procedure 3-7a). Conduct your ongoing assessment every 15 minutes for stable patients, every 5 minutes for unstable patients. Compare your findings to the baseline findings and note any trends.

Mental Status

You must steadfastly reassess mental status, ABCs, and any areas already compromised.

Any deterioration in mental status is cause for great concern.

Recheck your patient's mental status by performing the AVPU exam frequently during transport. Any deterioration in mental status is cause for great concern. The brain demands a constant supply of oxygen and glucose and a constant elimination of waste products. When it is deprived of either, even briefly, expect rapid mental status changes. A falling level of response indicates either a direct or indirect brain pathology. For example, following a head injury, your patient who was alert and oriented at the scene gradually becomes sleepy and eventually unarousable. You should suspect a life-threatening increase in intracranial pressure (pressure inside the enclosed skull) and expedite transport to the appropriate medical facility. Or your patient with an intra-abdominal hemorrhage becomes increasingly less arousable due to the decreased oxygenated blood flow to the brain (indirect pathology). Or sometimes patients improve following your interventions. After you administer 50 percent dextrose to your hypoglycemic diabetic patient, for instance, he becomes alert and begins talking.

Airway Patency

The patency of your patient's airway can change instantly. Bleeding, vomiting, and even secretions can suddenly obstruct the upper airway. Be prepared to suction your patient quickly. Respiratory burns and anaphylaxis can cause life-threatening swelling in a matter of minutes. Croup and epiglottitis also can quickly deteriorate into total upper airway occlusion.

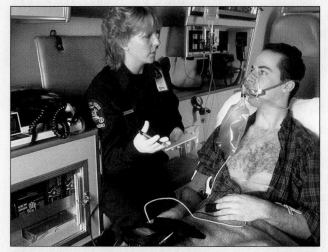

3-7a   Reevaluate the ABCs.

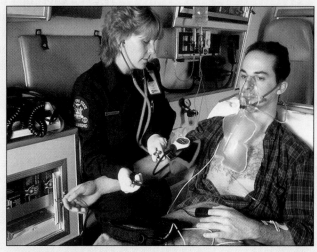

3-7b   Take all vital signs again.

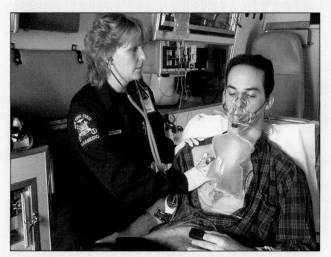

3-7c   Perform your focused assessment again.

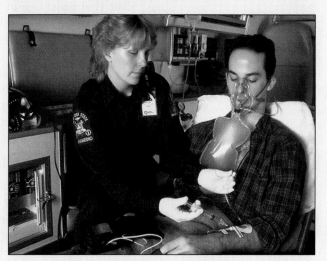

3-7d   Evaluate your interventions' effects.

Endotracheal intubation is the best way to secure the airway in patients with no gag reflex. But endotracheal tubes can become dislodged easily during transport. Recheck for tube placement frequently during transport and every time you move your patient onto a backboard, onto the stretcher, or onto the hospital gurney.

The price of proper airway management is eternal vigilance and a pessimistic outlook—anything that can go wrong will go wrong. Be prepared for the worst.

Breathing Rate and Quality

A change in respiratory rate or quality might indicate improvement or deterioration. A sudden increase in rate or respiratory effort suggests deterioration. For example, if your patient suddenly begins to gasp for air, has retractions, and uses his accessory neck muscles, he has a serious problem. Sometimes the signs are not so obvious. Subtle increases in respiratory rate can suggest a developing problem. A decrease in rate and effort could mean that your treatments are effective and your patient is improving. For example, after you administer an albuterol treatment, your patient breathes easier and his lung sounds improve. In infants and young children, however, a decrease in rate and effort may mean that your patient is exhausted and requires aggressive intervention. If, while assisting ventilation with a bag-valve mask, your partner suddenly complains that squeezing the bag is becoming more difficult, consider the possibility that a tension pneumothorax is developing or that bronchospasm or laryngospasm may be occurring. Airway and breathing management requires constant reevaluation.

Pulse Rate and Quality

Check central and peripheral pulses and compare the findings to earlier measurements. A rising pulse rate could indicate shock, hypoxia, or cardiac dysrhythmia. A falling rate could mean the terminal stage of shock or a rise in intracranial pressure. A sudden change in rate or regularity may suggest a cardiac dysrhythmia. The loss of peripheral pulses could mean decompensating shock.

Skin Condition

Similar to mental status, the skin quickly reflects the body's hemodynamic status. Reevaluate your patient's skin color, temperature, and condition. Cyanosis suggests decreased oxygenation. Lip cyanosis indicates central hypoxia (overall oxygen status), whereas peripheral cyanosis indicates decreased oxygen to the tissues. Pallor and coolness suggest decreased circulation to the skin, as seen in shock. If your patient suddenly develops hives after you administer a medication, suspect an allergic reaction. A localized redness and warmth could indicate bleeding under the skin or vasodilation. Cyanosis and coolness in a lower extremity suggest a peripheral vascular problem such as an arterial occlusion. A deep venous thrombosis will result in redness, swelling, and warmth in the lower leg.

Transport Priorities

Sometimes stable patients suddenly deteriorate en route to the hospital. For example, the formerly conscious and alert head injury patient now responds only to pain. Or your stable cardiac patient suddenly develops a life-threatening dysrhythmia. Or your patient suddenly cannot breathe because his simple pneumothorax has developed into a tension pneumothorax. In these cases, while you provide lifesaving treatments, change your transport decision to a higher priority. By the same token, if your unstable patient becomes stable, you may wish to downgrade your priority transport decision and decrease the danger and liability of driving with lights and siren on.

Vital Signs

Reassessing vital signs reveals trends clearly (Procedure 3-7b). A rising pulse rate combined with a falling blood pressure indicates shock. A decreasing pulse rate combined with a rising blood pressure, associated with an irregular respiratory pattern, suggests a rise in intracranial pressure. Any change in heart rate could indicate a cardiac dysrhythmia. A narrowing pulse pressure with a weakening pulse indicates cardiac tamponade, a tension pneumothorax, or hypovolemic shock. Reevaluate your critical patient's vital signs every 5 minutes and look for changes.

Reevaluate your critical patient's vital signs every 5 minutes.

Focused Assessment

Elicit your patient's chief complaint again to determine if the problem still exists or if other problems have arisen. Often following trauma your patient will develop more complaints en route to the hospital as the excitement of the incident begins to wear off. Patients often focus on their major injuries and might not even be aware of other problems. Repeat your focused assessment as your patient's chief complaint dictates (Procedure 3-7c).

Effects of Interventions

Evaluate the effects of any interventions (Procedure 3-7d). Did the albuterol treatment help open the lower airways? Did the oxygen and nitroglycerin relieve the chest pain? What are the effects of the fluid challenge? Is the pneumatic antishock garment inhibiting your patient's breathing? Did your intervention help or harm your patient? Is he getting better or worse? Know the expected therapeutic benefits of your interventions, and then evaluate whether they worked. For example, you administer lidocaine to convert ventricular tachycardia. Following administration, observe your patient's electrocardiogram for changes while noting any harmful side effects such as nausea, vomiting, or seizures.

Management Plans

Evaluate whether your care is working. If it is not, consider another management plan. Develop the courage to admit when your plan is not working and the flexibility to change your course of action. For example, your patient, an elderly man with a history of congestive heart failure (CHF) and chronic obstructive pulmonary disease (COPD), presents with severe difficulty breathing and audible wheezing. You suspect he is having an exacerbation of his COPD and administer two nebulizer treatments and begin transporting. En route, however, he is not improving, and now you also can hear crackles bilaterally. At this point, you suspect he is in CHF and change your management to administering nitroglycerin, furosemide, morphine, and continuous positive airway pressure (CPAP).

Patients often present with multiple complaints, symptoms, and histories. Formulating a definitive diagnosis is difficult without the hospital's labs, X-rays, and other assessment tools. Your ability to reassess your patient, reevaluate your field diagnosis, and alter your management plan will optimize patient care.

Have the courage to admit it if your plan is not working and the flexibility to change it.

Your ability to reassess your patient, reevaluate your field diagnosis, and alter your management plan will optimize patient care.

▶ Summary

Patient assessment is the key to providing effective prehospital emergency medical care. Its components include the initial assessment, the focused history and physical exam, vital signs, ongoing assessment, and the detailed physical exam. The initial assessment is designed to identify life-threatening airway, breathing, and circulation problems. The focused history and physical exam is designed to identify the signs and symptoms surrounding your patient's chief complaint. It is a problem-oriented approach that is easily modified to match your patient's clinical situation. The ongoing assessment is designed to reevaluate your patient for changes in status en route to the hospital. The detailed physical exam is a comprehensive head-to-toe evaluation designed to identify any conditions not already found. Although more suited to a clinical setting, it is intended to be done en route to the hospital if time allows.

The four general types of patients require distinctly different assessment approaches. The trauma patient with a significant mechanism of injury should receive an initial assessment, a rapid trauma assessment, and rapid transport. The patient with isolated, minor trauma, such as a cut finger or sprained ankle, should receive a physical exam focused on his particular problem or area. The responsive medical patient requires an initial assessment, a history and physical exam that focuses on his chief complaint, and vital signs. The unresponsive medical patient requires an initial assessment, followed by a rapid head-to-toe medical assessment and rapid transport. You will perform detailed history and physical exam techniques en route to the hospital if time and your patient's condition allow.

The assessment templates in this chapter are only guidelines. They do not dictate an exact procedure for assessing every patient. Instead, they provide general chronological guidelines to help you make critical transport and management decisions. As a paramedic you will be expected to use clinical judgment when deciding which assessment tools to use for your particular patient and situation. With time and experience, you will become adept at assessing real patients in crisis. The more effective and efficient you become with this process, the better your patient care will be.

▶ You Make the Call

You are sitting at the station reading the latest EMS journals when the call comes in for "difficulty breathing" at the VFW post on Wheatley Drive. You quickly recognize the address as a club where your unit responds at least once a week to a variety of medical problems among its membership of elderly veterans. Preliminary dispatch information reveals a man in his 80s with a history of "breathing problems" in severe distress. Because the patient is in acute respiratory distress, prearrival instructions are in progress.

En route to the scene, you begin to formulate a list of differential field diagnoses for acute respiratory distress. As you arrive on the scene you notice nothing unusual and no potential hazards. The scene appears safe to enter. As you walk through the door, you can hear obvious wheezing coming from the barroom. Mentally you begin to modify your differential field diagnosis. When you finally meet your patient, he sits upright on a barstool with his elbows on the bar. He appears very thin, with pursed lips, and is struggling to breathe effectively. He is in obvious distress, as evidenced by bulging neck muscles, retractions, and noisy respirations.

1. Outline each phase of your patient assessment for this patient.

See Suggested Responses at the back of this book.

▶ Review Questions

1. In all cases, you will perform a/an _____ _____ en route to the hospital to detect changes in patient condition.
   a. focused history
   b. initial assessment
   c. ongoing assessment
   d. detailed physical

2. The initial assessment's goal is to identify and correct immediately life-threatening conditions. These include all of the following EXCEPT:
   a. airway compromise.
   b. inadequate ventilation.
   c. major hemorrhage.
   d. minor/moderate bleeding.

3. The components of a scene size-up include:
   a. scene safety.
   b. mechanism of injury.
   c. body substance isolation.
   d. all of the above.

4. The most effective method of preventing disease transmission between patients and their health care workers is:
   a. masks.
   b. gowns.
   c. gloves.
   d. hand washing.

5. The National Institute of Occupational Safety and Health has designed _____ respirators to filter out the tuberculosis bacillus (TB).
   a. VENTI
   b. HEPA
   c. SCBA
   d. NIOH

6. The top priority at any emergency scene is the personal safety of:
   a. yourself.
   b. the crew.
   c. the patient.
   d. bystanders.

7. When considering the mechanism of injury for your trauma patient who was involved in a motor vehicle collision, you realize that which of the following is a predictor for serious injuries?
   a. intact windshield
   b. bent steering wheel
   c. intact passenger compartment
   d. single passenger in the vehicle

8. The goal of the _____ _____ is to identify and correct immediately life-threatening patient conditions.
   a. physical exam
   b. focused physical
   c. initial assessment
   d. ongoing assessment

9. The initial assessment should take less than _____ minute(s), unless you have to intervene with lifesaving measures.
   a. one
   b. two
   c. three
   d. five

10. A patient who is awake, as evidenced by open eyes, will register a/an _____ on the AVPU scale.
    a. A
    b. V

c. P

d. U

11. To assess your patient's airway, you should:

    a. look for chest rise.

    b. listen for air movement.

    c. feel for air movement.

    d. all of the above.

12. The _____ fracture more frequently than any other bone in the human body.

    a. scapulae

    b. femurs

    c. clavicles

    d. fibulae

13. Solid organs can bleed enough blood into the abdominal cavity to cause profound shock. All of the following are examples of solid organs EXCEPT:

    a. kidneys.

    b. stomach.

    c. spleen.

    d. liver.

14. This handy mnemonic is especially useful for eliciting a quick history from your trauma patient.

    a. AVPU

    b. PQRS

    c. DCAP

    d. SAMPLE

15. Generally, if your patient's pulse oximetry reading is below _____ percent, you should suspect shock, hypoxia, or respiratory compromise.

    a. 95

    b. 96

    c. 97

    d. 99

See Answers to Review Questions at the back of this book.

▶ Further Reading

Bates, Barbara, Lynn S. Bickley, and Robert A. Hoekelman. *A Guide to Physical Examination and History Taking.* 9th ed. Philadelphia: Lippincott, Williams & Wilkins, 2005.

Bledsoe, Bryan E., Robert S. Porter, and Richard A. Cherry. *Intermediate Emergency Care: Principles and Practice.* Upper Saddle River, N.J.: Pearson/Prentice Hall, 2004.

Bledsoe, Bryan E., Robert S. Porter, and Richard A. Cherry. "Twenty-five Tricks and Pearls of Physical Examination." *Journal of Emergency Medical Services (JEMS),* March 2005.

Campbell, John E. *Basic Trauma Life Support for Paramedics and Advanced EMS Providers.* 5th ed. Upper Saddle River, N.J.: Pearson/Prentice Hall, 2004.

Dalton, Alice, et al. *Advanced Medical Life Support.* 2nd ed. Upper Saddle River, N.J.: Pearson/Prentice Hall, 2003.

Dickinson, E. T., D. Limmer, M. O'Keefe, et al. *Emergency Care.* 9th ed., Fire Service Edition. Upper Saddle River, N.J.: Pearson/Prentice Hall, 2003.

Eichelberger, Martin R., et al. *Pediatric Emergencies: A Manual for Prehospital Care Providers.* 2nd ed. Upper Saddle River, N.J.: Pearson/Prentice Hall, 1998.

Foltin, George, et al. *Teaching Resource for Instructors in Prehospital Pediatrics for Paramedics.* New York: Center for Pediatric Medicine, 2002.

Hafen, Brent Q., et al. *Prehospital Emergency Care.* 7th ed. Upper Saddle River, N.J.: Pearson/Prentice Hall, 2004.

O'Keefe, Michael F., et al. *Emergency Care.* 10th ed. Upper Saddle River, N.J.: Pearson/Prentice Hall, 2005.

▶ Media Resources

See the Student CD at the back of this book for quizzes, animations, video skills clips, and other features related to this chapter. In particular, take a look at the Video Overview of Patient Assessment. Also, visit companion Website for Brady's paramedic series at **www.prenhall.com/bledsoe,**where you will find additional reinforcement and links to other resources.

Clinical Decision Making

Objectives

After reading this chapter, you should be able to:

1. Compare the factors influencing medical care in the out-of-hospital environment to other medical settings. (p. 249)
2. Differentiate between critical life-threatening, potentially life-threatening, and non-life-threatening patient presentations. (pp. 249–250)
3. Evaluate the benefits and shortfalls of protocols, standing orders, and patient care algorithms. (p. 250)
4. Define the components, stages, and sequences of the critical thinking process for paramedics. (pp. 250–258)
5. Apply the fundamental elements of critical thinking for paramedics. (pp. 256–258)
6. Describe the effects of the "fight-or-flight" response and its positive and negative effects on a paramedic's decision making. (p. 255)
7. Summarize the "six *R*s" of putting it all together: **R**ead the patient, **R**ead the scene, **R**eact, **R**eevaluate, **R**evise the management plan, **R**eview performance. (p. 258)
8. Given several preprogrammed and moulaged trauma and medical patients, demonstrate clinical decision making. (pp. 248–258)

Key Terms

acuity, p. 249
algorithm, p. 250
autonomic nervous
   system, p. 255
clinical judgment, p. 248
convergent, p. 254

critical thinking, p. 256
differential field diagnosis,
   p. 252
divergent, p. 254
field diagnosis, p. 248
impulsive, p. 254

protocol, p. 250
pseudo-instinctive,
   p.255
reflective, p. 253
standing orders, p. 250

Case Study

On a hot, muggy Friday evening the call comes in for a car vs. pedestrian collision. Reports from the scene are that a 14-year-old girl was struck by a car while in-line skating and lies in the street with blood coming from her mouth. First to arrive, Assistant Chief Tom Shoemaker secures the scene, confirms the initial report, and calls for Air-One, the county medevac helicopter. As the fire department rescue rolls out the door, the ambulance follows with paramedic Sue Bauer and EMT-Basic Jim Parent.

Upon arrival, Sue instructs Carl Coffee from the rescue team to immobilize the patient's head and neck while she begins an initial assessment. Her patient's name is Marcie. She is alert and oriented but does not remember what happened to her. She presents with obvious trauma to the mouth—all of her front teeth are missing or loose and she has minor bleeding. After the initial assessment and a rapid trauma assessment, Marcie appears hemodynamically stable. Sue decides to transport her by ground to a local community hospital. The rescue team immobilizes Marcie on a full backboard and quickly transports her.

En route to the hospital, Carl rides along to maintain verbal contact with Marcie and evaluate her mental status for changes. Sue begins her ongoing assessment and notes a declining mental status. Within minutes, Marcie becomes sleepy but is easily arousable by verbal stimuli. Sue decides to transport her to University Hospital, a level-1 trauma center with a specialized pediatric emergency department. This is a longer transport, but Sue believes her patient may be developing increasing intracranial pressure.

Marcie begins complaining of wanting to vomit. Sue and Carl quickly log roll her onto her side, but her nausea subsides. In the ED, Marcie vomits the frank blood she swallowed from her dental trauma, and her level of consciousness deteriorates further. Within minutes she becomes responsive only to deep pain. The emergency physician, Dr. Olsson, asks Sue for a chronological report on Marcie's mental status. Sue reports that she was alert and oriented 30 minutes earlier, then became responsive only to verbal commands approximately 15 minutes ago. They quickly transfer Marcie for a computerized tomography (CT) scan, which reveals an epidural hematoma from lacerating the middle meningeal artery and some minor bleeding from the middle cerebral artery.

INTRODUCTION TO CRITICAL THINKING

As a paramedic you eventually will face your moment of truth—a critical decision that can mean the difference between life and death.

As a paramedic you eventually will face your "moment of truth." You will confront a situation that requires you to make a critical decision. Often, you will have several options, but choosing the best one may mean the difference between life and death. And you will be all alone. Others may be at the scene, but as the paramedic, you will be responsible for that decision. That you someday will have to make a decision on which your patient's life hinges is a sobering thought.

In the 1970s, with rare exceptions, the first paramedics made few critical decisions. They usually worked under rigidly written protocols developed by their medical director. Mostly, they were required to contact the medical direction physician who, after hearing their report, would diagnose the patient's problem and order treatment. They were no more than technicians who needed only good psychomotor skills to conduct patient assessments and follow orders. As prehospital care has evolved, paramedics now do much more than collect data for the physician to evaluate. You not only will have to gather information, but analyze it, form a field diagnosis, and devise a management plan. In most cases you will do these things before contacting your medical direction physician.

Twenty-first-century paramedics are prehospital practitioners of emergency medicine—not field technicians.

Twenty-first-century paramedics are prehospital practitioners of emergency medicine—not field technicians. To fill this role, you will need to develop your critical decision-making skills—to be able to think rationally about what you are doing. Because patients seldom present with the classic textbook signs and symptoms, you will encounter situations that appear totally unfamiliar. These cases will call for you to use sound judgment in devising a management plan that meets your patient's needs. Making such decisions requires **clinical judgment**, using your knowledge and experience to make critical decisions regarding patient care. No one can teach you clinical judgment; you must develop it from experience. Unfortunately, experience often includes making bad decisions. We learn from our mistakes, if someone points them out and explains them to us. Your hospital and field preceptors will do this for you during this program.

clinical judgment
the use of knowledge and experience to diagnose patients and plan their treatment.

During this program, your instructors also will place you in as many problem-solving situations as possible to begin developing your clinical judgment. The number and type of supervised patient contacts you make during this program will determine how much clinical judgment you develop as a student. The more types of cases you see during your clinical rotations, the more clinically competent you will be when you complete your education.

PARAMEDIC PRACTICE

As a paramedic, you must gather, evaluate, and synthesize much information in very little time. You will obtain this information using your senses (sight, smell, hearing, and touch) during the history and physical exam. Analyzing these data will involve the total of your education, training, and clinical experience. For example, as you enter a patient's home, the sound of his gasping for breath with audible wheezes startles you. Having heard wheezing before and having learned in class that it results from a variety of problems will help you to make what is called a differential diagnosis. The differential diagnosis is a preliminary list of possible causes for your patient's problem. For example, a differential diagnosis for diffuse wheezing might include asthma, emphysema, bronchitis, and acute pulmonary edema. Now you conduct a history and physical exam and arrive at a **field diagnosis**, or impression.

field diagnosis
prehospital evaluation of the patient's condition and its causes.

Your next step will involve applying your clinical experience and exercising independent decision making as you develop and implement a management plan.

For example, your gasping and wheezing patient is an elderly male who presents with severe difficulty breathing. He has a history of cardiac and pulmonary disease, and you are not sure which problem precipitates this episode. You gather information and make an initial field diagnosis of congestive heart failure. You immediately administer medications (nitroglycerin, CPAP, morphine) to reduce cardiac preload, ease the workload of the heart, and increase tissue oxygenation. You prepare for endotracheal intubation and mechanical ventilation in case CPAP fails. This decision to administer potentially life-threatening drugs requires you to think clearly and work effectively under pressure. Few prehospital situations create more pressure than a patient struggling to breathe.

The prehospital emergency medical setting is unlike any other medical care environment. Paramedics carry out the same tasks as other clinicians. They assess patients, obtain vital signs, start IVs, manage airways, and perform many other invasive procedures. The difference is that paramedics perform these procedures in various uncontrolled and unpredictable environments under circumstances that do not exist in other clinical settings and without information gathered from laboratory results and X-rays. For example, starting an IV line in a well-lit, quiet hospital room is not a major challenge. Starting one while balancing yourself in the back of a rapidly moving ambulance is. Often you will use your skills in seemingly unmanageable circumstances. The key is to block out the distractions and focus on the task. Experienced paramedics do this better than anyone.

Patient Acuity

Not everyone who calls 911 has a life-threatening emergency. Just the opposite is true. The vast majority of our patients are people who want transportation to the hospital for non-life-threatening problems. For others, the emergency department is their only health care option, even for a sore throat. The spectrum of care in the prehospital setting includes three general classes of patient **acuity**: those with obvious critical life threats, those with potential life threats, and those with non-life-threatening presentations. Patients with obvious life-threatening conditions include major multisystem trauma; devastating single system trauma; end-stage disease presentations such as liver or renal failure when the patient is in the last days of his terminal illness and is close to death; and acute presentations of chronic diseases such as asthma or emphysema. These patients present with serious airway, breathing, circulation, or neurologic problems and often require aggressive resuscitation. Potential life-threatening conditions include serious multisystem trauma and multiple disease etiologies such as a diabetic with cardiac complications. Non-life-threatening presentations include isolated minor illnesses and injuries. You will be expected to manage cases in all three categories. In a typical 12-hour shift you may manage a patient in cardiac arrest; deliver a baby; control a lacerated, spurting artery; and transfer an elderly woman back to her nursing home. The wide range of patient types, degrees of severity, and complicating environmental factors makes prehospital care a unique form of emergency medicine.

Arriving at a management plan for patients with minor medical and traumatic events requires little critical thinking or clinical judgment. For example, if your patient has a fractured tibia, you will splint the leg and transport him to the emergency department for X-rays and casting. You have no real lifesaving decisions to make. On the opposite end of the acuity spectrum, patients with obvious life threats such as cardiac arrest and major trauma also require few critical decisions because caring for them is largely rote and standardized. For cardiac arrest, you perform CPR and work through the protocol associated with your patient's cardiac rhythm. For major trauma, you manage the ABCs while providing rapid transport to a trauma center.

acuity
the severity or acuteness of your patient's condition.

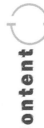

Review
Classes of Patient Acuity

- Critically life-threatening
- Potentially life-threatening
- Non-life-threatening

Patients who fall between minor medical and life threatening on the acuity spectrum pose the greatest challenge to your critical thinking abilities.

Patients who fall between minor medical and life threatening on the acuity spectrum pose the greatest challenge to your critical thinking abilities. These patients might become unstable at any moment. For example, if your patient is an infant with signs of respiratory distress, you must recognize the signs of early respiratory failure and take precautionary measures to keep him from deteriorating to respiratory arrest. In these cases, you use your knowledge of pediatric respiratory assessment, your skills in airway and breathing management, and your clinical judgment to determine how and when to intervene. You will constantly reassess and revise your interventions as needed.

Protocols and Algorithms

protocol
standard that includes general and specific principles for managing certain patient conditions.

Paramedics function in an emergency medical services system under the license of a medical director. Every state has enacted legislation allowing paramedics to practice medicine in the field and describing the scope of their practice. Within these laws, state and local EMS medical directors devise **protocols** that detail exactly what paramedics can do. Protocols are standards that include general and specific procedures for managing certain patient conditions. For example, every system will develop standards for managing asthma, congestive heart failure, and tension pneumothorax. Each will also develop protocols for special situations such as physician-on-scene, radio failure, and termination of resuscitation. **Standing orders** authorize you to perform certain procedures before contacting your medical direction physician. For example, you may administer oxygen, start an IV, and administer aspirin and nitroglycerin to a patient with cardiac chest pain. For repeat nitro orders, you may have to consult the physician. Patient care **algorithms** are flowcharts with arrows, lines, and boxes arranged schematically (Figure 4-1 ▶). To use them, you simply start at the top and follow wherever your patient's signs and symptoms lead.

standing orders
treatments you can perform before contacting the medical direction physician for permission.

algorithm
schematic flowchart that outlines appropriate care for specific signs and symptoms.

Protocols, standing orders, and patient care algorithms provide a standardized approach to emergency patient care. However, they address only "classic patients." Unfortunately, many patients present with atypical signs and symptoms, often requiring you to use clinical judgment and instinct to develop a management plan. Patients frequently present with nonspecific complaints that do not match any specific algorithm. Sometimes your patients just do not clearly describe what is bothering them. Another limitation of protocols is that they cannot adequately cover multiple disease etiologies such as the patient with chronic obstructive pulmonary disease and congestive heart failure. When your patient with this multiple history presents with severe difficulty breathing, you must quickly identify the underlying condition that is causing the present problem and follow the appropriate protocol. Nor do protocols deal with managing more than one patient problem at a time in possible multiple treatment situations. For example, your stroke patient also presents with shock and with bilateral Colles' fractures and a fractured hip from a fall. Protocols are standards designed to promote consistent patient care in common situations. They are written also to allow you, in consultation with the medical direction physician, to use clinical judgment to provide optimum care in unusual situations. The linear thinking, or "cookbook medicine," that protocols promote should not restrict you from consulting with your medical direction physician in difficult or unusual cases.

Do not allow the linear thinking, or "cookbook medicine," that protocols promote to restrain you from consulting with your medical direction physician.

CRITICAL THINKING SKILLS

The ability to think under pressure and make decisions cannot be taught; it must be developed. As a paramedic, you will be a team leader on emergency scenes. In that role you must make sound, reasonable decisions regarding your patient's care. Several

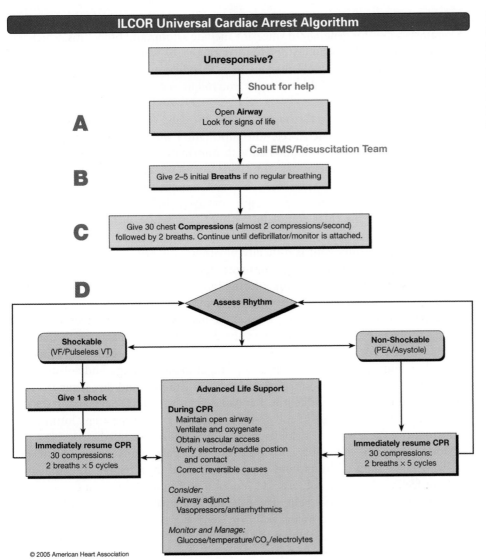

ILCOR Universal Cardiac Arrest Algorithm

Unresponsive?

Shout for help

A

Open Airway
Look for signs of life

Call EMS/Resuscitation Team

B

Give 2–5 initial **Breaths** if no regular breathing

C

Give 30 chest **Compressions** (almost 2 compressions/second)
followed by 2 breaths. Continue until defibrillator/monitor is attached.

D

Assess Rhythm

Shockable
(VF/Pulseless VT)

Non-Shockable
(PEA/Asystole)

Give 1 shock

Advanced Life Support

During CPR
  Maintain open airway
  Ventilate and oxygenate
  Obtain vascular access
  Verify electrode/paddle postion
    and contact
  Correct reversible causes

Consider:
  Airway adjunct
  Vasopressors/antiarrhythmics

Monitor and Manage:
  Glucose/temperature/CO_2/electrolytes

Immediately resume CPR
30 compressions:
2 breaths × 5 cycles

Immediately resume CPR
30 compressions:
2 breaths × 5 cycles

© 2005 American Heart Association

Figure 4-1 To use a patient care algorithm, follow the arrows to your patient's symptoms and provide care as indicated. (Reproduced with permission from "2005 American Heart Association Guidelines for Cardiopulmonary Resuscitation and Emergency Cardiovascular Care." *Circulation 2005,* Volume 112, II-3. *(© 2005 American Heart Association)*

aspects of this program will help you to develop this essential skill. In the classroom you will work on case histories. In the labs you will practice patient scenarios on moulaged victims. In the hospital you will assess and help manage real patients in the emergency department and critical care units. In the field internship, you will assess and manage patients in the streets. In all of these settings you will begin developing clinical judgment.

Fundamental Knowledge and Abilities

First, you must have an excellent working knowledge of anatomy and physiology and of the pathophysiology of your patient's disease or injury. To assess and manage a patient with difficulty breathing, for instance, you must know which organs and body systems are involved in breathing. You must understand the process of normal breathing and each body system's role in that effort. You must recall the factors that inhibit normal breathing and recognize the signs and symptoms of respiratory distress. For example, a patient might wheeze because of lower airway obstruction from secretions, bronchoconstriction, edema, or any combination of these conditions. All reduce the inner diameter of the airways, restricting airflow and making movement of air in and out of the lungs difficult. Managing this patient would require a knowledge of the respiratory

Review

Content

Decision-Making Requirements

- Knowing anatomy, physiology, and pathophysiology
- Focusing on large amounts of data
- Organizing information
- Identifying and dealing with medical ambiguity
- Differentiating between relevant and irrelevant data
- Analyzing and comparing similar situations
- Explaining decisions and constructing logical arguments

and cardiovascular causes of wheezing, because their treatments are vastly different. Respiratory causes for generalized wheezing include asthma and bronchitis, which you would manage with bronchodilators. Cardiac causes for wheezing include congestive heart failure, which you would manage with vasodilators and diuretics. Without a good working knowledge of these diseases, you might make a mistaken and potentially devastating field diagnosis.

You also must be able to focus on many specific data. When you conduct a patient assessment, you will evaluate all relevant information while focusing on specific important findings. You will be inundated with information requiring you to establish relationships and form conclusions. Your patient who presents with difficulty breathing and wheezing in the previous example would require an in-depth history and focused examination of his cardiac and respiratory systems. You also would assess other systems relative to his chief complaint (HEENT, musculoskeletal, neurologic, and lymphatic), while remaining focused on the primary problem (cardiorespiratory). Although his chief complaint is difficulty breathing, his primary problem might be cardiac, muscular, infectious, allergic, or neurologic.

You must be able to organize the information you obtain and form concepts from it. Initially you elicit your patient's chief complaint and begin to formulate a **differential field diagnosis**. As you conduct the history and a clearer picture of your patient's problem emerges, you narrow your differential field diagnosis to the most probable disease. For example, your patient has severe difficulty breathing and inspiratory stridor. Your differential field diagnosis might include foreign body obstruction, epiglottitis, respiratory burns, anaphylaxis, laryngeal trauma, and throat cancer. Then you learn that he is hoarse and febrile, has had a sore throat for 2 days, and in the past 6 hours has had increasing difficulty swallowing. You now suspect epiglottitis. This ability to formulate a working field diagnosis is essential for paramedics.

You must be able to identify and deal with medical ambiguity. Many patients present with vague signs and symptoms. It is not unusual for a patient to complain of "just not feeling right." He will provide you with an imprecise story and you will be unable to arrive at a specific field diagnosis. In these cases, your field diagnosis will have to be generalized: "abdominal pain" or "general illness." Often it will be almost impossible to definitively determine the underlying problem without laboratory results, X-rays, and other tests.

You must be able to differentiate between relevant and irrelevant data. You will have to sift the important data from the many bits of information you receive during your patient assessment. A positive family history for sudden cardiac death is relevant for your patient with chest pain; for your patient with a fractured arm it is not. Pupil and extraocular movement exams are relevant for trauma and for patients with an altered mental status; for a patient with asthma or arthritis they are not. When you radio the medical direction physician, you will report critical information only. Likewise, in your written documentation you will record relevant information and omit the rest.

You must be able to analyze and compare similar and contrasting situations. What were the similarities between your last three stroke patients? Did all three have facial drooping, slurred speech, and unilateral paralysis? Did they all have a history of hypertension? Can you depend on any patterns of presentation for future calls like this? Have some patient presentations been unusual? Have any patients presented with signs of stroke but ultimately had a different diagnosis? For example, your patient is a 45-year-old woman who presents with right-sided facial drooping. Your initial impression may be stroke, but further investigation reveals no other neurologic deficits. You now change your impression to Bell's palsy, caused by inflammation of the facial nerve (CN-VII). You must be able to recall the factors that help rule in or rule out a particular disease or injury.

You must be able to explain your decisions and construct logical arguments. Often, the emergency physician will want to know what you were thinking when you

differential field diagnosis
the list of possible causes of your patient's symptoms.

made your field diagnosis. You must be able to express yourself rationally while you make your case. These are the times when you demonstrate your professionalism to other health care providers. Observe the following conversation:

Physician: Why did you think your patient had Bell's palsy and not a stroke? How can you rule out a stroke in the field?

Paramedic: Well, she had paralysis on the entire right side of her face, indicating a lesion of the 7th cranial nerve, rather than the lower facial paralysis of a stroke. All other neuro tests were negative.

Physician: OK, I agree, good job!

Through interactions such as this, you establish credibility with the emergency physician. The next time you contact him regarding a patient, he is more apt to trust your assessment and judgment.

Useful Thinking Styles

As a paramedic, you will face confusing emergencies that would challenge even the most knowledgeable, analytical care provider. You must be able to stay calm and not panic. Your self-control in the face of extreme chaos will set the example for other team members to follow. Even when you are struggling to maintain your composure—especially then—never let others know. The key is focusing on the task and blocking out the distractions. Be like the duck—cool and calm on the water's surface, while paddling feverishly underneath.

Assume and plan for the worst, and always err on the side of benefiting your patient. For example, if you are deliberating whether to immobilize your patient, initiate advanced life support procedures, or administer oxygen, just do it! It is better to err by providing care than by withholding it. Be pessimistic! Anticipate all potential bad side effects of your treatments and prepare "plan B." For example, as you deliver a bronchodilating drug to your severe asthmatic patient, anticipate that it will not work and mentally prepare to intubate him and perform positive-pressure ventilation. Or while you are administering atropine to your patient with symptomatic bradycardia, plan ahead for external cardiac pacing and dopamine, if atropine therapy fails to restore adequate circulation.

Establish and maintain a systematic assessment pattern. Practice your assessments until they become second nature, and you will avoid skipping and missing steps. Be disciplined and stay focused, especially when you are confronted with a complex emergency scene. For example, your patient lies moaning on the ground in a pool of blood. Bystanders are screaming at you to help him; others are trying to tell you what happened. The police are gathering the story and trying unsuccessfully to talk with your patient. You must gain control of this scene. You do so by focusing on your patient and performing a systematic assessment. Use common acronyms (MS-ABC, OPQRST, SAMPLE) or make up your own to help you remember the key elements of your assessment. Except for safety concerns, never allow anything to distract you from your most important job—assessing and caring for your patient.

The different situations you encounter will require a variety of management styles. Adapting your styles of situation analysis (reflective vs. impulsive), data processing (convergent vs. divergent), and decision making (anticipatory vs. reactive) to each situation will enable you to provide the best possible care in every case.

Reflective vs. Impulsive   Some situations call for you to be **reflective**, take your time, and figure out what is wrong with your patient. You have a patient who complains of "not feeling well." She has a long history of cardiac, renal, respiratory, and diabetic problems. Because she is in no real distress and is hemodynamically stable, you can take your time to determine her primary problem. Other situations call for immediate action.

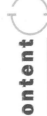

Review

Facilitating Behaviors

- Stay calm
- Plan for the worst
- Work systematically
- Remain adaptable

Be like the duck—cool and calm on the water's surface, while paddling feverishly underneath.

Except for safety concerns, never allow anything to distract you from your most important job—assessing and caring for your patient.

reflective
acting thoughtfully, deliberately, and analytically.

impulsive
acting instinctively without stopping to think.

divergent
taking into account all aspects of a complex situation.

convergent
focusing on only the most important aspect of a critical situation.

Whenever possible, anticipate problems and act before they occur.

They require you to make an instinctive, **impulsive** decision and manage your patient's life-threatening condition. For example, if your patient presents apneic and pulseless, you will immediately begin CPR and prepare for rapid defibrillation. If he presents with a spurting artery, you will at once take measures to control the hemorrhage. If he is choking and has a weak, ineffective cough, you will quickly perform abdominal thrusts. You have to think fast in these situations.

Divergent vs. Convergent   To process the data you receive from your patient and the scene, you can use either a divergent approach or a convergent approach. The **divergent** approach considers all aspects of a situation before arriving at a solution. It is insightful and works well when you are confronted with complex scenarios. For example, your emotionally distraught, stable patient presents with multiple problems and a long, complicated medical history. You need to consider the physical, emotional, and psychological aspects of his condition before making a field diagnosis and management plan. Likewise, extricating a victim from a wooded scene requires you to weigh a variety of environmental and medical factors before selecting a mode of transport.

On the other hand, the **convergent** approach focuses narrowly on a situation's most significant aspects. This technically oriented approach relies heavily on step-by-step problem solving and is best suited for simple, uncomplicated situations that require little thought or reflection. For example, you have an unresponsive, apneic, pulseless patient who presents in ventricular fibrillation. Your immediate concern is simple and straightforward—you manage the ABCs and defibrillate him as quickly as possible. Experienced paramedics employ both approaches effectively in the appropriate situations.

Anticipatory vs. Reactive   Your decision-making process can be either anticipatory or reactive. You either anticipate the possible ramifications of your actions in a proactive way or you react to events as you encounter them. For example, your patient presents with a severe laceration and severe blood loss. The bleeding is controlled. Now you can either anticipate his going into shock and begin measures before it happens, or you can wait until he shows signs of shock and then act. Unfortunately, by then it is often too late to do anything about it. Whenever possible, it is best to anticipate problems and act before they occur.

Patho Pearls

Knowing When *Not* to Act   In EMS education, emphasis is placed on when and where to apply an emergency intervention or administer a drug. With experience, you will learn that it is equally important to determine when *not* to apply an intervention or administer a drug. This is a trait that all skilled paramedics must develop.

Above all, trauma is a surgical disease. Definitive care of the trauma patient often must occur in the operating room. Despite our best attempts and technology, certain trauma patients will benefit only from rapid transport to a trauma center followed by emergency surgery to correct the problem. Attempts at stabilization in the field often delay the patient from receiving what he actually needs—rapid transport and surgical intervention.

It is easy to get caught up in the technology and care practices of modern EMS. However, it is important to realize that EMS, like many things in medicine, has its limitations. Sometimes, as the saying goes, discretion is the better part of valor. When faced with a critical trauma patient, the best care sometimes may simply be rapid immobilization and transport with any prehospital interventions provided en route. Making this decision will become easier with experience.

THINKING UNDER PRESSURE

When you must make a critical decision, physical influences may help or hinder your ability to think clearly. Your **autonomic nervous system**, which controls your involuntary actions, may respond by secreting "fight-or-flight" hormones. These hormones will enhance your visual and auditory acuity and will improve your reflexes and muscle strength. However, they may also impair your ability to think critically and diminish your ability to assess and concentrate. In these instances you will revert to your most basic instincts. Many an inexperienced paramedic has been "mentally paralyzed" by a complicated, critical call. With experience, you will learn to manage your nervousness and maintain a steadfast, controlled demeanor.

One way to enhance your ability to remain in control is to raise your technical skills to a **pseudo-instinctive** level. This means that you do not have to concentrate on them to perform them. For example, you do not think about tying your shoes, you just tie them. Such "muscle memory" is essential when performing emergency medical skills. When you set up for an albuterol nebulizer treatment, for instance, you automatically fit together the pieces of the device and administer the treatment without hesitation. This way you can concentrate on your patient's condition, controlling the scene, and managing the multitude of items that usually complicate any emergency call. Concentrating on more than one thing simultaneously is difficult, if not impossible.

autonomic nervous system
part of the nervous system that controls involuntary actions.

pseudo-instinctive
learned actions that are practiced until they can be done without thinking.

Mental Checklist

Thinking under pressure is not easy. Maintaining your composure, especially during a chaotic, complicated call is key to developing a management plan for the best patient outcome. Developing a routine mental checklist is a good way to stay focused and systematic. Pilots work through their preflight checklists routinely before ever turning over their engines. Medical clinicians develop acronyms and mnemonics to remember critical elements during stressful incidents. For example, when conducting an initial assessment, use the acronym MS-ABC. Use OPQRST to elicit your patient's present history, or use SAMPLE when time is critical. You can adopt the following checklist any time you must make a critical decision.

Maintaining your composure, especially during a chaotic, complicated call is key to developing a management plan for the best patient outcome.

Scan the Situation Stand back and scan the situation. Sometimes you can miss subtle signs if you focus too narrowly on one aspect of your patient's problem. Look for environmental factors and other not-so-obvious clues. For example, your patient lies unconscious on the floor. You rule out any airway, breathing, or circulation problems. No medical history is available and no medication bottles are present. When you detect a fruity odor on your patient's breath, you suspect diabetic ketoacidosis.

Stop and Think Do not do anything without stopping and weighing your actions. Consider all of your options before you act. Remember that for every action there is a reaction. Know what reactions to expect, and anticipate their possible harmful effects. For example, after administering lidocaine, monitor your patient closely for the expected benefits (eradication of ventricular tachycardia) and early signs of toxicity (numbness and tingling of the lips, drowsiness, nausea).

Decide and Act Once you have assessed the situation, make your decision and act confidently. Announce your management plan to your crew with a combination of authority, confidence, and respect. Convey the feeling that you know your actions are correct and will work. This confidence helps reassure your patient, his family, your crew, and other responders even in the most stressful situations.

Maintain Control To maintain clear, efficient control of the scene and everyone involved, you must first control yourself. Many situations will challenge your inner

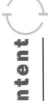

Review

Mental Checklist

- Scan the situation
- Stop and think
- Decide and act
- Maintain control
- Reevaluate

Content

strength and self-control. You will eventually be in charge of a scene where everyone seems out of control. These chaotic incidents can occur anywhere and anytime. Your job is to remain steadfast under fire.

Reevaluate Regularly reevaluate your plan's effects and revise it accordingly. Never assume that your plan is working to perfection. Anticipate ways your patient might deteriorate and devise alternate plans. Conduct an ongoing assessment en route to the hospital and be prepared to revise your management plan. For example, if you note increased lung congestion after administering fluids, stop the infusion.

THE CRITICAL DECISION PROCESS

critical thinking

thought process used to analyze and evaluate.

Understanding the **critical thinking** process is essential for a paramedic. Your ability to analyze data effectively and devise a practical management plan optimizes patient care. You may be able to conduct the most comprehensive history and physical exam, but if you cannot analyze the data and devise the proper management plan, your efforts will be fruitless. The critical thinking process has five steps: forming a concept, interpreting the data, applying the principles, evaluating the results, and reflecting on the incident. To explain the critical decision-making process, we will consider a 19-year-old female patient with a sudden onset of sharp pain to her right lower quadrant with some vaginal bleeding.

Form a Concept

The first step in critical decision making is to gather information and form a concept of your patient and the scene. You will get this information by assessing the general environment and the immediate surroundings. Note the mechanism of injury, if applicable. Then observe your patient's mental status, skin color, positioning, and note any deformities or asymmetry. In our sample case, your patient presents at home, sitting on a sofa. At first glance, she appears pale, diaphoretic, and anxious. Next you conduct an initial assessment, focusing on the MS-ABCs. Your initial goal is to identify and manage critical life threats. In this case, your general impression is of an alert and oriented but anxious young woman in moderate distress who presents with a clear airway; good air movement, as evidenced by her ability to converse in complete sentences; a strong, rapid, regular pulse; and cool, moist skin.

Now you ascertain your patient's chief complaint, history of present illness, past history, and current health status, while observing her affect (her general demeanor and attitude) and her degree of distress. You determine that her chief complaint is lower right quadrant pain that began suddenly 30 minutes ago. She also states she began bleeding at around the same time. She denies any nausea, vomiting, or diarrhea. You learn she has a past history of pelvic inflammatory disease and an active, unprotected sex life with multiple partners. Her last menstrual period was 6 weeks ago. She has had four pregnancies but no viable births. She appears in moderate distress.

Finally, you conduct a focused physical exam of the appropriate areas. This includes any diagnostic testing, such as an electrocardiogram, pulse oximetry, and blood glucose testing. You take a full set of vital signs, which can help you identify most life-threatening conditions. Remember that your patient's age, underlying physical and medical condition, and current medications can influence her vital signs. For example, the use of beta blockers could cause a general decrease in her pulse and blood pressure. Your patient has some deep palpation tenderness in the lower right quadrant but no rebound tenderness, and the rest of her abdomen is soft and nontender. She has minor bleeding at this time and has used only one sanitary pad since the bleeding began. Her vital signs are HR—110 and regular; respirations 20, not labored; BP—120/86.

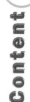

Review

Steps in Critical Decision Making

- Form a concept
- Interpret the data
- Apply the principles
- Evaluate the results
- Reflect on the incident

Interpret the Data

After you assess the patient you will interpret all of your data in light of your knowledge and experience. In this case, your knowledge base includes female reproductive anatomy, the physiology of a normal pregnancy, and the pathophysiology of pregnancy complications along with their classic signs and symptoms. It also involves the anatomy, physiology, and pathophysiology of the cardiovascular system and the signs and symptoms of shock. Your experience base includes every patient you have assessed and managed with a similar presentation. Your attitude toward managing patients with these symptoms also becomes a factor, because your experience may prejudice you. Consider all of the data and determine the most common and statistically probable conditions that fit your patient's initial presentation. This is your differential field diagnosis. Then, consider the most serious condition that fits your patient's situation. In our example, a field diagnosis of a ruptured ectopic pregnancy is obvious. When a clear medical diagnosis is elusive, base your treatment on the presenting signs and symptoms.

Apply the Principles

With your field diagnosis in mind, you devise a management plan that covers all contingencies. You will use written protocols, standing orders, and all the interventions at your disposal to manage your patient's particular problem. Sometimes patients present with atypical signs and symptoms. For example, a patient who presents with a sore throat and cough may actually be having a heart attack and congestive heart failure. Other times a protocol for your patient's problem simply may not exist. For example, your system may not have a protocol for facilitated intubation in head injuries. In these cases, consult with your medical direction physician for guidance in providing optimum care to your patient. The physician's emergency medical expertise and experience can be invaluable to you and your patient in unusual and difficult cases.

In our example, although your patient presents with relatively normal vital signs and is fully alert and oriented, you are very concerned. A basic principle of medicine is that all females of childbearing age with lower abdominal pain are pregnant until proven otherwise. You initiate advanced life support precautions en route to the hospital, including high-flow, high-concentration oxygen and two large-bore intravenous lines. Her presentation has led you to expect the worst. If her fallopian tube ruptures and begins to hemorrhage, she will need rapid fluid resuscitation and general shock management. Your experience includes similar patients who suddenly suffered a life-threatening hemorrhage from a ruptured fallopian tube. Again, your attitude becomes a factor in that you will not allow her stable presentation to undermine your initial instinct—that she is potentially in serious trouble.

Evaluate the Results

During the ongoing assessment, you reassess your patient's condition and the effects of your standing order/protocol interventions. In other words, you determine if your treatment is improving your patient's condition and status. For example, has the albuterol helped your patient's breathing? Did the nitro and oxygen relieve the chest pain? Is the hemorrhage under control? Reflect on your actions and either continue your original plan, discontinue treatment, or take a completely different approach. You may alter your initial impression if your patient's condition worsens or if you discover new information. If time and circumstances allow a detailed exam, you may discover less obvious problems.

In our sample case, your patient remains in potentially unstable condition. Your repeat assessment shows her vital signs are holding with the infusion of IV fluids. She is alert and not as anxious as before, and her skin is becoming warm and normal in color. You deliver her to the emergency department in stable, but guarded, condition.

Reflect on the Incident

After the call, discuss your field diagnosis and care with the emergency physician. Compare your field diagnosis with his diagnosis. Conduct a run critique with your crew and discuss ways to improve your assessment and management of this case and future cases. Add these data to your information and experience base for future calls. Make every patient contact a learning experience. In this case, the emergency physician confirms your field diagnosis with lab tests and an ultrasound.

Putting It All Together

A helpful mnemonic for the critical decision-making process is the "six *R*s":

1. **R**ead the scene—Observe the general environmental conditions, the immediate surroundings, and any mechanism of injury.
2. **R**ead the patient—Identify any life threats with the ABCs. Observe the patient's level of consciousness, skin color, position, location, and any obvious deformity or asymmetry. Talk to him to determine the chief complaint and whether it is a new problem or a worsening of a preexisting condition. Touch him to evaluate skin temperature and condition, pulse rate, and quality. Auscultate for problems with the upper and lower airways. Take a full set of vital signs.
3. **R**eact—Address any life threats as found, determine the most common and serious existing conditions, and treat him accordingly.
4. **R**eevaluate—Conduct a focused and detailed physical assessment, note any response to your initial management interventions, and discover other less obvious problems.
5. **R**evise the management plan—Change or stop interventions that are not working or are causing your patient's condition to worsen, or try something new.
6. **R**eview your performance by conducting a run critique—Be honest and critically evaluate your performance, always looking for better ways to manage a particular case presentation.

Making every patient contact a learning experience.

Content

Review

The Six *R*s

1. **R**ead the scene
2. **R**ead the patient
3. **R**eact
4. **R**eevaluate
5. **R**evise the management plan
6. **R**eview your performance

▶ Summary

Clinical decision making is an essential paramedic skill that you will develop with time and experience. The prehospital environment is unlike any other medical care setting and you will have to make decisions in less-than-optimal and sometimes dangerous conditions. Most times you will have the benefit of consulting with your medical direction physician in difficult and unusual situations; other times you may not. Your ability to gather information, analyze it, and make a critical decision may someday make the difference between your patient's life and death. This is inevitable. How well you prepare for that challenge will determine your ultimate success. The process begins in your paramedic training program. You must develop a good working knowledge of anatomy, physiology, pathophysiology, and the principles of emergency medicine. In time, through repeated patient contacts, you will develop the clinical judgment you need to make effective patient care decisions.

The critical decision-making process involves a series of steps that experienced clinicians do almost unconsciously. First you gather information (history and physical exam) to form an initial impression and then interpret it against your knowledge and experience to develop a working field diagnosis. You next apply the principles of emergency medicine to devise and implement a management plan and evaluate the effects of your treatments. Then you reevaluate and revise your plan as necessary. Finally you compare your findings with the emergency physician's diagnosis and discuss alternate ways to manage similar patients. With every patient contact, your experience grows and your clinical judgment improves. This is the essence of paramedic practice.

▶ You Make the Call

You are on your lunch break at a local fast-food restaurant when a middle-aged man comes up to you and says, "I have a terrible headache. Do you have any aspirin?" The man fully expects you to simply give him what he asks for. After all, you represent the health care industry and two aspirin seem like a simple request. But you notice that his left hand appears to be shaking. You ask him if this is normal and he replies, "What shaking?" You then ask him his name, and he has trouble remembering it. You also notice a slight slurring of his speech and his gait seems unstable.

1. Would you give him the aspirin?
2. Describe the knowledge base needed to manage this situation.
3. How would you proceed from this point?

See Suggested Responses at the back of this book.

▶ Review Questions

1. The use of knowledge and experience to diagnose patients and to plan their treatment is called:
   a. a field diagnosis.
   b. clinical judgment.
   c. written protocols.
   d. initial impression.

2. The severity or acuteness of your patient's condition is described as:
   a. acuity.
   b. criticality.
   c. life threatening.
   d. immediacy.

3. State and local EMS medical directors devise standards that include general and specific principles for managing certain patient conditions. These standards are known as:
   a. licenses.
   b. algorithms.
   c. protocols.
   d. standing orders.

4. Prior to contacting your medical director, you may be allowed to administer oxygen, start an IV, and administer aspirin and nitroglycerin to a patient with cardiac chest pain. This practice is based on a/an:
   a. protocol.
   b. direct order.
   c. algorithm.
   d. standing order.

5. The thinking style that mandates your focus on the most important aspect of a critical situation is referred to as:
   a. anticipatory.
   b. divergent.
   c. convergent.
   d. reactive.

6. One way to enhance your ability to remain in control is to raise your technical skills to a pseudo-instinctive level. This means that you:
   a. must utilize written notes to perform a skill correctly.
   b. do not have to concentrate on the skill in order to perform it.
   c. must perform the particular skill in concert with your partner.
   d. must concentrate only on the skill being performed and nothing else.

7. All of the following are components of the mental checklist EXCEPT:
   a. reevaluate.
   b. document.
   c. decide and act.
   d. scan the situation.

8. As you begin to determine if your treatment is improving your patient's condition, you are using this step in the critical decision-making process.
   a. Form a concept.
   b. Apply the principles.
   c. Evaluate.
   d. Reflect.

See Answers to Review Questions at the back of this book.

▶ Further Reading

Bates, Barbara, Lynn S. Bickley, and Robert A. Hoekelman. *A Guide to Physical Examination and History Taking*. 9th ed. Philadelphia: J.B. Lippincott, Williams & Wilkins, 2005.

Dalton, Alice L. "Enhancing Critical Thinking in Paramedic Continuing Education." *Prehospital and Disaster Medicine* 11 (October–December 1996): 246–253.

Farrell, Marian. "Planning for Critical Outcomes." *Journal of Nursing Education* 35 (September 1996): 278–281.

Janing, Judy. "Critical Thinking: Incorporation into the Paramedic Curriculum." *Prehospital and Disaster Medicine* 9 (October–November 1994): 238–242.

Seidel, Henry M., et al. *Mosby's Guide to Physical Examination*. 6th ed. St. Louis: Mosby, 2006.

▶ Media Resources

See the Student CD at the back of this book for quizzes, animations, video skills clips, and other features related to this chapter. In particular, take a look at the skills videos on the medical exam and trauma exam. Also, visit the Companion Website for Brady's paramedic series at **www.prenhall.com/bledsoe**, where you will find additional reinforcement and links to other resources.

Communications

Objectives

After reading this chapter, you should be able to:

Part 1

1. Identify the role and importance of verbal, written, and electronic communications in the provision of EMS. (pp. 266–275)
2. Describe the phases of communications necessary to complete a typical EMS response. (pp. 269–275)
3. List factors that impede and enhance effective verbal and written communications. (pp. 265–268)
4. Explain the value of data collection during an EMS response. (p. 267)
5. Recognize the legal status of verbal, written, and electronic communications related to an EMS response. (pp. 266–268)
6. Identify current technology used to collect and exchange patient and/or scene information electronically. (pp. 276–280)
7. Identify the various components of the EMS communications system and describe their function and use. (pp. 269–275)
8. Identify and differentiate among the following communications systems:
   - Simplex (p. 276)
   - Duplex (p. 276)
   - Multiplex (p. 277)
   - Trunked (p. 277)
   - Digital communications (pp. 277–278)
   - Cellular telephone (p. 278)
   - Facsimile (p. 278)
   - Computer (p. 279)
9. Describe the functions and responsibilities of the Federal Communications Commission. (p. 282)
10. Describe the role of emergency medical dispatch and the importance of prearrival instructions in a typical EMS response. (pp. 269–274)

11. List appropriate caller information gathered by the emergency medical dispatcher. (pp. 269, 273)
12. Describe the structure and importance of verbal patient information communication to the hospital and medical direction. (pp. 280–281)
13. Diagram a basic communications system. (pp. 266–267)
14. Given several narrative patient scenarios, organize a verbal radio report for electronic transmission to medical direction. (pp. 264–282)

Key Terms

automatic collision notification (ACN) system, p. 272
cellular telephone system, p. 278
communication, p. 265
digital communications, p. 277
duplex, p. 276
echo procedure, p. 282
emergency medical dispatcher (EMD), p. 273
facsimile machine (fax), p. 278

Federal Communications Commission (FCC), p. 282
libel, p. 280
mobile data terminal, p. 278
multiplex, p. 277
prearrival instructions, p. 273
prehospital care report (PCR), p. 267
priority dispatching, p. 273
protocol, p. 280

public safety answering point (PSAP), p. 269
radio band, p. 266
radio frequency, p. 266
semantic, p. 266
simplex, p. 276
slander, p. 280
10-code, p. 266
touch pad, p. 280
trunking, p. 277
ultrahigh frequency (UHF), p. 266
very high frequency (VHF), p. 282

Case Study

On a dry, warm Sunday afternoon, a 31-year-old male loses control of his motorcycle and strikes a highway sign. Several people witness the incident. The first bystander to reach the patient rushes to his automobile to dial 911 on his cellular telephone. Emergency medical dispatcher Vern Holland takes the necessary information and dispatches a basic life support engine company and an advanced life support ambulance. As Holland dispatches the emergency units, his partner, paramedic dispatcher Fred Hughes, instructs the caller in basic emergency care. The units receive the call via a computer printout of essential information.

They quickly arrive at the scene and initiate the appropriate care. Because the patient has a severe head injury, the paramedic performs only a limited assessment and immediately initiates transport. As the ambulance departs, he relays the following to Dr. Doyle, the medical direction physician:

Paramedic: Depew Ambulance to Mercy Hospital.

Dr. Doyle: Go ahead, Depew.

Paramedic: We are leaving the scene of a motorcycle collision on I-90. We have one patient, a male who is in his 30s, the rider of a motorcycle that went off the roadway and struck a sign. He responds to pain only, with obvious facial and chest trauma. There is a large laceration above the right eye with an exposed skull fracture. There is also blood draining from the right ear. Vital signs are blood pressure 110/60, pulse 110 and regular, respirations 10 and labored. Pupils are dilated and minimally reactive, yet equal. Palpation of

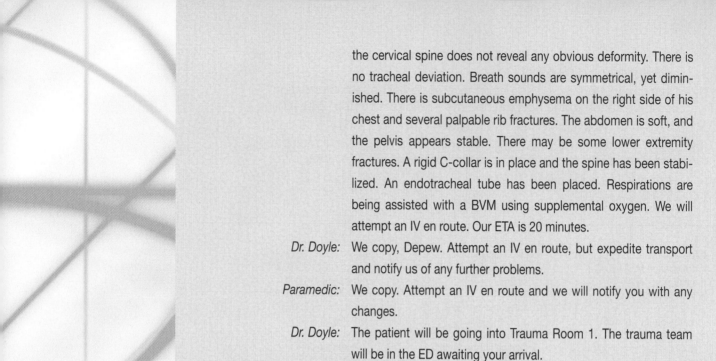

the cervical spine does not reveal any obvious deformity. There is no tracheal deviation. Breath sounds are symmetrical, yet diminished. There is subcutaneous emphysema on the right side of his chest and several palpable rib fractures. The abdomen is soft, and the pelvis appears stable. There may be some lower extremity fractures. A rigid C-collar is in place and the spine has been stabilized. An endotracheal tube has been placed. Respirations are being assisted with a BVM using supplemental oxygen. We will attempt an IV en route. Our ETA is 20 minutes.

Dr. Doyle: We copy, Depew. Attempt an IV en route, but expedite transport and notify us of any further problems.

Paramedic: We copy. Attempt an IV en route and we will notify you with any changes.

Dr. Doyle: The patient will be going into Trauma Room 1. The trauma team will be in the ED awaiting your arrival.

Paramedic: Copy that, Mercy. Depew clear.

Upon arrival, the trauma team and a neurosurgeon meet the patient. Despite comprehensive care, the patient dies as a result of his head injury. However, at the family's request, the patient's organs are harvested. They are sent to cities more than 1,500 miles away and used in two transplant operations.

INTRODUCTION TO COMMUNICATION

Knowledge of communications plays an important role in your paramedic training. All aspects of prehospital care require effective, efficient communications. During a routine transfer or a life-threatening emergency run, you will communicate with a wide variety of people, including the following:

- The emergency medical dispatcher (EMD) whose job it is to manage an entire system of EMS response and readiness, not just your call. You will transmit administrative information such as "responding," "arrived," "transporting," and "back-in-service." The EMD must know the location of all his resources to manage the system effectively. On a serious emergency call, the EMD can be your best ally by securing for you the resources you need to manage your incident.

- Your patient, his family, bystanders, and others who may, at times, not understand what you are doing and become obstructive. Quite often, people misconstrue your actions and words. You must try to keep them well informed.

- Personnel from other responding agencies, such as the police department, fire department, or mutual aid ambulances who may not share your priorities at the scene. You must communicate effectively with other responders to coordinate and implement your treatment plan. You will accomplish this face to face and via the radio. These communications require you to exhibit confidence and authority.

▶ Health care staff from physicians' offices, health care facilities, and nursing homes who usually do not understand the extent of your training or abilities. Often, uninformed staff may think you are just "ambulance drivers." In these cases, you must exhibit professionalism and a calm demeanor while you ask pertinent questions and discuss the case intelligently.

▶ The medical direction physician who has extended his license to you in the field. The physician's expertise and advice can be a tremendous resource for you during the call. You will need to communicate patient information and scene assessment effectively to him. He can prepare for your arrival if you have communicated to him the needs of your patient. For example, you are transporting a patient with a serious head injury who exhibits a decreasing level of consciousness. By reporting this information, the emergency department can arrange for the trauma team, including a neurosurgeon, to meet you in the ED on arrival. In such cases, good communication results in good patient care.

You must interact effectively with everyone involved in the call to coordinate a unified effort resulting in top-quality patient care. EMS is the ultimate team endeavor. Your performance as a paramedic is just one component in a series of interactions that ensure continuous first-rate care. From the call taker to the rehabilitation specialist, every player in this continuum is equally important—only their roles differ. Communication is not merely one aspect of an EMS response; it is the key link in the chain that results in the best possible patient outcome. Effective communication optimizes patient care during every phase of the EMS response.

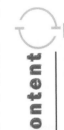

Communication is the key link in the chain that results in the best possible patient outcome.

BASIC COMMUNICATION MODEL

Communication is the process of exchanging information between individuals. It begins when you have an idea, or message, you would like to convey to someone else. You then encode that information in the language best suited for the situation. This might include words, numbers, symbols, or special codes. For instance, if you wanted to describe a collision scene to the medical direction physician, you would choose words that "paint a clear picture" of what you saw. In some systems, we communicate via code words. For example, 10-80 might mean a motor vehicle crash.

After you have encoded your message, you select the medium for sending it. You can speak face to face, send a fax, leave a voice message, send a letter or electronic mail (e-mail), or speak directly via telephone or radio. You might encode your message and send it via a paging system that posts either words or numbers; some pagers allow you to speak your message. Next, the intended receiver must decode and understand your message. Finally, he must give you feedback to confirm that he received your message and understood it. Consider the following example of an effective radio communication:

Dispatcher: Control to Unit 192, respond priority 1 to 483 County Route 22, cross street Canfield Road, on a possible heart.

Unit 192: Control, Unit 192 copy, responding priority 1 to 483 County Route 22.

Dispatcher: Unit 192 responding, 1228 hours.

In this simple example, the sender (dispatcher) encodes his message in a language that he knows the receiver (Unit 192) will understand. Unit 192 receives the message and

communication
the process of exchanging information between individuals.

Review

Basic Communications Model

1. Sender has an idea, or message.
2. Sender encodes message.
3. Sender sends message.
4. Receiver receives message.
5. Receiver decodes message.
6. Receiver gives feedback to sender.

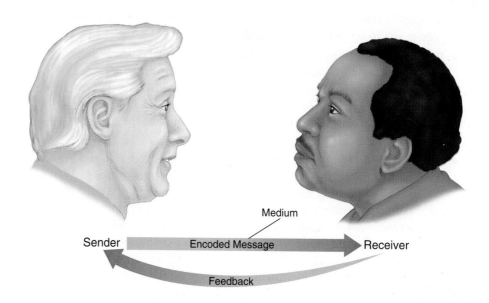

▶ **Figure 5-1** Communication occurs when individuals exchange information through an encoded message.

Medium

Sender   Encoded Message   Receiver

Feedback

acknowledges by repeating the key data. Finally, the sender confirms and concludes the communication (Figure 5-1 ▶).

VERBAL COMMUNICATION

semantic
related to the meaning of words.

10-code
radio communications system using codes that begin with the word ten.

Factors that can enhance or impede effective communication may be either **semantic** (the meaning of words) or technical (communications hardware). Communication requires a mutual language. For example, a city unit and a county unit that use different **10-code** systems will find it difficult to communicate effectively. A 10-10 may mean a working fire in one system and a cardiac emergency in another. Thus, many EMS systems have changed from using 10-codes to plain English.

When reporting your patient's condition to the medical direction physician, you should use terminology that is widely accepted by both the medical and emergency services communities. Using a 10-code system with which the ED staff is unfamiliar would be inappropriate. Telling the medical direction physician that you have a victim of a 10-21-Golf (assault with a gun) may be meaningless. Conversely, if the medical direction physician asks you for your pregnant patient's EDC (due date) or her LMP (last menstrual period) and you do not know those acronyms, you have failed to communicate. The receiver must be able to decode the sender's message.

Your communication network must consist of reliable equipment designed to afford clear communication among all agencies within the system.

Your communication network must consist of reliable equipment designed to afford clear communication among all agencies within the system. This becomes a challenge in systems that cover large geographical areas or where terrain interferes with transmission and reception. If you want to communicate with a unit clear across the county but your radio is not powerful enough to transmit that far, communication will be difficult, if not impossible. A system that covers a large geographical expanse can place repeaters strategically throughout its service area. These devices receive transmissions from a low-powered source and rebroadcast them at a higher power (Figure 5-2 ▶).

radio band
a range of radio frequencies.

radio frequency
the number of times per second a radio wave oscillates.

ultrahigh frequency (UHF)
radio frequency band from 300 to 3,000 megahertz.

Your regional EMS system may consist of many agencies that have conducted business for decades on different **radio bands** and **frequencies.** City units may transmit on **ultrahigh frequency (UHF)** radio waves because they penetrate concrete and steel well and are less susceptible to interference. County units may use a low band frequency because those waves travel farther and better over varied terrain. In any event, communicating among agencies will be difficult unless all units share a common

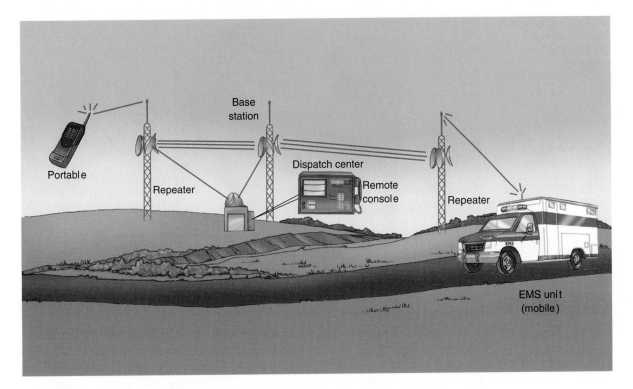

▶ **Figure 5-2** Example of an EMS system that uses repeaters.

frequency. This is rarely the case. The spectrum of communications equipment currently ranges from antiquated radios to mobile data terminals mounted inside emergency vehicles. Geographically integrating communications networks would enable routine and reliable communication among EMS, fire, law enforcement, and other public safety agencies. This would in turn facilitate coordinated responses during both routine and large-scale operations. Developing the necessary hardware (equipment and network) and software (language) will be essential to improving emergency communications.

WRITTEN COMMUNICATION

Written records are another important aspect of EMS communications. Your **prehospital care report (PCR)** is a written record of events that includes administrative information such as times, location, agency, and crew, as well as medical information. It will be used by hospital staff, agency administrators, system quality assurance/improvement committees, insurance and billing departments, researchers, educators, and lawyers. The data collected from your PCR can help to monitor and improve patient care through medical audits, research, education, and system policy changes. Furthermore, your written documentation becomes a legal record of the incident and may become part of your patient's permanent medical record. All legal rules regarding confidentiality and disclosure pertain to your PCR.

The same factors that influence verbal communication also affect written communication. Be objective, write legibly, thoroughly document your patient's assessment and care, and use terminology that is widely accepted in the medical community (Figure 5-3 ▶). Finally, your PCR illustrates your professionalism. A sloppy, incomplete PCR suggests sloppy, inefficient care. Chapter 6, Documentation, deals with PCRs and other written communications in much greater detail.

prehospital care report (PCR)
the written record of an EMS response.

Figure 5-3 The prehospital care report is as important as the run itself. Complete it promptly, accurately, and legibly.

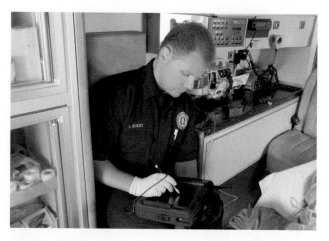

Terminology

Every industry develops its own terminology. Doing so makes communication within the industry more clear, concise, and unambiguous. The airline industry, for example, uses the term *payload* to describe the total weight of everything (passengers, fuel, luggage, and other items) on an airplane. Musical composers and arrangers use words like *fortissimo, allegro,* and *a cappella* to describe a specific tempo or style.

The medical field also uses an extensive list of terms, acronyms, and abbreviations that allow quick, accurate communication of complex information. (Chapter 6 includes an extensive table of standard charting abbreviations.) An emergency physician may request a CBC (complete blood count), ABGs (arterial blood gases), or a CIP (cardiac injury profile)—common terms describing diagnostic tests run on acutely ill patients. The emergency services industry has further developed its own terms for radio communication (Table 5–1). These words or phrases shorten air time and transmit thoughts and ideas quickly. For example, *copy, 10-4,* and *roger* mean "I heard you and I understand what you said." Using industry terminology appropriately is an important part of effective communication. It provides a common means of communicating with other emergency care professionals.

Using industry terminology appropriately provides a common means of communicating with other emergency care professionals.

Table 5–1	Common Radio Terminology
Term	**Meaning**
Copy, 10-4, roger	I understand
Affirmative	Yes
Negative	No
Stand by	Please wait
Repeat	Please repeat what you said
Landline	Telephone communications
Rendezvous	Meet with
LZ	Landing zone (helicopter)
ETA	Estimated time of arrival
Over	I am finished with my transmission
Mobile status	On the air, driving around
Stage	Wait before entering a scene
Clear	End of transmission
Unfounded	We cannot find the incident/patient
Be advised	Listen carefully to this

THE EMS RESPONSE

Your ability to communicate effectively during a stressful EMS response will determine the success or failure of your efforts. A brilliant assessment and management plan will be futile if you cannot communicate it to others. Dealing effectively with your patient and bystanders requires a variety of communication skills such as empathy, confidence, self-control, authority, and patience. Your clinical experience will suggest which skills to use in any particular situation. For example, you might use confidence and an authoritative posture when dealing with unruly bystanders. On the other hand, you would need to be gentle and empathetic with a child or an elderly grandmother. If you were in charge of an incident, you would have to communicate your authority within the structure of the emergency scene to providers from other responding agencies. Delegating tasks, listening to initial reports, and coordinating the scene require effective communication and interpersonal skills.

The sequence of an EMS response illustrates the importance of communications in prehospital care. A typical EMS response includes the following chain of events.

Detection and Citizen Access   To begin the response to any emergency once it has occurred, someone must detect the problem and summon EMS (Figure 5-4 ▶). Any citizen with an urgent medical need should have a simple and reliable mechanism for accessing the EMS system. In the United States, most people access EMS by telephone; thus, a well-publicized universal telephone number such as 911 provides direct citizen access to the communications center. At Enhanced 911 (E-911) communication centers, a computer displays the caller's telephone number and location. The centers also have instant call-back capabilities, should the caller hang up too soon. The 911 system has been available since the late 1960s. Currently, 96 percent of the population in the United States and 93 percent of the nation's geographic area enjoy a 911 system. There is no more reliable, and protected, communications system than our 911 system. Highway call boxes, citizens band (CB) radio, and amateur radio all provide alternate means of accessing emergency help in some regions.

Calls to 911 usually connect the caller to a **public safety answering point (PSAP)**, which then directs the caller to the appropriate agency for dispatch and response. (A public safety answering point is any agency that takes emergency calls from citizens in a given region and dispatches the emergency resources necessary to respond to individual calls for help. PSAPs are also considered 911 centers in those areas covered by 911 service.) In some systems, the PSAP call taker will elicit the information and determine the nature of the response. In others, he will simply answer with the question "Is this a police, fire, or medical emergency?" and transfer the caller to the appropriate dispatcher,

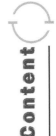

A brilliant assessment and management plan will be futile if you cannot communicate it to others.

Review

EMS Response Communications

- Detection and citizen access
- Automatic collision notification
- Call taking and emergency response
- Prearrival instructions
- Call coordination and incident recording
- Discussion with medical direction physician
- Transfer communications
- Back in service, ready for next call

public safety answering point (PSAP)

any agency that takes emergency calls from citizens in a given region and dispatches the emergency resources necessary to respond to individual calls for help.

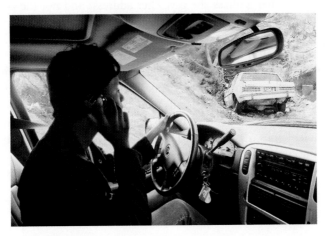

▶ **Figure 5-4**   The response begins when someone detects an emergency and summons EMS support. (© On Scene Photography/Michael Grill)

who will then elicit the information. Many systems use computerized technology at the PSAP to connect the caller automatically with the appropriate agency. Some even provide language translation. Future global positioning systems will allow the dispatcher to pinpoint a cellular phone caller's location. Additionally, automakers are installing communications computers in some automobiles. When involved in a collision, these "black boxes" automatically will provide the dispatcher with the location, speed, type of collision, projected damage, and suspected severity of injury.

Under a new rule issued by the U.S. Department of Transportation's National Highway Traffic Safety Administration (NHTSA) (**www.NHTSA.dot.gov**) automakers will be required, for the first time ever, to tell new car buyers if an event data recorder (EDR) has been installed in a vehicle. Event data recorders are electronic devices that capture crash data in the few seconds before, during, and after a crash. EDRs do not capture any data unless there is a collision that is severe enough to cause the air bag to deploy.

The NHTSA also expects the new rule, which takes effect with model year 2011 cars, will enhance the value of automatic crash notification (ACN) systems (discussed in the following section), including the Enhanced 911 emergency response system currently under development, by making it easier for vehicles equipped with ACN features to provide accurate and immediate information to emergency personnel.

In some systems, all public safety agencies are located within the same facility. In others, they are connected electronically. No one way is best. If the public receives timely, appropriate responses to all emergency calls, the system is effective.

The rapidly expanding popularity of wireless phones in the late twentieth century had a negative impact on the Enhanced 911 system. The E-911 system associated with wire-line telephones automatically provides emergency dispatchers with automatic number identification (ANI) and automatic location identification (ALI). The automatic provision of ANI and ALI data enables emergency dispatchers to dispatch an emergency response while EMD prearrival instructions are being given. Few EMS providers would disagree that E-911 coupled with EMD saves many lives each year.

Until recently, wireless phones were not able to provide emergency dispatchers with E-911 data such as ANI and ALI. Dispatchers were reliant on the caller's ability to communicate his location and phone number. Many cases have occurred where the caller had a decreased level of consciousness or was incapacitated, could not provide his location and number, and could not be found. These cases are almost always associated with bad patient outcomes.

In many cases the caller is simply too excited to provide the emergency dispatcher with the correct information. One such case involved a 19-year-old female in a rural New York State community who called 911 to report an oven fire. She was cooking dinner at her grandmother's home when the fire began. She assisted her grandmother out of the home and dialed 911 on her wireless telephone. When the dispatcher asked her for her address she gave "her address" and not the address of her grandmother's home. The resulting confusion over the location of the emergency was responsible for total loss of the structure. Cases like this were common in the years prior to the installation of E-911—it's hard to imagine, but true, that this event took place in the year 2002.

Further complicating the problem is the issue of "call routing." Typically, wire-line 911 calls are routed via a trunk line and a specialized address database to the nearest 911 center. Wireless 911 calls that do not carry address database data with them cannot be automatically routed to the nearest 911 center. Thus, emergency calls from wireless telephones may be routed out of your region, your county, your state, or even out of the country.

At the height of the rise in sales, 46,000 new wireless phone subscriptions were made each day. The rise in sales, in turn, caused a relative increase in 911 calls. Unfortunately, the largest percentage of this increase came from nonenhanced wireless phones.

Many 911 centers, in conjunction with wireless phone carriers, are putting technologies in place that allow for transmission and acceptance of ANI and ALI from wireless phones. The cost for the specialized telephone trunk lines, computer hardware and software, call routing equipment, and database managers necessary to make this possible is very high. Fortunately, progress has been steady and many 911 centers are receiving the necessary data. Currently, about 29 percent of U.S. PSAPs are able to gather location and call-back number information from wireless telephones.

Wireless phones can be located by terrestrial-based triangulation, global positioning systems (GPS), or a combination of the two. Triangulation of a wireless signal involves the use of three cellular phone towers. Based on the strength of telephone signal and time of signal arrival at each of the towers, the signal location can be calculated to within several meters. This calculated location is identified as a longitude/latitude that is then translated to a map location and street address in a specialized database. Because the call is recognized as having come from a phone with a unique identifier, another specialized database assigns the correct call-back number associated with that specific phone. This packet of information—a phone call with a 911 prefix, ALI data, and ANI data—is then transmitted digitally through selective routers and trunk lines to the closest public safety answering point, or 911 center. Geographic regions such as individual counties have had to decide to which PSAP they prefer to have these calls sent.

Once the call is received, the dispatcher is able to pinpoint the caller's location on a computerized map, speak directly to the caller, provide medical prearrival instructions, and start an emergency response. In cases of a disconnect, the dispatcher has enough information to recontact the person who dialed 911.

Systems that use global positioning location data require that the individual phones be fitted with hardware and software that allow them access to the GPS. Emergency 911 calls originating from such phones are still routed in the same manner and require access to the ANI database but not to an ALI database. Location information is transmitted automatically with the packet of data that comes from the phone when a 911 prefix is associated with the call. The data from these phones are transmitted to the appropriate PSAP. Call takers and dispatchers see the data in the same format as they see other 911 calls. In other words, the method of data transmission is transparent to the dispatch personnel, because ANI and ALI data are provided in identical formats with both methods. Putting these new communications technologies in place ensures the continuation of Enhanced 911 as cellular communications become more popular.

Patho Pearls

Calculating Force   One way to calculate the force involved in a motor vehicle crash (MVC) is to multiply the mass of the vehicle by the change in velocity divided by the time required for the change in velocity to occur: $F = M \times \Delta V/\Delta T$. If a 2,400-pound vehicle, as in the accompanying scenario, decelerates from 65 to 0 mph in 20 minutes, the force applied to the occupants does not exceed their ability to tolerate that force. However, if that same 2,400-pound vehicle decelerates from 65 to 0 mph over 0.8 second, as in our scenario, the force absorbed will far exceed the driver's ability to tolerate it. Consider also that few MVCs are comprised of a single impact. MVCs typically involve multiple forces, such as rolls and spins, that are applied to vehicle occupants from multiple directions or vectors. Each of these forces must be accounted for and contribute to the summation of total force applied to crash victims.

automatic collision notification (ACN) system
data collection and transmission system that can automatically contact a national call center or local public safety answering point and transmit specific crash data.

Automatic Collision Notification

Automatic collision notification (ACN) systems are data collection and transmission systems that may change the way we assess and treat victims of car crashes. As the name implies, ACN systems can automatically contact a national call center or local PSAP and transmit crash-specific data. For example, imagine a car containing a driver and one passenger that is traveling 45 mph along a highway. The driver loses control of the vehicle, exits the roadway, rolls over, and comes to rest against a tree. Because the ACN system in the vehicle contains special sensors called accelerometers, it can measure the change in total velocity (referred to as delta V—written as ΔV—for change in velocity), how quickly the car deceleration occurred (referred to as delta T—written as ΔT—for change in time), how many forces were applied to the vehicle, in which direction they were applied, how many times the car rolled over, and its final resting position. The sensor also has a GPS-enabled chip that can transmit the exact location of the vehicle. Other data available from the system can include the age and sex of the primary owner/driver of the vehicle, the crash-worthiness rating of the vehicle, and whether the air bags deployed in the crash.

Unfortunately, America's current 911 system is decades old, and was not built to handle the text, data, photos, and video that are increasingly common in personal communications. The current system is analog, not digital, and is landline based, not Internet based. This antiquated network cannot efficiently transmit the information available from new technologies.

ACN systems are just beginning to gain acceptance in the emergency care system. The usefulness of this technology will not be fully understood until ACN–to–PSAP transmissions become more common. The data, photos, and video provided by personal communication devices and ACN technology have the potential to improve emergency response, triage, and definitive care. That's assuming PSAPs are equipped to receive data, photos, and video, and that EMS providers know how to use this additional information to improve patient care.

Consider the following scenario that could typify an ACN application in a rural setting:

You're working the overnight shift in a county in northern New York State. This particular county is more than 2,800 square miles in area with a population of just over 100,000. Your particular volunteer agency services 340 square miles of area with one in-house advanced life support (ALS) duty crew and one ALS backup crew 24 hours per day. At 3 A.M. the county PSAP gets an ACN activation of a crash on a rural road several miles from your station. Once you're alerted and begin your response, county dispatch tells you that the ACN indicates a single-car MVC with a 65-mph delta V that occurred over 0.8 second. Based on your understanding of the mechanism of injury concept, you know that any occupants in the vehicle absorbed significant force. The ACN data show that the vehicle rolled twice and came to rest on its wheels. The VIN is traceable to a two-door sports car with a gross vehicle weight of 2,400 pounds, and the primary driver of the vehicle involved is a 20-year-old male.

You are the closest unit to the crash scene and you know that, as you leave your station, you'll have to make numerous critical decisions in the next several minutes. However, dispatch tells you that the crash data are being transmitted to the regional trauma center and, due to the incoming data, a helicopter has been placed on standby. Because of the crash data and a preestablished PSAP protocol, fire suppression, heavy-rescue unit, and extra manpower have already been dispatched and are responding. So some of your work has already been done. Some of your critical decisions have already been made, because the available technology assisted in

additional resources needed and record information about the call such as times, locations, and units involved. Your dispatcher can be your best friend. He can assign the resources you need to manage an incident: additional medical personnel to help with a cardiac arrest, for instance, or the fire department to provide specialized rescue. He also may facilitate communication with other agencies, hospitals, communication centers, and support services.

Discussion with the Medical Direction Physician   After conducting your assessment and initiating care as outlined by your local protocols, you will contact the medical direction physician to discuss the case. Following consultation, he may give you further orders for interventions such as medications or other medical procedures. The many ways to conduct this communication include the radio, telephone, and cellular phone. Taping these communications for use later is advisable. For example, if a discrepancy arose as to your orders, you could always refer to the tape, which never lies. At this point, you continue treatment and prepare your patient for transport. You will contact your dispatcher, who will record when you leave the scene and when you arrive at your destination.

Your professional relationship with your medical direction physicians must be based on trust. Transmission of clear, concise, controlled reports will encourage your medical direction physicians to accept your assessments and on-scene treatment plans. Your ability to communicate effectively on the radio will secure a large part of your professional reputation. The general radio procedures and standard format sections later in this chapter offer guidelines for communicating with your medical direction physician and transmitting patient information (Figure 5-7 ▶).

> Transmitting clear, concise, controlled reports will encourage your medical direction physicians to trust your assessments and on-scene treatment plans.

Transfer Communications   As you transfer care of your patient to the receiving facility staff, you must give the receiving nurse or physician a formal verbal briefing (Figure 5-8 ▶). This report should include your patient's vital information, chief complaint and history, physical exam findings, and any treatments rendered. Do not assume that the receiving nurse heard your radio report and knows of your patient. Some systems require the receiving nurse to sign the PCR to verify and document the transfer of care. In any case, never leave your patient until you have completed some type of formal transfer of care, because you may be charged with abandonment. Many systems likewise require the medical direction physician to sign the PCR for any medications administered by paramedics, especially if they included controlled substances such as morphine or diazepam. In all cases, end your documentation with transfer of care information on your PCR.

> Never leave your patient until you formally transfer responsibility for his care.

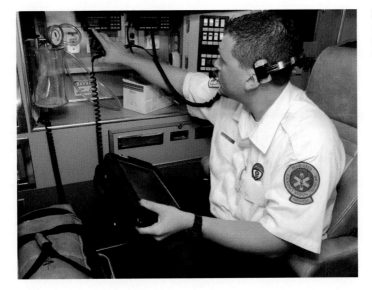

▶ **Figure 5-7**   You will discuss each case with the medical direction physician and follow his instructions for patient care. (© Jeff Forster)

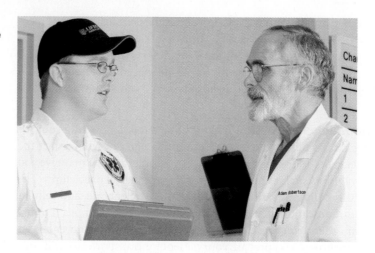

Figure 5-8 On arrival at the emergency department, you will give receiving personnel a formal, verbal briefing. (© Ken Kerr)

COMMUNICATION TECHNOLOGY

EMS systems can use all of today's various communication technologies. These include the more traditional forms of radio communication as well as innovations in radio technology and other media.

Radio Communication

Many types of radio transmission are possible, with new technologies being developed every day. Usage may vary from system to system. This section discusses some of the more common technologies in use today.

simplex

communications system that transmits and receives on the same frequency.

Simplex The most basic communications systems use **simplex** transmissions. These systems transmit and receive on the same frequency and thus cannot do both simultaneously (Figure 5-9 ▶). After you transmit a message, you must release the transmit button and wait for a response. This slows communication because you have to wait for all traffic to stop before you can speak. It also makes the system more formal and prevents open discussion. Simplex communications systems are most effective on the scene, when the incident commander or EMS dispatcher must transmit orders or directions without interruption. Most dispatch systems and on-scene communications use simplex transmissions.

duplex

communications system that allows simultaneous two-way communications by using two frequencies for each channel.

Duplex **Duplex** transmissions allow simultaneous two-way communications by using two frequencies for each channel (Figure 5-10 ▶). Each radio must be able to transmit and receive on each channel. For example, on channel 1, a hospital base station might transmit on 468.000 megahertz (MHz) and receive on 478.000 MHz. Field radios would

▶ **Figure 5-9** Simplex communications systems transmit and receive on the same frequency.

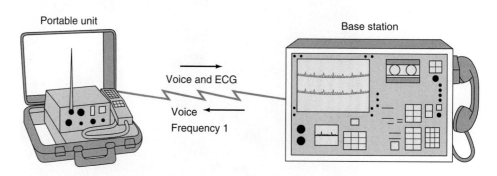

Portable unit

Voice and ECG

Voice
Frequency 1

Base station

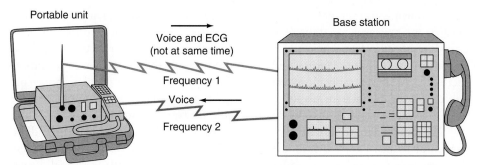

Portable unit

Voice and ECG
(not at same time)

Frequency 1

Voice

Frequency 2

Base station

▶ **Figure 5-10** Duplex communications systems use two frequencies for each channel.

then transmit on 478.000 MHz and receive on 468.000 MHz—just the opposite. Either party could then transmit and receive on the same channel simultaneously.

Duplex systems work like telephone communications. Many areas use them for communications between the field paramedic and the medical direction physician. The duplex system's major advantage is that one party does not have to wait to speak until the other party finishes his transmission. This allows a much freer discussion and consultation between physician and paramedic. For example, the medical direction physician can interrupt your report with an important question or concern. On the other hand, this ability to interrupt can be a disadvantage when abused.

Duplex systems all allow you to transmit either voice messages or data such as ECG strips.

Multiplex **Multiplex** systems are duplex systems with the additional capability of transmitting voice and data simultaneously (Figure 5-11 ▶). This enables you to carry on a conversation with the medical direction physician while you are transmitting an ECG strip. Speaking while you are transmitting the ECG strip, however, causes much interference on the ECG strip.

multiplex
duplex system that can transmit voice and data simultaneously.

Trunking Many communications systems operating in the 800-MHz range use **trunking** to hasten communications. Trunked systems pool all frequencies. When a radio transmission comes in, a computer routes it to the first available frequency. The computer routes the next transmission to the next available frequency, and so on. When a transmission terminates, that frequency becomes available and reenters the pool of unused frequencies. Trunking thus frees the dispatcher or field unit from having to search for an available frequency.

trunking
communications system that pools all frequencies and routes transmissions to the next available frequency.

Digital Communications Voice transmission can be time consuming and difficult to understand. The trend toward combining radio technology with computer technology has encouraged a shift from analog to **digital communications.** Digital radio equipment is becoming increasingly popular in emergency services communications systems. This technology translates, or encodes, sounds into digital code for broadcast.

digital communications
data or sounds translated into a digital code for transmission.

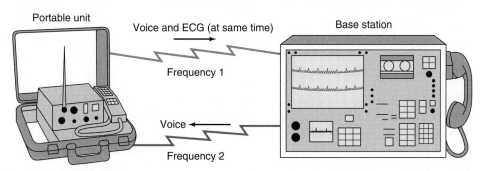

Portable unit

Voice and ECG (at same time)

Frequency 1

Voice

Frequency 2

Base station

▶ **Figure 5-11** Multiplex systems can transmit voice and data at the same time.

Digital transmission is much faster and much more accurate than analog transmission. Because the messages are transmitted in condensed form, they help to ease the overcrowding of radio frequencies. Also, because you need a decoder to translate digital transmissions back into voice, scanners cannot monitor them. Your communications, therefore, are considerably more secure than over the radio. Many cellular phone companies now use digital transmissions. Future technology will link patient-monitoring devices to a small computer equipped with a radio for transmission.

The **mobile data terminals** in many emergency vehicles are a basic form of digital communications. They are mounted in the vehicle cab and wired to the radio. When a data transmission such as the address of the incident comes in, the terminal displays the message on a screen or prints it in hard copy. Responders can reply by punching a button to send a message such as "en route," "arrived," or "transporting to the hospital." Though somewhat restrictive and primitive, these terminals have reduced on-air time to a minimum even in the busiest systems. It is important to remember, however, that voice communications will always have a place in emergency services. Crews will always need to speak to one another, to physicians and nurses, or to dispatchers.

Alternative Technologies

Among the more common alternatives to radio communications are the cellular telephone, the facsimile machine, and the computer.

Cell phone Many EMS systems have found that **cellular phone systems** (cell phones) provide a cost-effective way to transmit essential patient information to the hospital (Figure 5-12). Cellular technology is available in even the most remote areas. A cellular telephone service is divided into regions called *cells*. These cells are radio base stations, with which the mobile telephone communicates. When the transmission leaves one cell's range, another cell picks it up immediately, without interruption.

Like duplex radio transmissions, cellular phones make communication less formal, promote discussion, and reduce on-line times. They further allow the medical direction physician to speak directly with the patient and offer the additional advantages of being widely available and highly reliable. Because the ECG signal is digitized, it is easily transmitted on cell phone data channels. The hospital receives a better ECG signal than if it were transmitted over radio waves. The telephones themselves are inexpensive, but cell phone systems charge a monthly fee for their use. Their major disadvantage is that each cell can handle only a limited number of calls. Geography can interfere with the cell phone's signals, and in large metropolitan areas the cells often fill up and become unavailable, especially during peak hours. Cellular congestion frequently occurs in times of disaster when many local, state, and federal response agencies, news media, and citizens all require communications. Other disadvantages are that anyone with a scanner can monitor conversations on analog cell phones; cell phones require an external antenna; and the cell phone system will deny access to a cell if you do not know or forget the personal identification number (PIN). Despite their limitations, cell phones have become a popular medium for dispatching, on-scene, and medical direction communications. When using wireless phones for on-line medical direction, it is important to contact the base station physician on a recorded line. On-line medical direction recordings have been used as powerful allies in cases of litigation. Be sure to find out how to do this in your system.

Facsimile A **facsimile machine (fax)** provides a quick way to send printed information. This machine "reads" the printed information, digitizes it line by line, and transmits it to another machine, which then decodes it and prints a facsimile of the original. A fax machine enables health care agencies to exchange medical information immediately. Future systems will allow EMS responders to access a patient's medical record from a

mobile data terminal
vehicle-mounted computer keyboard and display.

cellular telephone system
telephone system divided into regions, or cells, that are served by radio base stations.

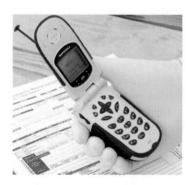

▶ **Figure 5-12** Cellular telephones have made it possible to transmit high-quality facsimiles, computer data, and 12-lead ECGs.

facsimile machine (fax)
device for electronically transmitting and receiving printed information.

general database; responders or database operators will be able to send the same information to the receiving facility. With some electronic run sheet systems, you will be able to transmit your patient information to the receiving hospital long before you arrive. This technology's one obvious limitation is that both the sending and the receiving agency must have access to a fax machine and a telephone line.

Computer   Computers have entered every aspect of our daily lives. In emergency services communications, they have revolutionized system management and incident data collection. Most dispatchers no longer enter data via pen and pencil, time-stamping machines, or typewriters. They can make a permanent record of any incident's events in real time. Computers also make research faster and easier. For example, if you wanted to determine the day of the week when most cardiac calls happen, or what time of day is busiest, or which area of a city needs more coverage, you could retrieve the pertinent data from your computerized records immediately. You can program your system to provide whatever type of data you want, in whatever format you desire. It also eliminates the need to enter retrospective data when conducting research. For example, the times, locations, and particulars of a call already will be in the computer files for immediate retrieval during a research project. A computer's limitations include its own power, speed, and capacity, as well as its operator's ability. Also, rigidly programmed machines that function only in certain restrictive ways can limit your flexibility.

New Technology

New technology is being developed every day. The National Aeronautics and Space Administration (NASA) has pioneered communications that allow television viewers to hear and see astronauts in space. Ground crews can monitor each astronaut's biologic function and maintain a permanent record throughout the trip—they have been doing this for decades.

In comparison to other industries, public safety communication systems are nearly archaic. Most EMS agencies still document patient assessment and care with handwritten run sheets, and some use radio equipment so old that replacement tubes are no longer available. But times are changing rapidly. Time constraints, storage space, and congested radio traffic necessitate developing new systems that will allow paramedics to transmit,

Legal Notes

Keeping It Private   Many modern EMS communications systems use encryption or similar technologies to ensure privacy and security. However, certain EMS communications, including some cell phone communications, can be monitored by persons with scanners or similar devices, which are becoming as sophisticated as the radios and phones themselves. It was once thought that radio communication was secure, but in fact it may not be. Furthermore, in many emergency departments, EMS radios are within earshot of patients, staff, and visitors. Thus, you should always assume that any EMS radio communication may be heard by someone other than the intended recipient. Because of this, you must carefully limit any information that might identify a particular patient. This includes such things as name, race, financial (insurance) status, and similar descriptors. Transmission of such information does not enhance patient care and may actually violate patient confidentiality laws including the Health Insurance Portability and Accountability Act and similar statutes. Always carefully plan your radio communications—especially when they deal with a particular patient.

receive, and store vital patient information quickly and reliably. Someday computer-based technology, digital satellite transmission, and electronic storage and retrieval of patient information will replace radio communications, written documentation, and file cabinets filled with EMS run sheets. These technologies are costly, but they already exist.

Current documentation systems already allow you to record all aspects of your EMS response electronically, by use of a **touch pad.** With pen-based reporting systems you can record patient information on a handheld computer. These systems do away with written documentation and capture information in real time, eliminating your need to estimate times after the call. Some systems integrate diagnostic technology and enable you to transmit ECG and pulse oximetry readings to the hospital before arrival. Such advanced knowledge of diagnostic test results from the field may radically change a medical direction physician's decisions and reduce the time needed to make an in-hospital diagnosis and begin therapy. Transmitting a 12-lead ECG, for example, will reduce the time before paramedics in transit or receiving emergency department personnel can begin cardiac muscle-saving fibrinolytic therapy for the patient with a suspected myocardial infarction. In some cases paramedics will be able to start therapy en route. Other systems allow you to receive important medical information from your patient's permanent record while on the scene or in transit. For instance, at the home of a patient with an altered mental status and no family to relate his history, you might access his medical records and attain his history via a computerized database. In this type of system, the transferring facility, the receiving hospital, and you can all access this information simultaneously.

A disadvantage of electronic recording systems is the absence of a "paper record" of the incident, should the information be accidentally erased or destroyed. The legal guidelines that apply to written and spoken communication also apply to electronic reporting. You must maintain patient confidentiality, you must be objective, and you must not **slander** or **libel** another person.

REPORTING PROCEDURES

As a paramedic, you must effectively relay all relevant medical information to the receiving hospital staff. Initially, you might do this over the radio or by cellular telephone. Later, when you deliver your patient to the emergency department, you can give additional information in person to the appropriate receiving hospital personnel.

One of your most important skills will be gathering essential patient information, organizing it, and relaying it to the medical direction physician. The medical direction physician will then issue appropriate orders for patient care. The amount and type of information you relay to the medical direction physician will depend on the type of technology you use, your patient's priority, and your local communication **protocols.** For example, if communications in your region are not secure (private), you must limit the type of information you can communicate without breaching patient confidentiality. The acuteness of your patient's clinical status and the amount of local radio traffic also may determine the length of your report. For a critical patient you may give a brief report while you tend to your patient's medical needs. For a complicated medical emergency, you may wish to communicate a greater share of the results of your history and physical exam to the medical direction physician.

Standard Format

Communicating patient information to the hospital or to the medical direction physician is a crucial function within the EMS system. Verbal communications, which may occur via radio or landline, give the hospital enough information on your patient's

---

touch pad
computer on which you enter data by touching areas of the display screen.

slander
to orally defame another person.

libel
to defame another person in writing.

One of your most important skills will be gathering essential patient information, organizing it, and relaying it to the medical direction physician.

protocol
predetermined, written guidelines for patient care.

condition to prepare for his care. These communications also should initiate the medical orders you need to treat your patient in the field. A standard format for transmitting patient assessment information helps to achieve those goals in several ways. First, it adds to the medical communication system's efficiency. Second, it helps the physician to assimilate information about the patient's condition quickly. Third, it ensures that medical information is complete. In general, your verbal reports to medical direction should include the following information:

- Identification of the unit and the provider
- Description of the scene
- Patient's age, sex, and approximate weight (for drug orders)
- Patient's chief complaint and severity
- Brief, pertinent history of the present illness or injury (OPQRST)
- Pertinent past medical history, medications, and allergies (SAMPLE)
- Pertinent physical exam findings
- Treatment given so far/request for orders
- Estimated time of arrival at the hospital
- Other pertinent information

The formats and contents of reports for medical and trauma patients differ to include only the information relevant to either type of emergency. Reports for medical patients emphasize the history in the beginning of the report; reports for trauma patients emphasize the injuries and the physical exam.

After transmitting your report, you will await further questions and orders from the medical direction physician. On arrival, your spoken report will give essential patient information to the provider assuming care. It should include a brief history, pertinent physical findings, treatment, and responses to that treatment.

General Radio Procedures

Proper use of the radio will make your communications skillful and efficient. All of your transmissions must be clear and crisp, with concise, professional content (Figure 5-13 ▶). Always follow these guidelines for effective radio use:

1. Listen to the channel before transmitting to ensure that it is not in use.
2. Press the transmit button for 1 second before speaking.
3. Speak at close range, approximately 2 to 3 inches, directly into, or across the face of, the microphone.
4. Speak slowly and clearly. Pronounce each word distinctly, avoiding words that are difficult to understand.
5. Speak in a normal pitch, keeping your voice free of emotion.
6. Be brief. Know what you are going to say before you press the transmit button.
7. Avoid codes unless they are part of your EMS system.
8. Do not waste air time with unnecessary information.
9. Protect your patient's privacy. When appropriate:
   - Use the telephone rather than a radio.
   - Turn off the external speaker.
   - Do not use your patient's name; doing so violates FCC regulations.
10. Use proper unit or hospital numbers and correct names or titles.

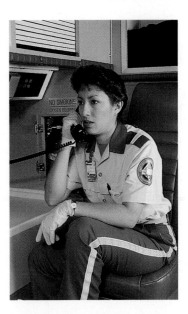

▶ **Figure 5-13** The professionalism of your communications reflects on the professionalism of your patient care.

11. Do not use slang or profanity.

12. Use standard formats for transmission.

13. Be concise in order to hold the attention of the person receiving your radio report.

14. Use the **echo procedure** when receiving directions from the dispatcher or orders from the physician. Immediately repeating each statement will confirm accurate reception and understanding.

15. Always write down addresses, important dispatch communications, and physician orders.

16. When completing a transmission, obtain confirmation that your message was received and understood.

Occasionally, communications equipment will not function properly. Even a weak battery can disrupt clear communication. If you are far from the base station, particularly if you have a portable radio, try to broadcast from higher terrain. Structures that contain steel and concrete can interfere with radio transmission. Simply moving outside the building or near a window may improve communications. If that does not work, try a telephone.

REGULATION

The **Federal Communications Commission (FCC)** controls and regulates all nongovernmental communications in the United States. This includes AM and FM radio, television, aircraft, marine, and mobile land frequency ranges. The FCC has designated frequencies within each radio band for special use. They include public safety frequencies in both the **very high frequency (VHF)** band and the ultrahigh frequency band (UHF). The FCC's primary functions include:

▶ Licensing and allocating radio frequencies

▶ Establishing technical standards for radio equipment

▶ Licensing and regulating the technical personnel who repair and operate radio equipment

▶ Monitoring frequencies to ensure appropriate usage

▶ Spot-checking base stations and dispatch centers for appropriate licenses and records

The FCC requires all EMS communications systems to follow appropriate governmental regulations and laws. You must stay abreast of and obey any FCC regulations that apply to your communications.

▶ Summary

As one of the fundamental aspects of prehospital care, accurate communications help ensure an EMS system's efficiency. Communications begin when the citizen accesses the EMS system and end when you complete your patient report. Your spoken messages must be understandable, and your written messages must be legible. All of your communications must be concise and complete and conform to national and local protocols. The more sophisticated and advanced your EMS system grows, the more sophisticated and advanced its communications—and, accordingly, your communications skills—must become.

▶ You Make the Call

A call comes into your unit for a "possible heart attack" on State Route 11. You and your partner climb into Palermo Rescue, a nontransport first-response vehicle. Your response time is about 10 minutes. Upon arrival, a family member meets you. He leads you into the den of a small farmhouse. Here you see your patient sitting in an overstuffed chair. You note that your patient is a 69-year-old male in obvious distress.

You begin questioning your patient to develop a history. As he speaks, you immediately notice that he has difficulty breathing. He complains of severe chest pain, which began about 30 minutes ago. With his hand, he indicates that the pain is pressure-like and substernal. He also indicates that it radiates to his left arm and jaw. He describes a history of heart disease, including two prior heart attacks. Three years ago, he had cardiac bypass surgery. He currently takes Lanoxin, Lasix, Capoten, and an aspirin a day. He is allergic to Mellaril.

You and your partner complete your assessment. Your patient says he weighs about 250 pounds. He is alert, but anxious. He exhibits jugular venous distention and bibasilar crackles. His abdomen is nontender. His distal pulses are good. Vital signs include blood pressure 210/110 mmHg, pulse of 70 per minute and regular, and respirations of 20 breaths per minute and mildly labored. Pulse oximetry is 93 percent on supplemental oxygen. During your assessment, your patient becomes progressively more dyspneic. The transporting ambulance arrives and the paramedic asks you to give a radio report to the receiving hospital based on your assessment while she prepares her patient for transport.

- Based on the preceding information, organize and prepare your radio report to inform the receiving hospital of your patient's condition.

See Suggested Responses at the back of this book.

▶ Review Questions

1. These devices receive transmission from a low-power source and rebroadcast them at a higher power.
   a. encoders
   b. 10-code systems
   c. repeaters
   d. decoders

2. The number of times per second a radio wave oscillates is the:
   a. band.
   b. frequency.
   c. dynamics.
   d. modulation.

3. At these communications centers, a computer displays the caller's telephone number and location.
   a. 911
   b. E-911
   c. UHF
   d. CB

4. Most commonly, the public's first contact with the EMS system is the:
   a. first responder.
   b. EMT-Basic.
   c. paramedic.
   d. emergency medical dispatcher.

5. In this type of communications system, only one-way transmission is possible. You either talk or listen. It is _____ transmission.
   a. simplex
   b. duplex
   c. trunking
   d. multiplex

6. An ECG can be transmitted during a conversation on the same frequency in a _____ system.
   a. simplex
   b. duplex
   c. trunking
   d. multiplex

7. All nongovernmental communications in the United States are controlled and regulated by the:
   a. Federal Bureau of Communications.
   b. Department of Health and Safety.
   c. Federal Communications Commission.
   d. Department of Transportation.

8. The process of immediately repeating each transmission received during radio communications is called the:
   a. patient report.
   b. echo procedure.
   c. auto feedback.
   d. repeater system.

See Answers to Review Questions at the back of this book.

▶ Further Reading

Clawson, Jeff J. "Emergency Medical Dispatch," in Roush, W. R., ed. *Principles of EMS Systems.* 2nd ed., pp. 263–289. Dallas: American College of Emergency Physicians, 1994.

Clawson, Jeff J., and Kate Dernocoeur. *Principles of Emergency Medical Dispatch.* Upper Saddle River, N.J.: Pearson/Prentice Hall, 1988.

Delbridge, Theodore R., and Paul Paris. "EMS Communications," in Roush, W. R., ed. *Principles of EMS Systems.* 2nd ed., pp. 245–261. Dallas: American College of Emergency Physicians, 1994.

Fitch J. "Benchmarking Your Comm Center." *Journal of Emergency Medical Services* (May 2006): 98–112.

Mackay, Michele. "Bandwidths, Frequencies, and Megahertz." *Journal of Emergency Medical Services* (*JEMS*) 22 (May 1997): 42–49.

Marshall, Loren. "Electronic Visions: The Future of EMS Communications Is Now." *Journal of Emergency Medical Services* (*JEMS*) 19 (March 1994): 54–63.

Stanford, Todd M. *EMS Report Writing: A Pocket Reference.* Upper Saddle River, N.J.: Pearson/Prentice Hall, 1992.

Steele, Susi B. *Emergency Dispatching: A Medical Communicator's Guide.* Upper Saddle River, N.J.: Pearson/Prentice Hall, 1993.

Stratton, Samuel J. "Triage by Emergency Medical Dispatchers." *Prehospital and Disaster Medicine* 7 (July–September 1992): 263–268.

▶ Media Resources

See the Student CD at the back of this book for quizzes, animations, video skills clips, and other features related to this chapter. Also, visit the Companion Website for Brady's paramedic series at **www.prenhall.com/bledsoe,** where you will find additional reinforcement and links to other resources.

Documentation

Objectives

After reading this chapter, you should be able to:

1. Identify the general principles regarding the importance of EMS documentation and ways in which documents are used. (pp. 288–290)
2. Identify and properly use medical terminology, medical abbreviations, and acronyms. (pp. 292–297)
3. Explain the role of documentation in agency reimbursement. (p. 289)
4. Identify and eliminate extraneous or nonprofessional information. (p. 302)
5. Describe the differences between subjective and objective elements of documentation. (pp. 302–305)
6. Evaluate a finished document for errors and omissions and proper use and spelling of abbreviations and acronyms. (pp. 299, 301–302)
7. Evaluate the confidential nature of an EMS report. (p. 311)
8. Describe the potential consequences of illegible, incomplete, or inaccurate documentation. (pp. 299, 301–302)
9. Describe the special documentation considerations concerning patient refusal of care and/or transport. (pp. 307–308)
10. Demonstrate how to properly record direct patient or bystander comments. (p. 298)
11. Describe the special considerations concerning multiple-casualty incident documentation. (pp. 309–311)
12. Demonstrate proper document revision and correction. (pp. 301–302)
13. Given a prehospital care report form and a narrative patient care scenario, record all pertinent administrative information using a consistent format; identify and record the pertinent, reportable clinical data for each patient; correct errors and omissions, using proper procedures; and note and record "pertinent negative" clinical findings. (pp. 288–312)

Key Terms

addendum, p. 301

against medical advice
(AMA), p. 307

bubble sheet, p. 290

field diagnosis, p. 304

jargon, p. 302

libel, p. 302

prehospital care report
(PCR), p. 288

response time, p. 289

slander, p. 302

triage tags, p. 310

Case Study

Tom Brewster is nervous. He has never been to a deposition before, and though everyone has assured him that he is not the target of any legal action, he has to wonder what the lawyers want from him.

As he sits outside the conference room, he goes over the call in his head. It was about 2:30 in the morning. He and Eric Billings, his partner, had just finished cleaning up from a GI bleeder when they were dispatched to the single-vehicle crash. The driver had gone off the left side of the road, crossed a ditch, and smashed into a tree. He had been lucky. He was out of the car, standing on the side of the road, and did not seem to have any serious injuries. He told Tom and Eric, "I think I'm fine, I just fell asleep and ran off the road." Still, they had performed an initial assessment followed by a rapid trauma assessment, immobilized the man, administered oxygen, and transported him to the emergency department. Tom rode in the back with the patient. On the way to the hospital he checked the glucose level, started an IV as a precaution, and applied a cardiac monitor.

"Everything was normal," Tom now thinks. "What did I miss?" He has reread his prehospital care report a hundred times. Though it has been 3 years, he now remembers almost every detail of the call. Until 2 weeks ago, he had almost completely forgotten about it.

All too soon, the lawyers call Tom into the conference room, introduce themselves, and swear him to honesty. One of the lawyers begins. "Do you recall the crash that occurred on the evening in question?"

"Yes, I do," Tom replies. He recounts that upon their arrival at the scene, the driver was out of the vehicle. Tom states that they managed him like any other trauma patient and he had no obvious injuries or indications of illness.

"Did the gentleman tell you he is diabetic?"

"No," Tom answers, "but we checked his blood sugar, and it was normal."

"Did he tell you he has heart problems?"

"No," Tom says again, "but we did put him on the heart monitor, and his rhythm was normal."

"Did he tell you he ran off the road because he passed out?"

"No, he told me he fell asleep." Tom feels better. He has the answer to every question, and he has the PCR to back him up.

After a few more questions, the lawyers dismiss Tom and allow him to leave. He has no idea what they were getting at, but he does know that he answered every question

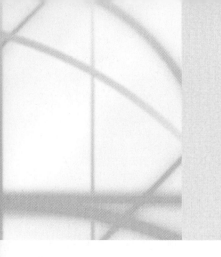

honestly. He wonders if he would have had all the answers if the case had been from 6 or 8 years ago. He has really worked on his documentation in the last few years, and he knows he would have never remembered all those details without the help of his PCR.

Six weeks later Tom gets a letter from the lawyer thanking him for his testimony. It turns out the patient was suing his private doctor for not "recognizing his obvious diabetes and heart problems. He claimed these illnesses caused him to be involved in the motor vehicle collision, and it resulted in serious injury." Tom's testimony—and his PCR—have been pivotal in getting the case dismissed.

INTRODUCTION

prehospital care report (PCR)
the written record of an EMS response.

Document exactly what you did, when you did it, and the effects of your interventions.

Your PCR reflects your professionalism.

In this age of litigation, treating your patient and documenting his care are separate but equally important duties. Your written **prehospital care report (PCR)** is the only truly factual record of events. When written correctly it accurately describes your assessment and care throughout the emergency call. It documents exactly what you did, when you did it, and the effects of your interventions. It can be your best friend or your worst enemy in a court proceeding.

Your PCR is your sole permanent, complete written record of events during the ambulance call. The dispatch center may have a record of the call times and audiotapes of radio transmissions, and your patient will have his memory of the call. You and other responders also may have some recollections about the call. Your PCR, however, will always be considered the most comprehensive and reliable record of the event. In addition, it reflects your professionalism. A well-written, thorough PCR suggests a thorough, efficient assessment and quality care. A sloppy, incomplete PCR suggests sloppy, inefficient care.

USES FOR DOCUMENTATION

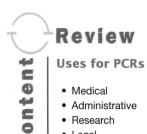

Review

Uses for PCRs

- Medical
- Administrative
- Research
- Legal

Your PCR will be a valuable resource for a variety of people. They include medical professionals, EMS administrators, researchers, and, occasionally, lawyers.

Medical

Hospital staff (nurses and physicians) may need more information from you than they can get before you have to take another call. For example, they may want a chronological account of your patient's mental status from the time you arrived on the scene. Your PCR can tell the emergency department staff of your patient's condition before he arrived at the hospital. It serves as a baseline for comparing assessment findings and detecting trends that indicate improvement or deterioration. The surgical staff will want to know the mechanism of injury and other pertinent findings during your initial assessment of your patient and the scene.

If your patient is admitted to the hospital, the floor or intensive care unit staff may need more information about his original condition than he can remember. In addition, your PCR provides them with information from people at the scene to whom they might not have access—family, bystanders, first responders, or other witnesses. Knowing about the circumstances that led to the event or the mechanism of injury may also help rehabilitation specialists to provide better therapy. Your PCR becomes

Prehospital Care Report

Agency Name	ARLINGTON RESCUE	MILEAGE		USE MILITARY TIMES

Agency Name ARLINGTON RESCUE

Dispatch Information CARDIAC

Call Location 124 CYPRUS ST 2nd FLOOR

MILEAGE
END 2 4 4 9 6
BEGIN 2 4 4 7 6
TOTAL 0 0 0 2 0

LOCATION CODE 0 1 2 4

CHECK ONE
☑ Residence ☐ Health Facility ☐ Farm ☐ Indus. Facility
☐ Other Work Loc. ☐ Roadway ☐ Recreational ☐ Other

USE MILITARY TIMES
CALL REC'D 0 7 0 5
ENROUTE 0 7 0 7
ARRIVED AT SCENE 0 7 1 9
FROM SCENE 0 7 3 8
AT DESTIN 0 7 5 4
IN SERVICE 0 8 1 0
IN QUARTERS 0 8 3 2

CALL TYPE AS REC'D
☑ Emergency
☐ Non-Emergency
☐ Stand-by

MECHANISM OF INJURY
☐ MVA (✓ seat belt used →) N/A
☐ Fall of _____ feet N/A
☐ Unarmed assault
☐ GSW
☐ Knife
☐ Machinery
☐ _____

▶ **Figure 6-1** The run data in a prehospital care report is vital to your agency's efforts to improve patient care.

an important document that helps ensure your patient's continuous effective care (Figure 6-1 ▶).

> Your PCR is an important document that helps ensure your patient's continuity of care.

Administrative

EMS administrators must gather information for quality improvement and system management. Information regarding **response times,** call location, the use of lights and siren, and date and time is vital to evaluating your system's readiness to respond to life-threatening emergencies. It also is essential to providing information about community needs. The quality improvement or quality assurance committee will use PCRs to identify problems with individual paramedics or with the EMS system. In some agencies, the billing department will need to determine which services are billable. Insurance carriers may need to know more about the illness or injury to process the claim. Some states will use your PCR data to allocate funding for regional systems.

> **response time**
> *time elapsed from when a unit is alerted until it arrives on the scene.*

Research

Your PCR may give researchers useful data about many aspects of the EMS call. For example, they may analyze your recorded data to determine the efficacy of certain medical devices or interventions such as drugs and invasive procedures. They also may use the data to cut costs, alter staffing, and shorten response times. Some systems use computerized or electronic PCRs and a computerized database to analyze the data (Figure 6-2 ▶). Regardless of the method you use, your written documentation provides the basis for continuously improving patient care in your EMS system.

> Your PCR provides the basis for continuously improving patient care in your EMS system.

Legal

Your PCR becomes a permanent part of your patient's medical record. Lawyers may refer to it when preparing court actions, and in a legal proceeding it might be your sole source of information about the case. You may be called on to testify in a case where your PCR becomes the central piece of evidence in your testimony. Or your PCR may serve as evidence in a criminal case and help determine the accused's innocence or guilt. Each state has its own laws regarding the length of time the hospital must keep its records.

Always write your PCR as if you knew you would have to refer to it someday in a court proceeding. Describe your patient's condition when you arrived and during your care, and note his status on arrival at the hospital. Always document his condition

Figure 6-2 The handheld electronic clipboard enables you to enter your prehospital care report directly into a computer. (© Jeff Forster)

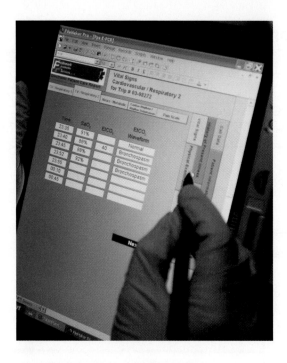

Assessment Pearls

Don't Write Patient Data on Your Gloves Many EMS providers write vital signs and other essential information on their medical exam gloves. There are several problems with this. First, unless the gloves are properly disposed of, you could be in store for a HIPAA violation. More important, if you're involved in direct contact with a patient, you should take off your gloves or change gloves before using such personal objects as a clipboard or a pen. Leaving the gloves on (or laying them on an ED countertop) to read the information you wrote can contaminate your personal materials.

Instead, use a whiteboard or piece of tape to record your information. If you use a whiteboard, use the pen only during patient care and clean it often. If you use a piece of tape or something similar, have a dedicated pen that you use only during the patient encounter (not the one you might stick in your mouth when contemplating where you'll eat later). Always remember to wipe the whiteboard or properly dispose of the tape after each call.

before and after any interventions, and avoid writing any subjective opinions such as "the patient is intoxicated, obnoxious, and looks like a crack addict." After your PCR is written, ask your partner to review it for completeness and accuracy. A complete, accurate, and objective account of the emergency call may be your best and only defense against a plaintiff's attorney who will try to find inconsistencies and ambiguities in your account.

A complete, accurate, and objective account of the emergency call may be your best and only defense in court.

GENERAL CONSIDERATIONS

Every EMS system has its own specific requirements for documentation. The type of call record used also varies from system to system. Some systems use reports with check boxes, some use **bubble sheets,** computer-scannable reports on which you record patient information by filling in boxes or "bubbles" (Figure 6-3). Still others may use

bubble sheet

scannable run sheet on which you fill in boxes or "bubbles" to record assessment and care information.

Do Not Staple or Fold

AGENCY CODE | **UNIT #** | **UNIT TYPE** | **DATE** | **PERSONNEL INFORMATION** | **RESPONSE/ TRANSPORT MODE** | **RESPONSE OUTCOME**

UNIT TYPE: AMBULANCE, RESCUE, OTHER

DATE: Jan, Feb, Mar, Apr, May, Jun, Jul, Aug, Sep, Oct, Nov, Dec — DAY — YR (91, 92, 93, 94, 95) RPT

PERSONNEL INFORMATION: ATTENDANT #1, ATTENDANT #2, ATTENDANT #3 (F, B, P, N, O) RPT

RESPONSE/TRANSPORT MODE:
To Scene: (2) Non-Emerg, (3) Emergency
From Scene: (2) Non-Emerg, (3) Emergency

RESPONSE OUTCOME:
Transported By This Unit
Care Transfer/Another Unit
Cancelled Enroute
Cancelled On Scene
False Call/No Patient Found
Dead on Scene
Refused Treatment
Treated, Refused Transport
P.O.V.
Standby
Unknown
Other

CALL RECEIVED | **ENROUTE** | **ARRIVE SCENE** | **DEPART SCENE** | **ARRIVE HOSPITAL** | **RETURN TO SERVICE** | **INCIDENT LOCATION** | **DISPATCH/INCIDENT TYPE**

(MILITARY TIME columns)

INCIDENT LOCATION:
Residence
Interstate
Highway
Street/Road
Public Access
Industrial/Off.
HMO/Clinic/Doctors Office
Hospital
Other

DISPATCH/INCIDENT TYPE:
Abdominal Pain — MVA
Asphyxiation/Choke — MVA - Motorcycle
Chest Pain — MVA - Ped/Bike
Diff. Breathing — Assault
Drowning — Assault - Sexual
Heat/Cold Problems — Bite/Sting
Ill Person — Burn/Elect.
OB/GYN — Fall
OD/Poison — Person Trapped
Person Down/Unconsc. — Stab/Gunshot
Psych/Behavioral — Other Trauma
Seizures — Standby
Other Medical — InterFacility Transfer

SUSPECTED MEDICAL ILLNESS | **INJURY SITE/TYPE** | **MECHANISM OF INJURY** | **GLASGOW COMA SCALE**

SUSPECTED MEDICAL ILLNESS: None
(P) (S) Abdom. Pain — Inhalation
(P) (S) Airway Obstr — OB/GYN
(P) (S) Allergic React — OD/Poison
(P) (S) Cancer Compli — Psych/Behv
(P) (S) Cardiac Arrest — Resp. Arrest
(P) (S) Cardiac Sympt. — Resp. Dist
(P) (S) Chest Pain — Seizures
(P) (S) Childbirth — Stroke
(P) (S) COPD — Syncope
(P) (S) Diabetes Comp. — Unconscious
(P) (S) Drug Reaction — Other
(P) (S) Heat/Cold Problems
P=Primary S=Secondary

INJURY SITE/TYPE: Amputate, Bite/Sting, Blunt-Major, Burn-Elec, Frac/Disloc, Penetrate, Soft-Closed, Soft-Open
None
Head, Face, Eye, Neck, Chest, Back, Upper Ext, Abdomen, Pelvis, Lower Ext

MECHANISM OF INJURY:
Flail Chest
Burns 10+%/face/arwy
Fall 20+ feet
Speed 40+ mph
20+ speed change
Deformity 20+"
Intrusion 12+"
Rollover
Ejection
Death same MV
Pedest. vs. MV 5+mph
Pedst. thrown/run over
Mtcycle 20+mph/sep.
Extrication >15 min.

GLASGOW COMA SCALE:
EYES: (4) Spontaneous, (3) To Voice, (2) To Pain, (1) Unresponsive
VERBAL: (5) Oriented, (4) Confused, (3) Inappropriate, (2) Garbled, (1) None
MOTOR: (6) Obeys Comm., (5) Pain-Local., (4) Pain-Withdraws, (3) Pain-Flexion, (2) Pain-Extends, (1) None

PRIOR AID: None, CPR, Extricate, Wound Mgt
Fire, Police, 1st Resp., Rescue, Bystander

THIS PATIENT LOCATION/PROTECTION:
Driver, Front Pass, Rear Pass, Other, Unknown
Shldr/Lap Belt, Shoulder Belt, Lap Belt, Safety Seat, Helmet
Not Used, Not Available, Unknown
Airbag (Deployed) Yes

SEX | **INITIAL VITAL SIGNS** | **BLS TREATMENT** | **CPR INFORMATION**

SEX: (F) (M)
AGE
Unable to Take, Not Taken, Pt. Refused
SYSTOLIC, DIASTOLIC, PULSE, RESP, PUPILS (L R)

This Patient Resident of:
Months, Apprx.
City, County, Arizona
Out of State, Unknown

BLS TREATMENT (A1 A2 A3 O):
Assessment, MAST Application
C-Spine Precautions, MAST Inflation
Oxygen, Monitor IV
CPR, Oral Care/Airway
Crisis Intervention, Oral Glucose
Defibrillation (AUTO), Restraints Applied
Extrication, Suction
Fracture Stabilize, Traction Splint
Hemorrhage Control, Wound Management
Ipecac/Charcoal Admin., Other

ALS TREATMENT (A1 A2 A3 O):
Cardiac Monitoring, Intubation - Nasal, NG Tube
Cardioversion, Intubation - Oral, Needle Thoracostomy
Cricothyroidotomy, IV-Central, Phlebotomy
Defibrillation, IV-Peripheral, SVN
EOA, Medication Admin,

CPR INFORMATION:
Time: Minutes (<4, 4-10, >10, Unk)
Arrest to CPR
Arrest to Defib
Arrest to ALS
Witnessed Arrest? (Y) (N) Unk
Pulse/Rhythm Restored? (Y) (N)
Traumatic Cardiac Arrest? (Y) (N)

ATTEMPTS:
IV, ET, OTH (1) (2) (3) (U)

MEDICATIONS | **EKG INITIAL/LAST** | **IV TYPE/RATE** | **# LINES** | **PT. RECEIVED BY** | **RESEARCH CODE** | **MISCELLANEOUS**

MEDICATIONS:
Albuterol — Lidocaine-Bolus
Aminoph. — Lidocaine Drip
Atropine 1/10 — Methylprednisone
Atropine 8/20 — Morphine
Bretylium — Naloxone
Calcium Chl. — Nifedipine
D50 — Nitrostat. Tab.
Diazepam — Nitrous Oxide
Diphenhydram. — Oxytocin
Dopamine — Phenobarbital
Epi 1:1000 — Sodium Bicarbonate
Epi 1:10,000 — Thiamine
Furosemide — Verapamil
Isoetharine — Other
Isoproterenol — HAZMAT

EKG INITIAL/LAST:
Nrml Sinus, Sinus Tach, Sinus Brady, Asystole, AV Block, Atrial Fib, Atrial Flut, EMD, Junctional, Paced, SV Tach, Vent Tach, Vent Fib, Other, PVC's, Unable

IV TYPE/RATE (TKO, Bolus, Wide, Other):
D5W, Normal Saline, Ringers Lact., Other

LINES: # Peripheral, # Central

MEDICAL CONTROL:
First / Hospital
Radio/Good
Radio/Poor
Protocol
Telephone
Radio/Phone Patch
Cellular
Phys On-Scene
None Required

ORDERS BY:
Protocol, Standing, Verbal

PATIENT DISPOSITION:
Improved, Worsened
Unchanged
Died in ER

MISCELLANEOUS:
If Multiple Pts On Scene, How Many?
If Transport to Level 1 Receiving Facility, Due to:
Pt. Condition
Mechanism

2002094

PLEASE DO NOT MARK IN THIS AREA

EMS FIRST CARE FORM - ARIZONA DEPARTMENT OF HEALTH SERVICES
Return to State EMS Office

SCANTRON® FORM NO. F-3087-EMS   0792-C 671-5 4 3 2 1
© 1992 EMS DATA SYSTEMS

Figure 6-3 This prehospital care report's format can be scanned into a computer.

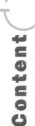

Review

Characteristics of a Well-Written PCR

- Appropriate medical terminology
- Correct abbreviations and acronyms
- Accurate, consistent times
- Thoroughly documented communications
- Pertinent negatives
- Relevant oral statements of witnesses, bystanders, and patient
- Complete identification of all additional resources and personnel

If you do not know how to spell a word, look it up or use another word.

computerized documentation. The particular type of operational data collected, such as time intervals, will also differ among systems. For example, proprietary EMS agencies may require more billing information than community-based volunteer agencies. The general characteristics of a well-written PCR, though, remain constant among all agencies and systems.

Medical Terminology

An essential component of good documentation is the appropriate use of medical terminology. Medical terms, though sometimes difficult to spell, transform your report into a universally accepted medical document. Learning the meanings and correct spellings of the medical terms that you will use in your PCRs is essential. Misused or misspelled words reflect poorly on your professionalism and may confuse the report's readers.

If you do not know how to spell a word, look it up or use another word. Many paramedics carry pocket-size medical dictionaries in their ambulances for this purpose. Using "plain English" is acceptable when you do not know the appropriate medical term or its correct spelling. *Chest* is just as accurate as *thorax* and better than "thoracks." *Belly* is not as professional as *abdomen*, but it is still better than "abodemin."

Abbreviations and Acronyms

Medical abbreviations and acronyms allow you to increase the amount of information you can write quickly on your report (Table 6–1). They also pose problems, however, because they can have multiple meanings. For instance, their meanings can vary in

Table 6–1	Standard Charting Abbreviations

Patient Information/Categories

Asian	A	Medications	Med
Black	B	Newborn	NB
Chief complaint	CC	Occupational history	OH
Complains of	c/o	Past history	PH
Current health status	CHS	Patient	Pt
Date of birth	DOB	Physical exam	PE
Differential diagnosis	DD	Private medical doctor	PMD
Estimated date of confinement	EDC	Review of systems	ROS
Family history	FH	Signs and symptoms	S/S
Female	♀	Social history	SH
Hispanic	H	Visual acuity	VA
History	Hx	Vital signs	VS
History and physical	H&P	Weight	Wt
History of present illness	HPI	White	W
Impression	IMP	Year-old	y/o
Male	♂		

Body Systems

Abdomen	Abd	Ear, nose, and throat	ENT
Cardiovascular	CV	Gastrointestinal	GI
Central nervous system	CNS	Genitourinary	GU

| Table 6-1 | Standard Charting Abbreviations *(Continued)* |

Gynecological	GYN	Obstetrical	OB
Head, eyes, ears, nose, and throat	HEENT	Peripheral nervous system	PNS
Musculoskeletal	M/S	Respiratory	Resp

Common Complaints

Abdominal pain	abd pn	Lower back pain	LBP
Chest pain	CP	Nausea/vomiting	n/v
Dyspnea on exertion	DOE	No apparent distress	NAD
Fever of unknown origin	FUO	Pain	pn
Gunshot wound	GSW	Shortness of breath	SOB
Headache	H/A	Substernal chest pain	sscp

Diagnoses

Abdominal aortic aneurysm	AAA	Inferior wall myocardial infarction	IWMI
Abortion	Ab	Insulin-dependent diabetes mellitus	IDDM
Acute myocardial infarction	AMI	Intracranial pressure	ICP
Adult respiratory distress syndrome	ARDS	Mass casualty incident	MCI
Alcohol	ETOH	Mitral valve prolapse	MVP
Atherosclerotic heart disease	ASHD	Motor vehicle crash	MVC
Chronic obstructive pulmonary disease	COPD	Multiple sclerosis	MS
Chronic renal failure	CRF	Non-insulin-dependent diabetes mellitus	NIDDM
Congestive heart failure	CHF	Organic brain syndrome	OBS
Coronary artery bypass graft	CABG	Otitis media	OM
Coronary artery disease	CAD	Overdose	OD
Cystic fibrosis	CF	Paroxysmal nocturnal dyspnea	PND
Dead on arrival	DOA	Pelvic inflammatory disease	PID
Delirium tremens	DTs	Peptic ulcer disease	PUD
Deep venous thrombosis	DVT	Pregnancies/births *(gravida/para)*	G/P
Diabetes mellitus	DM	Pregnancy-induced hypertension	PIH
Dilation and curettage	D&C	Pulmonary embolism	PE
Duodenal ulcer	DU	Rheumatic heart disease	RHD
End-stage renal failure	ESRF	Sexually transmitted disease	STD
Epstein-Barr virus	EBV	Transient ischemic attack	TIA
Foreign body obstruction	FBO	Tuberculosis	TB
Hepatitis B virus	HBV	Upper respiratory infection	URI
Hiatal hernia	HH	Urinary tract infection	UTI
Hypertension	HTN	Venereal disease	VD
Infectious disease	ID	Wolff-Parkinson-White syndrome (disease)	WPW

Medications

Angiotensin-converting enzyme	ACE	Lactated Ringer's, Ringer's lactate	LR, RL
Aspirin	ASA	Magnesium sulfate	$MgSO_4$
Bicarbonate	HCO_3^-	Morphine sulfate	MS
Birth control pills	BCP	Nitroglycerin	NTG
Calcium	Ca^{2+}	Nonsteroidal anti-inflammatory agent	NSAID

(Continued)

Table 6–1   Standard Charting Abbreviations *(Continued)*

Calcium channel blocker	CCB	Normal saline	NS
Calcium chloride	CaCl$_2$	Penicillin	PCN
Chloride	Cl$^-$	Phenobarbital	PB
Digoxin	Dig	Potassium	K$^+$
Dilantin (phenytoin sodium)	DPH	Sodium bicarbonate	NaHCO$_3$
Diphenhydramine	DPHM	Sodium chloride	NaCl
Diphtheria-pertussis-tetanus	DPT	Tylenol	APAP
Hydrochlorothiazide	HCTZ		

Anatomy/Landmarks

Abdomen	Abd	Lymph node	LN
Antecubital	AC	Medial collateral ligament	MCL
Anterior axillary line	AAL	Metacarpalphalangeal (joint)	MCP
Anterior cruciate ligament	ACL	Metatarsalphalangeal (joint)	MTP
Anterior-posterior	A/P	Midaxillary line	MAL
Distal interphalangeal (joint)	DIP	Posterior axillary line	PAL
Dorsalis pedis (pulse)	DP	Posterior cruciate ligament	PCL
Gallbladder	GB	Proximal interphalangeal (joint)	PIP
Intercostal space	ICS	Right lower lobe	RLL
Lateral collateral ligament	LCL	Right lower quadrant	RLQ
Left lower lobe	LLL	Right middle lobe	RML
Left lower quadrant	LLQ	Right upper lobe	RUL
Left upper lobe	LUL	Right upper quadrant	RUQ
Left upper quadrant	LUQ	Temporomandibular joint	TMJ
Left ventricle	LV	Tympanic membrane	TM
Liver, spleen, and kidneys	LSK		

Physical Exam/Findings

Arterial blood gas	ABG	Heel-to-shin (cerebellar test)	H → S
Bilateral breath sounds	BBS	Hemoglobin	Hgb
Blood sugar	BS	Inspiratory	Insp
Breath sounds	BS	Jugular venous distention	JVD
Cardiac injury profile	CIP	Laceration	Lac
Central venous pressure	CVP	Level of consciousness	LOC
Cerebrospinal fluid	CSF	Moves all extremities (well)	MAEW
Chest X-ray	CXR	Nontender	NT
Complete blood count	CBC	Normal range of motion	NROM
Computerized tomography	CT	Palpation	Palp
Conscious, alert, and oriented	CAO	Passive range of motion	PROM
Costovertebral angle	CVA	Point of maximal impulse	PMI
Deep tendon reflexes	DTR	Posterior tibial (pulse)	PT
Dorsalis pedis (pulse)	DP	Pulse	P
Electrocardiogram	EKG, ECG	Pupils equal and reactive to light	PEARL

Table 6-1 | Standard Charting Abbreviations *(Continued)*

Electroencephalogram	EEG	Pupils equal, round, reactive to light	PERRLA
Expiratory	Exp	and accommodation	
Extraocular movements (intact)	EOMI	Range of motion	ROM
Fetal heart tones	FHT	Respirations	R
Full range of motion	FROM	Tactile vocal fremitus	TVF
Full-term normal delivery	FTND	Temperature	T
Heart rate	HR	Unconscious	Unc
Heart sounds	HS	Urinary incontinence	UI

Miscellaneous Descriptors

After (post-)	$\bar{p}$	Not applicable	n/a
After eating	Pc	Number	No or #
Alert and oriented	A/O	Occasional	Occ
Anterior	ant.	Pack years	pk/yrs, p/y
Approximate	≈	Per	/
As needed	prn	Positive	+
Before (ante-)	$\bar{a}$	Posterior	post.
Before eating (*ante cibum*, before meal)	a.c.	Postoperative	PO
Body surface area (%)	BSA	Prior to arrival	PTA
Celsius	C	Radiates to	→
Change	Δ	Right	®
Decreased	↓	Rule out	R/O
Equal	=	Secondary to	2°
Fahrenheit	F	Superior	sup.
Immediately	stat	Times (for 3 hours)	× (×3h)
Increased	↑	Unequal	≠
Inferior	inf.	Warm and dry	W/D
Left	Ⓛ	While awake	WA
Less than	<	With (*cum*)	$\bar{c}$
Moderate	mod.	Within normal limits	WNL
More than	>	Without (*sine*)	$\bar{s}$
Negative	–	Zero	0
No, not, none	Ø		

Treatments/Dispositions

Advanced cardiac life support	ACLS	Nasogastric	NG
Advanced life support	ALS	Nasopharyngeal airway	NPA
Against medical advice	AMA	No transport—refusal	NTR
Automated external defibrillator	AED	Nonrebreather mask	NRM
Bag-valve mask	BVM	Nothing by mouth	NPO
Basic life support	BLS	Occupational therapy	OT
Cardiopulmonary resuscitation	CPR	Oropharyngeal airway	OPA
Carotid sinus massage	CSM	Oxygen	O_2
Continuous positive airway pressure	CPAP	Per square inch	psi

(Continued)

| Table 6-1 | Standard Charting Abbreviations (Continued) |

Do not resuscitate	DNR	Physical therapy	PT
Endotracheal tube	ETT	Positive end-expiratory pressure	PEEP
Estimated time of arrival	ETA	Short spine board	SSB
External cardiac pacing	ECP	Therapy	Rx
Intermittent positive-pressure ventilation	IPPV	Treatment	Tx
Long spine board	LSB	Turned over to	TOT
Nasal cannula	NC	Verbal order	VO

Medication Administration/Metrics

Centimeter	cm	Keep vein open	KVO
Cubic centimeter	cc	Kilogram	kg
Deciliter	dL	Liter	L
Drop(s)	gtt(s)	Liters per minute	lpm, L/min,
Drops per minute	gtts/min		liters/min
Every	Q	Microgram	mcg
Grain	gr	Milliequivalent	mEq
Gram	g, gm	Milligram	mg
Hour	h, hr, or °	Milliliter	mL
Hydrogen-ion concentration	pH	Millimeter	Mm
Intracardiac	IC	Millimeters of mercury	mmHg
Intramuscular	IM	Minute	min
Intraosseous	IO	Orally	PO
Intravenous	IV	Subcutaneous	SC, SQ
Intravenous push	IVP	Sublingual	SL
Joules	J	To keep open	TKO

Cardiology

Atrial fibrillation	AF	Paroxysmal supraventricular	PSVT
Atrial tachycardia	AT	tachycardia	
Atrioventricular	AV	Premature atrial contraction	PAC
Bundle branch block	BBB	Premature junctional contraction	PJC
Complete heart block	CHB	Premature ventricular contraction	PVC
Electromechanical dissociation	EMD	Pulseless electrical activity	PEA
Idioventricular rhythm	IVR	Supraventricular tachycardia	SVT
Junctional rhythm	JR	Ventricular fibrillation	VF
Modified chest lead	MCL	Ventricular tachycardia	VT
Normal sinus rhythm	NSR	Wandering atrial pacemaker	WAP
Paroxysmal atrial tachycardia	PAT		

You must be familiar with your local EMS system's acronyms and abbreviations.

different areas of medicine. Is *CP* chest pain, cardiovascular perfusion, or cerebral palsy? Is *CO* cardiac output or carbon monoxide? Is *BLS* basic life support or burns, lacerations, and swelling? These are all common abbreviations with more than one accepted meaning. Furthermore, many abbreviations are specific to one community. You must be familiar with those used in your local EMS system.

Abbreviations and acronyms can cause considerable confusion when someone unfamiliar with the call reads your report. Health care professionals who are not familiar with local customs or with emergency medicine might not understand them. One way to clarify the meaning of a new abbreviation or acronym is to write it out the first time you use it, followed by the abbreviation or acronym in parentheses. After that, you can use the abbreviation alone throughout the report. The following examples illustrate how abbreviations and acronyms can shorten your narratives. In standard English the report might be written:

> The patient is a 54-year-old conscious and alert male who complains of sudden onset of chest pain and shortness of breath that started 20 minutes ago. He has taken two nitroglycerin with no relief. He denies any nausea, vomiting, or dizziness. He has a past history of coronary artery disease, a heart attack 3 years ago, and high blood pressure. He takes nitroglycerin as needed, Procardia XL, hydrochlorothiazide, and potassium. He has no known drug allergies.

Using abbreviations and acronyms, the same report might be written:

> Pt. is 54 y/o CAO male c/o sudden onset CP/SOB × 20 min. Pt took NTG × 2 Ø relief. n/v, dizziness. PH: CAD, AMI × 3y, HTN. Meds: NTG prn, Procardia XL, HCTZ and K^+; NKDA.

Times

Incident times are another important but perilous part of the PCR. The times you record on your PCR are considered the official times of the incident. For medical and legal purposes, you must ensure their accuracy.

The PCR typically has spaces for the time the call was received, the dispatch time, the time of arrival at the scene, time of departure from the scene, time of arrival at the hospital, and time back in service (refer to Figure 6–1). Other time intervals are important as well. The time you and your crew arrived at the patient's side is often very different from the time the ambulance arrived at the scene—when your patient is on the fourth floor of a building without an elevator, for example, or in a field several hundred yards from the road. Whatever the reason, document in your report any significant discrepancies between your arrival at the scene and your arrival at the patient. The times of vital signs assessment, medication administration, certain medical procedures as local protocols require, and changes in patient condition are also important and require accurate documentation.

One common problem with documenting times is inconsistencies among the dispatch center clock, the ambulance clock, and your watch. Imagine a report that documents that the ambulance arrived on scene at 20:32 according to the dispatch time, that CPR was started at 20:29 according to your watch, and the first defibrillation was administered at 20:43 according to the defibrillator's internal clock. While we may recognize this phenomenon and tend to discount the accuracy of the recorded times, they are nonetheless the official, legal times. Whenever possible, therefore, record all times from the same clock. When that is not possible, be sure that all the clocks and watches you use are synchronized. If they cannot be synchronized and the documented times seem to conflict with each other, explain this in your narrative. A simple statement such as the following will suffice: "All time intervals on the scene were documented using my watch, all other times are those reported by the dispatch center."

Whenever possible, record all times from the same clock.

Communications

Your communications with the hospital are another important item to document. Though your system may make voice recordings of those communications, the recordings are usually not kept indefinitely. Again, the PCR will likely be the only permanent record of your discussion with the medical direction physician. Specifically, you should document any medical advice or orders you receive and the results of implementing that advice and those orders. In some situations you might need to document what you reported to the physician and/or discussed with him, so the reader will be able to understand the decision-making process. Finally, always document the physician's name on your PCR and, if possible, have him sign it to verify your treatments.

Pertinent Negatives

The patient assessment and medical interventions are the essence of the EMS event and become the core of your PCR. We will discuss specific approaches to documenting assessment and interventions later in this chapter, but some general rules apply regardless of the method.

Document all findings of your assessment, even those that are normal. Although the positive findings are usually of most interest, some negative findings—known as *pertinent negatives*—are also important. For example, if your respiratory distress patient does not have swollen ankles or crackles, that helps rule out a field diagnosis of congestive heart failure. Or if your patient with a broken leg does not have loss of sensory or motor function, it suggests he has no serious neurologic injury. You should include such information in your report.

The pertinent negatives vary for each chief complaint. In general, if a positive assessment finding for any given chief complaint would be important, a negative finding probably is pertinent. Even though these findings do not warrant medical care or intervention, your seeking them demonstrates the thoroughness of your examination and history of the event.

Oral Statements

Also essential to every PCR, regardless of approach, are the statements of witnesses, bystanders, and your patient. They help to document the mechanism of injury, your patient's behavior, the events leading up to the emergency, and any first aid or medical care others rendered before you arrived. They also may include information regarding the disposition of personal items such as wallets or purses. At crime scenes, document safety-related information such as weapons disposition. Your PCR may be the only written report of what happened to a murder weapon. Other details such as where you first saw a victim, what position he was in, and the time you arrived on the scene may someday be crucial evidence in a criminal proceeding.

Whenever possible, quote the patient—or other source of information—directly. Clearly identify the quotation with quotation marks, and identify its source. For example:

> Bystanders state the patient was "acting bizarre and threatening to jump in front of the next passing car."

Additional Resources

Document all of the resources involved in the event. If an air-medical service transported your patient, your documentation should include your assessment and all interventions up to the point when you transferred care. Identify the air-medical service and your patient's ultimate destination, if you know it. If other EMS, fire, rescue/extrication, or law enforcement agencies were involved in the call, document their roles. This can be particularly important in mutual aid calls, when many different agencies cooperate in your patient's care. Also include information about personnel from law enforcement and the coroner's or medical examiner's office for dead-on-arrival (DOA) scenes.

If a physician stops to help, identify him by name and document his qualifying credentials. If one of your medical direction physicians is on the scene and directs care, document his activities. Likewise document the names, credentials, and activities of any other medically qualified personnel present who offer to help. Your clinical experience and local protocols will determine how you integrate qualified health care workers into your emergency scene. Document that integration carefully.

ELEMENTS OF GOOD DOCUMENTATION

A well-written PCR is accurate, legible, timely, unaltered, and professional. Each of these traits is essential.

Completeness and Accuracy

The accurate PCR should be precise but comprehensive. Include all of the relevant information that anyone might be expected to want later, and exclude superfluous information. For example, if your patient's foot was run over by a lawn mower, reporting that his great toe on that foot had been amputated 6 years ago would be important; documenting that he had his tonsils removed when he was 3 years old probably would not. That you applied direct pressure to the bleeding foot is pertinent; that the lawn mower was a John Deere model 6354 is not.

Many PCRs provide check boxes and a space for written narratives (Figure 6-4 ▶). You should complete both the narrative and check-box sections of every PCR. All check-box sections of a document must show that you attended to them, even if you did not use a given section on a call. The check boxes can help to ensure that routine, common information is recorded for every call, but no PCR has a check box for every possible chief complaint, assessment finding, or intervention.

The narrative is the core of the documentation. Even if you document something in a check box, repeating that information in the narrative might be worthwhile. By doing so, you can expand on the yes-or-no limitations of the check box to explain the timing, the assessment findings, the circumstances, or the changes in patient condition associated with the indicated action. Always make sure that the information in your checked boxes and in your narrative are consistent. Inconsistencies will be extremely difficult to explain later on, especially in front of a jury.

Remember that proper spelling, approved abbreviations, and proper acronyms also affect your PCR's accuracy. Misspelled words lose their meaning; many abbreviations are not universally recognized; and several acronyms have more than one meaning. Make sure that the meaning of any abbreviation or acronym is clear.

Legibility

Poor penmanship and illegible reports lead to poor documentation. Some EMS providers say, "I wrote it, and I can read it. That's all that matters." This is simply not true. The PCR does not exist solely for its author's reference. It is a permanent record that many different people use. Your handwriting must be neat enough that other people can read and understand the report, especially the narrative. It must also be neat enough that you can read and understand it yourself many years from now, long after the event has faded

Review

Elements of Good Documentation

- Complete
- Accurate
- Legible
- Timely
- Without alterations
- Professional

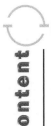

Your handwriting must be neat enough that other people can read and understand the report.

Prehospital Care Report

FOR BLS FR USE ONLY

Recycled Paper

M D Y		AGENCY CODE	VEH. ID.
DATE OF CALL	RUN NO.		

Name	Agency Name	MILEAGE		USE MILITARY TIMES
Address	Dispatch Information	END	CALL REC'D	
	Call Location	BEGIN	ENROUTE	
		TOTAL	ARRIVED AT SCENE	
Ph #	CHECK ONE ☐ Residence ☐ Health Facility ☐ Farm ☐ Indus. Facility ☐ Other Work Loc. ☐ Roadway ☐ Recreational ☐ Other	LOCATION CODE	FROM SCENE	

AGE	DOB M D Y	SEX M F	CALL TYPE AS REC'D. ☐ Emergency ☐ Non-Emergency ☐ Stand-by	COMPLETE FOR TRANSFERS ONLY	AT DESTIN
Physician				Transferred from ☐ No Previous PCR ☐ Unknown if Previous PCR	IN SERVICE

CARE IN PROGRESS ON ARRIVAL:
☐ None ☐ Citizen ☐ PD/FD/Other First Responder ☐ Other EMS

Previous PCR Number ☐-☐☐☐☐☐

IN QUARTERS

MECHANISM OF INJURY
☐ MVA (✓ seat belt used →) ☐ Fall of ___ feet ☐ GSW ☐ Machinery
☐ Struck by vehicle ☐ Unarmed assault ☐ Knife ☐ ___

☐ Extrication required ___ minutes

Seat belt used? ☐ Yes ☐ No ☐ Unknown

Seat Belt Use Reported By ☐ Crew ☐ Patient ☐ Police ☐ Other

CHIEF COMPLAINT   SUBJECTIVE ASSESSMENT

PRESENTING PROBLEM
If more than one checked, circle primary

☐ Allergic Reaction ☐ Unconscious/Unresp. ☐ Shock ☐ Major Trauma ☐ OB/GYN
☐ Syncope ☐ Seizure ☐ Head Injury ☐ Trauma-Blunt ☐ Burns
☐ Airway Obstruction ☐ Stroke/CVA ☐ Behavioral Disorder ☐ Spinal Injury ☐ Trauma-Penetrating Environmental
☐ Respiratory Arrest ☐ General Illness/Malaise ☐ Substance Abuse (Potential) ☐ Fracture/Dislocation ☐ Soft Tissue Injury ☐ Heat
☐ Respiratory Distress ☐ Gastro-Intestinal Distress ☐ Poisoning (Accidental) ☐ Amputation ☐ Bleeding/Hemorrhage ☐ Cold
☐ Cardiac Related (Potential) ☐ Diabetic Related (Potential) ☐ Hazardous Materials
☐ Cardiac Arrest ☐ Pain ☐ Other ___ ☐ Obvious Death

PAST MEDICAL HISTORY

☐ None
☐ Allergy to ___
☐ Hypertension ☐ Stroke
☐ Seizures ☐ Diabetes
☐ COPD ☐ Cardiac
☐ Other (List) ☐ Asthma

Current Medications (List)

VITAL SIGNS	TIME	RESP	PULSE	B.P.	LEVEL OF CONSCIOUSNESS	GCS	R PUPILS L	SKIN	STATUS
		Rate: ☐ Regular ☐ Shallow ☐ Labored	Rate: ☐ Regular ☐ Irregular		☐ Alert ☐ Voice ☐ Pain ☐ Unresp.		☐ Normal ☐ Dilated ☐ Constricted ☐ Sluggish ☐ No-Reaction	☐ Unremarkable ☐ Cool ☐ Pale ☐ Warm ☐ Cyanotic ☐ Moist ☐ Flushed ☐ Dry ☐ Jaundiced	C U P S
		Rate: ☐ Regular ☐ Shallow ☐ Labored	Rate: ☐ Regular ☐ Irregular		☐ Alert ☐ Voice ☐ Pain ☐ Unresp.		☐ Normal ☐ Dilated ☐ Constricted ☐ Sluggish ☐ No-Reaction	☐ Unremarkable ☐ Cool ☐ Pale ☐ Warm ☐ Cyanotic ☐ Moist ☐ Flushed ☐ Dry ☐ Jaundiced	C U P S
		Rate: ☐ Regular ☐ Shallow ☐ Labored	Rate: ☐ Regular ☐ Irregular		☐ Alert ☐ Voice ☐ Pain ☐ Unresp.		☐ Normal ☐ Dilated ☐ Constricted ☐ Sluggish ☐ No-Reaction	☐ Unremarkable ☐ Cool ☐ Pale ☐ Warm ☐ Cyanotic ☐ Moist ☐ Flushed ☐ Dry ☐ Jaundiced	C U P S

OBJECTIVE PHYSICAL ASSESSMENT

COMMENTS

TREATMENT GIVEN

☐ Moved to ambulance on stretcher/backboard
☐ Moved to ambulance on stair chair
☐ Walked to ambulance
☐ Airway Cleared
☐ Oral/Nasal Airway
☐ Esophageal Obturator Airway/Esophageal Gastric Tube Airway (EOA/EGTA)
☐ EndoTracheal Tube (E/T)
☐ Oxygen Administered @ ___ L.P.M., Method ___
☐ Suction Used
☐ Artificial Ventilation Method ___
☐ C.P.R. in progress on arrival by: ☐ Citizen ☐ PD/FD/Other First Responder ☐ Other
☐ C.P.R. Started @ Time ▶ ___ Time from Arrest Until C.P.R. ▶ ___ Minutes
☐ EKG Monitored (Attach Tracing) [Rhythm(s) ___]
☐ Defibrillation/Cardioversion No. Times ___ ☐ Manual ☐ Semi-automatic

☐ Medication Administered (Use Continuation Form)
☐ IV Established Fluid ___ Cath. Gauge ___
☐ Mast Inflated @ Time ___
☐ Bleeding/Hemorrhage Controlled (Method Used: ___)
☐ Spinal Immobilization Neck and Back
☐ Limb Immobilized by ___ ☐ Fixation ☐ Traction
☐ (Heat) or (Cold) Applied
☐ Vomiting Induced @ Time ___ Method ___
☐ Restraints Applied, Type ___
☐ Baby Delivered @ Time ___ In County ___
   ☐ Alive ☐ Stillborn ☐ Male ☐ Female
☐ Transported in Trendelenburg position
☐ Transported in left lateral recumbent position
☐ Transported with head elevated
☐ Other ___

DISPOSITION (See list)   DISP. CODE   CONTINUATION FORM USED YES

CREW	IN CHARGE	DRIVER'S NAME	NAME	NAME
	☐ EMT ☐ AEMT #	☐ CFR ☐ EMT ☐ AEMT #	☐ CFR ☐ EMT ☐ AEMT #	☐ CFR ☐ EMT ☐ AEMT #

© COPYRIGHT 1986 NEW YORK STATE DEPARTMENT OF HEALTH

EMS 100 (11/86) provided by NYS-EMS PROGRAM
DOH 3822 (6/94)

AGENCY COPY/WHITE

> **Figure 6-4** Complete both the narrative and check-box sections of every PCR.

from your memory. Your writing must be heavy enough to transfer to any carbon copies. Using a ballpoint pen whenever possible makes carbon copies more legible and makes it difficult for someone to tamper with the document. Clearly mark the check boxes to eliminate any doubt that a check mark is not just a meaningless scratch. Always remember that other members of the health care team may use the report for medical information, research, or quality improvement.

Timeliness

As a rule, you should avoid writing your report in the ambulance during transport of your patient for two reasons. First, the bumpy ride makes it difficult to write neatly. More importantly, your time is better spent communicating with your patient and conducting ongoing assessments. Most hospitals have an area where you can sit and complete your paperwork once patient care has been transferred.

Ideally, you should complete your report immediately after you complete the emergency call, when the information is fresh in your mind and you can check with your partner or patient if you have any questions about the events. At times you may be too busy to complete the entire documentation immediately following a call. If so, make notes on scratch paper and write enough of the report that you will be able to finish it completely and accurately later. The sooner you finish it, the more details you are likely to recall and the better the report will be.

> Ideally, you should complete your report immediately after you complete the emergency call.

Absence of Alterations

Mistakes happen. During a busy shift or in the middle of the night you will check the wrong box, misspell a word, or omit important information. You will be thinking of one medication and write another's name on your report. If you make a mistake writing your report, simply cross through the error with one line and initial it (Figure 6-5 ▶). Some systems may expect you to date the correction as well. Do not scribble over or blacken out any area of the call report. Never try to hide an error. Such foolish tactics only raise the reader's curiosity about what you wrote originally. After crossing out the error, continue with the correct information. If you find the error after you've already written several more sentences, submit an **addendum.**

> Never try to hide an error.

addendum
addition or supplement to the original report.

Whenever possible, have everyone involved in the call read or reread the PCR before you submit it. Make all corrections before you submit the report to the hospital or to the EMS administrative offices. Do not make changes on the original report after you have submitted it. If for any reason you need to make corrections after you have submitted the report, or some portion of it, place an addendum. Simply note on the original report, "See addendum," and attach the addendum to the original report. Write the addendum on a separate sheet of paper or on an official form if one exists. Likewise, if more information comes to your attention after you have submitted the report, write a supplemental narrative on a separate report form.

Write any addendum to your report as soon as you realize that you made an error or that additional information is needed. Note the purpose of the revision and why the information did not appear on your original report. The addendum should document

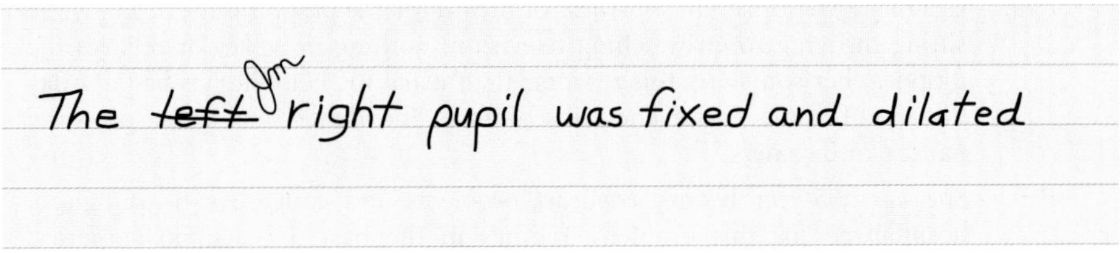

> **Figure 6-5** The proper way to correct a prehospital care report is to draw a single line through the error, write the correct information beside it, and initial the change.

the date and time that it was written, the reason it was written, and the pertinent information. Only the original author of a report should attach an addendum, as it is part of the official call record. Agencies should have separate forms for other EMS personnel, supervisors, or citizens who, for some reason, want to contribute to the documentation.

Professionalism

Write your report in a professional manner. Remember that someday it may be scrutinized by hospital staff, quality improvement committees, supervisors, lawyers, and the news media. Your patient's family may request, and is entitled to, a copy of your report from your agency. Write cautiously and avoid any remarks that might be construed as derogatory. **Jargon** can be confusing and does little to enhance your image. Do not describe a patient well known to EMS providers as a "frequent flyer." Never include slang, biased statements, or irrelevant opinions. Include only objective information. "The patient smelled of beer and had slurred speech and difficulty walking" are factual statements. "The patient was very drunk" is an inference; even if accurate, it is still just your opinion. **Libel** and **slander** are, respectively, writing or speaking false and malicious words intended to damage a person's character. Always write and speak carefully. A seemingly innocent phrase or comment can come back to haunt you.

NARRATIVE WRITING

The narrative is the part of the written report in which you depict the call at length. Less structured than the check-box or fill-in sections of your report, the narrative allows you the freedom to describe your assessment findings in detail. When other people read your report, they usually will rely on your written narrative for the most relevant information. For example, as you transfer care to the emergency nurse, she will usually scan your PCR for information concerning your patient's history, vital signs, and physical exam.

Narrative Sections

Any patient documentation includes three sections of importance: the subjective narrative, the objective narrative, and the assessment/management plan.

Subjective Narrative

The subjective part of your narrative typically comprises any information that you elicit during your patient's history. This includes the chief complaint (CC), the history of present illness (HPI), the past history (PH), the current health status (CHS), and the review of systems (ROS). In trauma, this also includes the mechanism of injury, as told to you by your patient or bystanders. The following is a typical subjective narrative on a patient complaining of shortness of breath:

CC: The patient is a 74-year-old conscious black female who complains, "I can't catch my breath."

HPI: Gradual onset of severe shortness of breath for the past 3 hours; began while sitting in living room watching television; nothing provokes or relieves the dyspnea; her son states this is worse than usual for her. She has had a 3-day history of some vague chest discomfort. She denies any chest pressure, nausea, or dizziness.

PH: She has a 5-year history of heart problems and congestive heart failure; hospitalized for this problem 3 times in the past 5 years; no surgeries.

Write cautiously and avoid any remarks that might be construed as derogatory.

jargon
language used by a particular group or profession.

libel
writing false and malicious words intended to damage a person's character.

slander
speaking false and malicious words intended to damage a person's character.

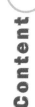**Review**

Approaches to the Physical Exam

- Head-to-toe approach
- Body systems approach

Content

CHS: Meds: Isosorbide, nitroglycerin, furosemide, digoxin, potassium; no known drug allergies; 50 pack/year smoker; nondrinker; non-drug abuser.

ROS: Resp: Unproductive cough for 1 day; audible wheezing; no hx of COPD or asthma; last chest X-ray 1 year ago. Card: no palpitations, pressure, or pain; + orthopnea; + paroxysmal nocturnal dyspnea; + edema for past few days; past ECG 1 year ago. GU: No changes in urinary patterns. Per. Vasc: + pitting edema for few days; cold feet.

Objective Narrative

The objective part of your narrative usually includes your general impression and any data that you derive through inspection, palpation, auscultation, percussion, and diagnostic testing. This includes vital signs, physical exam, and tests such as cardiac monitoring, pulse oximetry, and blood glucose determination.

To document your physical exam, you can use either of two approaches: head-to-toe or body systems. Although the medical community accepts both extensively, emergency medical services more often use the head-to-toe approach.

Head-to-Toe Approach   The head-to-toe approach is well suited for any call when you perform an entire physical exam, because you document your findings in the same order in which you conducted the exam—from head to toe. However, even though you may have conducted your pediatric assessment from toe to head, you should document it in head-to-toe order. This style encourages you to be systematic and thorough. It is appropriate for major trauma and serious medical emergencies, when you examine every body area and system. Include all circulatory and neurologic findings within the body area you are documenting. For example, when recording findings in the extremities, include distal neurovascular function. When documenting the head, include the results of cranial nerve testing. The following illustrates the head-to-toe approach for a patient who has been in a collision:

General: The patient presents in the front seat of the car, in moderate distress with bruises to his forehead and some facial lacerations. Pt. is alert and oriented to self, time, and place.

Vital signs: Pulse—100 strong, regular radial; BP—110/88; resp—24 nonlabored; skin pale and cool.

HEENT: Depression to right frontal bone, minor bleeding controlled prior to arrival; no drainage from ears, nose. No periorbital ecchymosis or Battle's sign; pupils equal and reactive to light; extraocular movements intact, cranial nerves II–XII intact.

Neck: Trachea midline; no jugular vein distention; + cervical spine tenderness.

Chest: Equal expansion; bruises across the chest wall; no deformities; equal bilateral breath sounds.

Abdomen: Soft, nontender, nondistended.

Pelvis: Unstable pelvic ring; pain upon palpation.

Extremities: + Circulation, sensory, and motor function in all four extremities; no deformities noted.

Posterior: No obvious injuries noted.

Diagnostics: Sinus tachycardia, no ectopy, pulse oximetry 97% on supplemental oxygen.

Body Systems Approach   The body systems approach focuses on body systems instead of body areas. It is best suited to screening and preadmission exams in which you conduct a comprehensive exam involving all body systems. Each body system has different key components that you should assess and document.

When you use the body systems approach in emergency medicine, you usually will focus only on the system, or systems, involved in the current illness or injury. For example, a patient having an asthma attack would require an in-depth evaluation of the respiratory system. Another patient with lower abdominal pain would need a close examination of the gastrointestinal system. Neither patient would require a full head-to-toe physical exam but, instead, intensive documentation of the affected body system or systems. The body systems approach can be one of the most comprehensive approaches to documentation. The following illustrates a body systems approach for a patient with chest pain and shortness of breath:

General:	Patient is a healthy-looking female who presents sitting upright in her chair, able to speak in phrases only.
Vital Signs:	Pulse—irregular, 90; BP—170/80; resp—28 labored; skin—warm and diaphoretic.
HEENT:	+ Lip cyanosis and pursing; some nasal flaring; pink, frothy sputum; jugular veins distended.
Respiratory:	Labored respiratory effort; accessory neck muscle use; trachea midline; + intercostal, supraclavicular, suprasternal retractions; = chest expansion; diffuse crackles and wheezing in all lung fields, decreased breath sounds.
Per. Vasc.:	+ Ascites fluid wave; + 2 pitting edema in lower extremities; strong peripheral pulses.
Labs:	Sinus tachycardia with occasional unifocal premature ventricular contractions. Pulse oximetry—92% room air; 97% on supplemental oxygen.

Assessment/Management Plan

In the assessment/management section, you document what you believe to be your patient's problem. This is also known as your **field diagnosis,** or impression. For example, your field diagnosis for a patient with chest pain may be "possible angina or rule out myocardial infarction." You do not have to make an exact diagnosis. When you are not sure, simply document what you suspect is the general problem. Sometimes, for instance, your field impression might be "rule out acute abdomen, or seizures." *Rule out* identifies possible diagnoses that you believe the emergency physician should evaluate.

Record your complete management plan from start to finish. This includes how you packaged and moved your patient to the ambulance. Did you carry him on a stair-chair or on a backboard fully immobilized or did he walk? List any interventions you completed before contacting your medical direction physician. For example, did you control bleeding with direct pressure? Did you start an IV? Then describe any orders from the medical direction physician, and always include his name. Describe how you transported your patient and the effects of any interventions such as drug administration or other invasive procedures. Include the results of ongoing assessments and any changes in your patient's condition. Finally, describe your patient's condition when you transferred care to the emergency staff. The following example is a management plan for a trauma patient with a pelvic fracture whose condition deteriorates en route to the hospital:

On-Scene

Extrication:	Rapid extrication from vehicle, placed supine on backboard.
Airway:	Airway cleared with suctioning, nasopharyngeal airway inserted.
Breathing:	Oxygen @ 15 liters/min via nonrebreather mask.
Circulation:	Bleeding from arm laceration controlled with dry sterile dressing and direct pressure; IV—16 ga. left antecubital area—normal saline run KVO per Dr. Johnson.

field diagnosis

what you believe to be your patient's problem, based on your history and physical exam.

Record your complete management plan from start to finish.

Transport

Transported by ground ambulance to University Hospital with full body immobilization supine on long spine board; ETA 10 minutes.

Ongoing: Patient becomes restless and anxious; VS: pulse—120 weak carotid only, BP—50 palpated, resp—28, skin: cool, pale, clammy with some mottling; PASG inflated; initial IV run wide open; second IV 16 ga. right antecubital normal saline—run wide open.

Arrival

Patient transferred to ED staff; restless; VS: pulse 120, BP—80 palpated, resp—26, skin—mottled and cool.

General Formats

The mnemonics SOAP and CHART identify two common patterns for organizing a narrative report. These acronyms provide templates for most medical and trauma reports. They help you to arrange your history, physical exam, and management plan into a logical, readable structure. They are widely used because they group information in categories that differentiate between subjective and objective information. For example, someone wanting only to determine your patient's medications can find that list easily in either the SOAP or CHART format. Either pattern is acceptable and effective when used consistently.

Review

Narrative Formats

- SOAP
- CHART
- Patient management
- Call incident

SOAP Format

SOAP stands for *S*ubjective, *O*bjective, *A*ssessment, and *P*lan. The detailed SOAP format includes:

Subjective:
- Chief complaint
- History of present illness
- Past history
- Current health status
- Family history
- Psychosocial history
- Review of systems

Objective:
- Vital signs
- General impression
- Physical exam
- Diagnostic tests

Assessment:
- Field diagnosis

Plan:
- Standing orders
- Physician orders
- Effects of interventions
- Mode of transportation
- Ongoing assessment

Review

SOAP

- Subjective
- Objective
- Assessment
- Plan

CHART Format

CHART stands for *C*hief complaint, *H*istory, *A*ssessment, *R*x (treatment), and *T*ransport. The detailed CHART format includes:

Chief Complaint

History:
- History of present illness
- Past history

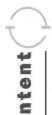

Review

CHART

- Chief complaint
- History
- Assessment
- Rx (treatment)
- Transport

- Current health status
- Review of systems

Assessment:
- Vital signs
- General impression
- Physical exam
- Diagnostic tests
- Field diagnosis

Rx:
- Standing orders
- Physician orders

Transport:
- Effects of interventions
- Mode of transportation
- Ongoing assessment

Other Formats

No single narrative format is ideal for all situations.

Like patient assessment itself, documentation is not "one-size-fits-all." No one narrative format is ideal for all situations. Two additional formats—patient management and call incident—are appropriate in certain circumstances.

Use the patient management format for critical patients when you focus on immediately managing a variety of patient problems.

Patient Management The patient management format is preferred for some critical patients, such as those in cardiac arrest, when you focus on immediately managing a variety of patient problems and not on conducting a thorough history and physical exam. This format is a chronological account from the time you arrived on the scene until you transferred care to someone else. It emphasizes your assessment and management of the conditions you found. Simply begin your chart with a description of the event and any other pertinent information and then document your management, starting with your airway, breathing, and circulation (ABC) assessment. Record everything in real time and in absolute chronological order, and always include the results of your interventions. A patient management chart would look like this:

Patient is an 89-year-old Hispanic male who was found by his wife unconscious on the floor immediately after collapsing. He presents pulseless and apneic.

Time	Intervention
1320	Airway cleared with suctioning; quick look—ventricular fibrillation.
1321	Defibrillation @ 360 joules—no change.
1322	CPR begun; oropharyngeal airway inserted, ventilation with BVM @ 12/min with supplemental oxygen.
1324	IV 18-gauge left antecubital area—normal saline KVO; epinephrine 1:10,000 1 mg IVP.
1325	Defibrillation @ 360 joules—no change.
1327	Defibrillation @ 360 joules—patient converts to normal sinus rhythm rate of 72 with strong peripheral pulses, BP—110/76, no spontaneous respirations. ET tube inserted. + lung sounds bilaterally with BVM.
1328	Ventilation continued @ 12/min via BVM; lidocaine infusion 2 mg/min.
1332	Patient transferred to ambulance on stretcher—transported to University Hospital.
1335	Patient has spontaneous respirations @ 20/min, + bilateral breath sounds; becoming more awake; HR—72, BP—120/76.
1340	Arrived at UH—Patient is conscious, alert, and oriented with retrograde amnesia.

Call Incident The call incident approach simply emphasizes the mechanism of injury, the surrounding circumstances, and how the incident occurred. Use this approach to begin documenting a trauma call with a significant mechanism of injury. It is most suitable when the events surrounding the call might be significant. It would be inappropriate for a man sitting in his living room with chest pain or for someone who simply cut his finger with a carving knife. You may use this style in both the subjective and objective sections of your PCR. The following example shows call incident documentation for a motor vehicle crash:

Use the call incident approach to begin documenting a trauma call with a significant mechanism of injury.

Subjective: The patient is a 46-year-old conscious and alert white male who was an unrestrained driver in a low-speed, head-on, two-car motor vehicle crash, moderate front-end damage, no passenger compartment intrusion, deformity to windshield, dashboard, and steering wheel. Patient states he "reached for cigarette on floor and when he looked up, there was another vehicle in front of him." He denies any loss of consciousness and can recall all details prior to and immediately following the crash. Patient complains of pain to the head, neck, chest, and hip from being thrown against the dashboard and windshield.

Objective: The patient presents in the front seat of the car, appears in moderate distress with bruises to his forehead, facial lacerations, and a deformed left leg. His left leg is pinned underneath the dashboard with his left foot hooked around the brake pedal. Upon arrival, fire department rescue personnel were holding manual stabilization of his head and neck and stabilizing the vehicle.

These are not the only systems of documentation. Indeed, you may use some combination of these systems or develop a unique format for your regional system. The important thing is for your documentation to be complete, accurate, and consistent. By using the same system to document every call, you will be less likely to accidentally overlook or omit something.

SPECIAL CONSIDERATIONS

Some circumstances create special problems for EMS documentation. Patient refusals, calls where transport is unnecessary, multiple patients, and mass casualties are among the more common examples. In these and other unusual circumstances, take extra care to document everything that happened during the call.

Patient Refusals

Two types of patients might refuse care. The first type is the person who is not seriously ill or injured and simply does not want to go to the hospital. For example, the belted driver of a minor automobile crash has an abrasion on his knee from striking the dashboard. He is alert and oriented, has no other injuries, and claims he will seek medical attention if it bothers him later. This type of patient usually signs your PCR in a special place marked "Refusal of Care," and you return to service.

The second type of patient is more worrisome. This patient refuses care even though you feel he needs it. This is known as **against medical advice (AMA).** Some legal experts regard AMA as your failure to convince your patient to accept necessary treatment and transport. Such patient refusals are particularly troublesome because they have the most potential to end badly. Still, patients retain the right to refuse treatment or transportation if they are competent to make that decision and are not actively suicidal. Although you cannot make a legal determination of competence (sometimes it takes a court decision),

against medical advice (AMA)
your patient refuses care even though you feel he needs it.

Table 6-2	Refusal of Care Documentation Checklist

- Thorough patient assessment
- Competency of the patient
- Your recommendation for care and transport
- Explanation to the patient about possible consequences of refusing care, including possibility of death, if appropriate
- Other suggestions for accessing care
- Willingness to return if the patient changes his mind
- Patient's understanding of statements and suggestions and apparent competence to refuse care based on that understanding

Patients retain the right to refuse treatment or transportation if they are competent to make that decision.

document that you believe your patient was competent to refuse care. Though specific laws vary from state to state, your patient will demonstrate competence by his understanding of the circumstances and the risks associated with refusing care and by accepting those risks and the responsibility for refusing care. Assess your patient as thoroughly as possible, with special emphasis on his mental status and behavior. Pay extra attention to any patient suspected of being under the influence of drugs or alcohol. Clearly document that your patient has an adequate mental status and understands your field diagnosis, alternative treatments, and the consequences of refusing care. Also record his reason for refusing care (Table 6–2).

Even after you document your patient's competence, most patient refusals require more thorough documentation than the typical EMS run because the opportunity for and consequences of abandonment charges are tremendous. Simply having your patient sign your PCR is not sufficient. Again, document that you described your patient's injuries to him and that he understood the risks of refusing treatment and transport. Inform him of potential complications from injuries that might not be obvious. Discuss those associated risks also, and document this discussion. Also document any involvement of your patient's family or friends. Because ruling out serious injury is all but impossible in the field, you may need to make clear the possibility of your patient's dying. Although this might seem extreme, it plainly conveys that the risks are serious. A patient who was informed that he was at risk of dying, refused care, and subsequently had his leg amputated because of an infection would have a hard time convincing a jury that he did not think the risks were serious.

In many systems, you must contact the medical direction physician before allowing a patient to refuse transport. If you confer with a physician, document any information, advice, or orders that the physician gives you. If your patient speaks directly to the physician, document that as well. Once more, document that your patient understands the circumstances and the risks and still chooses to refuse transport. Note that you instructed him to call an ambulance or go to the emergency department if his condition worsens, or if he just changes his mind. You can ask a bystander or law enforcement officer to witness the patient refusal, although this is not always required.

Your documentation also should include a complete narrative with quotations and statements from others on the scene. For example, if your patient's wife and son plead with him to go to the hospital, include their comments in your report. If your system uses a specific form for patient refusals, complete that paperwork as well (Figure 6-6 ▶). The additional form, however, is not a substitute for a complete documentation of the circumstances.

RELEASE FROM RESPONSIBILITY

DATE _____ 19 _____ TIME _____ a.m.
                                              p.m.

This is to certify that _____

is refusing   ☐ TREATMENT   ☐ TRANSPORTATION

against the advice of the attending Emergency Medical Technician and of the Phoenix Fire Department, and when applicable, the base hospital and the base hospital physician.

I acknowledge that I have been informed of the following:

1. The nature and potential of the illness or injuries.
2. The potential risks of delaying treatment and transportation, up to and including death.
3. The availability of ambulance transportation to a hospital for treatment.

Nevertheless, I assume all risks and consequences of my decision, including further physical deterioration, loss of limb, paralysis, and even death, and hereby release the attending Emergency Medical Technician and the Phoenix Fire Department, and when applicable, the base hospital and the base hospital physician from any ill effects which may result from my refusal.

Witness _____   Signed: **X** _____

Witness _____   Relationship to Patient _____

Refusal must be signed by the patient; or by the nearest relative or legal guardian in the case of a minor, or when patient is physically or mentally incompetent.

☐ Patient refuses to sign release despite efforts of attending Emergency Medical Technician to obtain such signature after informing patient of concerns listed in numbers 1, 2, and 3 above.

GUIDELINES — Patient Refusal Documentation

In addition to those items normally documented (chief complaint, history of present illness, mechanism of injury, physical assessment, etc.) the following items should be recorded, regardless of patient's cooperation:

- Mental Status (orientation, speech, etc.)

- Suspected presence of alcohol or drugs

- Patient's exact words (as much as possible) in the refusal of care OR the signing of the release form

- Circumstances or reasons (including exact words of patient, if possible) for INCOMPLETE ADVISEMENT (risk of injury, abusiveness, unruliness, risk of injury other than from patient, etc.)

- Advice given to patients' guardian(s)

Figure 6-6   One example of a refusal of care form.

Services Not Needed

Some systems allow you to determine that your patient does not need ambulance transport. Although such policies help to reduce ambulance utilization rates, the risks of denying transport are even greater than those of patient refusals. In these cases, the documentation must clearly demonstrate that transport was unnecessary. As with patient refusals, document any discussion you have with the emergency physician and any advice you give to your patient.

Transportation may not be needed for other reasons as well. Ambulances are often called to minor collisions where no injuries have occurred. When this happens, first responders such as the fire department rescue unit or a police agency might cancel the ambulance. If the ambulance is canceled en route, document the canceling authority and the time of notification. If you arrive on the scene and find no patients, document that. If, when you arrive, you are canceled by on-scene personnel, document that you made no patient contact and record the person and agency who canceled you. The difference is considerable between "no patients found" and "only minor injuries, patients refusing transport." Although they might refuse transport, evaluate people with even the most minor injuries. Consider them patients and document them accurately.

The risks of denying transport are even greater than those of patient refusals.

Multiple-Casualty Incidents

Multiple patients, mass casualties, and disasters all present special documentation problems. The number of patients needing care and transport during such situations may overwhelm you. Often, more than one ambulance crew cares for the many patients. Some EMS personnel may fill only support roles and never actually provide patient care. Obtaining complete patient information might be impossible, and completing documentation for one patient before going on to care for others might be impractical.

In these situations, you must weigh your patients' needs against the demand for complete documentation. Document as much as possible—as quickly as possible—on your PCR. You can complete the documentation later as an addendum. If you cannot remember the particulars of a specific patient or transport, do not guess. Document only what you know to be factual and accurate. A simple note at the end of the documentation explaining the circumstances will account for any missing information.

Some EMS agencies use special forms for multiple-patient events, and most provide a general incident report form or record that anyone connected with the call may complete. You should become familiar with local policies and procedures for documenting these situations. Many systems use **triage tags** to record vital information on each patient quickly (Figure 6-7 ▶). A triage tag has just enough room for your

triage tags

tags containing vital information, affixed to your patient during a multiple-patient incident.

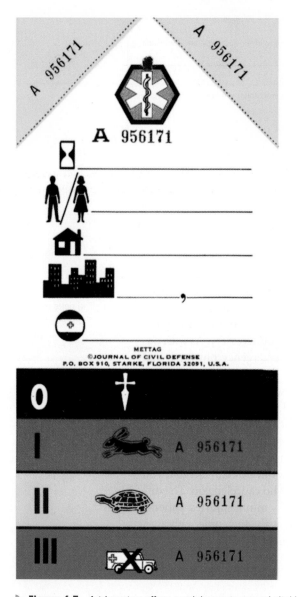
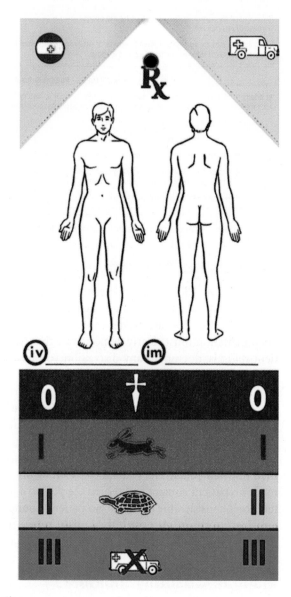

▶ **Figure 6-7** A triage tag offers a quick way to record vital information.

patient's vital information—name, major injuries, vital signs, treatment, and priority (urgent, nonurgent). You affix it to your patient, and it remains there throughout the event; you can transfer its information to your PCR later. Whatever your local policies, document as completely and accurately as possible without detracting from patient care.

CONSEQUENCES OF INAPPROPRIATE DOCUMENTATION

Inappropriate documentation can have both medical and legal consequences. The medical consequences of inadequate documentation are potentially the most serious. Health care providers across several disciplines may refer to your PCR in planning their care for a patient. Do not guess about your patient's medical problems if you are not certain. An inaccurate or incomplete report can affect patient care for many hours, even days, after the ambulance call ends. Failing to document a medication allergy or documenting an incorrect medical history could have grave effects. If no one can read your sloppy report, it is useless despite the importance of its information. Good documentation now enables good care later.

The potential legal consequences of inadequate documentation are enormous. If poor documentation results in inappropriate care, you may be held responsible. Or if the documentation does not make it clear that you informed a patient of the risks when he refused transport, you may be legally accountable for any harmful consequences. If the documentation does not explicitly say the patient in ventricular fibrillation was defibrillated immediately, you might be accused of providing inadequate care. Even though you did everything appropriately, poor, incomplete, or inaccurate documentation will encourage anyone who is pursuing a frivolous lawsuit. Good documentation discourages such actions. Always remember that if it is not documented, you did not do it.

Inaccurate, incomplete, illegible documentation also reflects poorly on the EMS provider writing the report. Missing information, misspelled words, and poor penmanship give the impression of a sloppy, incompetent provider. Good documentation, on the other hand, enhances the EMS provider's professional stature.

CLOSING

As a paramedic you will assume responsibility for your documentation. Although documentation is often a begrudged task, it is one of the most important parts of an EMS call. Ensuring that your documentation is complete, accurate, legible, and appropriate is one of your professional responsibilities. As a professional, you should recognize this responsibility and set a positive example for others as you fulfill it.

Your report's confidentiality cannot be overemphasized. Confidentiality is your patient's legal right. Do not discuss your report with anyone not medically connected directly with the case. Generally, you are allowed to share patient information with another health care provider who will continue care, with third-party billing companies, with the police if it is relevant to a criminal investigation, and with the court if it issues a subpoena. Your report also may be used for quality assurance or research. In these cases, block out the patient's name.

The PCR: Your Best Friend or Your Worst Enemy   It is often difficult to sit and write a prehospital care report (PCR) after a long and difficult call. However, the importance of this record cannot be overemphasized. Years later, when the call is nothing but a distant memory, the PCR will be there to provide the facts and details of the patient encounter. Thus, for accuracy and clarity, the PCR must be completed as soon as possible after the call when all of the facts are known. Waiting even a few hours may result in a PCR that is less than complete or inaccurate.

The PCR is a valuable document. Not only does it provide medical personnel with the details of care provided in the prehospital setting, but it can also protect prehospital providers from negligence claims and malpractice allegations. In a court of law, it has been said, what is not documented in the patient record was not performed. Although this may not always be the case, it is difficult to prove that a certain prehospital procedure was performed if it was not documented in the PCR.

Although still relatively uncommon, malpractice suits against EMS personnel are on the rise. Most claims of negligence include such things as failure to secure and maintain an airway, failure to follow accepted protocols, failure to transport when care was necessary, and failure to properly restrain a combative or dangerous patient. You should be aware of the various aspects of EMS practice that can result in allegations of negligence and document these accurately. For example, proper placement of an endotracheal tube should be verified by at least three methods and documented in the PCR. In addition, you should document that the tube remained in proper position by repeated patient evaluations and through use of monitoring systems such as capnography and pulse oximetry. Also you must document care to show that you followed appropriate protocols and standing orders. If you deviated from these, you must document in detail why this occurred and whether medical direction was contacted.

Patient refusal is a difficult area for EMS. Competent patients have the right to refuse medical care, even when the failure to obtain medical care may result in harm. However, paramedics cannot adequately determine which patients are competent and which are not (competency is a finding of law). Thus, when faced with a nontransport situation, document the circumstances well and obtain a statement from a third-party witness to the refusal.

Patient restraint poses a significant risk for both the patient and rescuers. Always follow local protocols regarding patient restraint and document that these were followed. Try to involve law enforcement personnel in any situation where restraint may be needed.

In the event you are sued for negligence, the PCR can be either your best friend or your worst enemy. If you prepared it well and documented details of the call, then you have little to worry about. If you prepared it sloppily or incompletely, then be prepared to answer a lot of difficult questions. Always take the time to prepare an accurate patient report—you will not regret it when it is needed.

Computer charting will certainly become common in the future. Several systems now on the market allow you to enter data electronically, transmit that information to the receiving facility, and immediately receive a printed report. When you use such systems, remember that the principles of effective documentation still apply.

▶ Summary

Regardless of the system you use for documentation, all EMS records should possess the same basic attributes. Appropriate terminology, proper spelling, accepted abbreviations and acronyms, and accurate times are essential. A description of the patient assessment and interventions, including pertinent negatives and communications with on-line physicians, is equally important. Finally, all of the personnel and resources involved in a call must be documented. The record must be accurate and precise, free of jargon, and neatly written. Corrections should be made properly, including the use of an addendum when appropriate.

Prehospital care providers may use many systems of documentation, including the CHART and SOAP formats. Whatever system you use, it is best if you use the same one consistently. This results in more reliable, complete documentation and reduces the chances of omitting important information. Any of the existing documentation systems can incorporate a head-to-toe assessment of the patient. Special situations such as multiple patients and refusals of transportation require extra attention. They are often the most difficult calls to document, yet they are also the calls for which good documentation can be most valuable. A complete narrative—in addition to any check boxes or filled-in "bubble" sheets—is the best way to ensure that all the necessary information is documented.

Although EMS providers frequently dislike documentation, it is one of the most important parts of the EMS call. Ensuring that the documentation is complete, accurate, legible, and appropriate is one of an EMS provider's professional responsibilities. Your PCR is the only permanent record of the ambulance call and the only permanent reflection of your professionalism.

▶ You Make the Call

While helping the quality assurance officer in your agency, you come across the following narrative: "We were dispatched to a 10-48, coroner Main/Spice. Vehicle is upside down. PMD on scene reports no serious injuries. Patient is nasty and abusive. Looks like a drug abuser. Is walking around acting abnoctious. Minor injuries identified and treated per protocol. Police arrested patient. EMS transport not needed."

1. What is wrong with this narrative? (You should be able to identify at least ten faults.)
2. What will you do to make sure your documentation is better than this?

See Suggested Responses at the back of this book.

▶ Review Questions

1. Your prehospital care report will be a valuable resource for:
   a. medical professionals.
   b. EMS administrators.
   c. researchers.
   d. all of the above.

2. You should always attempt to complete your PCR:
   a. at the scene.
   b. en route to the hospital.
   c. immediately after the call.
   d. at the end of your duty shift.

3. The proper way to correct an error in your prehospital care report is to:
   a. completely and immediately blacken out the error.
   b. draw a single line through the error, correct, and initial.
   c. highlight the error and place quotation marks around it.
   d. erase the error completely and enter the correct information.

4. The call incident approach to documentation emphasizes:
   a. the mechanisms of injury.
   b. the surrounding circumstances.
   c. how the incident occurred.
   d. all of the above.

5. If your patient refuses transport and care, simply having him sign your PCR is not sufficient.
   a. true
   b. false

6. Of the following abbreviations, which one means "drops"?
   a. Gtts
   b. Dps
   c. Drps
   d. Gms

7. The medical abbreviation that means "hypertension" is _____.
   a. HBV
   b. H/A
   c. HPI
   d. HTN

8. The medical abbreviation that means your patient has difficulty breathing during exertion is _____.
   a. CHF
   b. MOI
   c. DOE
   d. DOA

See Answers to Review Questions at the back of this book.

▶ Further Reading

Bevelacqua, Armando S. *Prehospital Documentation: A Systematic Approach.* Upper Saddle River, N.J.: Pearson/Prentice Hall, 1992.

Brown-Nixon, Candace. "Field Documentation Myths." *Emergency Medical Services* 19 (August 1990): 18–21, 68.

Strange, Julie. "Does Your Documentation Reflect Your Care?" *Emergency Medical Services* 19 (August 1990): 23–29.

▶ Media Resources

See the Student CD at the back of this book for quizzes, animations, video skills clips, and other features related to this chapter. In particular, take a look at the video "Explaining Medical Terminology." Also, visit the Companion Website for Brady's paramedic series at **www.prenhall.com/bledsoe**, where you will find additional reinforcement and links to other resources.

Precautions on Bloodborne Pathogens and Infectious Diseases

Prehospital emergency personnel, like all health care workers, are at risk for exposure to bloodborne pathogens and infectious diseases. In emergency situations it is often difficult to take or enforce proper infection control measures. However, as a paramedic, you must recognize your high-risk status. Study the following information on infection control carefully.

Infection control is designed to protect emergency personnel, their families, and their patients from unnecessary exposure to communicable diseases. Laws, regulations, and standards regarding infection control include:

- *Centers for Disease Control and Prevention (CDC) Guidelines.* The CDC has published extensive guidelines on infection control. Proper equipment and techniques that should be used by emergency response personnel to prevent or minimize risk of exposure are defined.

- *The Ryan White Act.* The Ryan White Act of 1990 allows emergency personnel to find out if they were exposed to an infectious disease while rendering patient care. Employers are required to name a "designated officer" to coordinate communications with the treating hospital.

- *Americans with Disabilities Act.* This act prohibits discrimination against individuals with disabilities, including those with contagious diseases. It guarantees equal employment opportunities and job protection if the infected individual can perform essential job functions and does not pose a threat to the safety and health of patients and coworkers.

- *Occupational Safety and Health Administration (OSHA) Regulations.* OSHA has enacted a regulation entitled Occupational Exposure to Bloodborne Pathogens that classifies emergency response personnel as being at the greatest risk of occupational exposure to communicable diseases. This regulation requires employers to provide hepatitis B (HBV) vaccinations free of charge, maintain a written exposure control plan, and provide personal protective equipment. These requirements primarily apply to private employers. Applicability to local and state governmental employees varies by locality. Many states have developed their own OSHA plans.

- *National Fire Protection Association (NFPA) Guidelines.* This is a national organization that has established specific guidelines and requirements regarding infection control for emergency response agencies, particularly fire departments and EMS services.

STANDARD PRECAUTIONS AND PERSONAL PROTECTIVE EQUIPMENT

Emergency response personnel should practice Standard Precautions by which ALL body substances are considered to be potentially infectious. To practice Standard Precautions, all emergency personnel should utilize personal protective equipment (PPE). Appropriate PPE should be available on every emergency vehicle. The minimum recommended PPE includes the following:

- *Gloves.* Disposable gloves should be donned by all emergency response personnel BEFORE initiating any emergency care. When an emergency incident involves more than one patient, you should attempt to change gloves between patients. When gloves have been contaminated, they should be removed as soon as possible. To properly remove contaminated gloves, grasp one glove approximately 1 inch from the wrist. Without touching the inside of the glove, pull the glove halfway off and stop. With that half-gloved hand, pull the glove on the opposite hand completely off. Place the removed glove in the palm of the other glove, with the inside of the removed glove exposed. Pull the second glove completely off with the ungloved hand, only touching the inside of the glove. Always wash hands after gloves are removed, even when the gloves appear intact.

- *Masks and Protective Eyewear.* Masks and protective equipment should be present on all emergency vehicles and used in accordance with the level of exposure encountered. Masks and protective eyewear should be worn together whenever blood spatter is likely to occur, such as during arterial bleeding, childbirth, endotracheal intubation, invasive procedures, oral suctioning, and cleanup of equipment that requires heavy scrubbing or brushing. Both you and the patient should wear masks whenever the potential for airborne transmission of disease exists.

- *HEPA and N-95 Respirators.* Due to the resurgence of tuberculosis (TB), prehospital personnel should protect themselves from TB infection through use of an N-95 or a high-efficiency particulate air (HEPA) respirator, as approved by the National Institute of Occupational Safety and Health (NIOSH). It should fit snugly and be capable of filtering out the tuberculosis bacillus. An N-95 or HEPA respirator should be worn when caring for patients with confirmed or suspected TB. This is especially true when performing "high-hazard" procedures such as administration of nebulized medications, endotracheal intubation, or suctioning on such a patient.

- *Gowns.* Gowns protect clothing from blood splashes. If large splashes of blood are expected, such as with childbirth, wear impervious gowns.

- *Resuscitation Equipment.* Disposable resuscitation equipment should be the primary means of artificial ventilation in emergency care. Such items should be used once, then disposed of.

Remember, the proper use of personal protective equipment ensures effective infection control and minimizes risk. Use ALL protective equipment recommended for any particular situation to ensure maximum protection.

Consider ALL body substances potentially infectious and ALWAYS practice Standard Precautions.

Suggested Responses to "You Make the Call"

The following are suggested responses to the "You Make the Call" scenarios presented in each chapter of Volume 2, Patient Assessment. Each represents an accepted response to the scenario and should not be interpreted as the only correct response.

Chapter 1—The History

1. *List some nonverbal communication techniques that will facilitate open discussion of your patient's problems.*
   Eye contact; body language; a calm, controlled voice; touch; active listening.
2. *Outline the components of the interview that you would use for this patient in the following categories:*
   a. *History of present illness*—Use the mnemonic OPQRST–ASPN to gather information concerning Mr. Harmon's current problem. What were you doing when the chest pain started? Did it begin suddenly or gradually? Does anything make the pain better or worse? Can you describe the pain in your own words? How bad is it? Can you rate it on a scale of one to ten? How long have you had the pain? Do you have any shortness of breath, nausea, or dizziness?
   b. *Past history*—Do you have a history of heart problems? Are you being treated for any other medical problems? Have you ever been hospitalized? Have you had any surgeries?
   c. *Current health status*—Are you taking any medications (including over-the-counter medications)? Do you have any allergies to medications? Do you smoke? If so, how many packs per day and for how many years? How much alcohol do you drink in a week? Do you take any recreational drugs such as marijuana, cocaine, or amphetamines? Have you had your cholesterol or triglyceride levels checked? Any other screening tests?
   d. Review of systems
   Cardiac—Have you ever had heart trouble, high blood pressure, rheumatic fever, heart murmurs, chest pain or discomfort, palpitations, shortness of breath, shortness of breath while lying flat, or peripheral edema? Have you ever been awakened from sleep with shortness of breath? Have you ever had an ECG or other heart tests?
   e. *Respiratory*—Have you ever had any of the following: wheezing, coughing up blood, asthma, bronchitis, emphysema, pneumonia, TB, or pleurisy? When was your last chest X-ray? Are you coughing now? If so, can you describe the sputum?
   f. *Gastrointestinal*—Have you ever had any of the following: trouble swallowing, heartburn, loss of appetite, nausea/vomiting, regurgitation, vomiting blood, indigestion? Have you had abdominal pain, food intolerance, excessive belching or passing of gas? Have you had any black, tarry stools or chronic diarrhea?

Chapter 2—Physical Exam Techniques

1. *How would you begin the exam?*
   As with any other patient in any other situation, begin with an initial assessment. Make sure your patient has a patent airway, is breathing effectively, has circulatory

integrity, and is alert and oriented. Identify and correct any abnormalities in his airway, breathing, and circulation (ABCs). Only then should you continue with a history and physical exam.

2. What is your differential field diagnosis?

A differential field diagnosis is a list of possible reasons for your patient's complaint. In this case, you would suspect a distal bone fracture, a ligament sprain, a joint dislocation, or a muscle or tendon strain.

3. What elements of the history are appropriate to ask this patient?

Has your patient ever experienced muscle or joint pain, stiffness, arthritis? If so, ask her to describe the location or symptoms. Has she ever sprained her ankle before? Previous sprains weaken ligaments surrounding the ankle joint and are prone to further sprains.

4. Outline your physical exam.

First remove both shoes and inspect the foot and ankle for obvious deformities, redness, and swelling. Compare your findings to the uninjured ankle. Then feel around the entire joint and pinpoint any areas of tenderness and swelling. Now test for range of motion. If your patient is in significant pain, or these movements cause further pain, do not perform them in the field. Ask your patient to bring her foot upward (dorsiflexion). Normal dorsiflexion is 20°. Then have her point it downward (plantar flexion). Normal plantar flexion is 45°. Now provide some resistance and ask her to repeat both movements. Note any difficulties or pain. While stabilizing the ankle with one hand, grasp the heel with the other hand and invert the foot, then evert it. Normal inversion is 30°, normal eversion 20°. Now ask her to perform the same movements against resistance. These four procedures test the stability of the ankle joint. A sprained ankle will cause your patient pain when the injured ligament is stretched or torn. Because the lateral ligaments are smaller and weaker than the medial ligaments, lateral sprains are more common, causing severe pain upon inversion and plantar flexion.

Chapter 3—Patient Assessment in the Field

1. Outline each phase of your patient assessment for this patient.

Scene size-up: Survey the scene for hazards and ensure it is safe to enter. Form a general impression from the first look at your patient. Note his posture, facial expressions, skin color, and degree of distress.

Initial assessment: Assess his airway, breathing, and circulation; provide immediate oxygen therapy as you ascertain the history.

Focused history and physical exam: Ascertain chief complaint, history of present illness, past history, and current health status. Assess for lip cyanosis and pursing, accessory muscle use, and retractions. Note the respiratory rate and quality. Observe the inspiratory and expiratory phases. Inspect, palpate, auscultate, and percuss the chest. Obtain baseline vital signs.

Ongoing exam: Re-evaluate airway, breathing, and circulation. Reassess the chief complaint and the effects of interventions. Reassess vital signs every 5 minutes. Alter priority determinations and management plans as necessary.

Chapter 4—Clinical Decision Making

1. Would you give him the aspirin?

No, never. This patient obviously has a neurologic problem, not a simple headache. His clinical condition requires a full history and physical exam with emphasis on the neurologic exam.

2. Describe the knowledge base necessary to manage this situation.

You would need to know the anatomy and physiology of the brain, the pathophysiology and classic signs and symptoms of neurologic diseases. You would also need to recall the principles of emergency management of acute neurologic disease.

3. *How would you proceed from this point?*

At this point, convince the man to be evaluated and transported to the hospital. Conduct a full history and physical exam and treat him accordingly.

Chapter 5—Communications

"This is Palermo Rescue, paramedic Randy Griffin. We have a 69-year-old, 115-kg male with chest pain and difficulty breathing that began approximately 1:00 P.M. He describes the pain as pressure-like, and it radiates to the left arm and jaw. He suffered immediate dyspnea and orthopnea. He has a history of heart disease, including two prior MIs and a bypass 3 years ago. He currently takes Lanoxin, Lasix, Capoten, and aspirin. He is allergic to Mellaril.

On physical exam, we find him to be morbidly obese and in moderate distress. He is diaphoretic and pale. He has bilateral basilar crackles and prominent JVD. His distal pulses are strong and he has +2 pitting edema. Vital signs are as follows: BP, 210/110; pulse, 70; respirations, 20; pulse ox, 93 percent on supplemental O_2. ECG shows sinus rhythm with no ectopy. We are administering oxygen via nonrebreather mask, we have started an IV of normal saline running KVO, we have administered 2 baby aspirin, 3 nitro, and 4 mg of morphine without relief of the pain."

Chapter 6—Documentation

1. *What is wrong with this narrative?*

What is a "10–48"? Is this the same in every EMS system?

Was the ambulance dispatched to the corner of Main and Spice?

Was the ambulance dispatched to the coroner, at Main and Spice?

Was the ambulance dispatched to the main coroner, whose name is Spice?

What is "PMD"?

"Patient is nasty and abusive" is judgmental.

"Looks like a drug abuser" is judgmental.

"Abnoctious" should be spelled "obnoxious."

"Obnoxious" is judgmental.

What exactly are the injuries?

Exactly what treatment, if any, was rendered?

Was EMS transport not needed because the patient was not hurt, or because the police transported him?

Did the patient go to the hospital or to jail?

2. *What will you do to make sure your documentation is better than this?*

Avoid using codes.

Practice spelling and use only words you can spell correctly.

Do not use abbreviations that are unclear; spell out terms the first time you use them, followed by the abbreviation in parentheses.

Do not be judgmental.

Describe the head-to-toe assessment completely.

Be particularly careful and complete in no-transport situations.

Answers to Review Questions

Below are answers to the Review Questions presented in each chapter of Volume 2, *Patient Assessment.*

Chapter 1
1. d
2. d
3. d
4. d
5. a
6. c
7. d
8. c
9. c
10. c

Chapter 2
1. c
2. b
3. c
4. c
5. d
6. a
7. d
8. b
9. d
10. c
11. a
12. b
13. d
14. a

15. c
16. b
17. d
18. c
19. b
20. d

Chapter 3
1. c
2. d
3. d
4. d
5. b
6. a
7. b
8. c
9. a
10. a
11. d
12. c
13. b
14. d
15. a

Chapter 4
1. b
2. a

3. c
4. d
5. c
6. b
7. b
8. c

Chapter 5
1. c
2. b
3. b
4. d
5. a
6. d
7. c
8. b

Chapter 6
1. d
2. c
3. b
4. d
5. a
6. a
7. d
8. c

Glossary

10-code radio communications system using codes that begin with the word *ten*.

active listening the process of responding to your patient's statements with words or gestures that demonstrate your understanding.

acuity the severity or acuteness of your patient's condition.

addendum addition or supplement to the original report.

advanced life support (ALS) life-support activities that go beyond basic procedures to include adjunctive equipment and invasive procedures.

against medical advice (AMA) your patient refuses care even though you feel he needs it.

algorithm schematic flowchart that outlines appropriate care for specific signs and symptoms.

ascites bulges in the flanks and across the abdomen, indicating edema caused by congestive heart failure.

auscultation listening with a stethoscope for sounds produced by the body.

automatic collision notification (ACN) system data collection and transmission system that can automatically contact a national call center or local public safety answering point and transmit specific crash data.

autonomic nervous system part of the nervous system that controls involuntary actions.

Babinski's response big toe dorsiflexes and the other toes fan out when sole is stimulated.

Battle's sign black and blue discoloration over the mastoid process.

blood pressure force of blood against arteries' walls as the heart contracts and relaxes.

borborygmi loud, prolonged, gurgling bowel sounds indicating hyperperistalsis.

bradycardia pulse rate lower than 60.

bradypnea slow breathing.

bronchophony abnormal clarity of patient's transmitted voice sounds.

Broselow tape a measuring tape for infants that provides important information regarding airway equipment and medication doses based on your patient's length.

bruit sound of turbulent blood flow around a partial obstruction.

bubble sheet scannable run sheet on which you fill in boxes or "bubbles" to record assessment and care information.

capnography real-time measurement of exhaled carbon dioxide concentrations.

cardiac monitor machine that displays and records the electrical activity of the heart.

cardiac output the amount of blood the heart ejects each minute, measured in milliliters.

cellular telephone system telephone system divided into regions, or cells, that are served by radio base stations.

chief complaint the pain, discomfort, or dysfunction that caused your patient to request help.

circulation assessment evaluating the pulse and skin and controlling hemorrhage.

clinical judgment the use of knowledge and experience to diagnose patients and plan their treatment.

closed-ended questions questions that elicit a one- or two-word answer.

communication the process of exchanging information between individuals.

convergent focusing on only the most important aspect of a critical situation.

crackles light crackling, popping, nonmusical sounds heard usually during inspiration, also called rales.

crepitus crunching sounds of unlubricated parts in joints rubbing against each other.

critical thinking thought process used to analyze and evaluate.

Cullen's sign discoloration around the umbilicus (occasionally the flanks) suggestive of intra-abdominal hemorrhage.

decerebrate arms and legs extended.

decorticate arms flexed, legs extended.

delirium an acute alteration in mental functioning that is often reversible.

dementia a deterioration of mental status that is usually associated with structural neurologic disease.

depression a mood disorder characterized by hopelessness and malaise.

detailed physical exam careful, thorough process of eliciting the history and conducting a physical exam.

diastole phase of cardiac cycle when ventricles relax.

diastolic blood pressure force of blood against arteries when ventricles relax.

differential field diagnosis   the list of possible causes for your patient's symptoms.

digital communications   data or sounds translated into a digital code for transmission.

diuretic   a medication that stimulates the kidneys to excrete excess water.

divergent   taking into account all aspects of a complex situation.

duplex   communications system that allows simultaneous two-way communications by using two frequencies for each channel.

dysmenorrhea   difficult or painful menstruation.

dyspnea   the sensation of having difficulty breathing.

echo procedure   immediately repeating each transmission received during radio communications.

egophony   abnormal change in tone of patient's transmitted voice sounds.

emergency medical dispatcher (EMD)   the person who manages an EMS system's response and readiness.

end-tidal carbon dioxide (ETCO$_2$) detector   a device used in capnography to measure exhaled carbon dioxide concentrations.

facsimile machine (fax)   device for electronically transmitting and receiving printed information.

Federal Communications Commission (FCC)   agency that controls all nongovernmental communications in the United States.

field diagnosis   prehospital evaluation of the patient's condition and its causes.

focused history and physical exam   problem-oriented assessment process based on initial assessment and chief complaint.

general impression   your initial, intuitive evaluation of your patient.

glucometer   tool used to measure blood glucose level.

Grey Turner's sign   discoloration over the flanks suggesting intra-abdominal bleeding.

HEENT   head, eyes, ears, nose, and throat.

hematemesis   vomiting of blood.

hematuria   blood in the urine.

hemoptysis   coughing up of blood.

hypertension   blood pressure higher than normal.

hyperthermia   increase in body's core temperature.

hypotension   blood pressure lower than normal.

hypothermia   decrease in body's core temperature.

impulsive   acting instinctively without stopping to think.

index of suspicion   your anticipation of possible injuries based on your analysis of the event.

initial assessment   prehospital process designed to identify and correct life-threatening airway, breathing, and circulation problems.

inspection   the process of informed observation.

intermittent claudication   intermittent calf pain while walking that subsides with rest.

jargon   language used by a particular group or profession.

Korotkoff sounds   sounds of blood hitting arterial walls.

lesion   any disruption in normal tissue.

libel   writing false and malicious words intended to damage a person's character.

major trauma patient   person who has suffered significant mechanism of injury.

manometer   pressure gauge with a scale calibrated in millimeters of mercury (mmHg).

mechanism of injury   combined strength, direction, and nature of forces that injured your patient.

mobile data terminal   vehicle-mounted computer keyboard and display.

multiplex   duplex system that can transmit voice and data simultaneously.

nocturia   excessive urination at night.

open-ended questions   questions that allow your patient to answer in detail.

ophthalmoscope   handheld device used to examine interior of eye.

orthopnea   difficulty breathing while lying supine.

otoscope   handheld device used to examine interior of ears and nose.

palpation   using your sense of touch to gather information.

paroxysmal nocturnal dyspnea   sudden onset of shortness of breath at night.

patient assessment   problem-oriented evaluation of patient and establishment of priorities based on existing and potential threats to human life.

percussion   the production of sound waves by striking one object against another.

perfusion   passage of blood through an organ or tissue.

periorbital ecchymosis   black and blue discoloration surrounding the eye sockets.

personal protective equipment (PPE)   equipment designed to protect against infection. The minimum recommended personal protective equipment includes protective gloves, masks and protective eyewear, HEPA and N-95 respirators, gowns, and disposable resuscitation equipment.

pitting   depression that results from pressure against skin when pitting edema is present.

pleural friction rub   the squeaking or grating sound of the pleural linings rubbing together.

polyuria   excessive urination.

prearrival instructions   dispatcher's instructions to caller for appropriate emergency measures.

prehospital care report (PCR)   the written record of an EMS response.

priapism   a painful and prolonged erection of the penis.

primary problem   the underlying cause for your patient's symptoms.

priority dispatching   system that uses medically approved questions and predetermined guidelines to determine the appropriate level of response.

protocol   predetermined, written guidelines for patient care.

pseudo-instinctive   learned actions that are practiced until they can be done without thinking.

public safety answering point (PSAP)   any agency that takes emergency calls from citizens in a given region and dispatches the emergency resources necessary to respond to individual calls for help.

pulse oximeter   noninvasive device that measures the oxygen saturation of blood.

pulse pressure   difference between systolic and diastolic pressures.

pulse quality   strength, which can be weak, thready, strong, or bounding.

pulse rate   number of pulses felt in 1 minute.

pulse rhythm   pattern and equality of intervals between beats.

quality of respiration   depth and pattern of breathing.

radio band   a range of radio frequencies.

radio frequency   the number of times per second a radio wave oscillates.

rapid trauma assessment   quick check for signs of serious injury.

referred pain   pain that is felt at a location away from its source.

reflective   acting thoughtfully, deliberately, and analytically.

respiration   exchange of oxygen and carbon dioxide in the lungs and at the cellular level.

respiratory effort   how hard patient works to breathe.

respiratory rate   number of times patient breathes in 1 minute.

response time   time elapsed from when a unit is alerted until it arrives on the scene.

review of systems   a list of questions categorized by body system.

rhonchi   continuous sounds with a lower pitch and a snoring quality.

scene safety   doing everything possible to ensure a safe environment.

semantic   related to the meaning of words.

semi-Fowler's position   sitting up at 45°.

simplex   communications system that transmits and receives on the same frequency.

slander   speaking false and malicious words intended to damage a person's character.

sphygmomanometer   blood pressure measuring device comprising a bulb, a cuff, and a manometer.

Standard Precautions   a strict form of infection control that is based on the assumption that all blood and other body fluids are infectious.

standing orders   treatments you can perform before contacting the medical direction physician for permission.

stethoscope   tool used to auscultate most sounds.

stridor   predominantly inspiratory wheeze associated with laryngeal obstruction.

stroke volume   the amount of blood the heart ejects in one beat.

subcutaneous emphysema   crackling sensation caused by air just underneath the skin.

systole   phase of cardiac cycle when the ventricles contract.

systolic blood pressure   force of blood against arteries when ventricles contract.

tachycardia   pulse rate higher than 100.

tachypnea   rapid breathing.

tenderness   pain that is elicited through palpation.

thrill   vibration or humming felt when palpating the pulse.

tidal volume   amount of air one breath moves in and out of lungs.

tinnitus   the sensation of ringing in the ears.

touch pad   computer on which you enter data by touching areas of the display screen.

triage tags   tags containing vital information, affixed to your patient during a multiple-patient incident.

trunking   communications system that pools all frequencies and routes transmissions to the next available frequency.

turgor   normal tension in the skin.

ultrahigh frequency (UHF)   radio frequency band from 300 to 3,000 megahertz.

very high frequency (VHF)   radio frequency band from 30 to 300 megahertz.

visual acuity wall chart/card   wall chart or handheld card with lines of letters used to test vision.

vital statistics   height and weight.

wheezes   continuous, high-pitched musical sounds similar to a whistle.

whispered pectoriloquy   abnormal clarity of patient's transmitted whispers.

Index

The paramedic index includes entries for all five volumes in the Paramedic Care series. Each reference presents volume number followed by page reference in that volume. The sample entry Abdominal cavity, 4:437 refers to Volume 4, page 437.

Air medical transport, 4:521–527
Abandonment, 1:137
ABCs, 1:551
Abdomen, 2:97–103, 4:74–75, 4:455–464
Abdominal anatomy and physiology, 4:455–464
Abdominal aorta, 3:76, 3:414, 4:462
Abdominal arteries, 2:102, 4:462
Abdominal cavity, 4:455–464, 4:463
Abdominal quadrants, 2:98
Abdominal trauma, 4:452–483
 abdominal wall injury, 4:466
 accessory organs, 4:456–458
 anatomy/physiology, 4:455–464
 blunt trauma, 4:465–466
 digestive tract, 4:456, 457
 genitalia, 4:459–460
 hollow organ injury, 4:466–467
 mesentery/bowel injury, 4:468–469
 pediatric patients, 4:472
 pelvic injury, 4:469
 penetrating trauma, 4:464–465
 peritoneum, 4:463
 peritonitis, 4:469
 pregnancy, 4:470–471, 4:477, 4:479–481
 pregnant uterus, 4:461

rapid trauma assessment, 4:475–477
scene size-up, 4:472–474
solid organ injury, 4:467
spleen, 4:458
urinary system, 4:458–459
vascular structure injury, 4:468
vasculature, 4:461–462
Abdominal wall injury, 4:466
Abducens nerve, 2:148, 4:290
Aberrant conduction, 5:149
ABO blood groups, 1:244
Abortion, 3:727–728
Abrasions, 4:144–145
Abruptio placentae, 3:731–732, 4:471
Absence seizure, 3:303
Absent rhythm, 5:110
Absolute refractory period, 3:100
Absolute zero, 3:548
Absorbent dressings, 4:159
Absorption, 5:468
Abstract, 1:658
Abuse and assault, 5:218–235
 child abuse. See Child abuse and neglect
 elder abuse, 5:223–225
 partner abuse, 5:220–223
 sexual assault, 5:231–235
Academic Emergency Medicine, 1:68

Accelerated idioventricular, 5:136
Accelerated junctional rhythm, 5:133–134
Acceleration, 4:25
Accessory nerve, 2:153
Accessory organ diseases, 3:401–407
Accidental Death and Disability: The Neglected Disease of Modern Society, 1:53, 4:5
Acclimatization, 3:552
Accurate information, 5:311
ACE, 1:222, 3:337
ACE inhibitors, 1:356–357, 5:203
Acetabulum, 4:233
Acetaminophen, 3:481–482, 5:206
Acetaminophen poisoning treatment algorithm, 3:483
Acetylcholine, 3:82
Acetylcholinesterase (AChE), 5:466
AChE, 5:466
Acid, 3:473
Acid-base balance, 1:202–207
Acidosis, 1:203
Acini, 3:333
ACLS pulseless arrest algorithm, 5:146
ACN systems, 2:272
Acoustic nerve, 2:151, 4:290
Acquired immune deficiencies, 1:273

Acquired immune deficiency syndrome (AIDS), 1:25
Acquired immunity, 1:239, 3:360
Acquired immunodeficiency syndrome (AIDS), 1:236, 1:273–274
ACS, 5:183–187
ACTH, 1:278, 3:332
Action potential, 3:87
Activase, 5:170
Activated charcoal, 3:452
Active immunity, 3:360, 3:606
Active internal rewarming, 3:564
Active listening, 2:8
Active rescue zone, 5:414
Active transport, 1:195, 1:304, 3:417
Actual damages, 1:127
Acuity, 2:249
Acute anterior wall infarct, 3:241
Acute arterial occlusion, 3:217
Acute carbon monoxide poisoning, 3:463
Acute coronary syndrome (ACS), 5:183–187
Acute effects, 5:464
Acute gastroenteritis, 3:387–388
Acute idiopathic thrombocytopenia purpura (ITP), 3:538
Acute infections, 5:298

Acute inferior wall (diaphragmatic) infarct, 3:243

Acute inflammatory response, 1:255–256

Acute lymphocytic leukemia (ALL), 3:536–537

Acute mountain sickness (AMS), 3:580–581

Acute myelogenous leukemia (AML), 3:536

Acute myocardial infarction, 3:236–245

Acute pulmonary embolism, 3:217

Acute renal failure (ARF), 3:426–429

Acute respiratory distress syndrome (ARDS), 5:210, 5:289

Acute retinal artery occlusion, 4:315

Acute tubular necrosis, 3:427

Addendum, 2:301

Addictions, 1:20–21, 3:499

Addisonian crisis, 3:352

Addison's disease, 1:374, 3:351, 3:352

Adduction/abduction, 4:228

Adenocarcinoma, 3:52

Adenosine, 5:89, 5:168

Adenosine triphosphate (ATP), 1:175, 1:219

ADH, 1:180, 1:197, 3:331, 4:114

Adherent dressings, 4:159

Adhesion, 3:399

Adhesive bandage, 4:160

Adjunct medications, 1:319

Adjunctive RSI agents, 1:598

Administration, 5:377–378

Administration of drugs. See Medication administration

Administration tubing, 1:435–439

Administrative documentation, 2:289

Administrative law, 1:121

Adolescence, 1:518–519, 5:50–51. See also Pediatrics

physical examination, 2:169

Adrenal cortex, 1:374, 3:334

Adrenal glands, 3:334–335, 3:414, 4:459

Adrenal insufficiency, 3:352

Adrenergic, 1:333

Adrenergic agonists, 1:344–345

Adrenergic antagonists, 1:345

Adrenergic receptor specificity, 1:345

Adrenergic receptors, 1:341–344

Adrenocorticotropic hormone (ACTH), 1:278, 3:332, 4:115

Adult respiratory distress syndrome (ARDS), 3:35, 3:570–571

Advance directive, 1:139, 5:155

Advanced life support (ALS), 1:50, 1:86, 2:187, 5:266, 5:267, 5:312

Aerobic metabolism, 1:219, 4:108

Aeromedical evacuations, 5:350

Affect, 3:665

Afferent, 3:277

Affinity, 1:312

Africanized honey bees (AHBs), 3:488–489

Afterbirth, 3:716

Afterload, 1:214, 3:80, 4:87

Against medical advice (AMA), 2:307

AGE, 3:573, 3:576–577

Age. See Life-span development

Age-related conditions, 3:680–681

Ageism, 5:152

Aggregate, 4:91

Agonal respirations, 1:554

Agonist, 1:313

Agonist-antagonist (partial agonist), 1:313

Agricultural emergencies, 5:511–518

AHBs, 3:488–489

Aid, 5:437

AIDS, 1:25, 1:236, 1:273–274

Air and gas monitor, 5:458

Air bags, 4:31–33, 5:431, 5:514

Air embolism, 1:451

Air-purifying respirator (APR), 5:473

Air splint, 4:257–258

Airborne, 3:601

Airway, 4:325–331

Airway assessment, 2:201–205

Airway management, 1:529–641

advanced airway management, 1:572–627

Ambu laryngeal mask, 1:613

approach to the difficult airway, 1:620–627

basic airway management, 1:564–572

basic mechanical airways, 1:568–572

children, 5:70–86, 5:124–125

Cobra perilaryngeal airway, 1:613

documentation, 1:639–641

EGTA/EOA, 1:614

endotracheal intubation, 1:604–606

esophageal tracheal combitube, 1:607–609

field extubation, 1:606–607

foreign body removal under direct laryngoscopy, 1:615

gastric distention/decompression, 1:632

King LT airway, 1:614

laryngeal mask airway, 1:611–614

manual airway maneuvers, 1:565–568

nasotracheal intubation, 1:604–606

newborn, 5:11–12

oxygenation, 1:633–634

patients with stoma sites, 1:627–629

pediatric patients, 5:70–86, 5:124–125

pharyngotracheal lumen airway, 1:609–611

respiratory problems, 1:549–551

respiratory system, 1:534–549

respiratory system assessment, 1:551–564. See also Respiratory system assessment

suctioning, 1:629–631

surgical airways, 1:615–620

ventilation, 1:635–639. See also Ventilation

Airway resistance, 3:12

Airway thermal burn, 4:195–196

Albumin, 1:200

Alcohol abuse, 5:207

Alcoholism, 3:503

Aldosterone, 4:115

Algorithms, 2:250

Alimentary canal, 4:455–464

Alkali, 1:203, 3:473

Alkalinizing agents, 5:172

Alkalosis, 1:203

ALL, 3:536–537

Allergens, 1:270, 3:361

Allergic reaction, 3:358, 3:362

Allergies and anaphylaxis, 3:356–371
    airway protection, 3:368
    allergies, 3:361–363
    anaphylaxis, 3:363–364
    delayed hypersensitivity, 3:361
    immediate hypersensitivity, 3:361–363
    immune system, 3:359–361
    management, 3:366–370
    medication administration, 3:368–369
    patient assessment, 3:364–366
    patient education, 3:371
    psychological support, 3:369
    signs/symptoms, 3:370

Allergy, 1:209, 1:267, 1:270–271, 3:361

Allied health professions, 1:92

Alloimmunity, 1:268

Alpha adrenergic receptors, 1:179

Alpha error, 1:652

Alpha radiation, 4:193, 5:462

Alpha receptors, 3:82

Alpha$_1$ antagonists, 1:356

ALS, 1:50, 1:86, 2:187, 3:315, 5:266, 5:267, 5:312

ALS intervention, 5:301–302

ALS skills, 5:442

Alteplase, 5:170

Altered mental status, 5:168–169

Alternative fuel systems, 5:431

Alternative pathway, 1:258

Alternative response, 1:50

Alternative time sampling, 1:651

Alveolar dead space, 3:13, 4:412

Alveolar duct, 3:4

Alveolar epithelium, 3:9

Alveolar minute volume (V_{A-min}), 1:548

Alveolar volume (V_A), 1:548

Alveoli, 1:539, 3:4, 3:8–9

Alzheimer's disease, 1:212, 3:313, 5:190

AMA, 2:307

AMA Drug Evaluation, 1:295

Ambu laryngeal mask, 1:613

Ambulance crashes, 1:41–42

Ambulance escort, 1:42

Ambulance operations, 5:335–356
    air medical transport, 5:350–356
    ambulance design, 5:337
    checking ambulances, 5:339–341
    deadly intersection, 5:348–350
    due regard, 5:345–346
    educating providers, 5:343
    employment and staffing, 5:341–342
    escorts, 5:347
    lights & siren, 5:346–347
    medical equipment standards, 5:338
    multi-vehicle responses, 5:347–348
    operational staffing, 5:342
    parking/loading the ambulance, 5:348
    reducing collisions, 5:343–344
    safety, 5:342–350
    SOPs, 5:345

standards, 5:337–339
    traffic congestion, 5:341–342

Ambulance volante, 1:53

Amebiasis, 1:381

Amidate, 4:335

Amiodarone, 5:89, 5:168

AML, 3:536

Amniotic fluid, 3:716

Amniotic sac, 3:715, 3:716

Ampere, 4:189

Amphetamine actions, 1:325

Amphiarthroses, 4:227

Ampule, 1:416

Amputations, 4:148, 4:172

AMS, 3:580–581

Amyotrophic lateral sclerosis (ALS), 3:315

Anabolism, 1:178, 1:186, 3:338

Anaerobic, 4:93

Anaerobic metabolism, 1:219, 4:108

Analgesia, 1:319

Analgesics, 1:319, 5:205

Analysis of variance (ANOVA), 1:656

Anaphylactic response, 1:185

Anaphylactic shock, 1:223, 1:228–230, 4:119, 5:106

Anaphylaxis, 1:229, 3:358. *See* Allergies and anaphylaxis

Anastomoses, 3:77

Anatomical dead space, 3:13, 4:412

Anatomy, 1:178

Anchor, 5:437

Anchor time, 1:37

Androgenic hormones, 3:335

Anectine, 1:597, 4:334, 5:83

Anemia, 1:211, 3:532, 3:533–534, 4:97

Anesthesia, 1:319

Anesthetic, 1:321

Aneurysm, 3:215–216, , 4:434, 5:184–185

Anger, 3:672

Angina pectoris, 3:184–187, 5:182–183

Angiocatheter, 1:440

Angioedema, 3:362

Angioneurotic edema, 3:362

Angiotensin converting enzyme (ACE), 1:222, 3:337

Angiotensin converting enzyme (ACE) inhibitors, 1:356–357

Angiotensin I, 1:222, 3:337

Angiotensin II, 3:337

Angiotensin II receptor antagonists, 1:357

Angiotensinogen, 3:337

Angiotensin, 4:115

Angle of Louis, 4:408

Angry patients, 2:21

ANH, 3:336–337

Anion, 1:192

Ankle injuries, 4:269–270

Ankles, 2:120–123, 2:125

Ankylosing spondylitis (AS), 4:377, 5:197–199

Annals of Emergency Medicine, 1:68

Annulul fibrosus, 4:347

Anorexia nervosa, 3:676

ANOVA, 1:656

Anoxia, 1:554

Anoxic hypoxemia, 5:173

ANP, 1:216, 3:85

Antacid, 1:368

Antagonist, 1:313

Anterior axillary line, 4:408

Anterior cerebral artery, 3:276

Anterior communicating artery, 3:276

Anterior cord syndrome, 4:371

Anterior descending artery, 3:76

Anterior fascicles, 3:89

Anterior great cardiac vein, 3:77

Anterior infarct, 3:238

Anterior longitudinal ligament, 4:348

Anterior medial fissure, 4:357

Anterior pituitary, 3:332

Anterior pituitary drugs, 1:373

Anterior pituitary gland, 3:330

Anterograde amnesia, 4:308

Anterolateral infarct, 3:238, 3:242

Anterpartum, 5:4

Anti-inflammatory agents, 5:205–206

Antiasthmatic medications, 1:363–365

Antibiotics, 1:235, 1:380

Antibody, 1:238, 3:359, 3:603

Anticholinergics, 1:337–338, 1:365, 1:369

Anticoagulant, 1:361–362, 1:451

Anticoagulant therapy, 5:293

Antidiuresis, 3:418

Antidiuretic hormone (ADH), 1:180, 1:197, 3:331, 4:114

Antidote, 3:452

Antidotes for toxicological emergencies, 3:453

Antidysrhythmic, 1:351–353

Antiemetic, 1:370

Antiepileptic drugs, 1:323–324

Antigen-antibody complexes, 1:247

Antigen-binding sites, 1:245

Antigen-presenting cells (APCs), 1:252

Antigen processing, 1:251

Antigens, 1:238, 1:241–243, 3:359, 3:524, 3:603

Antihistamine, 1:366, 3:368–369

Antihyperlipidemic, 1:363

Antihypertensives, 1:353–360, 5:202

Antineoplastic agent, 1:379

Antiplatelet, 1:361

Antiseizure medications, 1:323–324, 5:205

Antiseptica, 1:398

Antitussive, 1:367

Anuria, 3:426

Anus, 2:107–108, 3:384, 3:694, 3:696

Anxiety, 3:671–672

Anxiety disorder, 3:671

Anxious avoidant attachment, 1:513

Anxious patients, 2:20–21

Anxious resistant attachment, 1:513

Aorta, 3:77, 3:386

Aortic dissection, 5:184

Aortic dissection and rupture, 4:434–435, 448

Aortic stenosis, 5:9

APCs, 1:252

Apgar, Virginia, 3:746

APGAR score, 3:746, 5:11

Aphasia, 5:189, 5:245

Apnea, 1:598

Apnea monitors, 5:136

Apneustic center, 1:546, 4:413

Apneustic respiration, 3:19, 3:286

Apoptosis, 1:187

Appeal, 1:123

Appellate courts, 1:122

Appendicitis, 3:401–402

Appendicular skeleton, 4:231

Appendix, 3:384, 3:400

APR, 5:473

Apresoline, 1:358

Aqueous humor, 4:294

Arachnoid membrane, 3:270, 3:278, 4:286, 4:358

ARDS, 3:35, 3:570–571, 5:210, 5:289

Area trauma center, 4:11

ARF, 3:426–429

Arginine vasopressin (AVP), 4:114

Arm, 2:113

Arrhythmia, 3:103

Arrows, 4:69

Arterial gas embolism (AGE), 3:573, 3:576–577

Arterial system, 3:79

Arteries, 4:87

Arteriole, 3:4, 3:79, 3:416, 4:88

Arteriosclerosis, 3:215

Arteriovenous malformations, 5:194

Artery, 3:416

Arthritis, 4:247–248

Arthrus reaction, 1:270

Articular surface, 4:226

Articulation disorders, 5:245

Artifact, 3:91

Artificial pacemaker rhythm, 5:145–148

Artificially acquired immunity, 3:360

Aryepiglottic fold, 1:612

Arytenoid cartilage, 1:536

AS, 5:197–199

Ascending aorta, 3:75

Ascending colon, 3:384, 3:400

Ascending limb of the Loop of Henle, 3:416

Ascending loop of Henle, 3:415

Ascending reticular activating system, 4:288, 4:290

Ascending tracts, 4:358

Ascites, 2:101

ASD, 5:8

Asepsis, 1:397

ASHD, 5:187

Asherman chest seal, 4:445

Asphyxia, 3:22

Aspiration, 1:537

Aspirin, 5:170

Assault, 1:137. See Abuse and assault

Assault rifle, 4:68

Assay, 1:297

Assessment-based management, 5:306–322

assessment/management choreography, 5:314–315

BLS/ALS, 5:312

common complaints, 5:322

distracting injuries, 5:313

environmental/personnel considerations, 5:314

equipment, 5:315–316

history, 5:318–319

initial assessment, 5:317–318

patient care provider, 5:315

patient compliance, 5:313

patient's history, 5:311

pattern recognition, 5:311–312

personal attitudes, 5:312

physical exam, 5:311, 5:318–319

presenting the patient, 5:320–322

team leader, 5:314–315

uncooperative patients, 5:312–313

Assessment from the doorway, 5:56

Assessment pearls

abused patient, 2:19

cerebrospinal fluid, 2:234

chest pain, 2:11

child's weight, 2:169

closer look, 2:37

congestive heart failure, 2:92

crossover test, 2:47

deep tendon reflexes, 2:163

Dugas' sign, 2:119
fingernails, 2:57
gestational age, 2:18
glucometer reading, 2:225
hip fracture, 2:127
impaired peripheral perfusion, 2:138
pediatric breath sounds, 2:172
pulsus paradoxus, 2:46
respiratory rate, 2:44
skin abnormalities in dark-skinned people, 2:53
spinal disk disease, 2:132
standard examination system, 2:30
testicular torsion, 2:107
ticklish patient, 2:102
two-point sensory discrimination, 2:160
Assisted living, 1:524
Asthma, 1:209, 1:363, 1:364, 3:42–45, 5:100–101, 5:282
Astramorph, 4:336
Asystole, 5:110, 5:143–145
Ataxic (Biot's) respirations, 3:19, 3:286
Atelectasis, 1:539, 4:414
Atherosclerosis, 3:215
Atherosclerotic heart disease (ASHD), 5:187
ATP, 1:175, 1:219
Atracurium, 1:597, 4:335
Atria, 3:74
Atrial enlargement, 3:254
Atrial fibrillation, 5:122–123
Atrial flutter, 5:121–122
Atrial natriuretic hormone (ANH), 3:336–337
Atrial natriuretic peptide (ANP), 1:216, 3:85
Atrial septal defect (ASD), 5:8
Atrial syncytium, 3:85

Atrioventricular (AV) bundle, 3:85
Atrioventricular valves, 3:74
Atrophy, 1:182
Atropine, 4:336
Atropine sulfate, 5:89
Atypical angina, 5:185
Augmented limb leads, 3:92, 3:224
Aural medications, 1:403
Auscultation, 2:34–35
Authoritarian, 1:516
Authoritative, 1:516
Auto anatomy, 5:432–433
Auto rollover, 4:39
Autoimmune disease, 3:519
Autoimmunity, 1:268, 1:271, 3:605
Automatic collision notification (ACN) systems, 2:272
Automaticity, 3:89
Automobile collisions. See Motor vehicle collisions
Autonomic dysfunction, 5:186
Autonomic ganglia, 1:331
Autonomic hyperreflexia syndrome, 4:372
Autonomic nervous system, 1:331, 1:332, 2:255, 3:268, 3:280, 3:327
Autonomic neuropathy, 3:552
Autonomy, 1:154
Autoregulation, 4:289
AV blocks, 3:245–246
AV bundle, 3:85
Avian influenza, 3:632–633
AVP, 4:114
AVPU levels, 2:200–201
Avulsions, 4:147–148
Axial loading, 4:35
Axial skeleton, 4:231
Axial stress, 4:366–367
Axillary nerve, 3:277

Axis deviation, 3:227–229
Axons, 3:269, 4:358

B lymphocytes, 1:239, 1:245
Babinski's response, 2:164
Babinski's sign, 4:381
Back boarding/extrication from the water, 5:425
Back pain, 3:316–318
Back safety, 1:21–23
Bacteria, 1:235, 3:597–598
Bacterial peritonitis, 4:469
Bactericidal, 3:598
Bacteriostatic, 3:598
Bag-valve mask, 1:636
Ball-and-socket joints, 4:228
Ballistics, 4:63
Bamboo spine, 4:377, 5:197
Bandage, 4:158–160, 171
Baptism, 5:36
Bare lymphocyte syndrome, 1:272
Bariatric devices, 5:248
Baroreceptors, 1:179, 4:113
Barotrauma, 1:511, 1:616, 3:573
Barton, Clara, 1:53
Basal metabolic rate (BMR), 3:550
Base, 1:203
Basement lamina, 3:9
Basic life support (BLS), 1:50, 5:312
Basic mechanical airways, 1:568–572
Basilar artery, 3:276
Basophil, 1:198, 1:262, 3:361, 3:517, 3:518
Battery, 1:137, 5:220–223
Battle's sign, 2:232, 4:300, 4:301
Beck's triad, 4:433
Bed sores, 5:195
Bedside manner, 5:316
Behavior, 3:662

Behavioral disorders. See Psychiatric and behavioral disorders
Behavioral emergency, 3:662
Belay, 5:437
Bell's palsy, 3:314
Bend fractures, 5:129
Beneficence, 1:154
Benign prostatic hyperplasia, 1:378, 3:413
Benzodiazepines, 5:205
Bereavement, 3:673
Beta adrenergic antagonists, 1:355
Beta adrenergic receptors, 1:179
Beta-agonists, 3:369
Beta-blocker poisoning treatment algorithm, 3:473
Beta-blockers, 5:171–172, 5:202
Beta-blockers (class II), 1:352
Beta-endorphins, 1:279
Beta error, 1:652
Beta radiation, 4:193, 5:462
Beta receptors, 3:82
Beta specific agents, 1:364
Biaxial joints, 4:228
Bicarbonate (HKO), 1:193
Bicarbonate buffer system, 1:203
B.I.G., 1:468
Bilateral periorbital ecchymosis, 4:301
Bile duct, 3:384
Bilevel positive airway pressure (BiPAP), 5:281, 5:289
Bioassay, 1:298
Bioavailability, 1:307
Bioequivalence, 1:298
Biologic half-life, 1:316
Biological, 3:664
Biological agents, 5:535–539

Biotoxin, 5:533

Biotransformation, 1:308, 5:465

Biot's respirations, 1:554, 3:19, 3:286

BiPAP, 5:281, 5:289

Bipolar disorders, 1:213, 3:673–674

Bipolar frame traction splint, 4:260

Bipolar limb leads, 3:91, 3:224

Birth injuries, 5:35–36

Black widow spider bites, 3:491

Bladder, 4:459

Blast injuries, 4:45–52
  abdomen, 4:52
  assessment, 4:49–51
  blast wind, 4:48
  burns, 4:49, 4:52
  confined face explosions/structural collapses, 4:48–49
  ears, 4:52
  explosion, 4:45
  lungs, 4:51–52
  penetrating wounds, 4:52
  personal displacement, 4:48
  pressure wave, 4:47–48
  projectiles, 4:48

Blast wind, 4:48

Blastocyst, 3:715

Blebs, 3:38

Blepharospasm, 4:215

Blinding, 1:651

Blistering agents, 5:532

Blood, 1:198, 1:434

Blood-brain barrier, 1:308, 4:289

Blood disorders. See Hematology

Blood flow, 3:75

Blood group antigens, 1:243–244

Blood groups, 1:244

Blood loss/transfusion, 4:509

Blood pressure, 2:44

Blood products, 3:524–526

Blood spatter evidence, 5:496

Blood supply to spine, 4:350

Blood transfusion, 3:525

Blood tube, 1:461

Blood tube sequence, 1:462

Blood tubing, 1:438–439, 1:446, 1:448–449

Blood typing, 3:524–526

Blood vessels, 1:215, 4:140

Bloodborne, 3:601

BLS, 1:50, 5:312

Blunt cardiac injury, 4:431–432, 447

Blunt trauma, 4:20–59
  blast injuries. See Blast injuries
  compression, 4:26
  crush injuries, 4:55–56
  energy conservation, 4:24
  falls, 4:53–54
  force, 4:25
  inertia, 4:23–24
  kinetic energy, 4:24–25
  motor vehicle collisions. See Motor vehicle collisions
  motorcycle collisions, 4:42
  pedestrian collisions, 4:42–44
  recreational vehicle collisions, 4:44–45
  shear, 4:27
  sports injuries, 4:54–55
  stretch, 4:26

BMR, 3:550

BNP, 1:216, 3:85

Body armor, 5:492

Body collision, 4:28–29

Body fluid, 1:188–191

Body of uterus, 3:696

Body splinting, 4:510

Body substance isolation (BSI), 1:24

Body surface area (BSA), 4:197–198

Body temperature, 2:47–48

Bohr effect, 3:515

Boiling point, 5:461

Bolus, 1:413

Bonding, 1:513

Bone, 4:74

Bone aging, 4:234

Bone classification, 4:227

Bone Injection Gun (B.I.G.), 1:468

Bone injury, 4:242–246

Bone repair cycle, 4:246–247

Bone structure, 4:225–227

Bony fish poisoning, 3:485, 3:498

Borborygmi, 2:103

Borrowed servant doctrine, 1:129

Botulinum, 5:533

Bowel obstruction, 3:399–401, 5:194

Bowman's capsule, 3:415, 3:416

Boyle's law, 3:571

BPD, 5:283

Brachial plexus, 3:277, 4:362

Bradycardia, 2:41, 3:101
  children, 5:110, 5:111
  newborn, 5:29

Bradycardia algorithm, 3:106

Bradydysrhythmia, 5:110

Bradykinin, 1:260

Bradypnea, 2:42, 3:28

Brain, 2:143, 3:274, 4:287–288

Brain abscess, 3:312

Brain injury, 4:302–310

Brain ischemia, 5:187

Brain natriuretic peptide (BNP), 1:216, 3:85

Brainstem, 3:274, 4:288

Branches, 5:378, 5:379

Braxton-Hicks contractions, 3:736

Breach of duty, 1:126

Breast cancer, 1:209

Breathing, 4:331–332

Breathing assessment, 2:206–207

Breathing patterns, 2:45

Breech presentation, 3:747

Broad ligament, 3:696

Bronchi, 1:538, 3:8, 4:410

Bronchial vessels, 3:9

Bronchiectasis, 5:284

Bronchioles, 3:4

Bronchiolitis, 5:101–102

Bronchitis, 3:40–41, 5:281–282

Bronchophony, 2:91

Bronchopulmonary dysplasia (BPD), 5:283

Bronchospasm, 3:12

Broselow tape, 2:40

Broviac catheters, 5:291

Brown recluse spider bites, 3:490–491

Brown-Séquard syndrome, 4:371

Brudzinski's sign, 3:630

Bruit, 2:95, 3:118, 3:287

Bruton agammaglobulinemia, 1:272

BSA, 4:197–198

BSI, 1:24

Bubble sheets, 2:290

Buccal, 1:400

Buckle fractures, 5:129

Buffer, 1:193

Buffer system, 1:203

Bulimia nervosa, 3:676

Bundle branch blocks, 3:246–250, 5:149

Bundle of His, 3:89

Bundle of Kent, 5:150

Burden Nasoscope, 1:573

Burette chamber, 1:438

Burn severity, 4:206

Burnout, 1:37

Burns, 4:182–220, 5:228
  airway thermal, 4:195–196
  body surface area (BSA), 4:197–198

burn severity, 4:206
carbon monoxide
    poisoning, 4:195
chemical, 4:191,
    213–215
children, 5:123,
    5:129–130
elderly persons, 5:214
electrical, 4:189–191,
    4:212–213
eschar, 4:199
focused and rapid
    trauma assessment,
    4:204–207
full thickness, 4:197,
    4:204, 4:205
hypothermia,
    4:198–199
hypovolemia, 4:199
infection, 4:199–200
inhalation injury, 4:195,
    4:210
local and minor, 4:208
moderate to severe,
    4:208–210
organ failure, 4:200
partial thickness, 4:196,
    204, 4:205
physical abuse, 4:200
radiation injury,
    4:191–194, 4:215–217
rule of nines, 4:197–198
rule of palms, 4:198
scene size-up,
    4:201–202
skin, 4:185–187
special factors, 4:200
superficial, 4:196, 205
thermal, 4:187–189, 4:
    4:200–211
toxic inhalation, 4:195
transportation, 4:207
BURP maneuver, 1:586
Bursa, 4:230
Bursitis, 4:247

C-FLOP, 5:369
Ca, 1:193
CAAMS, 5:354
CAAS, 5:339
CABG, 5:190
Calcaneus, 4:234

Calcitonin, 3:332
Calcium (Ca), 1:193
Calcium channel blocker
    poisoning treatment
    algorithm, 3:472, 5:172
Calcium channel
    blockers (class IV),
    1:352, 1:357
Calcium chloride, 5:89
Caliber, 4:64
Callus, 4:246
CAMEO, 5:458
Cancellous, 4:226
Cancer, 1:209–210
    challenged patient,
    5:253–255
Cancer drugs, 1:379–380
Cannabinoids, 1:370
Cannula, 1:435
Cannulation, 1:430
Capillaries, 1:539, 3:8,
    3:79, 4:88
Capillary endothelium,
    3:9
Capillary refill, 4:528–529
Capillary washout, 4:117
Capnogram, 1:562, 3:32
Capnography, 1:558–564,
    2:49, 3:29–33, 4:121
Capnometry, 3:29
Caput succedaneum, 5:35
Carbaminohemoglobin,
    3:16
Carbon dioxide, 1:534
Carbon dioxide
    concentration in
    blood, 1:545–546
Carbon dioxide levels,
    1:543–546
Carbon monoxide,
    3:457–458
Carbon monoxide
    poisoning, 3:291,
    4:195
Carbon monoxide (CO)
    poisoning treatment
    algorithm, 3:466
Carbonic acid, 1:203
Carbonic anhydrase,
    1:203
Carboxyhemoglobin,
    3:54

Cardiac arrest, 3:209–215
    newborn, 5:36–37
Cardiac contractile force,
    1:214
Cardiac contractility, 4:87
Cardiac cycle, 3:79–82
Cardiac decompensation,
    5:269
Cardiac depolarization,
    3:86–87
Cardiac emergencies,
    3:163–219
    acute arterial occlusion,
    3:217
    acute coronary
    syndrome, 3:183–184
    acute pulmonary
    embolism, 3:217
    ALS, 3:163
    aneurysm, 3:215–216
    angina pectoris,
    3:184–187
    atherosclerosis, 3:215
    BLS, 3:163
    cardiac arrest,
    3:209–215
    cardiac tamponade,
    3:202–205
    cardiogenic shock,
    3:206–209
    carotid sinus massage,
    3:179–181
    defibrillation,
    3:172–175
    ECG monitoring,
    3:163–166
    heart failure,
    3:196–202
    hypertensive
    emergencies,
    3:205–206
    myocardial infarction,
    3:187–196
    pharmacological
    management,
    3:167–172
    precordial thump, 3:167
    support/communicatio
    n, 3:181–182
    synchronized
    cardioversion,
    3:175–176

    transcutaneous cardiac
    pacing, 3:176–179
    vagal maneuvers, 3:166
    vasculitis, 3:217
Cardiac glycosides, 1:359
Cardiac medications,
    3:471–473
Cardiac monitor, 2:50
Cardiac muscle, 1:176
Cardiac notch, 3:4
Cardiac output, 1:214,
    2:94, 3:80, 4:87
Cardiac plexus, 3:82
Cardiac sphincter, 3:384
Cardiac syncope, 5:186
Cardiac tamponade,
    3:202–205
Cardioaccceleratory
    center, 4:113
Cardiogenic shock, 1:223,
    1:224–225, 3:206–209,
    4:119–120, 5:105–107
Cardioinhibitory center,
    4:113
Cardiology, 3:64–260
    anatomy, 3:73–79
    AV blocks, 3:245–246
    axis deviation,
    3:227–229
    bundle branch blocks,
    3:246–250
    cardiac cycle, 3:79–82
    cardiac emergencies,
    3:163–219. *See also*
    Cardiac emergencies
    chamber enlargement,
    3:250–255
    conduction
    abnormalities,
    3:245–255
    disease findings,
    3:230–245
    dysrhythmias,
    3:103–153 *See also*
    Dysrhythmia
    ECG, 3:90–103. *See also*
    Electrocardiogram
    (ECG)
    electrolytes, 3:85
    electrophysiology,
    3:85–90
    heart, 3:73–77

Cardiology, (contd.)
myocardial ischemia, 3:230
nervous control of the heart, 3:82, 3:84
patient assessment, 3:153–163
physiology, 3:79–90
prehospital ECG monitoring, 3:256–260
QRS axis, 3:227
12-lead ECG, 3:230
Cardiomyopathy, 1:211, 5:107–108
Cardiovascular disease (CVD), 3:71
Cardiovascular disorders, 1:211
Cardiovascular inquiries, 4:430–435
Cardiovascular system, 1:177, 1:346–363, 2:92–97
geriatrics, 5:173
infants, 1:510
late adulthood, 1:522
pediatric patients, 5:55
pregnancy, 3:716–717
toddlers/preschoolers, 1:514–515
Cardizem, 5:168
Carina, 1:538, 3:7, 3:8
Carotid sinus massage, 3:179–181
Carpal bones, 4:232
Carrier-mediated diffusion, 1:304
Cartilage, 4:227
Cascade, 1:258
Case-control studies, 1:649
Caseous necrosis, 1:187
Catabolism, 1:178, 1:186, 3:338
Cataracts, 5:166, 5:167
Catatonia, 3:670
Catecholamines, 1:214, 1:277–279, 4:97
Catheter inserted through the needle, 1:441
Cation, 1:192

Cauda equina, 4:371, 4:357
Causes of death, 4:7
Cave-ins, 5:428–429
Cavitation, 4:64, 4:420
CBT, 3:551
CDC, 3:596
Cecum, 3:400
Cell and cellular environment, 1:173–201
cell, defined, 1:173
cell structure, 1:174–176
cellular adaptation, 1:182–183
cellular death, 1:187
cellular injury, 1:183–187
electrolytes, 1:191–193
intravenous therapy, 1:197–202
organs/organ systems/organism, 1:177–178
osmosis/diffusion, 1:193–197
system integration, 1:178–181
tissues, 1:176
water, 1:188–191
Cell body, 3:269
Cell-mediated immunity, 1:239, 1:240, 1:249, 3:519, 3:604
Cell-mediated issue reactions, 1:270
Cell membrane, 1:173, 1:174
Cellular components, 1:261–263
Cellular immunity, 3:359, 3:361
Cellular products, 1:263
Cellular swelling, 1:186
Cellular telephone systems, 2:278
Cellulitis, 5:270
Celox, 4:104
Center for Pediatric Medicine (CPEM), 5:44

Centers for Disease Control and Prevention (CDC), 3:596
Central cord syndrome, 4:371
Central IV lines, 5:136–137
Central nervous system (CNS), 3:268–279
bones of the skull, 3:271
brain, 3:272–276
dysfunction, 3:59
medications, 1:319–331
neuron, 3:269–270
protective structures, 3:270–272
spinal cord, 3:276–278
stimulants, 1:324
Central neurogenic hyperventilation, 1:554, 3:19, 3:286
Central pain syndrome, 3:314
Central sulcus, 4:287
Central venous access, 1:432
Centrally acting adrenergic inhibitors, 1:355
Centriole, 1:173
Cephalopelvic disproportion, 3:750–751
Cerebellum, 3:274, 3:275, 3:276, 4:288
Cerebral contusion, 4:303
Cerebral hemisphere, 3:274
Cerebral homeostasis, 3:282
Cerebral palsy, 5:255
Cerebral perfusion pressure (CPP), 4:289
Cerebrospinal fluid (CSF), 2:234, 3:14, 3:272, 4:286
Cerebrum, 2:143, 3:273, 3:274, 4:287
Certification, 1:64, 1:124
Cervical collar application, 4:388

Cervical concavity, 4:348
Cervical immobilization device (CID), 4:396
Cervical nerves, 4:361
Cervical plexus, 3:277, 4:362
Cervical spine, 4:351–352
Cervical spine exam reminder, 4:379
Cervical spine trauma, 4:316
Cervical vertebrae, 4:347, 4:351
Cervix, 3:696, 3:715, 4:460
Cervix of uterus, 3:696
CF, 5:255–256, 5:282
Chain of evidence, 5:234
Challenged patient, 5:238–260
arthritis, 5:253
cancer, 5:253–255
cerebral palsy, 5:255
communicable diseases, 5:260
culturally diverse patients, 5:258–259
cystic fibrosis, 5:255–256
developmental disabilities, 5:250–252
Down syndrome, 5:251
FAS, 5:251–252
hearing impairment, 5:241–243
multiple sclerosis, 5:256
muscular dystrophy, 5:256–257
myasthenia gravis, 5:258
obesity, 5:246–249
paralysis, 5:249
pathological challenges, 5:252–258
patients with financial challenges, 5:260
physical challenges, 5:240–249
poliomyelitis, 5:257
speech impairments, 5:245–246
spina bifida, 5:258

terminally ill patients, 5:259–260

visual impairments, 5:243–245

Chamber enlargement, 3:250–255

Chancroid, 3:651

CHART format, 2:305–306

CHD, 3:71

Chemical agents, 5:530–535

Chemical asphyxiants, 5:466–467

Chemical burns, 4:191, 4:213–215

Chemical injury, 1:184

Chemical peritonitis, 4:469

Chemical restraint, 3:687

Chemoreceptors, 1:179, 4:113

Chemotactic factors, 1:257, 4:150

Chemotaxis, 1:257, 3:516

Chemotherapy, 1:379–380

CHEMTEL, Inc., 5:458

CHEMTREC, 5:458

Chest compression newborn, 5:22, 5:23

Chest discomfort, 5:182

Chest/lungs, 2:84–92

Chest wall abnormalities, 2:87

Chest wall contusion, 4:420

Chest wall injuries, 4:420–424

Chest wounds, 4:79–80

Cheyne-Stokes respirations, 1:554, 3:19, 3:286, 4:309

CHF, 5:198

Chi square test, 1:656

Chickenpox, 1:25, 3:626–629

Chief complaint, 2:3, 2:11, 2:222

Child abuse and neglect, 5:131–134, 5:225–231
abdominal injuries, 5:229

burns/scalds, 5:228

characteristics of abused children, 5:226–227

characteristics of abusers, 5:226

emotional abuse, 5:230

fractures, 5:229

head injuries, 5:229

maternal drug abuse, 5:229

neglect, 5:229–230

physical examination, 5:228

shaken baby syndrome, 5:229

Child safety seats, 4:33

Childhood development by age, 1:495–499

Children, 1:499–501
bag-valve ventilation, 1:637

communication, 1:499–501

dosage calculations, 1:481

illness/injury prevention, 1:110

medication administration, 1:302–303

needs/expectations regarding death, 1:33

physical examination, 2:167–174

temperament, 1:514

therapeutic communication, 1:498

Children. *See also,* Pediatrics

Chitosan, 4:105

Chlamydia, 3:650

Chloride (Cl), 1:193

Choanal atresia, 5:10

Cholecystitis, 1:212, 3:402–404

Cholera, 5:538

Cholinergic, 1:333, 1:336–337

Chordae tendoneae, 3:75

Chromatin, 1:173, 1:175

Chromosomes, 1:186

Chronic alcohol ingestion, 3:504–506

Chronic alcoholic, 3:505

Chronic ambulatory peritoneal dialysis (CPAD), 3:434–435

Chronic bronchitis, 3:40–41

Chronic carbon monoxide poisoning, 3:463

Chronic gastroenteritis, 3:389

Chronic hypertension, 3:733

Chronic lymphocytic leukemia (CLL), 3:536

Chronic mucocutaneous candidiasis, 1:273

Chronic myelogenous leukemia (CML), 3:536–537

Chronic obstructive pulmonary disease (COPD), 3:3–4, 3:23–24, 5:179–180

Chronic renal failure (CRF), 3:430–435

Chronotropy, 3:82

Chyme, 4:456

CID, 4:396

Ciguatera (bony fish) poisoning, 3:485, 3:498

Cilia, 1:173, 3:5

Cincinnati Prehospital Stroke Scale (CPSS), 3:299–300

Circadian rhythms, 1:37

Circle of Willis, 3:275, 3:276

Circular muscle, 3:387

Circulation assessment, 2:207–210

Circulatory overload, 1:450

Circulatory system, 1:213–216, 2:137

Circumcision, 3:421

Circumduction, 4:228

Circumflex artery, 3:76

Cirrhosis, 3:386

CISD, 1:40

CISM, 1:40, 5:393

Citizen involvement in EMS, 1:91

Civil law, 1:122

Civil rights, 1:129

CK, 5:195

Cl, 1:193

Clamp, 1:436–437

Clan labs, 5:487

Clandestine drug laboratories, 5:487–488

Class IA drugs, 1:351

Class IB drugs, 1:351

Class IC drugs, 1:352

Classic pathway, 1:258

Claudication, 3:215

Clavicle, 4:232, 4:267

Cleaning, 1:29

Cleft lip, 5:10

Cleft palate, 5:10

Clinical decision making, 2:246–258
clinical judgment, 2:248

critical decision process, 2:256–258

critical thinking skills, 2:250–254

paramedic practice, 2:248–250

patient acuity, 2:249–250

protocols/algorithms, 2:250

thinking under pressure, 2:255–256

Clinical judgment, 2:248

Clitoris, 3:694, 3:695, 3:696

CLL, 3:536

Clonal diversity, 1:245, 1:249

Clonal selection, 1:245, 1:249

Clonic phase, 3:303

Closed-ended questions, 2:6

Closed fracture, 4:243

Closed incident, 5:371

Closed pneumothorax, 4:425–426

Closed questions, 1:495
Closed stance, 1:493
Clostridium botulinum, 1:235
Clostridium tetani, 1:235
Clot formation, 3:522
Clotting system, 1:258
CML, 3:536–537
CN-I, 2:146
CN-II, 2:149
CN-III, 2:149, 2:150
CN-IV, 2:150
CN-IX, 2:154
CN-V, 2:150–153
CN-VI, 2:150
CN-VII, 2:153
CN-VIII, 2:153
CN-X, 2:154
CN-XI, 2:154
CN-XII, 2:154
CNS. *See* Central nervous system (CNS)
    circulation, 4:288
    dysfunction, 3:59
    medications, 1:319–331
    stimulants, 1:324
Co-morbidity, 4:406
CO-oximetry, 3:464
CO poisoning, 3:291
CO poisoning treatment algorithm, 3:466
Coagulation, 4:91
Coagulation cascade, 1:259
Coagulation necrosis, 4:191
Coagulation system, 1:258
Coagulative necrosis, 1:187
Coarctation of the aorta, 5:9
Cobra perilaryngeal airway (PLA), 1:613
Coccygeal nerve, 4:361
Coccygeal spine, 4:356
Coccyx, 4:347, 4:356
Code of Ethics, 1:93, 1:153
Code of Hammurabi, 1:51
Cognitive disorders, 3:669

Cohort studies, 1:650
Cold diuresis, 3:565
Cold-protective response, 5:422–423
Cold (green) zone, 5:461
Cold (safe) zone, 5:460
Colic, 3:394
Collagen, 4:151
Collagen synthesis, 4:151
Collateral circulation, 3:77
Collecting duct, 3:415, 3:416
Colles' fracture, 4:267
Collision evaluation, 4:41
Colloids, 1:200, 1:433
Colorectal cancer, 1:210
Colorimetric end-tidal CO_2 detector, 1:560, 3:30
Colormetric tubes, 5:458
Colostomy, 5:249, 5:296
Column injury, 4:368
Coma, 3:281
Combined alpha/beta antagonists, 1:356
Command, 5:369–378
Command staff, 5:375
Comminuted fracture, 4:244
Commission on Accreditation of Air Medical Services (CAAMS), 5:354
Commission on Accreditation of Ambulance Services (CAAS), 5:339
Common bile duct, 3:384
Common law, 1:121
Commotio cordis, 4:432
Communicable, 3:602
Communicable period, 3:603
Communication, 1:96, 2:8–9, 2:262–282
    defined, 2:265
    EMS response, 2:269–275
    regulation, 2:282
    reporting procedures, 2:280–282

technology, 2:276–280
    terminology, 2:268
    verbal, 2:266–267
    written, 2:267–268
Community-acquired infections, 3:440
Community involvement, 1:90–91
Community trauma center, 4:11
Comorbidity, 5:160
Comparative negligence, 1:128
Compartment syndrome, 4:154–155, 4:240, 5:514, 5:156
Compassionate touch, 1:494
Compensated shock, 1:222, 4:117–118, 5:103–104
Compensation, 1:222
Compensatory mechanisms, 1:215
Competent, 1:132
Competitive antagonism, 1:313
Complement system, 1:258
Complete abortion, 3:728
Complete cord transection, 4:370
Complex partial seizures, 3:304
Compliance, 1:556
Compression, 4:26
Concealment, 5:490
Concentration, 1:477
Conception, 3:718
Concussion, 4:305
Concussion of the cord, 4:369
Conduction, 3:548
Conduction abnormalities, 3:245–255
Conductive deafness, 5:241
Conductivity, 3:89
Condyloid joints, 4:228
Confidence interval, 1:656

Confidentiality, 1:130–132, 1:160–162
Confined-space hazards, 5:425–427
Confined-space protections in the workplace, 5:428
Conflict resolution, 1:155–158
Confounding variable, 1:650
Confusion, 3:665
Congenital, 5:107
Congenital heart disease, 5:107
Congestive heart failure (CHF), 5:198
Congregate care, 5:154
Conjunctiva, 4:295
Connective tissue, 1:176, 4:73
Consensual reactivity, 4:321
Consensus standards, 5:366
Consent, 1:132, 1:162
Consequentialism, 1:153
Constipation, 5:164
Constitutional law, 1:121
Contact and cover, 5:491
Contained incident, 5:371
Contaminated food, 3:485–486
Contamination, 3:602
Contamination zone, 5:460
Contemplative approach, 5:318
Continuing education, 1:98
    pediatrics, 5:43–44
Continuous positive airway pressure (CPAP), 1:86, 3:201–202, 3:203, 5:281, 5:289
Continuous quality improvement (CQI), 1:73
CONTOMS, 5:493
Contraceptives, 3:701

Contractility, 3:89
Contraction, 1:266
Contracture, 1:267
Contralateral, 4:358
Contrecoup injuries, 4:303
Contributory negligence, 1:128
Control study, 1:651
Control zone, 5:460
Controlled breathing, 1:39
Contusion, 4:239–240
Contusions, 4:143–144
Convection, 3:548
Convenience sampling, 1:651
Conventional reasoning, 1:518
Convergent, 2:254
Coordination of transport, 1:58
COPD, 3:3–4, 3:23–24, 5:179–180
Copperhead bite, 3:494
Cor pulmonale, 3:38, 5:282
Coral snake bite, 3:494, 3:496–497
Cord injury, 4:368–370
Cord laceration, 4:369
Cord transection, 4:369
Cordarone, 5:168
Core body temperature (CBT), 3:551
Core temperature, 3:549
Cormack and LeHane classification system, 1:625
Cornea, 4:295
Coronary arteries, 3:76, 4:416
Coronary arteriogram, 5:190
Coronary artery bypass grafting (CABG), 5:190
Coronary artery disease, 1:211
Coronary circulation, 3:78
Coronary heart disease (CHD), 3:71

Corpus luteum, 3:715
Corrected QT (QTc), 3:95
Corrosives, 5:465
Cortex, 3:414
Corticosteroids, 3:369, 5:206
Corticotropin-releasing factor (CRF), 1:277, 1:278
Cortisol, 1:280
Cough reflex, 4:410
Cough suppressants, 1:367
Coughing, 1:554
Counseling, 1:108
Counter-current heat exchange, 3:550
Coup injuries, 4:302
Coupling interval, 5:139
Cover, 5:490
Coxsackie virus, 5:107
CPAP, 1:86, 3:201–202, 3:203, 5:281, 5:289
CPEM, 5:44
CPK, 5:195
CPSS, 3:299–300
CQI, 1:73
Crackles, 1:556, 2:88, 3:27
Cramping, 4:241
Cranial injury, 4:300–302
Cranial nerves, 2:146–155, 3:279, 4:289–290
Cranium, 4:284–285
Cravat, 4:160
Creatine kinase (CK), 5:195
Creatine phosphokinase (CPK), 5:195
Creatinine, 3:418
Crepitus, 2:111, 3:25
Crew assignments, 5:407
CRF, 1:277, 1:278, 3:430–435
Cribbing, 5:514
Cricoid cartilage, 1:534, 1:536, 1:617, 3:5
Cricoid pressure, 1:537, 1:566–567, 4:325–326
Cricothyroid membrane, 1:534, 1:537, 1:617, 3:5

Cricothyrotomy, 4:70, 4:330–331
Crime scene awareness, 5:478–497
    body armor, 5:492
    clandestine drug laboratories, 5:487–488
    contact/cover, 5:491
    cover/concealment, 5:490
    dangerous scenes, 5:481–482, 5:483–488
    distraction/evasion, 5:490
    domestic violence, 5:488
    drug-related crimes, 5:486–487
    EMS and police operations, 5:494
    evidence preservation, 5:495–497
    highway encounters, 5:484
    retreat, 5:489
    safety tactics, 5:488–491
    scene approach, 5:480–483
    tactical considerations, 5:488–494
    tactical EMS, 5:492–494
    tactical patient care, 5:491–494
    violent street incidents, 5:484–486
    warning signals/communications, 5:491
Criminal abortion, 3:729
Criminal law, 1:122
Critical care transport, 1:9–10
Critical Incident Stress Debriefing (CISD), 1:40
Critical Incident Stress Management (CISM), 1:40, 5:393
Critical thinking, 2:256
Crohn's disease, 1:212, 3:394–396

Cross-sectional study, 1:649
Cross-trained individuals, 1:6
Croup, 3:638, 5:96–97
Crowning, 3:725
Crumple zone, 4:36
Crush injuries, 4:55–56, 4:144, 4:156
Crush points, 5:515
Crush syndrome, 4:144, 4:157–158
Crux, 5:456
Crystalloids, 1:200, 1:433
Crystodigin, 1:359
CSF, 2:234, 3:14, 3:272
Cullen's sign, 2:101, 2:218, 3:382
Cultural considerations
    blood loss/transfusion, 4:509
    cardiovascular disease, 3:72
    cultural responses to illness/injury, 1:152
    diabetes, demographics, 3:337
    eye contact, 1:494
    geriatrics, 5:153
    immunizing at-risk populations, 1:111
    infant baptism, 5:36
    medicinal practices of the Hmong, 5:227
    metric system, 1:473
    prenatal care, 3:723
    race/sex risk factors, 3:404
    racial bias and analgesia, 3:534
    religious/cultural beliefs, 1:133
    respecting patient's beliefs/customs, 2:30
    responses to death, 5:31
    smoking, 3:37
    therapeutic communications, 1:502
Cultural imposition, 1:502
Cumbersome PPE, 5:442

Current, 4:189

Current of injury, 3:232

Cushing's disease, 1:374

Cushing's reflex, 4:308

Cushing's syndrome, 3:350, 3:351

Cushing's triad, 3:289, 4:309

Customer satisfaction, 1:74

Cutting the umbilical cord, 5:13–14

CVD, 3:71

Cyanide, 3:468–471

Cyanokit, 4:211, 4:212

Cyanosis, 1:553, 3:21, 5:30–31, 5:61

Cyanotic spell, 5:107

Cystic duct, 3:384

Cystic fibrosis (CF), 5:255–256, 5:282

Cystic medial necrosis, 3:216

Cystitis, 3:439, 3:705

Cytochrome oxidase, 5:466

Cytokine, 1:174, 1:251, 1:263

Cytoplasm, 1:174, 1:175

Cytoskeleton, 1:173, 1:174, 1:175

Cytosol, 1:173, 1:174

Cytotoxic, 1:174, 1:250

Cytotoxin, 1:174

D_5W, 1:201, 1:434

$D_{50}W$, 1:377

DAI, 4:305

Daily stress, 1:39

Dalton's law, 3:571–572

Dams, 5:421

DAN, 3:578

Dangerous materials incidents. See Hazardous materials incidents

Dangerous scenes, 5:481–482, 5:483–488

Date rape drugs, 5:232

Dead space volume, 4:412

Dead space volume (V_D), 1:548

Deadly intersection, 5:348–350

Deafness, 5:241, 5:242

Death, 1:526

Death and dying, 1:31–35

Death in the field, 1:142–143

Debridement, 1:265

Deceleration, 4:25

Decerebrate, 2:201

Decerebrate posturing, 3:288

Decision making. See Clinical decision making

Decode, 1:490

Decompensated shock, 1:222, 4:118, 5:104

Decompensation, 1:180, 1:222–223

Decompression, 1:632

Decompression illness, 3:573, 3:574–576

Decontamination, 3:451, 3:511

Decontamination of equipment, 1:28–31

Decorticate, 2:201

Decorticate posturing, 3:288

Decubitus ulcers, 5:195–196

Deep tendon reflexes (DTRs), 2:163

Deep venous thrombosis, 3:218

Defamation, 1:131

Defendant, 1:122

Defibrillation, 3:172–175

Degenerative neurologic disorders, 3:313

Degloving injury, 4:147

Degranulation, 1:256

Dehydration, 1:190, 3:557–558

Delayed effects, 5:464

Delayed hypersensitivity, 1:250

Delayed hypersensitivity reactions, 1:268, 3:361

DeLee suction trap, 5:12

Delirium, 2:22, 3:669, 5:188–189

Delirium tremens (DTs), 3:505–506

Delta wave, 5:150

Deltoid, 1:427

Delusions, 3:670

Demand valve device, 1:637

Dementia, 2:22, 3:669, 5:189–190

Demifacets, 4:354

Demobilized, 5:375

Demographic, 5:341

Demyelination, 5:283

Denature, 4:187

Dendrites, 3:269

Dens, 4:351

Deontological method, 1:153

Deoxyhemoglobin, 3:15

Department of Health and Human Services (DHHS), 3:596

Depersonalization, 3:675

Deployment, 5:337

Depolarization, 3:87

Depression, 3:672, 5:208

Dermatologic drugs, 1:382

Dermatome, 3:277

Dermatome chart, 2:161

Dermatomes, 3:278, 4:362

Dermis, 4:139–140, 4:185–186

Descending colon, 3:384, 3:400

Descending limb of the Loop of Henle, 3:416

Descending loop of Henle, 3:415

Descending tracts, 4:358

Descriptive statistics, 1:654–655

Descriptive studies, 1:649

Desensitization, 3:371

Desired dose, 1:476

Detailed physical exam, 2:231–238

Devascularization, 4:225

Dextran, 1:200, 1:433

Dextrose, 4:336–337

DHHS, 3:596

Diabetes insipidus, 3:331

Diabetes mellitus, 1:210, 1:374–375, 3:337, 3:338, 5:192

Diabetic ketoacidosis, 3:341–346, 5:117

Diabetic retinopathy, 5:243

Dialysate, 3:434

Dialysis shunts, 5:292–293

Diapedesis, 1:261

Diaphoresis, 3:21

Diaphragm, 3:4, 3:10, 4:409, 4:463

Diaphragmatic hernia, 5:10, 5:28–29

Diaphragmatic infarct, 3:243

Diaphragmatic perforation, 4:435–436

Diaphysis, 4:225

Diarrhea, 1:369
  newborn, 5:35

Diastole, 2:93, 3:79

Diastolic blood pressure, 2:45, 4:110

Diazepam, 4:273–274, 4:335, 5:171

DIC, 3:540

Diencephalon, 3:273

Diet-induced thermogenesis, 3:548

Dietary supplements, 1:382–386

Differential field diagnosis, 2:3, 2:252

Differentiation, 1:176

Difficult airway, 1:620

Difficult child, 1:514

Diffuse axonal injury (DAI), 4:305

Diffusion, 1:194, 1:195, 1:305, 1:306, 1:544, 3:14–15, 3:19

DiGeorge syndrome, 1:272

Digestion aid drugs, 1:370

Digestive system, 2:99

Digestive tract, 4:456, 4:457
Digital communications, 2:277
Digital intubation, 1:590–594, 4:328
Digitalis, 5:171, 5:203
Digitoxin, 1:359
Digoxin, 1:353, 1:359, 5:171, 5:203
Digoxin toxicity, 5:203–204
Diltiazem, 5:168
Dilution, 5:468
Diplomacy, 1:97
Diplopia, 4:312
Direct pressure, 4:93
Direct vasodilators, 1:358
Directed intubation, 4:328–329
Dirty bomb, 5:530
Disaster management, 5:391
Disaster mental health services, 1:40, 5:393–394
Disasters, 5:377
Discovery, 1:123
Disease period, 3:603
Disentanglement, 5:409, 5:414–415
Disinfectant, 1:397
Disinfecting, 1:29
Disinfection, 3:611
Dislocation, 4:242
Dislocation at the sternoclavicular joint, 4:423
Dislodged teeth, 4:340
Disposal, 5:468
Disposal of contaminated materials, 4:521
Disruption of the trachea, 4:436
Dissecting aortic aneurysms, 3:216
Disseminated intravascular coagulation (DIC), 3:540
Dissociate, 1:192
Dissociative disorders, 3:675

Distal tubule, 3:415, 3:416
Distance factor, 5:508–509
Distracting injuries, 5:313
Distraction, 5:490
Distributive shock, 1:223, 4:119, 5:105
Diuresis, 3:340, 3:418
Diuretic, 1:207, 1:354, 2:14, 5:202–203
Diuretics, 4:334
Divergent, 2:254
Diver's Alert Network (DAN), 3:578
Diverticula, 3:396
Diverticulitis, 3:396–397
Diverticulosis, 3:396, 5:193
Diving injury immobilization, 4:397–398
Dizziness, 5:188
Do Not Attempt Resuscitation (DNAR) orders, 5:279
Do Not Resuscitate (DNR) order, 1:139, 1:141–142, 1:158–159, 5:156
Dobutamine, 5:90, 5:169
Dobutrex, 5:169
Documentation, 1:89, 1:144–145, 2:286–312
    abbreviations/acronyms, 2:292–297
    administrative, 2:289
    airway management, 1:639–641
    alterations, 2:301–302
    closing, 2:311–312
    completeness/accuracy, 2:299
    inappropriate documentation, 2:311
    incident times, 2:297
    legal, 2:289–290
    legibility, 2:299–301
    medical, 2:288
    multiple-casualty incidents, 2:309–311

    narrative writing, 2:302–307
    oral statements, 2:298
    patient refusals, 2:307–309
    professionalism, 2:302
    research, 2:289
    special considerations, 2:307–311
    terminology, 2:292
    timeliness, 2:301
Documented danger, 5:483
Domestic abuse, 5:223
Domestic violence, 5:488
Dopamine, 5:25, 5:90, 5:169
Dopamine antagonists, 1:370
Dorsal gluteal, 1:427
Dorsal root, 3:278
Dorsiflexors, 2:124
Dosage on hand, 1:477
Dose packaging, 1:301
Dosimeter, 4:194, 5:530
DOT paramedic curriculum, 1:8
Double blinding, 1:651
Down-and-under pathway, 4:35
Down-regulation, 1:313
Down syndrome, 5:251, 5:252
Downed lines, 5:430
Downtime, 3:212
Drag, 4:63
Dressings/bandage, 4:158–160, 4:171
Drip chamber, 1:435
Drip rate, 1:435
Driving safety, 1:108
Dromotropy, 3:82
Drop former, 1:436
Drowning, 3:567–571, 5:123
Drug, 1:293, 1:395. See also Pharmacology
Drug abuse, 5:206–207
Drug Information, 1:294
Drug overdose, 3:500
Drug-related crimes, 5:486–487

Drug-response relationship, 1:316
Drugs, 1:395
Dry dressings, 4:159
Dry drowning, 3:568
Dry gangrene, 1:187
Dry lime, 4:214
Dry mouth syndrome, 3:504
DTRs, 2:163
DTs, 3:505–506
Ductus arteriosus, 3:722, 5:5
Ductus venosus, 3:722, 5:5
Due regard, 5:345–346
Dugas' sign, 2:119
Duodenal colic adhesion, 3:400
Duodenum, 3:384, 3:386, 3:400, 4:456, 4:457
Duplex, 2:276
Dura mater, 3:270, 3:278, 4:286, 4:358
Duramorph, 4:336
Duration of action, 1:316
Duty to act, 1:126
Duty to report, 1:143
Dynamic steady state, 1:276
Dysmenorrhea, 2:18, 3:700
Dyspareunia, 3:700
Dysphagia, 5:160
Dysphoria, 5:208
Dysplasia, 1:183
Dyspnea, 1:554, 2:17, 3:23, 4:51
Dysrhythmia, 1:349–350, 3:103–153
    atria, 3:113–123
    AV junction, 3:123–124
    children, 5:108–110
    classification, 3:104
    conduction disorders, 3:149–151
    elderly persons, 5:184
    electrolyte abnormalities, 3:151–153
    hypothermia, 3:153
    impulse formation, 3:103–104

Dysrhythmia, *(contd.)*
pulseless electrical
activity, 3:148–149
SA node, 3:105–113
sick sinus syndrome,
3:112–113
sinus arrest, 3:108–110
sinus block, 3:110–111
sinus bradycardia,
3:104–105, 3:106
sinus dysrhythmia, 3:108
sinus pause, 3:111
sinus tachycardia,
3:105–107
ventricles, 3:134–148
Dystonias, 3:213
Dysuria, 3:705

Ear injury, 4:313
Ear medications, 1:371
Early adulthood,
1:519–520
Early discharge, 1:111
Ears, 2:72–77
Easy child, 1:514
Eating disorders, 3:676
EBM, 1:75
EBV, 3:636
Ecchymosis, 4:143
ECF, 1:189
ECG. *See*
Electrocardiogram
(ECG)
ECG leads, 3:91–92,
3:222–226
augmented, 3:92,
3:224–225
bipolar, 3:91, 3:224
Einthoven's triangle,
3:91, 3:224
lead aVF, 3:101, 3:224,
3:226
lead aVL, 3:101, 3:224,
3:226
lead aVR, 3:101, 3:224,
3:226
lead I, 3:101, 3:224, 3:226
lead II, 3:101, 3:224,
3:226
lead III, 3:101, 3:224,
3:226
lead V_1, 3:101, 3:225

lead V_2, 3:101, 3:226
lead V_3, 3:101, 3:226
lead V_4, 3:101, 3:226
lead V_5, 3:101, 3:226
lead V_6, 3:101, 3:226
precordial, 3:92,
3:225–226
12-lead angles, 3:226
unipolar, 3:92,
3:224–225
Eclampsia, 3:733, 3:734
Ecstasy, 3:503
Ectopic beat, 3:103
Ectopic focus, 3:103
Ectopic pregnancy, 3:706,
3:729–730
EDC, 3:719
EDD, 1:563
Eddies, 5:421
Edema, 1:196–197, 2:141,
4:308
Education, 5:310
certification levels,
1:65–66
EMS providers,
5:105–106, 5:343
initial, 1:64
professional journals,
1:68
rural EMS, 5:504–505,
5:506
Effacement, 3:736
Effector, 1:179
Efferent, 3:277
Efficacy, 1:312
Egg cell, 3:696
Egophony, 2:91, 3:49
EGTA, 1:614
Einthoven, Willem, 3:90,
3:222
Einthoven's triangle,
3:91
Ejaculatory duct, 3:420
Ejection fraction, 3:80
Elastic bandage, 4:160
Elastin fibers, 1:539, 3:8
Elbow, 2:115, 2:118
Elbow extensors, 2:116
Elbow injuries, 4:271
Elderly patients. *See*
Geriatrics; Late
adulthood

therapeutic
communication, 1:501
Elderly persons. *See*
Geriatrics
Elective abortion, 3:729
Electric power, 5:431
Electrical alternans, 4:434
Electrical burns,
4:189–191, 4:212–213
Electricity, 5:427
Electrocardiogram
(ECG), 3:90–103
axis deviation,
3:227–229
corrected QT, 3:95
defined, 3:90
ECG recording,
3:220–222
graph paper, 3:93–94
leads, 3:91–92, 3:100,
3:222–226. *See also*
ECG leads
prehospital ECG
monitoring,
3:256–260
prolonged QT interval,
3:99
QRS axis, 3:227
QT interval, 3:95
rhythm strips,
3:101–103
routine ECG
monitoring, 3:92–93
12-lead ECG, 3:230
Electrolytes, 1:191–193,
3:85
Electromechanical pump
tubing, 1:437
Electronic $ETCO_2$
detectors, 1:560,
3:31–32
Electrophysiology,
3:85–90
Elimination problems,
5:164
Ellipsoidal joints, 4:228
Emancipated minor,
1:133
Emboli, 1:450,4:51
Embolic strokes, 3:296
Embryonic stage, 3:719
EMD, 1:63, 2:273

Emergency department
closures, 1:68
Emergency doctrine,
1:133
*Emergency Medical
Abstracts,* 1:664
Emergency medical
dispatcher (EMD),
1:63, 2:273
*Emergency Medical
Services: At the
Crossroads,* 1:57
*Emergency Medical
Services (EMS),* 1:68
Emergency Medical
Services for Children
(EMSC), 5:44
Emergency medical
services (EMS) system,
1:49. *See also* EMS
system
Emergency Medical
Services Systems Act,
1:54
Emergency medical
technician-basic (EMT-
B), 1:65
Emergency medical
technician-
intermediate (EMT-
Intermediate), 1:66
Emergency Medical
Technician-Paramedic
(EMT-Paramedic),
1:66
*Emergency Response
Guidebook* (ERG),
5:457, 5:533
Emergent phase, 4:189
Emesis, 1:369–370, 5:276
Empathy, 1:95, 1:489
Emphysema, 3:38–40,
5:281–282
*EMS Agenda for the
Future,* 1:55–56
EMS communications
officer, 5:390
EMS dispatch, 1:63–64
EMS Level 1 training,
5:451
EMS Level 2 training,
5:451

EMS patient refusal
 checklist, 1:136
EMS stresses, 1:39–40
EMS system, 1:47–77
 communications,
  1:62–64
 education/certification,
  1:64–68
 future directions,
  1:55–57
 history, 1:51–55
 local/state-level
  agencies, 1:59
 medical direction,
  1:59–61
 patient transportation,
  1:68–71
 public information and
  education, 1:61–62
 quality assurance and
  improvement, 1:72–74
 receiving facilities,
  1:71–72
 research, 1:75–76
 system financing,
  1:76–77
 twenty-first century,
  1:57–59
EMS timeline, 1:52
EMSC, 5:44
EMT-B, 1:65
EMT Code of Ethics, 1:93
EMT-Intermediate, 1:66
EMT-Paramedic, 1:66
EMT-Paramedic:
 National Standards
 Curriculum, 1:7, 1:8,
 1:64
EMT-Tacticals (EMT-Ts),
 5:493
EMT-Ts, 5:493
Encephalitis, 3:641–642
Encephalitis-like agents,
 5:538
Encode, 1:489
End-diastolic volume,
 3:80
End-stage renal failure,
 3:430
End-tidal carbon dioxide
 (ETCO$_2$) detector,
 2:49–50

End-tidal CO$_2$ (ETCO$_2$),
 1:558–563, 3:30
End-tidal CO$_2$ detector,
 1:561
Endocardium, 3:74, 4:417
Endocrine glands, 1:179,
 3:326
Endocrine signaling, 1:179
Endocrine system, 1:178
 geriatrics, 5:174–175
 late adulthood, 1:523
Endocrine system
 medications,
 1:371–379
 adrenal cortex, 1:374
 estrogens/progestins,
  1:377
 female reproductive
  system, 1:377–378
 hypoglycemic agents,
  1:377
 infertility agents, 1:378
 insulin preparations,
  1:375–376
 male reproductive
  system, 1:378–379
 oral contraceptives,
  1:377–378
 oral hypoglycemic
  agents, 1:376–377
 pancreas, 1:374–377
 parathyroid/thyroid
  glands, 1:373–374
 pituitary gland,
  1:372–373
 sexual behavior, 1:379
 uterine
  stimulants/relaxants,
  1:378
Endocrinology,
 3:323–353
 Addison's disease,
  3:352–353
 adrenal glands,
  3:334–335
 anatomy/physiology,
  3:326–337
 blood glucose
  determination,
  3:344–345
 Cushing's syndrome,
  3:351–352

diabetes mellitus,
 3:338–341
diabetic emergencies,
 3:342, 3:343
diabetic ketoacidosis,
 3:341–346
endocrine
 disorders/emergencies,
 3:337–353
endocrine system,
 3:328–329
gonads, 3:335–336
HHNK coma,
 3:346–347
hypothalamus,
 3:327–330
hypothyroidism/myxed
 ema, 3:349–350
pancreas, 3:333–334
parathyroid glands,
 3:333
pineal gland, 3:336
pituitary gland,
 3:330–332
thymus gland, 3:333
thyroid gland, 3:332
thyroid gland disorders,
 3:347
thyrotoxic crisis,
 3:348–349
Endogenous pyrogen,
 1:263
Endometriosis,
 3:705–706
Endometritis, 3:705
Endometrium, 3:696,
 3:697, 3:715
Endoplasmic reticulum,
 1:175
Endorphins, 1:319–320
Endotoxins, 1:235–236,
 3:598
Endotracheal intubation,
 1:604–606, 4:327–330
children, 5:78–83
Endotracheal tube
 (ETT), 1:407, 1:563,
 1:575–577
Enema, 1:413
Energy-absorbing
 bumpers, 5:431
Energy conservation, 4:24

Engine compartment,
 5:432
Engulfment, 5:427
Enrollment shortages,
 5:504
Enteral drug
 administration,
 1:407–414
gastric tube, 1:410–412
oral, 1:408–410
rectal, 1:412–414
Enteral route, 1:310
Enterotoxin, 3:485
Entrance wound, 4:76–77
Enucleation, 5:243
Environmental
 considerations, 5:314
Environmental
 emergencies,
 3:544–586
defined, 3:547
diving emergencies,
 3:571–578
drowning, 3:567–571
fever, 3:558
frostbite, 3:566–567
heat/cold, 3:548
heat disorders,
 3:551–558
heatstroke, 3:556–557
high altitude illness,
 3:578–582
homeostasis, 3:547–548
hyperthermia,
 3:551–552
hypothermia,
 3:559–566
nuclear radiation,
 3:582–586
pressure disorders,
 3:574–578
thermogenesis (heat
 gain), 3:548
thermolysis (heat loss),
 3:548–549
thermoregulation,
 3:549–551
trench foot, 3:567
EOA, 1:614
Eosinosphil, 1:198, 1:262,
 3:517, 3:518
Ephephysis, 4:226

Epicardium, 3:74, 4:416
Epidemiology, 1:104, 4:6
Epidermis, 4:139, 4:185
Epidermoid carcinoma, 3:52
Epididymis, 3:420
Epidural hematoma, 4:304
Epidural space, 3:278
Epiglottis, 1:534, 1:536, 1:612, 1:617, 3:4, 3:5, 3:637–638, 5:98–99
Epilepsy, 3:302
Epinephrine, 1:277–278, 3:334, 3:368, 5:25, 5:89, 5:90, 5:168
Epiphyseal fracture, 4:245
Epiphyseal plate, 4:226
Epistaxis, 4:96, 5:185
Epithelial tissue, 1:176
Epithelialization, 1:266, 4:151
EPS, 1:326
Epstein-Barr virus (EBV), 3:636
Equipment decontamination, 1:28–31
disposal of contaminated equipment/sharps, 1:398
essential, 5:337
hazardous materials incidents, 5:471–473
IV access, 1:433–441
level A hazmat protective equipment, 5:471
level B hazmat protective equipment, 5:471–473
level C hazmat protective equipment, 5:473
level D hazmat protective equipment, 5:473
malfunction, 5:272
PPE, 1:24, 2:188, 5:403–407
rescue awareness and operations, 5:403–407

resuscitation, 1:26
standards, 5:338
take-in, 5:316
transportation, 5:442
vehicle stabilization, 5:435
Equipment decontamination, 1:28–31
Equipment malfunction, 5:272
ERG, 5:457, 5:533
ERV, 1:549, 3:12–13
Erythema, 4:143, 5:532
Erythroblastosis fetalis, 3:525
Erythrocyte, 1:174, 1:198, 3:514, 4:89
Erythropoiesis, 3:515
Erythropoietin, 3:419, 3:513, 4:115
Eschar, 4:199
Escorts, 5:347
Esophageal detector device (EDD), 1:563
Esophageal gastric tube airway (EGTA), 1:614
Esophageal obturator airway (EOA), 1:614
Esophageal tracheal combitube, 1:607–609, 2:205
Esophageal varices, 3:386–387, 4:97, 5:193
Esophagus, 1:534, 1:612, 3:5, 3:384, 3:386, 3:400, 4:417
Essential equipment, 5:337
Estimated date of confinement (EDC), 3:719
Estrogens, 1:377
ETCO$_2$, 1:558–563, 3:30
ETCO$_2$ detector, 2:49–50
Ethical relativism, 1:152
Ethics, 1:74, 1:149–166
code of ethics, 1:153
confidentiality, 1:160–162
conflict resolution, 1:155–158

consent, 1:162
decision making, 1:152–153
fundamental principles, 1:154
fundamental questions, 1:153–154
impact on individual practice, 1:153
obligation to provide care, 1:163–164
professional relations, 1:164–166
relationship to law and religion, 1:151–152
research, 1:151
resource allocation, 1:162–163
resuscitation attempts, 1:158–160
teaching, 1:164
Ethmoid air cells, 3:6
Ethnocentrism, 1:502
Etomidate, 4:335
ETT, 1:407, 1:563, 1:575–577
ETT size, 1:600
Eukaryotes, 1:173
Eustachian tubes, 1:535
Evaporation, 3:549
Evasion, 5:490
Evidence base, 1:58
Evidence-based medicine (EBM), 1:75
Evidence preservation, 5:495–497
Evisceration, 4:466
evisceration care, 4:480
Exam techniques. See Physical examination
Excitability, 3:89
Excited delirium, 3:681–682
Exclusionary zone, 5:460
Exertional metabolic rate, 3:550, 3:551
Exit wound, 4:77
Exocrine, 5:282
Exocrine glands, 1:179, 3:326
Exotoxins, 1:235, 3:485, 3:597

Expectorant, 1:367
Experimental studies, 1:650
Expiration, 3:11
Expiratory reserve volume (ERV), 1:549, 3:12–13, 4:411
Explosion, 4:45
Explosives, 5:527–528
Exposure, 1:30
Expressed consent, 1:132–133
Extended, remote, or wilderness protection, 5:406
Extension tubing, 1:437
External jugular vein IV access, 1:444–446
External respiration, 4:109
Extracellular compartment, 1:189
Extracellular fluid (ECF), 1:189
Extramedullary hematopoiesis, 3:512
Extrapyramidal symptoms (EPS), 1:326
Extrauterine, 5:5
Extravasation, 1:449
Extravascular, 1:459
Extravascular space, 4:189
Extremities, 4:74
Extrication, 5:389, 5:413
Extrinsic ligament, 1:536
Extrinsic risk factors, 3:4
Extubation, 1:550
Exudate, 1:261
Eye contact, 1:494
Eye injury, 4:314–315, 4:338–399
Eye protection, 5:405, 5:406
Eyes, 2:62–72
Eyewear, 1:25
EZ-IO, 1:469

Facial bones, 2:62, 4:291
Facial injury, 4:310–312
Facial nerve, 2:150, 4:290

Facial soft-tissue injury, 4:311

Facial trauma. *See* Neck, facial, and neck trauma

Facial wounds, 4:79

Facilitated diffusion, 1:195, 1:304, 3:417

Facilities Unit, 5:378

Facsimile machine (fax), 2:278

Factitious disorders, 3:675

Fail-safe franchise, 1:76

Fainting, 5:185

Fallopian tube, 3:696, 3:697, 4:460

Fallout, 5:529

Falls, 4:53–54, 5:162

False imprisonment, 1:137

Falx cerebri, 4:287

Family history, 1:209

Farm machinery, 5:511, 5:512

FAS, 5:229, 5:251–252

Fascia, 4:94

Fasciae, 4:141

Fasciculations, 4:334, 5:531

Fasciculus, 4:235

Fast-break decision making, 5:469

F.A.S.T.1, 1:469

Fatigue, 4:240

Fatigue fracture, 4:245

Fatty change, 1:186

Fatty necrosis, 1:187

Fax, 2:278

FBAO
 children, 5:48, 5:71, 5:77–78, 5:99–100, 5:102–103

FCC, 2:282

FDA pregnancy categories, 1:302

Fear, 3:665

Febrile seizures, 5:113

Fecal-oral route, 3:601

Federal Communications Commission (FCC), 2:282

Federal court system, 1:122

Federal Emergency Management Agency (FEMA), 3:596

Feedback, 1:490

Feet, 2:120–123, 2:125

FEMA, 3:596

Female genitalia, 2:103–105

Female reproductive system, 1:377–378, 2:100

Femoral arteries, 4:462

Femoral nerve, 3:277

Femur, 4:233

Femur fractures, 4:264–266

Fentanyl, 4:274, 4:336, 5:170

Fertilized ovum, 3:715

Fetal alcohol syndrome (FAS), 5:229, 5:251–252

Fetal circulation, 3:720–722

Fetal development, 3:718–720

Fetal heart tones (FHTs), 3:719

FEV, 1:549, 3:13

Fever, 3:558
 newborn, 5:32–33

FHTs, 3:719

Fibrin, 1:258, 4:91

Fibrinolysis, 3:523

Fibrinolytic, 1:362

Fibrinolytic agents, 5:170–171

Fibroblasts, 1:264, 4:151

Fibrosis, 5:173

Fibrous pericardium, 4:416

Fibula, 4:234

Fibular fractures, 4:266

Fick Principle, 1:218

Field diagnosis, 2:248, 2:304

Field examination, 2:183–245
 airway assessment, 2:201–205

AVPU levels, 2:200–201

breathing assessment, 2:206–207

circulation assessment, 2:207–210

comprehensive exam, 2:232–238

isolated-injury trauma patient, 2:221

location of all patients, 2:195–196

major trauma patient, 2:211–220

mechanism of injury, 2:196–197

mental status, 2:200

nature of illness, 2:197–198

ongoing assessment, 2:238–241

priority determination, 2:210–211

responsive medical patient, 2:222–229

scene safety, 2:190–194

standard precautions, 2:188–190

unresponsive medical patient, 2:230–231

Field extubation, 1:606–607

Field pronouncements, 1:34

Fight-or-flight, 1:36

Filtrate, 3:416

Filtration, 1:196, 1:305

Fimbriae of fallopian tube, 3:696

Finance, 5:377–378

Financing EMS system, 5:76–77

Finger fractures, 4:272

FiO₂, 1:545

Fire and fuel, 5:430–431

Firewall, 5:432

First-degree burn, 4:196

First-pass effect, 1:309

First responder, 1:65

Fitness, 1:107–108

5 percent dextrose in water (D_5W), 1:201, 1:434

Fixed facilities, 5:453

Fixed-wing aircraft, 5:351. *See also* Air medical transport

Flagella, 1:175

Flail chest, 1:552, 3:18, 4:423–424, 4:444–445

Flame/flash protection, 5:405–406

Flammable/explosive limits, 5:461

Flanks, 3:414

Flash point, 5:461

Flashback chamber, 1:440

Flat effect, 3:670

Flat water, 5:421–425

Flechettes, 4:48

Flight-or-fight response, 4:511

Flow regulator, 1:437

Fluency disorders, 5:246

Fluid shift phase, 4:189

Focal clonic seizures, 5:32

Focused history and physical exam, 2:211

Follicle-stimulating hormone (FSH), 1:518, 3:332

Fontanelles, 1:512

Food poisoning, 3:640–641

Foot injuries, 4:270

Foot protection, 5:405

Foramen ovale, 5:5

Force, 4:25

Forced expiratory volume (FEV), 1:549, 3:13

Forebrain, 3:273

Foreign bodies, 1:550

Foreign body airway obstruction. *See* FBAO

Formable splints, 4:257

Fossa ovalis, 5:5

Fractured humerus, 4:267

Fractures, 4:242–246

Frank-Starling mechanism, 1:214

FRC, 1:549, 3:13

Free drug availability, 1:303

French, 1:568

Freshwater drowning, 3:569

Frontal impact, 4:34–36

Frontal sinuses, 3:4, 3:6

Frostbite, 3:566–567

FSH, 1:518, 3:332

Fugue state, 3:675

Full-body vacuum mattress, 4:397

Full-body vacuum splint, 4:397

Full thickness burn, 4:197, 4:204, 4:205

Functional impairment, 5:160

Functional residual capacity (FRC), 1:549, 3:13, 4:412

Fundus of uterus, 3:696

Fungus, 3:599

Furosemide, 5:171

GABA, 1:322–323

Gaffiti, 5:486

Gag reflex, 1:536

Galea aponeurotica, 4:284

Gallbladder, 3:384, 3:403, 4:457, 4:458

Gamma-aminobutyric acid (GABA), 1:322–323

Gamma globulin therapy, 1:274

Gamma-hydroxybutyrate (GHB), 5:232

Gamma radiation, 4:193, 5:463

Ganglionic blocking agents, 1:338, 1:359

Ganglionic stimulating agents, 1:339

Gangrene, 4:153, 5:270

Gangrenous necrosis, 1:187

Gangs, 5:485–486

GAS, 1:275–276

Gas gangrene, 1:187, 4:153

Gastric arteries, 3:386

Gastric distention, 1:632

Gastric feeding tubes, 5:137

Gastric lavage, 3:452

Gastric tube administration, 1:410–412

Gastritis, 5:193

Gastrocolic adhesion, 3:400

Gastroenteritis, 3:639–640, 5:115

Gastroenterology, 3:375–407

accessory organ diseases, 3:401–407

acute gastroenteritis, 3:387–388

appendicitis, 3:401–402

bowel obstruction, 3:399–401

cholecystitis, 3:402–404

chronic gastroenteritis, 3:389

Crohn's disease, 3:394–396

diverticulitis, 3:396–397

esophageal varices, 3:386–387

hemorrhoids, 3:397–398

hepatitis, 3:405–407

lower GI bleeding, 3:392

lower GI diseases, 3:391–401

pancreatitis, 3:404–405

pathophysiology, 3:378–380

patient assessment, 3:380–383

peptic ulcers, 3:389–391

treatment, 3:383

ulcerative colitis, 3:392–394

upper GI bleeding, 3:384–386

upper GI diseases, 3:383–391

Gastrointestinal bleeding, 5:193–194

Gastrointestinal disorders, 1:212

Gastrointestinal system, 1:177

geriatrics, 5:175

late adulthood, 1:523

pregnancy, 3:717–718

Gastrointestinal system drugs, 1:367–370

Gastroepiploic artery, 3:386

Gastrostomy tubes, 5:137

Gauge, 1:415

Gauze bandages, 4:160

GBS, 3:59, 5:269, 5:283–284

GCS. *See* Glasgow Coma Scale (GCS)

Geiger counter, 3:583, 4:194, 5:530

General adaptation syndrome (GAS), 1:275–276

General impression, 2:198

Generalized seizures, 3:302, 3:303

Genes, 1:186

Genetics, 1:207–213

Genital warts, 3:649

Genitalia, 4:459–460

Genitofemoral nerve, 3:277

Genitourinary system, 1:177, 3:413

geriatrics, 5:176–177

Geriatric abuse, 5:210–211

Geriatrics, 1:110, 1:501, 5:146–217. *See also* Late adulthood

abuse/neglect, 5:210–211

alcohol abuse, 5:207

altered mental status, 5:168–169

Alzheimer's disease, 5:190

angina pectoris, 5:182–183

aortic dissection/aneurysm, 5:184–185

AS, 5:197–199

bowel obstruction, 5:194

burns, 5:214

cardiomuscular system, 5:173

communication, 1:501

communication difficulties, 5:162, 5:163, 5:166–169

COPD, 5:179–180

defined, 5:152

delirium, 5:188–189

dementia, 5:189–190

depression, 5:208

diabetes mellitus, 5:192

dizziness, 5:188

drug abuse, 5:206–207

dysrhythmias, 5:184

elder abuse, 5:223–225

elimination problems, 5:164

endocrine system, 5:174–175

falls, 5:162

gastrointestinal system, 5:175

genitourinary system, 5:176–177

GI hemorrhage, 5:193–194

head/spinal injuries, 5:214–215

heart failure, 5:183–184

hematology, 5:177

hypertension, 5:185

hyperthermia, 5:201

hypothermia, 5:200

illness/injury prevention, 1:110

immune system, 5:177

incontinence, 5:163–164

inflammation, 1:267

integumentary system, 5:175–176

lung cancer, 5:182

medication administration, 1:303–304

mesenteric infarct, 5:194

multiple-system failure, 5:160

musculoskeletal system, 5:176

myocardial infarction, 5:183

nervous system, 5:174

orthopedic injuries, 5:212–214

osteoarthritis, 5:196

osteoporosis, 5:196–197

Parkinson's disease, 5:190–191, 5:205

patient assessment, 5:165–166

physical exam, 5:169

pneumonia, 5:178–179

pressure ulcers, 5:195–196

prevention/self-help, 5:157–159, 5:163

pulmonary edema, 5:182

pulmonary embolism, 5:180–182

renal disorders, 5:199

renal system, 5:176

respiratory system, 5:170–173

seizure, 5:188

shock trauma resuscitation, 4:517–519

skin disease, 5:194–195

stroke, 5:187

suicide, 5:209–210

syncope, 5:185–186

thermoregulatory system, 5:175

thyroid disorders, 5:192

toxicological emergencies, 5:201–206

urinary disorders, 5:199–200

vertigo, 5:188

German measles, 1:25, 3:634

Gerontology, 5:152

Gestational diabetes, 3:735

GFR, 3:416

GH, 1:280, 3:332

GHB, 5:232

GHIH, 3:330

GHRH, 3:330

GI/GU crisis, 5:270, 5:294–298

GI hemorrhage, 5:193–194

GI system infections, 3:639–641

Glans, 3:420

Glasgow Coma Scale (GCS), 3:289, 4:322–323, 4:505

adult, 3:290

children, 3:290, 5:66, 5:67–68

Glass ampules, 1:416, 1:417

Glaucoma, 1:371, 5:166, 5:243

Gliding joints, 4:228

Global aphasia, 5:245

Glomerular filtration, 3:416

Glomerular filtration rate (GFR), 3:416

Glomerulonephritis, 5:199

Glomerulus, 3:415, 3:416

Glossopharyngeal nerve, 2:151, 4:290

Glottic function, 5:22

Glottic opening, 1:534, 3:5, 3:7

Glottis, 1:537

Gloves, 1:25, 5:405

Glucagon, 1:375, 3:333, 4:110

Glucocorticoids, 1:365, 3:335, 4:115

Glucometers, 2:51

Gluconeogenesis, 1:220, 3:334

Glucose, 5:89

Glucose intolerance, 3:431

Gluteus muscles, 2:132

Glycogen, 4:115

Glycogenolysis, 1:220, 3:333, 4:115

Glycolysis, 4:108

Glycosuria, 3:340

Gold standard, 5:337

Golden Hour, 5:508

Golden Period, 4:13–14

Golgi apparatus, 1:173, 1:175

Gonadotropin, 1:518

Gonads, 3:335–336

Gonorrhea, 3:646–647

Good Samaritan laws, 1:125, 1:128

Gout, 1:211, 4:248

Governmental immunity, 1:128

Gram-negative bacteria, 1:235

Gram-positive bacteria, 1:235

Gram stains, 1:235, 3:597

Granulation, 1:265

Granulocyte maturation, 3:518

Granulocytes, 1:174, 1:262, 3:517 4:150

Granuloma, 1:264

Graves' disease, 1:271, 3:347–348

Gray matter, 4:358

Great vessels, 4:414, 4:417

Greater auricular nerve, 3:277

Greater curvature of stomach, 3:386

Green treatment unit, 5:387

Green zone, 5:461

Greenstick fractures, 4:245, 5:129

Grey Turner's sign, 2:101, 2:218, 3:382

Grief, 1:32

Groshong catheters, 5:291

Growth hormone (GH), 1:280, 3:332, 4:115

Growth hormone inhibitory hormone (GHIH), 3:330

Growth hormone releasing hormone (GHRH), 3:330

Growth plate, 5:54

Guarding, 4:469

Guillain-Barré syndrome (GBS), 3:59, 5:269, 5:283–284

Gunshot wounds, 4:464

Gurgling, 1:555

Gynecology, 3:691–709

anatomy/physiology, 3:693–698

female reproductive organs, 3:694–698

gynecological abdominal pain, 3:703–707

menstrual cycle, 3:698–699

patient assessment, 3:699–702

sexual assault, 3:707–709

H. pylori, **1:368, 3:391**

H_2 receptor antagonists, 1:368

Habbits, 1:20–21

Habitual abortion, 3:729

HACE, 3:581, 3:582

Haddon, William, 5:274

Haddon matrix, 4:6, 4:8

Hair, 2:55–58

Hairline fracture, 4:244

Hairy cell leukemia, 3:536

Half-life, 3:583

Hallucinations, 3:670

Halo test, 4:301

Hand, 2:112

Hand-held electronic CO_2 detector, 1:561

Hand injury, 4:272

Hand washing, 1:27

Handgun, 4:67

Hansen's disease, 1:381

Hantavirus, 3:638–639

HAPE, 3:581

Haptens, 1:242

Hashimoto's thyroiditis, 3:519

Hate crimes, 5:485

Haversian canals, 4:225

Hawking, Stephen, 5:246

Hawthorne effect, 1:651

Hazard control,
5:410–411
Hazardous atmosphere
rescues, 5:425–429
Hazardous cargoes, 5:431
Hazardous materials,
5:511
Hazardous materials
incidents, 5:446–474
approaches to
decontamination,
5:468–471
chemical asphyxiants,
5:466–467
contamination and
toxicology review,
5:463–467
corrosives, 5:465
hazardous materials
zones, 5:460–461
hazmat protection
equipment, 5:471–473
hydrocarbon solvents,
5:467
incident size-up,
5:451–461
medical monitoring and
rehabilitation,
5:473–474
NFPA 704 System, 5:456
pesticides, 5:466
practice, 5:474
pulmonary irritants,
5:465–466
role of the paramedic,
5:450–451
specialized terminology,
5:461–463
substance
identification,
5:456–459
terrorism, 5:453–454
Hazardous terrain
rescues, 5:436–443
*Hazardous Waste
Operations and
Emergency Response
Standard (2004)*, 5:450
Hazmat suits, 5:406
HBO therapy, 3:460,
3:468
HBOCs, 1:200, 1:434–435

hCG, 3:336
HCO₃, 1:193
HDLs, 1:362
Head, 2:60–62, 4:76
Head injury
children, 5:126–127,
5:127–128
Head rests, 4:33
Head-tilt, 5:59
Head-tilt/chin-lift, 1:565,
2:202, 5:59
Headache, 3:308–310
Health care professional,
1:66
Health Insurance
Portability and
Accountability Act
(HIPAA), 1:131
Health maintenance
organization (HMO),
1:163
Health of paramedic. *See*
Well-being of
paramedic
Hearing and respiratory
protection, 5:406
Hearing protection, 5:405
Heart, 2:93, 3:73–77,
4:415–417
Heart failure, 3:196–202,
5:183–184
Heart rate, 3:287
Heart rate calculator
rulers, 3:101
Heat cramps, 3:553, 3:554
Heat disorders,
3:551–558
Heat Escape Lessening
Position (HELP),
5:418
Heat exhaustion, 3:554,
3:555
Heat illness, 3:551
Heat loss, 3:548–549
Heat stress factors, 5:474
Heatstroke, 3:554, 3:556,
5:200, 5:201
HEENT, 2:17
Helicobacter pylori, 1:368,
3:391
Helicopter transport,
4:521–527

Helicopters, 1:69, 5:351.
See also Air medical
transport
rural EMS, 5:509
Helmet removal,
4:389–390
Helmets, 5:404–405,
5:406
Helminthiasis, 1:381
HELP, 5:418
Hematemesis, 2:18,
3:385, 4:467, 4:97
Hematochezia, 3:388,
4:103, 4:467
Hematocrit, 1:199, 3:516,
4:89
Hematologic disorders,
1:210–211
Hematology, 3:510–541
anemias, 3:533–534
blood products/blood
typing, 3:524–526
defined, 3:512
disseminated
intravascular
coagulation, 3:540
hemophilia, 3:538–539
hemostasis, 3:521–524
leukemia, 3:536–537
leukopenia/neutropenia
, 3:536
lymphomas, 3:537–538
multiple myeloma,
3:540
patient
assessment/manageme
nt, 3:526–532
plasma, 3:513–514
platelets, 3:520
polycythemia,
3:535–536
red blood cell diseases,
3:532–536
red blood cells,
3:514–516
sickle cell anemia,
3:534–535
thrombocytopenia,
3:538
thrombocytosis, 3:538
transfusion reactions,
3:526

Von Willebrand's
disease, 3:539–540
white blood cell
diseases, 3:536–538
white blood cells,
3:516–520
Hematoma, 4:94, 4:144
Hematopoiesis, 3:512
Hematuria, 2:18, 4:467
HemCon, 4:105
Hemochromatosis, 1:210
Hemoconcentration,
1:464
Hemodialysis, 3:434
Hemoglobin, 1:198, 3:15,
3:514, 4:89
Hemoglobin-based
oxygen-carrying
solutions (HBOCs),
1:200, 1:434–435
Hemolysis, 1:464, 3:516
Hemophilia, 1:210,
3:538–539
Hemopneumothorax,
4:428
Hemoptysis, 2:17, 3:23,
4:51, 4:96, 4:430, 5:282
Hemorrhage, 4:86–107
additional assessment
considerations, 4:103
arteries, 4:88
blood, 4:89
capillaries, 4:88–89
classification, 4:90
clotting, 4:90–92
defined, 4:86
direct pressure, 4:104
elevation, 4:105
external, 4:93–94
focused physical exam,
4:102
heart, 4:86–87
initial assessment, 4:101
internal, 4:94–96
ongoing assessment,
4:103
pressure points, 4:106
rapid trauma
assessment, 4:101–102
scene size-up, 4:99–101
specific wound
considerations, 4:107

stage 1, 4:97
stage 2, 4:98
stage 3, 4:98
stage 4, 4:98–99
topical hemostatic
agents, 4:104–105
tourniquets, 4:106
transport
considerations, 4:107
vascular system,
4:87–89
veins, 4:89
Hemorrhagic strokes,
3:296
Hemorrhoids, 3:397–398
Hemostasis, 1:360–361,
3:521–524, 4:149
Hemothorax, 1:545, 3:18,
4:428–429, 447
Henry's law, 3:572
Hepa respirator, 1:25,
1:27
Heparin lock, 1:456
Hepatic alteration, 1:412
Hepatic flexure, 3:400
Hepatitis, 3:405–407,
3:619–622
Hepatitis A, 3:620
Hepatitis B, 1:25, 3:610,
3:620–621
Hepatitis C, 1:25, 3:621
Hepatitis D, 3:621
Hepatitis E, 3:622
Hepatitis G, 3:622
Hepatomegaly, 5:184
Hereditary disorders,
1:210–211
Hering-Breuer reflex,
1:546, 3:14
Hernia, 3:399
Herniation, 5:28
Herpes simplex virus
type 1, 3:637
Herpes simplex virus
type 2, 3:649
Herpes zoster, 5:195
Hespan, 1:200, 1:433
Hetastarch, 1:200, 1:433
HEVs, 5:435
HF acid, 3:474–475
HHNK coma, 3:346
Hiatal hernia, 5:175

Hiccoughing, 1:554
Hiccups, 1:554
Hickman catheters, 5:291
High altitude, 3:578
High altitude cerebral
edema (HACE), 3:581,
3:582
High altitude illness,
3:578–582
High altitude pulmonary
edema (HAPE), 3:581
High-angle/low-angle
evacuation, 5:440
High-angle rescues,
5:436–437
High-density
lipoproteins (HDLs),
1:362
High-energy wounds,
4:420
High-pressure regulators,
1:633
High-pressure tool
injuries, 4:157
Highway encounters,
5:484
Highway operations,
5:429–436
Highway
operations/vehicle
rescues, 5:429–436
Hilum, 3:9, 3:414
Hinge joints, 4:227
Hip dislocation, 4:268
Hip flexors, 2:131
Hip joint, 2:130
HIPAA, 1:131
Hips, 2:126–128, 2:133
Hispanic families, 1:501
Histamine, 1:257, 1:366,
3:362, 4:111
Histamine poisoning,
3:485
Histocompatibility locus
antigens, 1:243
History taking, 2:1–23
angry patients, 2:21
anxious patients,
2:20–21
asking questions, 2:6–7
blindness, 2:23
chief complaint, 2:11

communication, 2:8–9
confusing behaviors,
2:22
crying, 2:21
current health status,
2:14–17
depression, 2:22
hearing problems, 2:23
intoxication, 2:21
introductions, 2:5–6
language, 2:8–9, 2:23
limited intelligence,
2:22–23
multiple symptoms,
2:20
overly talkative patients,
2:20
past history, 2:13–14
preliminary data,
2:10–11
present illness, 2:11–13
rapport, 2:4–10
reassurance, 2:21
review of systems,
2:17–19
sensitive topics, 2:9–10
sexually attractive
patient, 2:22
silence, 2:19–20
HIV, 1:236, 3:610,
3:615–619
HLA antigens, 1:243
HMO, 1:163
Hmong, 4:509
Hodgkin's lymphoma,
3:538
Hollow-needle catheter,
1:440
Hollow organ injury,
4:466–467
Home artificial
ventilators, 5:136
Home care, 5:263–302
acute infections, 5:298
ALS intervention, 5:301
artificial
airways/tracheostomie
s, 5:286–288
asthma, 5:282
bronchitis, 5:281–282
bronchopulmonary
dysplasia, 5:283

cardiac conditions,
5:294
cystic fibrosis, 5:282
emphysema, 5:281–282
epidemiology,
5:266–275
GI/GU crisis, 5:294–298
GI tract devices,
5:295–298
home oxygen therapy,
5:284–286
home ventilation,
5:288–289
hospice and comfort
care, 5:300–302
maternal care,
5:298–300
neuromuscular
degenerative diseases,
5:283–284
newborn care,
5:298–300
patient assessment,
5:275–280
respiratory disorders,
5:280–291
sleep apnea, 5:284
tracheostomy,
5:286–287
vascular access devices,
5:291–294
Home oxygen therapy,
5:284
Home safety inspection
form, 4:488
Home ventilation,
5:288–289
Homeostasis, 1:178,
3:326, 3:547–548, 4:86
Hookworms, 3:600
Hormone actions, 1:372
Hormone replacement
therapy (HRT), 5:174
Hormones, 3:326
Hospice, 5:273
Hostile/uncooperative
patients, 1:503
Hot (red) zone, 5:460
HPO_4, 1:193
HRT, 5:174
HSV-2, 3:649
Hub, 1:440

Huber needle, 1:458
Human chorionic
    gonadotropin (hCG),
    3:336
Human
    immunodeficiency
    virus (HIV), 1:236,
    1:273–274, 3:610,
    3:615–619
Human studies, 1:299
Humerus, 4:232, 4:267
Humoral immunity,
    1:239, 1:240, 1:249,
    3:359, 3:519, 3:604
Huntington's disease,
    1:212
Hurricane Katrina, 5:365
Hybrid electric vehicles
    (HEVs), 5:435
Hydralazine, 1:358
Hydration, 1:189–190
Hydrocarbon solvents,
    5:467
Hydrocarbons, 3:475–476
Hydroelectric intakes,
    5:421
Hydrofluoric (HF) acid,
    3:474–475
Hydrolysis, 1:309
Hydrostatic pressure,
    1:196, 4:116
Hydroxocobalamin,
    4:211, 4:212
Hymenoptera, 3:358,
    3:450
Hyoid, 1:538, 3:7
Hyoid bone, 1:536, 1:617
Hyperadrenalism, 3:351
Hyperbaric oxygen
    chamber, 3:575
Hyperbaric oxygen
    (HBO) therapy, 3:460,
    3:468
Hyperbilirubinemia, 5:14
Hypercalcemia, 5:152
Hypercarbia, 1:546
Hyperglycemia, 3:339
    children, 5:117–119
Hyperglycemic
    hyperosmolar
    nonketotic (HHNK)
    coma, 3:346

Hyperkalemia, 5:152
Hypermetabolic phase,
    4:189
Hypernatremia, 1:193
Hyperosmolar, 3:417
Hyperplasia, 1:182
Hypersensitivity, 1:185,
    1:267, 3:361
Hypertension, 1:211,
    2:45, 5:185
Hypertensive
    emergencies,
    3:205–206
Hypertensive
    encephalopathy,
    3:205
Hyperthermia, 2:48,
    3:551–552, 5:201
Hyperthyroidism, 3:347
Hypertonic, 1:193, 1:433
    solutions, 1:201
Hypertrophy, 1:182,
    3:250, 5:173, 5:269
Hyperventilation
    syndrome, 3:57–59
Hyphema, 4:314
Hypnosis, 1:322
Hypo-osmolar, 3:417
Hypocalcemia, 5:152
Hypochondriasis, 5:208
Hypodermic needle,
    1:415
Hypoglossal nerve, 2:153,
    4:290
Hypoglycemia, 3:339,
    3:346–347
    children, 5:116–117
    newborn, 5:33–34
Hypoglycemic agents,
    1:377
Hypoglycemic seizure,
    3:347
Hypokalemia, 5:151
Hyponatremia, 1:193
Hypoperfusion,
    1:213–234, 4:508
    anaphylactic shock,
    1:228–230
    cardiogenic shock,
    1:224–225
    hypovolemic shock,
    1:225–227

multiple organ
    dysfunction
    syndrome, 1:232–234
    neurogenic shock,
    1:227–228
    pathophysiology,
    1:218–223
    physiology, 1:213–218
    septic shock, 1:231–232
Hypopharynx, 1:534, 3:5
Hypophyseal portal
    system, 3:330
Hypoplastic left heart
    syndrome, 5:9
Hypotension, 2:46
Hypothalamus, 3:273,
    3:274, 3:327–330,
    3:550, 4:288
Hypothermia, 2:48,
    3:559–566, 5:153,
    5:200
    newborn, 5:33
Hypothermia algorithm,
    3:563
Hypothyroidism,
    1:373–374, 3:347,
    3:349–350
Hypotonic, 1:193, 1:434
Hypotonic solutions,
    1:201
Hypoventilation, 1:545
Hypovolemia, 4:333,
    4:508
    newborn, 5:31
Hypovolemic shock,
    1:223, 1:225–227,
    4:119, 5:105
Hypotension, 4:508
Hypothermia, 4:509–510
Hypoxemia, 1:547, 4:412
Hypoxia, 1:183, 1:554,
    1:582, 3:19, 4:333
Hypoxic drive, 1:547,
    4:412

IAFF, 3:596
Iatrogenic deficiencies,
    1:273
IC, 5:369
ICF, 1:189
ICP, 4:284, 5:372
ICS, 5:366

IDDM, 1:374–375, 3:340
Idiopathic epilepsy, 3:302
Idioventricular rhythm,
    5:135
IDLH, 5:463
IDLs, 1:362
IFPA, 1:67
Ig, 3:239, 3:359, 3:605
IgA, 1:248
IgD, 1:248
IgE, 1:248
IgE reactions, 1:268–269
IgG, 1:248
IgM, 1:248
Ignition temperature,
    5:461
ILCOR universal cardiac
    arrest algorithm,
    2:251, 5:145
Ileocecal valve, 3:384
Iliac crests, 4:233
Ilial volvulus, 3:400
Iliohypogastric nerve,
    3:277
Ilioinguinal nerve, 3:277
Ilium, 4:232
Illness/injury prevention,
    1:102–113
    early discharge, 1:111
    EMS provider
    commitment,
    1:107–109
    epidemiology,
    1:104–105
    geriatric patients,
    1:110
    implementation of
    prevention strategies,
    1:112–113
    infants/children,
    1:109–110
    medications, 1:111
    motor vehicle collisions,
    1:110
    organizational
    commitment,
    1:105–106
    prevention in the
    community,
    1:109–113
    prevention within EMS,
    1:105–109

work/recreation hazards, 1:111

ILs, 1:263

Immediate evacuation, 5:318

Immediate hypersensitivity reactions, 1:268, 3:361

Immediately dangerous to life and health (IDLH), 5:463

Immobilization children, 5:88–92, 5:125

Immune-complex-mediated reactions, 1:269–270

Immune response, 1:238–253, 3:359
aging, 1:253
allergy, 1:267
antigens/immunogens, 1:241–243
autoimmunity, 1:268
blood group antigens, 1:243–244
cell-mediated, 1:249–252
defined, 1:238
fetal/neonatal immune function, 1:252–253
histocompatibility locus antigens, 1:243
humoral, 1:245–249
humoral *vs.* cell-mediated immunity, 1:239–240
hypersensitivity, 1:267–272
immunity deficiencies, 1:272–275
isoimmunity, 1:268
lymphocytes and the lymph system, 1:240–241
natural *vs.* acquired immunity, 1:239
primary *vs.* secondary immune responses, 1:239
stress, and, 1:280–283

Immune senescence, 5:177

Immune system, 3:359
geriatrics, 5:177
infants, 1:511
infectious diseases, 3:604
toddlers/preschoolers, 1:515

Immune thrombocytopenic purpura (ITP), 1:272

Immunity, 1:125, 1:238, 1:381

Immunization schedule (0-6 years), 1:383

Immunization schedule (7-18 years), 1:384

Immunizing at-risk populations, 1:111

Immunogens, 1:241–243

Immunoglobulin (Ig), 1:239, 3:359, 3:605

Impacted fracture, 4:244

Impaired hemostasis, 4:154

Impaired peripheral perfusion, 2:138

Impaled objects, 4:80, 4:146, 4:340

Impartiality test, 1:158

Impetigo, 3:652

Implied consent, 1:133

Improvisation, 5:442–443

Impulse control disorders, 3:678

Impulsive, 2:254

IMS, 5:366

IMV, 5:283

In-line IV fluid heaters, 1:439–441

In-water patient immobilization, 5:423–425

In-water spinal immobilization, 5:423–425

Inadequate tissue perfusion, 5:188

Incapacitating agents, 5:534

Incendiary agents, 5:528

Incidence, 1:208

Incident command post (ICP), 5:372

Incident Command System (ICS), 5:366

Incident Commander (IC), 5:369

Incident management. *See* Medical incident management

Incident Management System (IMS), 5:366

Incisions, 4:146

Incomplete abortion, 3:728

Incontinence, 5:163–164

Incubation period, 1:24, 3:603

Incubator, 5:26

Indeterminate axis, 3:227

Index case, 3:595

Index of suspicion, 2:197, 4:13

Induced active immunity, 3:360

Induced passive immunity, 3:360

Induction agents, 1:598

Industrial medicine, 1:10

Inertia, 4:23

Inevitable abortion, 3:728

Infant baptism, 5:36

Infants, 1:509–514, 5:48. *See also* Pediatrics
dosage calculations, 1:481
illness/injury prevention, 1:110
physical examination, 2:167–174

Infarction, 1:184, 3:236, 3:399

Infarction localization grid, 3:236, 3:237

Infection, 3:602, 4:151–153, 5:270–271
children, 5:93–94

Infection injury, 4:158

Infectious disease exposure procedure, 1:30

Infectious diseases, 3:591–656
bacteria, 3:597–598
body's defenses, 3:603–606
chickenpox, 3:627–629
complement system, 3:605
contraction/transmission/ disease stages, 3:601–603
defined, 3:594
GI system infections, 3:639–641
hepatitis, 3:619–622
HIV, 3:615–619
immune system, 3:604–605
individual host immunity, 3:606
infection control, 3:607–613
lymphatic system, 3:605–606
meningitis, 3:629–631
microorganisms, 3:596–601
nervous system infections, 3:641–646
nosocomial infections, 3:654
patient assessment, 3:613–615
patient education, 3:654
personal protection, 1:24
pneumonia, 3:625–626
preventing transmission, 3:654–656
public health agencies, 3:596
public health principles, 3:595
SARS, 3:626–627
skin diseases, 3:651–654
STDs, 3:646–651
tuberculosis, 3:622–625
viruses, 3:598–599

Infectious injury, 1:184–185

Inferential statistics, 1:656

Inferior articular facets, 4:348

Inferior gluteal nerves, 3:277

Inferior infarct, 3:239

Inferior lobe, 3:4

Inferior nasal concha, 4:291

Inferior turbinate, 3:6

Inferior vena cava, 3:414, 4:462

Infertility agents, 1:378

Infestation, 3:652

Inflammation, 1:254–267
  acute inflammatory response, 1:255–256
  cellular components, 1:261–263
  cellular products, 1:263
  chronic inflammatory responses, 1:264
  defined, 1:254
  geriatric patients, 1:267
  immune response, contrasted, 1:254
  local inflammatory responses, 1:264–265
  mast cells, 1:256–257
  neonates, 1:267
  plasma protein systems, 1:258–261
  resolution and repair, 1:265–267
  systemic responses to acute inflammation, 1:263–264

Inflammatory process, 3:520

Influenza, 1:25, 3:631

Information officer (IO), 5:376–377

Informed consent, 1:132

Infranodal, 5:127–128

Infusion, 1:421

Infusion controller, 1:459

Infusion pumps, 1:460

Infusion rate, 1:479, 1:480

Ingested toxins, 3:453–455

Ingestion, 3:448

Inhalation, 1:404, 3:449

Inhalation injury, 4:195, 4:210

Inhaled toxins, 3:455–456

Initial assessment, 2:198, 5:317–318

Injected toxins, 3:487–499

Injection, 1:404, 3:449–450

Injury, 1:104

Injury current, 3:232

Injury risk, 1:105

Injury-surveillance program, 1:105

Innate immunity, 3:360

Innominate, 4:232

Inotropy, 3:82

Insect bites, 3:488–493

Insertion, 4:235

Inspection, 2:31–32

Inspiration, 3:11

Inspiratory capacity, 4:412

Inspiratory reserve volume (IRV), 1:548, 3:12–13, 4:411

Institutional elder abuse, 5:224

Insufflate, 1:583

Insulin, 1:375, 3:333, 3:334, 4:110

Insulin-dependent diabetes mellitus (IDDM), 1:374–375, 3:340

Insulin preparations, 1:375–376

Insulin shock, 3:346–347

Integrity, 1:95

Integumentary system, 4:138

Intentional injury, 1:104

Interarytenoid notch, 1:612

Interatrial septum, 3:74, 3:75

Interbrain, 3:273

Intercalated discs, 3:85

Intercostal muscles, 3:10, 4:409

Intercostal space, 4:408

Interferon, 1:263

Interleukins (ILs), 1:263

Intermediate-density lipoproteins (IDLs), 1:362

Intermittent claudication, 2:19

Intermittent mandatory ventilation (IMV), 5:283

Internal carotid artery, 3:276

Internal respiration, 4:109

International Association of Firefighters (IAFF), 3:596

International Flight Paramedics Association (IFPA), 1:67

Interpersonal justifiability test, 1:158

Interpersonal relations, 1:41

Interpersonal zones, 1:492

Interpolated beat, 5:138

Intersection, 5:348–350

Interspinous ligament, 4:350

Interstitial fluid, 1:189

Interstitial nephritis, 3:428

Interstitial space, 3:9, 4:88

Intervener physician, 1:60

Intervention development, 4:8

Intervention studies, 1:650–653

Interventricular septum, 3:74

Intervertebral disc, 4:347

Interview techniques, 1:495–498

Intestinal volvulus, 3:400

Intoxication, 4:40

Intracatheter, 1:441

Intracellular compartment, 1:189

Intracellular fluid (ICF), 1:189

Intracellular parasites, 1:236

Intracerebral hemorrhage, 3:296, 4:304, 5:187

Intracranial hemorrhage, 3:294–302, 4:303

Intracranial perfusion, 4:306

Intracranial pressure (ICP), 4:284

Intractable, 5:188

Intradermal injection, 1:422–424

Intramedullary hematopoiesis, 3:513

Intramuscular injection, 1:427–430

Intramuscular injection sites, 1:427

Intraosseous (IO) infusion. See IO infusion

Intraosseous needle, 1:467

Intrapartum, 5:4

Intrarenal abscesses, 3:440

Intravascular fluid, 1:189

Intravascular space, 4:189

Intravenous bolus, 1:452–453

Intravenous cannulas, 1:440–441

Intravenous drug administration. See IV access

Intravenous drug infusion, 1:452, 1:454–456

Intravenous fluids, 1:433

Intravenous (IV) therapy, 1:197–202

Intraventricular septum, 3:75

Intrinsic ligament, 1:536

Intrinsic pathway, 1:260

Intrinsic risk factors, 3:3

Introitus, 3:694

Intropin, 5:169

Intubation, 1:536

Intussusception, 3:399

Invasion of privacy, 1:132
Inverted pyramid of
    neonatal resuscitation,
    5:15–16
Involuntary consent,
    1:133
IO, 5:376–377
IO infusion, 1:465–473
    children, 5:85–87
Ion, 1:192
Ion transport, 1:307
Ionization, 4:192
Ionize, 1:306
Ionizing radiation, 3:583
Ipsilateral, 4:358
Iris, 4:294
Iron, 3:484
Irreversible antagonism,
    1:314
Irreversible shock, 1:223,
    4:118, 5:104
IRV, 1:548, 3:12–13
Ischemia, 1:183, 1:184,
    4:116
Ischemic colitis, 5:194
Ischial tuberositatis,
    4:233
Ischium, 4:232
Islets of Langerhans,
    3:333
Isoimmune neutropenia,
    1:272
Isoimmunity, 1:268
Isolated-injury trauma
    patient, 2:221
Isolation, 5:468
Isolette, 5:26
Isometric exercise, 1:17
Isosthenuria, 3:430
Isotonic, 1:193, 1:433
Isotonic exercise, 1:17
Isotonic solutions, 1:201
ITLS spinal clearance
    protocol, 4:383
ITP, 1:272, 3:538
IV access, 1:430–465
    administration tubing,
        1:435–439
    blood tubing,
        1:446–449
    central venous access,
        1:432

drug administration,
    1:451–461
equipment/supplies,
    1:433–441
external jugular vein,
    1:444–446
flow rates, 1:449
hand/arm/leg access,
    1:442–444
in-line IV fluid heaters,
    1:439–441
measured volume
    administration set,
    1:446
medical solutions, 1:421
peripheral IV access
    complications,
    1:450–451
peripheral venous
    access, 1:431–432
    types, 1:431–433
venous blood sampling,
    1:461–465
IV therapy, 1:197–202

J wave, 3:562
Jackson's theory of
    thermal wounds, 4:188
Jargon, 2:302
Jaundice, 3:529
Jaw thrust, 1:565–566,
    5:60
Jehovah's Witnesses, 4:509
JEMS, 1:68
Joint, 4:227
Joint capsule, 4:229–230
Joint injury, 4:241–242
Joint structure,
    4:227–230
Joule's law, 4:189
*Journal of Emergency
    Medical Services
    (JEMS),* 1:68
*Journal of Pediatric
    Emergency Medicine,*
    1:68
*Journal of Trauma: Injury,
    Infection and Critical
    Care,* 1:68
JRA, 5:253
Jugular venous distention
    (JVD), 3:287

JumpSTART Pediatric
    MCI Triage Tool,
    5:138–141
JumpSTART System,
    5:381–384
Junctional bradycardia,
    5:132–133
Justice, 1:154
Juvenile rheumatoid
    arthritis (JRA), 5:253
JVD, 3:287

K, 1:193, 1:355
Katrina, 5:365
Keloid, 4:155
Kernig's signs, 3:630
Ketamine, 5:233
Ketone bodies, 3:339
Ketosis, 3:339
Kevlar, 5:492
KI tablets, 5:530
Kidney failure, 1:211
Kidney stones, 1:211,
    3:435–438
Kidneys, 3:414–419,
    4:458, 4:467
Killer bees, 3:488–489
Kinetic energy, 4:24–25,
    4:63
Kinetics, 4:23
King LT airway, 1:614
Kinin system, 1:260
KKK-A-1822 Federal
    Specifications for
    Ambulances, 1:69–71
Knee dislocation, 4:242
Knee extensors, 2:128
Knee flexors, 2:127
Knee injuries, 4:268–269
Knees, 2:124, 2:126–129
Knives, 4:69
Korotkoff sounds, 2:45
Korsakoff's psychosis,
    3:294
Krebs cycle, 4:108
Kübler-Ross, Elisabeth,
    1:31
Kussmaul's respirations,
    1:554, 3:19, 3:286, 3:343
Kussmaul's sign, 4:433
Kyphosis, 4:375, 5:172,
    5:376

Labia, 3:694
Labia majora, 3:694,
    3:695, 3:696
Labia minora, 3:694,
    3:695,3:696
Labor, 3:738–740
Laboratory-based
    simulations, 5:322
Labyrinthitis, 5:241
Lacerations, 4:145–146
Lacrimal bone, 4:291
Lacrimal fluid, 4:295
Lacrimal sac, 3:6
Lactated Ringer's, 1:201,
    1:434
Lactic acid, 4:93
Lactic dehydrogenase
    (LDH), 5:195
Lactose intolerance,
    1:212
Lamina propria, 1:538,
    3:7
Laminae, 4:348
Landing zone, 5:354–356
Landsteiner, Karl, 3:524,
    3:525
Language, 2:8–9, 2:23
Language disorders,
    5:245
Lanoxin, 1:353, 1:359,
    5:171, 5:203
LAPSS, 3:298–299
Large cell carcinoma,
    3:52
Large intestine, 4:457
Larrey, Jean, 1:51, 1:53
Laryngeal inlet, 1:612
Laryngeal Mask Airway
    (LMA), 1:611–613, 5:84
Laryngopharynx, 1:534,
    3:5, 3:6
Laryngoscope, 1:574
Laryngoscope blades,
    1:575
Laryngotracheobronchiti
    s, 5:96
Larynx, 1:534, 1:536–537,
    1:538, 3:4, 3:5, 3:7,
    3:384
Lasix, 5:171
Late adulthood,
    1:522–526

Latent period, 3:603
Lateral femoral
    cutaneous nerve, 3:277
Lateral impact, 4:36
Lateral marginal veins,
    3:77
Lawsuits, 1:128
Laxative, 1:369
LCt/LD, 5:463
LDH, 5:195
LDLs, 1:362–363
Le Fort criteria, 4:311,
    4:312
Lead, 3:485
Leadership, 1:94
*Leadership Guide to
    Quality Improvement
    for Emergency Medical
    Services Systems, A,*
    1:72
Leading questions, 1:495
LeChetalier's Principle,
    1:203
Left anterior hemiblock,
    3:251
Left atrium, 3:75, 3:77
Left axis deviation, 1:227
Left bundle branch, 3:89
Left bundle branch block,
    3:248, 3:252
Left coronary artery, 3:76
Left lung, 3:4
Left mainstem bronchus,
    1:538, 3:7
Left posterior hemiblock,
    3:250
Left primary bronchus,
    3:4
Left pulmonary arteries,
    3:77
Left pulmonary veins,
    3:77
Left ventricle, 3:75, 3:77
Legal considerations,
    1:117–144
  advance directives,
    1:139
  anatomy of a civil
    lawsuit, 1:122–123
  confidentiality,
    1:130–132
  consent, 1:132–138

crime/accident scenes,
    1:143
death in the field,
    1:142–143
DNR order, 1:141–142
documentation,
    1:144–145
duty to report, 1:143
ethics, 1:151
laws affecting
    EMS/paramedic,
    1:123–125
legal system, 1:121–122
liability, 1:120
living will, 1:140–141
negligence, 1:125–129
organ donation, 1:142
patient transportation,
    1:138
reasonable force, 1:138
resuscitation issues,
    1:139–143
special liability
    concerns, 1:129–130
Legal documentation,
    2:289–290
Legal notes
accidental needlesticks,
    1:414
back injuries, 1:22
children, 5:56
cost of trauma care,
    4:10
crime, terrorism and
    you, 4:62
cross-trained
    individuals, 1:6
drawing blood for law
    enforcement, 1:461
emergency department
    closures, 1:68
evidence preservation at
    crime scenes, 5:495
field pronouncements,
    1:34
gatekeeper to the health
    care system, 1:87
gynecological physical
    exam, 1:702
high risk for lawsuits,
    1:128
HIPAA, 1:131

home care, 5:267
intervening outside
    your EMS system,
    1:163
National Incident
    Management System
    (NIMS), 5:367
negligence/malpractice,
    1:581
9/11 and beyond, 1:72
patient restraint, 1:683
PCR, 2:312
pediatric abdominal
    trauma, 4:472
privacy and security,
    2:279
reporting contagious
    diseases, 1:595
rescue calls, routine
    calls and safety, 5:410
risk management
    strategy, 1:73
safety first, 1:315
spinal motion
    restriction (SMR),
    4:376
substance abuse in
    EMS, 1:21
transporting a burn
    victim, 4:207
WMD attacks, 5:539
Legislative law, 1:121
Leprosy, 1:381
Lesion, 2:54
Lesser cornu, 1:536
Lesser curvature of
    stomach, 3:386
Lesser occipital nerve,
    3:277
Lethal
    concentration/lethal
    doses (LCt/LD), 5:463
Leukemia, 3:536–537
Leukocyte, 1:174, 1:198,
    3:516, 3:604, 4:89
Leukocytosis, 3:536
Leukopenia, 3:536
Leukopoiesis, 3:517
Leukotrienes, 1:257, 1:365
Level A hazmat
    protective equipment,
    5:471

Level B hazmat protective
    equipment, 5:471–473
Level C hazmat
    protective equipment,
    5:473
Level D hazmat
    protective equipment,
    5:473
Level IV trauma facility,
    4:11
Lex talionis, 1:51
LH, 1:518, 3:332
Liability, 1:120
Liaison officer (LO),
    5:376
Libel, 1:131, 2:280, 2:302
Lice, 3:652
Licensure, 1:64, 1:124
Lidocaine, 5:89, 5:90,
    5:168, 5:202
Life-care community,
    5:154
Life expectancy, 1:522
Life-span development,
    1:507–526
  adolescence, 1:518–519
  early adulthood,
    1:519–520
  infants, 1:509–514
  late adulthood,
    1:522–526
  middle adulthood,
    1:520–522
  school age, 1:517–518
  toddler/preschoolers,
    1:514–517
Ligament of Treitz, 3:384,
    4:469
Ligaments, 4:229
Ligamentum arteriosum,
    4:417, 5:5
Ligamentum flavum,
    4:350
Ligamentum teres, 5:7
Ligamentus venosum, 5:5
Lighting, 5:406
Lightning strikes, 4:212
Lights and siren, 5:346–347
Limb presentation, 3:748
Limbic system, 3:273
Limited patient access,
    5:442

Lip abnormalities, 2:82
Lipolysis, 1:220
Liquefaction necrosis, 1:187, 4:191
Liquid oxygen, 5:285
Lithium, 3:479–481
Litmus paper, 5:458
Liver, 3:384, 4:456–458, 4:468
Living will, 1:140–141
LMA, 5:84
LO, 5:376
Lobes, 3:9
Local, 1:397
Local agencies, 1:59
Local effects, 5:464
Lock-out/tag-out, 5:511
Log roll, 4:391–392
Logistics section, 5:378
Long spine board, 4:395–397
Long-term decision making, 5:469–470
Longitudinal muscle, 3:387
Loniten, 1:358
Los Angeles Prehospital Stroke Screen (LAPSS), 3:298–299
Lou Gehrig's disease, 3:315
Low-angle/high-angle evacuation, 5:440
Low-angle rescues, 5:437–438
Low back pain (LBP), 3:316
Low-density lipoproteins (LDLs), 1:362–363
Lower airway anatomy, 1:537–540, 3:7–10
Lower extremity, 4:232–234
Lower gastrointestinal bleeding, 3:392
Lower gastrointestinal diseases, 3:391–394
Lower GI bleeding, 3:392, 5:193–194
Lumbar concavity, 4:348
Lumbar nerves, 4:361
Lumbar plexus, 3:277, 4:362

Lumbar spine, 4:354–355
Lumbar vertebrae, 4:347, 4:355
Lumbosacral plexus, 3:277
Lumen, 1:607, 3:79, 4:140
Lung cancer, 1:210, 3:51–53
Lung capacities, 3:13
Lung compliance, 3:12
Lung parychema, 1:539
Lung tissue, 1:538, 3:7
Lung transplants, 5:284
Lung volumes, 3:12, 4:411–412
Lungs, 3:9, 4:74, 4:410
Luteinizing hormone (LH), 1:518, 3:332
Lyme disease, 3:645–646, 4:248
Lymph, 3:605
Lymph node exam, 2:86
Lymph system, 1:240–241
Lymphangitis, 4:152
Lymphatic system, 1:178, 2:139, 3:605
Lymphocyte, 1:174, 1:198, 1:239, 3:517, 3:519, 3:604, 3:605, 4:140
Lymphokine, 1:251, 1:263
Lymphoma, 3:536–537
Lysosome, 1:173, 1:175

Maceration, 5:195
Machinery entrapment, 5:427
Macrodrip administration tubing, 1:435
Macrophage-activating factor (MAF), 1:263
Macrophages, 1:251, 1:262, 3:604, 4:140
MAD, 1:403
MAF, 1:263
Magill forceps, 1:579
Magnesium (Mg), 1:193
Magnesium sulfate, 5:89
Maine spinal clearance protocol, 4:382

Major basic protein (MBP), 3:518
Major histocompatibility complex (MHC), 1:243
Major incidents, 5:377
Major trauma patient, 2:211–220
Malaria, 1:380
Male genitalia, 2:106–107
Male genitourinary system, 3:420
Male reproductive system, 1:378–379, 2:101, 2:106
Malfeasance, 1:126
Mallampati classification system, 1:624
Malleolus, 4:234
Mallory-Weiss tear, 3:384, 5:193
Malpractice, 1:581
Mammalian diving reflex, 3:570, 5:423
Management choreography, 5:314–315
Mandible, 4:290, 4:291
Mandibular dislocation, 4:311
Manic, 3:673
Manic-depressive illness, 1:212–213
Mannitol, 4:334
Manometer, 2:36
Manual airway maneuvers, 1:565–568
Manual cervical immobilization, 4:386–388
Manubrium, 4:408
MAOIs, 1:329, 3:477–478
MAP, 4:89
Marfan syndrome, 5:175
Marginal artery, 3:76
Margination, 1:261
Marine animal injection, 3:497–498
Mark I kit, 5:532
Masks, 1:25, 3:624
Mass, 4:24
Mass casualty incident (MCI), 5:364

MAST, 1:68, 4:127
Mast cells, 1:256–257, 3:361
MAT, 3:114–115
Material safety data sheets (MSDS), 5:458, 5:459
Maternal care, 5:298–300
Maternal drug abuse, 5:229
Mathematics, 1:473–481
Maturation, 1:176, 1:266
Maxilla, 4:290
Maxillary bone, 4:291
Maxillary sinus, 3:6
Maximum life span, 1:522
MBP, 3:518
McBurney point, 3:402
MCI, 5:364, 5:392–394
MCL$_1$, 3:92–93
MD, 3:313, 5:256–257, 5:283
MDI, 1:405
MDMA, 5:233
Mean arterial pressure (MAP), 4:89
Measles, 3:633
Measured volume administration set, 1:438, 1:446, 1:447
Measures of central tendency, 1:654
Meatus, 3:5
Mechanism of injury, 2:196–197
Mechanism of injury (MOI), 1:85, 5:317
Mechanism of injury analysis, 4:12–13
Meconium, 5:12
Meconium staining, 3:751–752
Median nerve, 3:277
Mediastinum, 3:4, 4:414
Medicaid, 5:155, 5:157
Medical anti-shock trouser (MAST), 4:127
Medical calculations, 1:477
Medical direction, 1:54, 1:129

Medical director, 1:59
Medical documentation, 2:288
Medical equipment standards, 5:338
Medical incident management, 5:360–394
  command, 5:369–378
  command procedures, 5:373–375
  command staff, 5:376–377
  communications, 5:373, 5:390–391
  disaster management, 5:391–392
  division of operations functions, 5:378–380
  extrication/rescue unit, 5:389
  finance/administration, 5:377–378
  functional groups, 5:380–391
  identifying staging area, 5:372
  incident size, 5:370–371
  logistics, 5:378
  morgue, 5:386
  multiple casualty incidents, 5:392–394
  on-scene physicians, 5:387
  operations, 5:378
  origins, 5:366–369
  planning/intelligence, 5:378
  regulations/standards, 5:366–368
  REHAB unit, 5:390
  resource utilization, 5:373
  singular vs. unified command, 5:371–372
  staging, 5:388
  termination of command, 5:375
  transport unit, 5:388–389
  treatment, 5:386–387
  triage, 5:380–386

Medical supply unit, 5:378
Medically clean, 1:397
Medicare, 5:155
Medicated solutions, 1:421
Medication, 1:111, 1:395. See also Pharmacology
Medication administration, 1:391–481
  disposal of contaminated equipment/sharps, 1:398
  documentation, 1:398
  enteral, 1:407–414. See also Enteral drug administration
  general principles, 1:395–399
  intraosseous infusion, 1:465–473
  IV access, 1:430–465. See also IV access
  mathematics, 1:473–481
  medical asepsis, 1:397–398
  medical calculations, 1:477
  medical direction, 1:396
  metric system, 1:473–476
  oral medications dosage calculations, 1:477–481
  parenteral, 1:414–430. See also Parenteral drug administration
  percutaneous, 1:399–404
  pulmonary, 1:404–407
  standard precautions, 1:396–397
Medication atomization device (MAD), 1:403
Medication injection ports, 1:437
Medication packaging, 1:415–421
Medicine cup, 1:409
Medicine dropper, 1:409

Medium-duty rescue vehicle, 5:338
Medulla, 1:546, 3:13, 3:276, 3:414
Medulla oblongata, 3:274, 4:288
Medullary canal, 4:227
Melatonin, 3:336
Melena, 3:385, 4:97, 5:194
Memory cells, 1:245
Menarche, 3:698
Meniere's disease, 5:167
Meninges, 3:270
Meningitis, 1:25, 3:629–631, 5:114–115
Menopause, 3:699
Menorrhagia, 3:706
Menstrual cycle, 3:698–699
Mental health services, 1:40, 5:377
Mental status examination (MSE), 3:665, 3:667, 5:278–279
Mercury, 3:485
Mesencephalon, 3:274
Mesenteric infarct, 5:193, 5:194
Mesentery, 3:387, 4:463
Mesentery/bowel injury, 4:468–469
Metabolic acidosis, 1:206
Metabolic alkalosis, 1:207
Metabolism, 1:178, 1:308, 3:326, 4:108
Metacarpals, 4:232
Metal stylet, 1:440
Metals, 3:482–485
Metaphysis, 4:226
Metaplasia, 1:183
Metatarsals, 4:234
Metered dose inhalers (MDI), 1:405
Methamphetamine, 5:487
Methylxanthines, 1:365
Metric equivalents, 1:475
Metric prefixes, 1:474
Metric system, 1:473–476
Mg, 1:193
MHC, 1:243
MI, 5:183, 5:187–196

Microangiopathy, 3:427
Microcirculation, 1:215, 4:88
Microdrip administration tubing, 1:435
Microorganisms, 3:596–601
Microvilli, 1:173, 1:175
Midaxillary line, 4:408
Midazolam, 4:336
Midbrain, 3:274, 3:276, 4:288
Midclavicular line, 4:408
Middle adulthood, 1:520–522
Middle cerebral artery, 3:276
Middle lobe, 3:4
Middle turbinate, 3:6
MIF, 1:263
Migration-inhibitory factor (MIF), 1:263
Military Assistance to Safety and Traffic (MAST), 1:68
Mineralocorticoids, 3:335
Minerals, 1:385
Minimum effective concentration, 1:316
Minimum standards, 5:337
Minor, 1:133
Minoxidil, 1:358
Minute alveolar volume, 3:13
Minute respiratory volume, 3:13
Minute volume (V_{min}), 1:548, 4:412
Miosis, 5:531
Miscarriage, 3:705, 3:727
Misfeasance, 1:126
Missed abortion, 3:729
Mistrust, 1:513
Mitochondria, 1:175
Mitochondrian, 1:173
Mitosis, 1:182
Mitral stenosis, 5:9
Mitral valve, 3:75, 3:77
Mitral-valve prolapse, 1:211

Mittelschmerz, 3:705
Mix-O-Vial, 1:419
Mobile data terminals, 2:278
Modeling, 1:517
Moderate diffuse axonal injury, 4:305
Modified chest lead 1 (MCL₁), 3:92–93
MODS, 1:234–236
MOI, 1:85, 5:317
Monaxial joints, 4:227
Monoamine oxidase inhibitors (MAOIs), 1:329, 3:477–478
Monoclonal antibody, 1:248
Monocyte, 1:174, 1:198, 1:262, 3:517, 3:519
Monokine, 1:251, 1:263
Mononeuropathy, 3:282
Mononucleosis, 3:636–637
Monroe-Kelly doctrine, 4:289
Mons pubis, 3:694
Monthly Prescribing Reference, 1:294
Mood disorders, 3:672–674
Morals, 1:151
Morbidity, 1:208
Morgue, 5:386
Morgue officer, 5:386
Moris pubis, 3:694
Moro reflex, 1:511
Morphine, 4:274, 4:336
Morphine sulfate, 5:170
Mortality, 1:208
Motor aphasia, 5:245
Motor system, 2:154–160
Motor vehicle collisions (MVC), 1:110, 4:28–41
  air bags, 4:31–33
  body collision, 4:28–29
  child safety seats, 4:33
  collision evaluation, 4:41
  frontal impact, 4:34–36
  head rests, 4:33
  intoxication, 4:40
  lateral impact, 4:36

organ collision, 4:29–30
  rear-end impact, 4:38–39
  restraints, 4:31
  rollover, 4:39
  rotational impact, 4:36–38
  seat belts, 4:31
  secondary collision, 4:30–31
  vehicle collision, 4:28
  vehicle collision analysis, 4:39–40
  vehicular mortality, 4:41
Motor vehicle laws, 1:124
Motorcycle collisions, 4:42
Mourning, 1:32
Mouth, 2:78–82
Mouth-to-mask ventilation, 1:635
Mouth-to-mouth ventilation, 1:635
Mouth-to-nose ventilation, 1:635
MS, 1:212, 3:313
MSDS, 5:458, 5:459
MSE, 3:667
Mucolytic, 1:367
Muconium-stained amniotic fluid, 5:27–28
Mucosa, 3:387
Mucous cartilage, 1:538, 3:7
Mucous membranes, 1:399, 1:535
Mucoviscidosis, 5:255–256
Mucus, 1:535
Multidraw needle, 1:462
Multifactorial disorders, 1:207–208
Multifocal atrial tachycardia (MAT), 3:114–115
Multifocal seizures, 5:32
Multiple births, 3:750
Multiple casualty incident (MCI), 2:309–311, 5:364, 5:392–394

Multiple myeloma, 3:540
Multiple organ dysfunction syndrome (MODS), 1:234–236
Multiple personality disorder, 3:675
Multiple sclerosis (MS), 1:212, 3:313, 5:256
Multiple-vehicle responses, 5:347–348
Multiplex, 2:277
Multisystem organ failure, 1:232
Mumps, 3:633–634
Murphy's sign, 3:404
Muscarinic acetylcholine receptors, 1:336
Muscarinic cholinergic antagonists, 1:338
Muscle cramp, 4:241
Muscle fatigue, 4:240
Muscle spasm, 4:241
Muscle strength scale, 2:159, 4:239
Muscle strength tests, 2:159
Muscle tissue, 1:176
Muscle tone, 2:159
Muscular dystrophy (MD), 3:313, 5:256–257, 5:283
Muscular injury, 4:239–241
Muscular system, 1:178
Muscular tissue and structure, 4:235–239
Musculocutaneous nerve, 3:277
Musculoskeletal system, 2:108–136
  geriatrics, 5:176
  toddlers/preschoolers, 1:515
Musculoskeletal trauma, 4:221–279
  ankle injuries, 4:269–270
  arthritis, 4:247–248
  bone aging, 4:234
  bone injury, 4:242–246
  bone repair cycle, 4:246–247

bone structure, 4:225–227
  bursitis, 4:247
  clavicle, 4:267
  compartment syndrome, 4:240
  contusion, 4:239–240
  detailed physical exam, 4:252–253
  dislocation, 4:242
  elbow injuries, 4:271
  fatigue, 4:240
  femur fractures, 4:264–266
  finger fractures, 4:272
  focused history and physical exam, 4:250–252
  foot injuries, 4:270
  fractures, 4:242–246
  hand injury, 4:272
  hip dislocation, 4:268
  humerus, 4:267
  immobilizing the injury, 4:255
  initial assessment, 4:248–249
  joint injury, 4:241–242
  joint structure, 4:227–230
  knee injuries, 4:268–269
  lower extremity, 4:232–234
  medications, 4:273–274
  muscle cramp, 4:241
  muscle spasm, 4:241
  muscular injury, 4:239–241
  muscular tissue and structure, 4:235–239
  neurovascular function, 4:256
  patient refusals/referrals, 4:275
  pediatrics, 4:274–275
  pelvic fractures, 4:263–264
  penetrating injury, 4:240
  positioning the limb, 4:255

Musculoskeletal trauma, (contd.)
protecting open wounds, 4:254
psychological support, 4:275
radius/ulna, 4:267
rapid trauma assessment, 4:249–250
scene size-up, 4:248
shoulder injuries, 4:270–271
skeletal organization, 4:230
soft and connective tissue injuries, 4:272–273
splinting devices, 4:256–262
sports injury considerations, 4:253–254, 4:275
sprain, 4:241
strain, 4:241
subluxation, 4:241–242
tendonitis, 4:247
tibial/fibular fractures, 4:266
upper extremity, 4:231–232
wrist injury, 4:272
Mushrooms, 3:486–487
Mutual aid agreements, 5:378
Mutual Aid Coordination Center (MACCs), 5:368
MVC, 1:110
Myasthenia gravis, 1:272, 5:258, 5:269, 5:284
Mycobacterium tuberculosis, 1:235
Mycoses, 1:237
Myocardial aneurysm/ rupture, 4:434
Myocardial infarction (MI), 5:183, 5:187–196
Myocardial injury, 3:232
Myocardial ischemia, 3:230, 3:236
Myocardium, 3:74, 4:417
Myoclonic seizures, 5:32

Myoclonus, 3:315
Myoglobin, 5:195
Myometrium, 3:696, 3:697
Myotomes, 4:363
Myxedema, 3:347, 3:349–350
Myxedema coma, 3:350

N-95 respirator, 1:25, 1:27
Na, 1:192
Nader pin, 5:433
NAEMSE, 1:67
NAEMSP, 1:67
NAEMT, 1:67
Nails, 2:58–60
Nalbuphine, 4:274
Naloxone, 4:336, 5:24, 5:89
Narcan, 4:336, 5:24
Narcan neonatal, 5:25
Narcotic analgesics, 5:205
Nares, 1:535, 4:292
NAS, 5:35
Nasal bones, 4:291
Nasal canula, 1:634
Nasal cavity, 1:534, 1:535, 3:4, 3:5, 4:292
Nasal decongestants, 1:366
Nasal flaring, 3:22
Nasal injury, 4:312–313
Nasal medications, 1:402
NASAR, 1:67
Nash, John, 3:670
Nasogastric (NG) tubes, 1:411, 5:22, 5:295
Nasolacrimal ducts, 1:535
Nasopharyngeal airway, 1:568–570
children, 5:76
Nasopharynx, 1:534, 3:4, 3:5, 3:6
Nasotracheal intubation, 1:604–606, 4:328
Nasotracheal intubation technique, 1:605–606
Nasotracheal route, 1:604
National Association of Emergency Medical Technicians (NAEMT), 1:67

National Association of EMS Educators (NAEMSE), 1:67
National Association of EMS Physicians (NAEMSP), 1:67
National Association of Search and Rescue (NASAR), 1:67
National Council of State EMS Training Coordinators (NCSEMSTC), 1:67
National EMS Education Standards, 1:57
National EMS Scope of Practice Model, 1:56–57
National Fire Protection Association (NFPA), 3:596, 5:338
National Highway Safety Act, 1:54
National Incident Management System (NIMS), 5:366, 5:367, 5:368
National Institute for Occupational Safety and Health (NIOSH), 3:596, 5:338
National Registry of Emergency Medical Technicians (NREMT), 1:67
National Report Card on the State of Emergency Medicine: Evaluating the Environment of Emergency Care Systems State by State, 1:59
Natriuretic peptides (NPs), 1:216
Natural immunity, 1:239, 3:360
Natural passive immunity, 3:360
Naturally acquired immunity, 3:360
Nature of the illness (NOI), 1:85, 5:317
NCSEMSTC, 1:67

Near-drowning, 3:567
Nebulizer, 1:404
Neck, 2:82–84, 4:76
Neck, facial, and neck trauma
airway, 4:325–331
ascending reticular activating system, 4:290
blood-brain barrier, 4:289
blood pressure maintenance, 4:333
brain, 4:287–288
brain injury, 4:302–310
breathing, 4:331–332
cerebral contusion, 4:303
cerebral perfusion pressure (CPP), 4:289
cerebrospinal fluid, 4:286
circulation, 4:332–333
CNS circulation, 4:288
concussion, 4:305
cranial injury, 4:300–302
cranial nerves, 4:289–290
cranium, 4:284–285
cricoid pressure, 4:325–326
cricothyrotomy, 4:330–331
detailed assessment, 4:324–325
dislodged teeth, 4:340
ear, 4:293
ear injury, 4:313
emotional support, 4:337–338
endotracheal intubation, 4:327–330
eye, 4:294–295
eye injury, 4:314–315, 4:338–399
face, 4:290–293
facial injury, 4:310–312
focused history and physical exam, 4:324
Glasgow Coma Scale, 4:322–323

hemorrhage control,
4:332–333
hypovolemia, 4:333
hypoxia, 4:333
impaled objects, 4:340
initial assessment,
4:317–319
intracranial
hemorrhage, 4:303
intracranial perfusion,
4:306
medications, 4:334–337
nasal injury, 4:312–313
neck injury, 4:315–316
ongoing assessment,
4:325
oropharyngeal/
nasopharyngeal
airways, 4:326–327
patient positioning,
4:326
pinna injury, 4:338
rapid trauma
assessment, 4:319–324
scalp, 4:284
scalp avulsion, 4:338
scalp injury, 4:298–300
scene size-up, 4:317
suctioning, 4:326
transport
considerations, 4:337
Neck injury, 4:315–316
Neck trauma. See Neck,
facial, and neck
trauma
Necrosis, 1:187, 1:451,
4:157
Needle adapter, 1:437
Needle cricothyrotomy,
1:615–619, 5:77
Negative feedback, 3:550
Negative feedback loop,
1:180
Negligence, 1:125–129,
1:581
Negligence per se, 1:127
Neoantigen, 1:270
Neonatal abstinence
syndrome (NAS), 5:35
Neonatal cardiac arrest,
5:36–37
Neonatal care, 3:744–747

Neonatal flow algorithm,
5:16
Neonatal seizures,
5:31–32
Neonatal transport, 5:26
Neonate, 3:744, 5:3
Neonatology, 5:1–39
airway management,
5:11–12
APGAR score, 5:11
apnea, 5:5, 5:28
baptism, 5:36
birth injuries, 5:35–36
bradycardia, 5:29
cardiac arrest, 5:36–37
chest compressions,
5:22, 5:23
circulatory system, 5:6,
5:7
congenital anomalies,
5:7–10
cutting the umbilical
cord, 5:13–14
cyanosis, 5:30–31
diaphragmatic hernia,
5:28–29
diarrhea, 5:35
epidemiology, 5:4
fever, 5:32–33
growth and
development, 5:47–48
heat loss, 5:12–13
hypoglycemia, 5:33–34
hypothermia, 5:33
hypovolemia, 5:31
intubation/tracheal
suctioning, 5:19
inverted pyramid for
resuscitation, 5:15,
5:16
maternal narcotic use,
5:24
meconium-stained
amniotic fluid, 5:27–28
neonatal flow
algorithm, 5:16
pathophysiology, 5:5–7
patient assessment,
5:10–11
prematurity, 5:29–30
respiratory distress,
5:30–31

resuscitation, 5:15–25
risk factors, 5:4
seizure, 5:31–32
supplemental oxygen,
5:20
transport, 5:26
venous access, 5:23–24
ventilation, 5:20–22
vital signs, 5:20
vomiting, 5:34
Neoplasm, 3:311–312
Neovascularization, 4:151
Nephrology. See Urology
and nephrology
Nephron, 3:414, 3:416,
5:176
Nerve agents, 5:531–532
Nerve tissue, 1:176
Nervous control of the
heart, 3:84
Nervous system, 1:178,
2:142–167, 3:18–19
geriatrics, 5:174
infants, 1:511
late adulthood, 1:524
pediatric patients, 5:55
toddlers/preschoolers,
1:515
Nervous system
infections, 3:641–646
Net filtration, 1:196
Neuroeffector junction,
1:333
Neurogenic shock, 1:223,
1:227–228, 4:120,
4:372, 5:106–107
Neuroleptanesthesia,
1:321
Neuroleptic, 1:326
Neuroleptic actions,
1:326
Neurology, 3:265–319
altered mental status,
3:293–294
anatomy/physiology,
3:268–280
autonomic nervous
system, 3:280
back pain/nontraumatic
spinal disorders,
3:316–318
brain, 3:272–276

brain abscess, 3:312
central nervous system
(CNS), 3:268–279. See
also Central nervous
system (CNS)
CNS disorders,
3:280–281
degenerative neurologic
disorders, 3:313–316
general assessment,
3:282–292
headache, 3:308–310
neoplasms, 3:311–312
nervous system
emergencies,
3:292–319
pathophysiology,
3:280–282
peripheral nervous
system, 3:279–280
peripheral neuropathy,
3:282
seizures/epilepsy,
3:302–307
stroke/intracranial
hemorrhage,
3:294–302
syncope, 3:307–308
"weak and dizzy,"
3:310–311
Neuromuscular blocking
agents, 1:338–339
Neuromuscular
disorders, 1:212
Neuron, 1:333, 3:269
Neurotransmitter, 1:333,
3:82, 3:270
Neutralization, 5:468
Neutron radiation, 4:193
Neutropenia, 3:519, 3:536
Neutropenic, 5:254
Neutrophil, 1:198, 1:262,
3:517, 3:518, 3:604
Newborn care, 5:298–300
Newton's first law,
4:23–24
Newton's second law of
motion, 4:25
NEXUS, 4:381
NFPA, 3:596, 5:338
NFPA 704 System, 5:456
NG tubes, 5:295, 5:411

Nicotinic acetylcholine receptors, 1:336
Nicotinic cholinergic antagonists, 1:338
NIDDM, 1:375–376, 3:340
NIMS, 5:366, 5:367, 5:368
NIOSH, 3:596, 5:338
Nipride, 1:358, 5:171
Nitrogen narcosis, 3:573, 3:577–578
Nitroglycerin, 1:360, 5:169–170
Nitronox, 4:273, 5:169
Nitrous oxide, 4:273, 5:169
Nocturia, 2:18, 5:184
NOI, 1:85, 5:317
Nominal data, 1:656
Non-Hodgkin's lymphoma, 3:538
Non-insulin-dependent diabetes mellitus (NIDDM), 1:375–376, 3:340
Non-ST-segment elevation myocardial infarction (NSTEMI), 5:188
Nonabsorbent dressings, 4:159
Nonadherent dressings, 4:159
Noncardiogenic shock, 5:105
Noncompensatory pause, 3:116
Noncompetitive antagonism, 1:314
Nonconstituted drug vial, 1:419–420
Nonfeasance, 1:126
Noninvasive respiratory monitoring, 1:556–564
Nonmaleficence, 1:154
Nonocclusive dressings, 4:159
Nonopioid analgesics, 1:320–321
Nonrebreather mask, 1:634

Nonselective sympathomimetics, 1:364
Nonsterile dressings, 4:159
Nonsteroidal anti-inflammatory drugs (NSAIDs), 1:321, 1:381, 3:482, 5:206
Nontraumatic spinal disorders, 3:316–318
Nontraumatic vaginal bleeding, 3:706–707
Nonverbal communication, 1:492–494
Norcuron, 1:597, 4:335
Norepinephrine, 1:277–278, 3:82, 3:334, 5:168–169
Normal flora, 3:596
Normal saline, 1:201, 1:434
Normal sinus rhythm, 3:103
Nose, 2:77–78
Nose breather, 1:511
Nosocomial, 3:654 infections, 3:440
NPs, 1:216
NREMT, 1:67
NSAIDs, 1:321, 1:381, 3:482, 5:206
NSTEMI, 5:188
Nuchal ligament, 4:350
Nuclear detonation, 5:528–530
Nuclear envelope, 1:173
Nuclear pores, 1:173
Nuclear radiation, 3:582–586, 4:191–194
Nucleolus, 1:173, 1:175
Nucleus, 1:175
Nucleus pulposus, 4:347
Nuisance variable, 1:650
Null hypothesis, 1:661
Nutrition, 1:18–20
Nutritional deficiencies, 1:273
Nutritional imbalances, 1:185

Oath of Geneva, 1:92
Obesity, 1:18, 1:212, 5:246–248
Obligate intracellular parasites, 3:598
Obligation to provide care, 1:163–164
Oblique fracture, 4:244
Observation bias, 1:651
Obstetrics
 abnormal delivery situations, 3:747–750
 abortion, 3:727–728
 abruptio placentae, 3:731–732
 APGAR scoring, 3:746
 bleeding, 3:727–732
 Braxton-Hicks contractions, 3:736
 breech presentation, 3:747
 cephalopelvic disproportion, 3:750–751
 complications of pregnancy, 3:726–737
 ectopic pregnancy, 3:729–730
 fetal circulation, 3:720–722
 fetal development, 3:718–720
 field delivery, 3:741–744
 gestational diabetes, 3:735
 hypertensive disorders, 3:732–734
 labor, 3:738–740
 limb presentation, 3:748
 maternal complications, 3:753–754
 meconium staining, 3:751–753
 medication administration, 1:302
 multiple births, 3:750
 neonatal care, 3:744–747
 neonatal resuscitation, 3:746–747
 patient assessment, 3:723–725

 patient management, 3:725–726
 placenta previa, 3:730–731
 precipitous delivery, 3:751
 prenatal period, 3:714–722
 preterm labor, 3:736–737
 prolapsed cord, 3:747–749
 puerperium, 3:737–747
 shoulder dystocia, 3:751
 supine hypotensive syndrome, 3:734–735
 trauma, 3:726–727
Obstructive lung disease, 3:37–38
Obstructive shock, 1:223, 4:119
Obturator nerve, 3:277
Occlusive dressings, 4:159
Occlusive strokes, 3:295
Occupational Safety and Health Administration (OSHA), 3:596, 5:338
Ocular medication, 1:401
Oculomotor nerve, 2:148, 4:287, 4:290
Odds ratio, 1:657
Odontoid process, 4:351
Off-duty paramedics, 1:129–130
Off-line medical direction, 1:61
Ohm, 4:189
Ohm's law, 4:189
Oklahoma City bombing, 5:365
Old age. See Geriatrics
Old-old, 5:151
Olecranon, 4:232
Olfactory nerve, 2:147, 4:290
Oliguria, 3:426
Omentum, 4:463
Omphalocele, 5:10
On-line medical direction, 1:60

On-scene physicians, 5:387
Oncotic force, 1:196
Onset of action, 1:316
Open cricothyrotomy, 1:615, 1:619–623
Open-ended questions, 1:495, 2:6
Open fracture, 4:243
Open incident, 5:371
Open pneumothorax, 4:426–427, 4:445
Open stance, 1:493
Operational staffing, 5:342
Operations level, 5:451
Operations Section, 5:378
Ophthalmic drugs, 1:371
Ophthalmoscope, 2:37
Opiate receptors, 1:320
Opioid agonist-antagonists, 1:321
Opioid agonists, 1:319–320
Opioid antagonists, 1:321
Opportunistic pathogens, 3:596
Opposition, 4:235
Optic nerve, 2:148, 4:290
Oral cavity, 1:535, 4:292
Oral contraceptives, 1:377–378
Oral drug administration, 1:408–410
Oral hypoglycemic agents, 1:376–377
Oral medications dosage calculations, 1:477–481
Oral statements, 2:298
Oral syringe, 1:410
Orbit, 4:294
Ordinal data, 1:656
Ordnance, 4:48
Organ, 1:177
Organ collision, 4:29–30
Organ donation, 1:142
Organ system, 1:177
Organelles, 1:175
Organic, 3:664

Organic brain syndrome, 5:189
Organism, 1:178
Organizational commitment, 1:105–106
Organophosphates, 3:449
Organs, 4:73–74
Origin, 4:235
Orogastric tube, 5:22
Oropharyngeal airway, 1:570–572
    children, 5:74–76
Oropharynx, 1:534, 3:5, 3:6
Oropharyngeal/nasopharyngeal airways, 4:326–327
Orotracheal intubation, 4:327
Orthopedic stretcher, 4:393
Orthopnea, 2:17, 3:23
Orthostatic hypotension, 4:103
Orthostatic syncope, 5:186
OSHA, 3:596, 5:338
Osmolarity, 1:195, 3:417
Osmosis, 1:193–197, 1:305, 3:417
Osmotic diuresis, 1:226, 3:340, 3:418
Osmotic gradient, 1:193
Osmotic pressure, 1:195
Osteoarthritis, 4:247, 5:196, 5:253
Osteoblast, 4:225
Osteoclast, 4:225
Osteocyte, 4:225
Osteoporosis, 4:245, 5:196–197
Ostia, 3:77
OTC medications, 1:296
Otitis media, 5:241
Otoscope, 2:37
Outline of lowest rib, 3:414
Ovarian ligament, 3:696
Ovaries, 3:336, 3:696, 3:697–698, 4:459
Ovary, 3:715

Over-the-counter (OTC) medications, 1:296
Over-the-needle catheter, 1:440–441
Overdoses, 1:386
Overdrive respiration, 4:124
Overhydration, 1:191
Overpressure, 4:47
Ovulation, 3:698, 3:714
Ovum, 3:715
Oxidation, 1:309
Oxygen, 1:534, 1:543–546, 3:368, 4:334, 5:169
Oxygen concentration in blood, 1:544–545
Oxygen concentrators, 5:285
Oxygen cylinders, 5:285
Oxygen-deficient atmospheres, 5:426
Oxygen dissociation curve, 3:15
Oxygen humidifier, 1:634
Oxygen saturation percentage (SpO_2), 1:557–558
Oxygen transport, 1:216–218, 3:514–515
Oxygenation, 1:633–634
Oxyhemoglobin, 3:15
Oxytocin, 3:331

P-Q interval (PQI), 3:94–95
P wave, 3:94, 3:96, 3:97
PA, 1:544
Pa, 1:544
$PaCO_2$, 1:559, 3:30
PACs, 3:115–117
Pallor, 3:21
Palmar grasp, 1:512
Palpation, 2:32–33
Pancolitis, 3:392
Pancreas, 1:374–377, 3:333–334, 3:384, 4:457, 4:458, 4:467
Pancreatic injury, 4:467
Pancreatitis, 3:404–405
Pancuronium, 1:597
Panic attack, 3:671

Papilla, 3:415
PAR, 5:341
Para-aminophenol derivatives, 1:321
Paracrine signaling, 1:179
Paradoxical breathing, 1:552
Paralysis, 5:249
Paralytic shellfish poisoning, 3:485
Paralytics, 4:334–335
Paramedic
    attributes, 1:6
    education, 1:6–8, 1:310
    EMT-Paramedic Curriculum, 1:8
    expanded scope of practice, 1:9–11
    nature of profession, 1:4–6
    role of. See Roles/responsibilities of the paramedic
    well-being, 1:14–43. See also Well-being of paramedic
Paramedic education, 5:310
Paranasal sinuses, 2:78, 3:5
Paraplegia, 4:370
Parasites, 1:237, 3:600
Parasympathetic nervous system, 1:333–339, 3:268, 4:86
Parasympatholytics, 1:334
Parasympathomimetics, 1:334
Parathyroid glands, 1:373–374, 3:333
Parathyroid hormone (PTH), 3:333
Parenchyma, 1:539
Parenteral drug administration, 1:414–430
    glass ampules, 1:416, 1:417
    hypodermic needle, 1:415
    intradermal injection, 1:422–424

Parenteral drug
administration, (contd.)
intramuscular injection,
1:427–430
medication packaging,
1:415–421
nonconstituted drug
vial, 1:419–420
prefilled/preloaded
syringe, 1:419–420
routes, 1:421–430
subcutaneous injection,
1:424–427
syringe, 1:414–415
vials, 1:416–1:418
Parenteral routes,
1:310–311
Parietal pericardium,
3:74, 4:416
Parietal pleura, 3:9
Parkinson's disease,
3:313–314, 5:190–191,
5:205
drugs, 1:329–331
Parotid gland, 3:384
Paroxysmal nocturnal
dyspnea (PND), 2:18,
3:23, 3:199
Paroxysmal
supraventricular
tachycardia (PSVT),
3:117–119
Partial agonist, 1:313
Partial pressure, 1:543,
1:544
Partial pressure of
oxygen, 1:217
Partial rebreather mask,
1:634
Partial seizures, 3:303
Partial thickness burn,
4:196, 4:204, 4:205
Particulate evidence, 5:496
Partner abuse, 5:220–223
Parts per million/parts
per billion (ppm/ppb),
5:463
PASG, 1:76, 4:127–130,
4:527–528
Passive immunity, 3:360,
3:606
Passive transport, 1:304

Patent ductus arteriosus
(PDA), 5:7–8
Patho pearls
adrenergic agonists,
1:344
allergic reactions, 3:364
behavioral emergencies,
3:664
biomechanics of
penetrating trauma,
4:70
bullet's travel, 4:64
calculating force, 2:271
compression, stretch,
and shear, 4:27
cost-benefit
considerations, 5:350
edema, 4:308
EMS evolution, 1:86
explosion, 4:46
hazmat and terrorism,
5:450
high-pressure tool
injuries, 4:157
kidney stones, 3:436
life span and disease,
1:521
listening to the patient,
2:7
medications that cross
the placenta, 1:301
obese patients, 5:247
obesity, 1:18
paramedic education,
5:310
patients with mental
disorders, 1:135
physiology, 1:181
quality considerations
in rural EMS, 5:503
rewarming, 3:564
"sixth sense," 2:199
stroke, 3:300
substance abuse, 3:499
when not to act, 2:254
science vs. dogma, 4:125
thoracic trauma, 4:437
traction splint, 4:259
trauma and the laws of
physics, 4:28
Pathogen, 1:24, 1:184,
1:381, 3:359, 3:596

Pathological fractures,
4:245–246
Pathology, 1:180
Pathophysiology, 1:83,
1:180
Patient access, 5:411–412
Patient advocacy, 1:97
Patient assessment, 1:85,
2:186
Patient care provider,
5:315
Patient care refusal, 4:507
Patient compliance, 5:313
Patient exposure, 5:442
Patient history. See
History taking
Patient interview, 1:491
Patient location, 5:317
Patient management,
1:86
Patient monitoring, 5:442
Patient packaging,
5:415–416
Patient protection,
5:406–407
Patient Self-
Determination Act,
1:139
Patient transfer, 1:89
Patient transportation,
1:138
Patient's history, 5:311
Pattern recognition,
5:311–312
Pavulon, 1:597
PCI, 5:190
PCR, 2:267, 2:288
PDA, 5:7–8
PDQ Statistics (Norman/
Streiner), 1:664
PE, 3:754, 5:197, 5:545
PEA, 5:110, 5:148–149
Peak expiratory flow rate
(PEFR), 3:29
Peak flow, 3:13
Peak load, 5:341
Pedestrian collisions,
4:42–44
Pediatric abdominal
trauma, 4:472
Pediatric airway,
1:540–541

Pediatric analgesia and
sedation, 5:126
Pediatric assessment
triangle, 5:57
Pediatric bradycardia
treatment algorithm,
5:111
Pediatric Glasgow Coma
Scale, 4:323, 4:516,
5:66, 5:67–68
Pediatric healthcare
provider BLS
algorithm, 5:64
Pediatric immobilization
system, 5:88–92
Pediatric intubation,
1:599–603
Pediatric laryngeal mask
airway (LMA), 5:84
Pediatric poisoning,
5:119–121
Pediatric-size suction
catheters, 5:72
Pediatric spinal injuries,
4:373–374
Pediatric tachycardia
algorithm, 5:109
Pediatric trauma score,
4:516, 5:66
Pediatrics, 5:40–145
abdomen, 5:54
abdominal injury, 5:128
abdominal trauma, 4:472
airway, 5:53–54
ALS skills, 5:45
analgesia/sedation,
5:126
anatomy/physiology,
5:51–56
asthma, 5:100–101
BLS algorithm, 5:64
bronchiolitis, 5:101–102
burns, 5:123, 5:129–130
car accidents, 5:121–123
cardiomyopathy,
5:107–108
cardiovascular system,
5:55
chest and lungs, 5:54
chest injuries, 5:128
child abuse and neglect,
5:131–134

communication/ psychological support, 5:46–47

congenital heart disease, 5:107

continuing education, 5:43–44

croup, 5:96–97

drowning, 5:123

dysrhythmia, 5:108–110

electrical therapy, 5:88

endotracheal intubation, 5:78–83

epiglottis, 5:98–99

extremities, 5:54

extremity injuries, 5:128–129

FBAO, 5:71, 5:77–78, 5:99–100, 5:102–103

fluid management, 5:126

fluid therapy, 5:88

general information, 4:513

Glasgow Coma Scale, 4:516, 5:66, 5:67–68

growth and development, 5:47–51

head, 5:52–53

head injury, 5:126–128

history, 5:65–67

hyperglycemia, 5:117–119

hypoglycemia, 5:116–117

immobilization, 5:88–92, 5:125

infection, 5:93–94

IO infusion, 5:85–87

JumpSTART, 5:138–141

LMA, 5:84

medication therapy, 5:88–90

meningitis, 5:114–115

metabolic differences, 5:55–56

nasogastric intubation, 5:84–86

nasopharyngeal airways, 5:76

nausea and vomiting, 5:115–116

needle cricothyrotomy, 5:77

nervous system, 5:55

oropharyngeal airways, 5:74–76

oxygenation, 5:74

penetrating injuries, 5:123

physical exam, 5:67–70

pneumonia, 5:102

poisoning, 5:119–121

rapid sequence intubation, 5:83–84

respiratory emergencies, 5:60–61, 5:62, 5:94–96

respiratory system, 5:55

scene size-up, 5:57

seizure, 5:113–114

shock, 5:103–107

shock trauma resuscitation, 4:512–517

SIDS, 5:130–131

skin and body surface area, 5:54–55

special needs children, 5:134–138

spinal injury, 4:373–374

suctioning, 5:72

transport, 5:65, 5:90–93

trauma score, 4:516, 5:66

vascular access, 5:85

ventilation, 5:76–77

vital signs, 5:62, 5:68–69

weight, 5:69

Pedicles, 4:348

PEDs, 5:406

PEEP, 3:37, 5:22, 5:281, 5:289

Peer review, 1:74

PEFR, 3:29

Pelvic fractures, 4:263–264

Pelvic inflammatory disease (PID), 3:703–704

Pelvic injury, 4:469

Pelvic space, 4:455–464

Pelvic splint, 4:264

Pelvis, 4:232

Penetrating thoracic trauma, 4:420

Penetrating trauma, 4:60–82

abdomen, 4:74–75

assault rifle, 4:68

assessment, 4:78

ballistics, 4:63

bone, 4:74

chest wounds, 4:79–80

connective tissue, 4:73

direct injury, 4:70

entrance wound, 4:76–77

exit wound, 4:77

expansion/fragmentation, 4:65–66

extremities, 4:74

facial wounds, 4:79

handgun, 4:67

head, 4:76

impaled objects, 4:80

knives/arrows, 4:69

low-velocity wounds, 4:72

lungs, 4:74

neck, 4:76

organs, 4:73–74

permanent cavity, 4:71

pressure shock wave, 4:71

profile, 4:64

rifle, 4:68

scene size-up, 4:77–78

secondary impacts, 4:66–67

shape, 4:67

shotgun, 4:68–69

stability, 4:65

temporary cavity, 4:71

thorax, 4:75

zone of injury, 4:72

Penile erectile tissue, 3:420

Peptic ulcer disease (PUD), 1:367–368, 5:193

Peptic ulcers, 1:212, 3:389–391

Percussion, 2:33–34

Percussion sounds, 2:33

Percutaneous coronary intervention (PCI), 5:190

Percutaneous transluminal coronary angioplasty (PTCA), 5:190

Perfluorocarbons, 1:434

Perforating canals, 4:225

Perfusion, 1:213, 2:45, 3:15, 3:19–20

Pericardial cavity, 3:74

Pericardial tamponade, 4:74, 4:432–434, 4:447

Pericardium, 3:74, 4:416

Perimetrium, 3:696, 3:697

Perinephric abscesses, 3:440

Perineum, 3:694

Periorbital ecchymosis, 2:232

Periosteum, 4:227

Peripheral adrenergic neuron blocking agents, 1:355–356

Peripheral arterial atherosclerotic disease, 3:217

Peripheral intravenous access, 1:443

Peripheral nerves, 2:156

Peripheral nervous system (PNS), 3:279–280, 3:268

Peripheral neuropathy, 3:282

Peripheral pulse sites, 2:42

Peripheral vascular resistance, 1:215, 4:88

Peripheral vascular system, 2:136–142

Peripheral venous access, 1:431–432

Peripheral vessels, 3:78

Peripherally inserted central catheter (PICC), 1:432, 5:291

Peristalsis, 4:456

Peritoneal space, 4:455–464

Peritoneum, 4:463

Peritonitis, 3:378, 4:469

Permanent cavity, 4:71

Permissive, 1:516

Permissive hypotension, 1:227

Peroxisomes, 1:175

Persistent ductus arteriosus, 5:8

Persistent fetal circulation, 5:5

Personal attitudes, 5:312

Personal care home, 5:154

Personal flotation devices (PFDs), 5:406, 5:422

Personal hygiene, 1:95–96

Personal protective equipment (PPE), 1:24, 2:188, 5:403–407

Personality disorders, 3:676–678

Personnel considerations, 5:314

Pertussis, 1:25, 3:635

Pesticides, 5:466

PETCO$_2$, 1:559, 3:30

Petechiae, 3:529

Petit mal seizure, 3:303

PFDs, 5:422

pH, 1:202–207, 3:14

pH scale, 1:202

Phagocyte, 1:174, 1:262

Phagocytosis, 1:174, 3:516, 3:604, 4:150

Phalanges, 4:232

Pharmacodynamics, 1:304, 1:312–318

Pharmacokinetics, 1:304–312

Pharmacology, 1:289–391

   antiasthmatic medications, 1:363–365

   autonomic nervous system medications, 1:331–346

   cancer drugs, 1:379–380

   cardiovascular drugs, 1:346–363

   CNS medications, 1:319–331

   constipation drugs, 1:369

   defined, 1:293

   dermatologic drugs, 1:382

   diarrhea drugs, 1:369

   diet supplement drugs, 1:382–386

   digestion and drugs, 1:370

   drug classifications, 1:318–386

   drug research, 1:298–300

   drug sources, 1:294

   drugs affecting ears, 1:371

   drugs affecting eyes, 1:371

   emesis drugs, 1:369–370

   endocrine system, 1:371–379. See also Endocrine system medications

   general aspects, 1:293–295

   infectious diseases/inflammation drugs, 1:380/382

   legal aspects, 1:296–298

   medication administration, 1:300–304. See also Medication administration

   minerals, 1:385

   new drug development timeline, 1:298

   overdoses, 1:386

   pharmacodynamics, 1:312–318

   pharmacokinetics, 1:304–312

   poisoning, 1:386

   PUD drugs, 1:367–369

   reference materials, 1:294–295

   respiratory system drugs, 1:363–367

   rhinitis/cough drugs, 1:365–367

   vitamins, 1:385

Pharyngitis, 3:638

Pharyngotracheal lumen airway, 1:609–611, 2:205

Pharynx, 1:536, 3:6, 3:384

Phenergan, 5:171

Phenol, 4:214

Phobia, 3:672

Phosphate (HPO$_4$), 1:193

Phototherapy, 5:35

Phrenic nerve, 3:277, 4:414

Physical agents, 1:185

Physical examination, 2:27–178, 5:311. See also Field examination

   abdomen, 2:97–103

   anus, 2:107–108

   cardiovascular system, 2:92–97, 3:159–163

   chest/lungs, 2:84–92

   ears, 2:72–77

   eyes, 2:62–72

   female genitalia, 2:103–105

   gastrointestinal system, 3:381–383

   general survey, 2:39–51

   geriatrics, 5:169

   hair, 2:55–58

   head, 2:60–62

   infants/children, 2:167–174

   male genitalia, 2:106–107

   mouth, 2:78–82

   musculoskeletal system, 2:108–136

   nails, 2:58–60

   neck, 2:82–84

   nervous system, 2:142–167, 3:284–289

   nose, 2:77–78

   peripheral vascular system, 2:136–142

   recording examination findings, 2:175–178

   respiratory system, 1:553–556, 3:24–27

   screening exam report, 2:176–178

   skin, 2:52–55

   techniques, 2:31–38

Physical fitness, 1:17–23, 1:107–108

Physical restraint, 3:685–687

Physician's Desk Reference, 1:294

Physiologic shunt, 3:9

Physiological dead space, 4:412

Physiological development

   adolescence, 1:518–519

   infants, 1:509–513

   late adulthood, 1:522

   school age, 1:517

   toddlers/preschoolers, 1:514–515

Physiological stress, 1:276, 1:282

Physiology, 1:169–283, 1:178, 1:181

   acid-base balance, 1:202–207

   cell and cellular environment, 1:187–202. See also Cell and cellular environment

   cells responding to change/injury, 1:181–187

   family history and associated risk factors, 1:209–213

   genetics/environment/ lifestyle/age/gender, 1:207–209

   hypoperfusion, 1:213–234. See also Hypoperfusion

   immune response, 1:238–253. See also Immune response

   normal cell, 1:173–181

   respiratory system, 1:541–549

   self-defense mechanisms, 1:234–238

PI, 1:662

Pia mater, 3:270, 3:278, 4:286, 4:358

PICC, 1:432, 5:291

PID, 3:703–704

Pierre Robin syndrome, 5:10

Pill-rolling motion, 5:191
Pillow splint, 4:258
Pinch points, 5:515
Pineal gland, 3:336
Pink puffers, 3:39
Pinna, 4:293
  injury, 4:338
Pinworms, 3:600
Pit viper bite, 3:495
Pitting, 2:141
Pitting edema scale, 2:142
Pituitary gland,
    1:372–373, 3:274,
    3:330–332
Pivot joints, 4:227
PJCs, 5:130–131
PLA, 1:613
Placard classifications,
    5:454–456
Placebo effect, 1:651
Placenta, 3:714, 3:715
Placenta previa,
    3:730–731
Placental barrier, 1:308
Plaintiff, 1:122
Planning/intelligence
    section, 5:378
Plantar flexors, 2:124
Plasma, 1:198, 3:513–514
Plasma kinin cascade,
    1:260
Plasma-level profile,
    1:316
Plasma membrane, 1:174
Plasma protein fraction,
    1:200, 1:433
Plasma protein systems,
    1:258–261
Plasmanate, 1:200
Platelet, 4:89
Platelet phase, 4:91
Platelets, 1:198, 1:262,
    3:520
Play, 1:516
Pleura, 1:539–540, 3:9,
    3:74
Pleural cavity, 3:74
Pleural friction rub, 2:90,
    3:27
Pleural membranes, 3:4
Pleural space, 3:4, 4:410
Pleuritic, 3:49

Plica, 3:387
Pluripotent stem cell,
    3:512
PMS, 3:699
PND, 2:18, 3:23, 3:199
Pneumatic anti-shock
    garment (PASG), 1:76,
    4:527–528, 4:127–130
Pneumomediastinum,
    3:573, 3:577
Pneumonia, 1:25,
    3:48–50, 3:625–626
  children, 5:102
  elderly persons,
    5:178–179
Pneumonia-like agents,
    5:537–538
Pneumotaxic center,
    1:546, 4:413
Pneumothorax, 1:545,
    1:583, 3:18, 3:573, 4:51
  closed, 4:425–426
  open, 4:426–427, 4:445
  simple, 4:425–426
  tension, 4:427–428,
    4:445–447
PNS, 3:268
POGO classification
    system, 1:625
Poiseuille's law, 3:79
Poisoning, 1:386
  children, 5:119–121
Poisonous plants,
    3:486–487
Poisons, 5:464–465
Poliomyelitis (polio),
    3:315, 5:257, 5:283
Polycythemia, 3:38,
    3:532, 3:535–536, 5:14,
    5:187
Polymerized
    hemoglobin, 1:200
Polyneuropathy, 3:282
Polypharmacy, 5:161
Polyuria, 2:18
Pons, 3:274, 3:276, 4:288
Portable mechanical
    ventilator, 1:639
Portal, 3:386
Portal system, 4:110,
    4:462
Positional asphyxia, 3:685

Positive end-expiratory
    pressure (PEEP), 3:37,
    5:22, 5:281, 5:289
Positive-pressure
    ventilators, 5:289
Post-traumatic stress
    disorder (PTSD),
    3:672
Postconventional
    reasoning, 1:518
Posterior axillary line,
    4:408
Posterior communicating
    artery, 3:276
Posterior descending
    artery, 3:76
Posterior fascicles, 3:89
Posterior longitudinal
    ligament, 4:348
Posterior medial sulcus,
    4:357
Posterior pituitary drugs,
    1:373
Posterior pituitary gland,
    3:330, 3:331–332
Posterior third of tongue,
    1:612
Postganglionic nerves,
    1:332
Postpartum depression,
    5:299
Postpartum hemorrhage,
    3:753
Postrenal ARF, 3:428
Posture, 1:22, 3:665
Potassium (K), 1:193,
    1:355
Potassium channel
    blockers (class III),
    1:352
Potassium iodide (KI)
    tablets, 5:530
PPD, 3:608
PPE, 1:24, 2:188,
    5:403–407
ppm/ppb, 5:463
PQI, 3:94–95
PR interval (PRI),
    3:94–95, 3:98
Practice sessions, 5:322
Pre-eclampsia, 3:732,
    3:733–734

Prearrival instructions,
    2:273
Precapillary sphincter,
    1:215
Precautions, 1:107
Precipitous delivery,
    3:751
Preconventional
    reasoning, 1:518
Precordial leads, 3:92,
    3:225–226
Precordial thump, 3:167
Precordium, 4:432
Preembryonic stage,
    3:719
Prefilled/preloaded
    syringe, 1:419–420
Preganglionic nerves,
    1:332
Pregnancy
  abdominal trauma,
    4:470–471, 4:477,
    4:479–481
  uterus, 4:461
Pregnant patients. See
    Obstetrics
Pregnant uterus, 4:461
Prehospital care report
    (PCR), 2:267, 2:288
Prehospital ECG
    monitoring,
    3:256–260
Prehospital Emergency
    Care, 1:68
Preload, 1:213, 3:80, 4:87
Premature atrial
    contractions (PACs),
    3:115–117
Premature junctional
    contractions (PJCs),
    5:130–131
Premature newborn,
    5:29–30
Premature ventricular
    contraction (PVC),
    5:137–140
Premenstrual syndrome
    (PMS), 3:699
Prenatal period,
    3:714–722
Prepuce, 3:420, 3:694
Prerenal ARF, 3:426–427

Presbycusis, 1:524, 5:242
Preschoolers, 1:514–517, 5:49. *See also* Preschoolers
physical examination, 2:168
Pressure disorders, 3:574–578
Pressure injuries, 4:155
Pressure shock wave, 4:71
Pressure ulcer, 5:194, 5:195–196
Pressure wave, 4:47–48
Preterm labor, 3:736–737
Prevalence, 1:208
Preventing illness/injury. *See* Illness/injury prevention
Preventive strategies, 3:414
PRI, 3:94–95, 3:98
Priapism, 2:106, 3:438
Primary apnea, 5:5
Primary areas of responsibility (PAR), 5:341
Primary bronchi, 1:538, 3:7
Primary care, 1:10, 1:88
Primary contamination, 5:463
Primary coronary stenting, 5:190
Primary immune response, 1:239
Primary intention, 1:265
Primary prevention, 1:105
Primary problem, 2:11
Primary response, 3:359
Primary skin lesions, 2:56–57
Primary Staging Area, 5:372
Primary triage, 5:380
Primum non nocere, 1:154
Principal investigator (PI), 1:662
Prinzmetal's angina, 5:185
Prions, 1:237, 3:599

Priority dispatching, 2:273
Privacy, 1:132, 2:279
PRL, 3:280, 3:332
Problem patient, 1:135–137
Procainamide, 5:89
Proctitis, 3:392
Prodrugs, 1:308
Profession, 1:64
Professional attitudes, 1:93–94
Professional attributes, 1:94–98
Professional behaviors, 1:490–491
Professional identity, 1:58
Professional journals, 1:68
Professional relations, 1:164–166
Professionalism, 1:73, 1:92–98, 2:302
Profile, 4:64
Progestins, 1:377
Progressive shock, 1:222
Projectiles, 4:48
Prokaryotes, 1:173
Prolactin (PRL), 1:280, 3:332
Prolapsed cord, 3:747–749
Prolongation of the QT interval, 1:211
Prolonged QT interval, 3:99
Promethazine, 5:171
Prompt care facilities, 5:507
Pronator-supinator muscles, 2:117
Property conservation, 5:371
Prospective research, 1:650
Prostaglandins, 1:257
Prostate, 3:420
Prostatitis, 3:439
Protective blankets, 5:407
Protective custody, 3:452
Protective gloves, 1:25
Protective shielding, 5:407

Protocols, 1:61, 2:250, 2:280
Prototype, 1:318
Protozoan, 3:599–600
Proximal tubule, 3:415, 3:416
Proximate cause, 1:127
Pruritus, 5:194
PSAP, 2:269
Pseudo-instinctive, 2:255
Pseudoseizures, 3:304
PSVT, 3:117–119
Psychiatric and behavioral disorders, 1:212–213, 3:660–687
age-related conditions, 3:680–681
anxiety, 3:671–672
behavioral emergencies, 3:662–663
chemical restraint, 3:687
cognitive disorders, 3:669
dissociative disorders, 3:675
eating disorders, 3:676
excited delirium, 3:681–682
factitious disorders, 3:675
impulse control disorders, 3:678
mood disorders, 3:672–674
pathophysiology, 3:663–664
patient assessment, 3:664–668
personality disorders, 3:676–678
physical restraint, 3:685–687
schizophrenia, 3:669–670
somatoform disorders, 3:674–675
substance-related disorders, 3:674
suicide, 3:679–680
verbal de-escalation, 3:684–685

violent patients and restraint, 3:684–687
Psychiatric disorders, 1:212–213. *See* Psychiatric and behavioral disorders
Psychiatric medications, 3:668
Psychogenic amnesia, 3:675
Psychological first aid, 1:40
Psychological stress, 1:282
Psychoneuroimmunologic regulation, 1:277
Psychosis, 3:679
Psychosocial, 3:664
Psychosocial development
adolescence, 1:519
infants, 1:513–514
late adulthood, 1:524
school age, 1:517–518
toddlers/preschoolers, 1:515–517
Psychotherapeutic medications, 1:325–329
PTCA, 5:190
PTH, 3:333
PTSD, 3:672
Pubic bone, 3:715
Pubis, 4:232
Public health agencies, 3:596
Public health principles, 3:595
Public safety answering point (PSAP), 2:269
Public utility model, 1:76
PUD, 1:367–368, 5:193
Pudendum, 3:694
Puerperium, 3:737–747
Pulmonary agents, 5:533
Pulmonary artery, 3:75
Pulmonary capillaries, 3:4
Pulmonary circulation, 1:542–543
Pulmonary contusion, 4:429–430

Pulmonary drug administration, 1:404–407
Pulmonary edema, 5:182
Pulmonary embolism (PE), 1:545, 3:55–57, 3:754, 5:180–182, 5:197
Pulmonary hilum, 4:410
Pulmonary injuries, 4:425–430
Pulmonary irritants, 5:465–466
Pulmonary overpressure, 3:573
Pulmonary overpressure accidents, 3:576
Pulmonary shunting, 3:20
Pulmonary stenosis, 5:9
Pulmonary system
  infants, 1:510–511
  toddlers/preschoolers, 1:514
Pulmonary trunk, 3:77
Pulmonary valve, 3:77
Pulmonary veins, 3:75
Pulmonary vessels, 3:9
Pulmonology, 3:1–60
  ARDS, 3:35–37
  asthma, 3:42–45
  capnography, 3:29–33
  carbon monoxide inhalation, 3:54–55
  chronic bronchitis, 3:40–41
  CNS dysfunction, 3:59
  COPD, 3:3
  diffusion, 3:19
  emphysema, 3:38–40
  GBS, 3:59
  hyperventilation syndrome, 3:57–59
  lower airway anatomy, 3:7–10
  lung cancer, 3:51–53
  obstructive lung disease, 3:37–38
  pathophysiology, 3:17–20
  perfusion, 3:19–20
  physical exam, 3:24–27

physiological processes, 3:10–17
pneumonia, 3:48–50
pulmonary embolism, 3:55–57
respiratory anatomy/physiology, 3:4–17
respiratory disorders, 3:33–60
respiratory system assessment, 3:20–33
SARS, 3:50–51
spontaneous pneumothorax, 3:57
toxic inhalation, 3:53
upper airway anatomy, 3:5–7
upper airway obstruction, 3:34–35
upper respiratory infection, 3:45–48
ventilation, 3:17–19
Pulse CO-oximeter, 3:466
Pulse oximeter, 2:48–49
Pulse oximetry, 1:557–558, 3:28
Pulse/perfusion, 5:381
Pulse pressure, 2:45, 4:97
Pulse quality, 2:41
Pulse rate, 2:41
Pulse rhythm, 2:41
Pulse sites, 2:42
Pulseless arrest algorithm, 5:146
Pulseless electrical activity (PEA), 5:110, 5:148–149
Pulseless ventricular tachycardia, 5:110
Pulsus alternans, 3:200, 4:434
Pulsus paradoxus, 1:554, 3:28, 3:200, 4:434
Punctures, 4:146
Pupil, 4:294
Pure Food and Drug Act of 1906, 1:296
Purkinje system, 3:89, 3:90
Pus, 1:264
PVC, 5:137–140

Pyelonephritis, 3:440
Pylorus, 3:386
Pyramids, 3:415
Pyrexia, 3:558
Pyriform fossae, 1:536, 1:612
Pyrogen, 1:450, 3:558

Q wave, 3:94
QA, 1:73
QI, 1:55, 4:16–17
QRS axis, 3:227
QRS complex, 3:94, 3:98
QRS interval, 3:95
QT interval, 3:95
QTc, 3:95
Quadriplegia, 4:370
Qualitative statistics, 1:656
Quality assurance (QA), 1:73
Quality improvement (QI), 1:55
Quality of care, 1:58
Quality of respiration, 2:44
Quantitative statistics, 1:656
Questioning techniques, 1:495–496
QuickClot, 4:105

R-R interval, 3:101–102
Rabies, 3:642–643
Raccoon eyes, 4:301
RAD, 3:583
Rad, 4:194
Radial nerve, 3:277
Radiation, 3:549, 3:582–586
Radiation absorbed dose (RAD), 3:583
Radiation injury, 4:191–194, 215–217
Radio bands, 2:266
Radio communication, 2:276–278
Radio frequency, 2:266
Radio terminology, 2:268
Radius, 4:232, 4:267
Rales, 1:556, 2:88
Rape, 5:231

Revised trauma score, 4:505, 4:506
Rapid intervention team, 5:390
Rapid isotonic infusion, 4:529
Rapid sequence intubation (RSI), 1:596, 4:329
  children, 5:83–84
Rapid transport, 4:510–511
Rapid trauma assessment, 2:213
Rappel, 5:437
Rapport, 1:490, 2:4–10
RAS, 3:275, 3:276
Rattlesnake bite, 3:493, 3:495
Raynaud's phenomenon, 1:270
Reabsorption, 3:416
Rear-end impact, 4:38–39
Reasonable force, 1:138
Rebleeding, 4:154
Rebound tenderness, 4:469
Receiving facilities, 1:87–88
Receptor, 1:312
Reciprocal, 3:239
Reciprocity, 1:64
Recirculating currents, 5:419–420
Recompression, 3:575
Recreation hazards, 1:111
Recreational emergencies, 5:518–520
Recreational vehicle collisions, 4:44–45
Rectal medication administration, 1:412–414
Rectum, 3:384, 3:400, 3:696
Rectus femoris, 1:429
Red blood cells, 1:198, 3:9, 3:514–516
Red bone marrow, 4:227
Red treatment unit, 5:387
Red zone, 5:460

Reduced nephron mass, 3:430

Reduced renal mass, 3:430

Reduction, 4:262

Reel splint, 4:259, 4:261

Reentrant pathways, 1:350

Referred pain, 2:12, 3:379, 3:421

Reflective, 2:253

Reflex arc, 4:363

Reflexes, 2:162–167, 3:277

Refractory period, 3:100

Reframe, 1:39

Refusal of service, 1:134–135

Regeneration, 1:265

Regional training center, 4:10–11

Registration, 1:64

Regulations, 5:366–368

Rehabilitation (REHAB) area, 5:390

Relative refractory period, 3:100

Release-from-liability, 1:128, 1:134

Religion, 1:151

Religious beliefs, 1:133

Reteplase, 5:170

REM, 3:583

Remodeling, 4:151

Renal, 3:413

Renal ARF, 3:427

Renal artery, 3:414

Renal calculi, 3:413, 3:435–438

Renal dialysis, 3:433

Renal (kidney) failure, 1:211

Renal pelvis, 3:415

Renal system
geriatrics, 5:176
infants, 1:511
late adulthood, 1:523
toddlers/preschoolers, 1:515

Renal vein, 3:414

Renin, 3:419

Renin-angiotensin-aldosterone system, 1:357

Renin-angiotensin system, 1:222

Repair, 1:265

Reperfusion, 5:186

Repolarization, 3:87

Reportable collisions, 5:343

Reporting procedures, 2:280–282

Reporting requirements, 1:124

Reproductive system, 1:178

Reproductive systems, 4:460

RES, 3:604

Res ipsa loquitur, 1:127

Rescue, 5:389

Rescue awareness and operations, 5:399–443
hazardous atmosphere rescues, 5:425–429
hazardous terrain rescues, 5:436–443
highway operations/vehicle rescues, 5:429–436
patient protection, 5:406–407
phase 1 (arrival/size-up), 5:409–410
phase 2 (hazard control), 5:410–411
phase 3 (patient access), 5:411–412
phase 4 (medical treatment), 5:412–414
phase 5 (disentanglement), 5:414–415
phase 6 (patient packaging), 5:415–416
phase 7 (removal/transport), 5:416
protective equipment, 5:403–407
rescue operations, 5:409–416

rescuer protection, 5:403–406
role of the paramedic, 5:402–403
safety procedures, 5:407–409
surface water rescues, 5:416–425

Rescuer protection, 5:403–406

Research, 1:75, 1:151, 1:647–664
applying study results, 1:661
case-control studies, 1:649
cohort studies, 1:650
descriptive statistics, 1:654–655
descriptive studies, 1:649
format, 1:657–658
inferential statistics, 1:656
intervention studies, 1:650–653
participating in research, 1:661–663
publishing the paper, 1:658
qualitative/quantitative statistics, 1:656
reference books, 1:663–664
what to look for when reviewing a study, 1:659–660

Research: The Who, What, Why, When, and How (Menegazzi), 1:663

Research documentation, 2:289

Reserve capacity, 5:342

Reservoir, 3:601

Residual volume (RV), 1:549, 3:12, 3:13, 4:411

Resiliency, 4:73

Resistance, 3:603, 4:189

Resolution, 1:265

Resolution phase, 4:189

Resource allocation, 1:162–163

Resource utilization, 5:373

Respect, 1:97

Respiration, 1:534, 2:42, 3:16, 3:549

Respirators, 3:624

Respiratory acidosis, 1:205

Respiratory alkalosis, 1:205, 1:206

Respiratory control, 4:412–414

Respiratory cycle, 1:541–542

Respiratory distress
children, 5:60–61, 5:62, 5:94–95
newborn, 5:30–31

Respiratory effort, 2:42

Respiratory epithelium, 1:538, 3:7

Respiratory failure, 5:269

Respiratory membrane, 3:9

Respiratory mucosa, 3:7

Respiratory problems, 1:549–551

Respiratory protection, 5:405

Respiratory rate, 1:546, 2:42, 2:206

Respiratory shock, 4:120

Respiratory syncytial virus (RSV), 3:635

Respiratory system, 1:177
alveoli, 1:539
bronchi, 1:538
carbon dioxide concentration in blood, 1:545–546
diffusion, 1:544
geriatrics, 5:170–173
inadequate ventilation, 1:551
larynx, 1:536–537
late adulthood, 1:522–523
lower airway anatomy, 1:537–540
lung parychema, 1:539
nasal cavity, 1:535
oral cavity, 1:535

oxygen/carbon dioxide levels, 1:543–546
oxygen concentration in blood, 1:544–545
patient assessment, 1:551–564. *See also* Respiratory system assessment
pediatric airway, 1:540–541
pediatric patients, 5:55
pharynx, 1:536
physiology, 1:541–549
pleura, 1:539–540
pregnancy, 3:716–717
pulmonary circulation, 1:542–543
regulation of respiration, 1:546–551
respiratory cycle, 1:541–542
trachea, 1:538
upper airway anatomy, 1:534–537
Respiratory system assessment, 1:551–564
capnography, 1:558–564
focused history, 1:553
initial assessment, 1:551–552
noninvasive respiratory monitoring, 1:556–564
physical examination, 1:553–556
pulse oximetry, 1:557–558
Respiratory system drugs, 1:363–367
Response times, 1:58, 2:289
Responsive medical patient, 2:222–229
Resting potential, 3:86
Resuscitation, 1:158–160, 3:212. *See* Shock trauma resuscitation
Resuscitation equipment, 1:26
Resuscitation fluids, 1:199
Resuscitation issues, 1:139–143

Resuscitative approach, 5:317–318
Retavase, 5:170
Reticular activating system (RAS), 3:275, 3:276
Reticular formation, 3:276
Reticuloendothelial system (RES), 3:604
Reticulospinal tract, 4:358
Retina, 4:294
Retinal detachment, 4:315
Retinopathy, 5:192
Retroauricular ecchymosis, 4:300, 4:301
Retrograde amnesia, 4:308
Retrograde intubation, 4:328
Retroperitoneal space, 4:455–464
Retrospective research, 1:649
Return of spontaneous circulation (ROSC), 3:212
Returning to service, 1:90
Review of systems, 2:17
Rewarming, 3:564
Rewarming shock, 3:564–565
Rh and ABO isoimmunization, 1:272
Rh blood group, 1:243
Rh factor, 1:243
Rhabdomyolysis, 4:157
Rheumatic disorders, 1:211
Rheumatic fever, 1:209
Rheumatoid arthritis, 1:272, 4:248, 5:253
Rhinitis, 1:365
Rhinorrhea, 5:531
Rhomboid muscles, 4:410
Rhonchi, 1:556, 2:90, 3:27
Rhythm strips, 3:90

Rib fracture, 4:421–423; 444
Ribosomes, 1:173, 1:175
Rifle, 4:68
Right atrium, 3:75, 3:77
Right axis deviation, 3:227
Right bundle branch, 3:89
Right bundle branch block, 3:247, 3:253
Right coronary artery, 3:76
Right kidney, 3:414
Right lung, 3:4
Right mainstem bronchus, 1:538, 3:7
Right primary bronchus, 3:4
Right ureter, 3:414
Right ventricle, 3:75, 3:77
Right ventricular infarctions, 3:240–245
Rigid cervical collar application, 5:425
Rigid splints, 4:257
Ring injury, 4:148
Riot control agents, 4:214
Risk analysis, 4:6–8
Risk factor analysis, 1:208
Risk management strategy, 1:73
Roadway safety, 1:41–43
Roentgen equivalent in man (REM), 3:583
Rohypnol, 3:503, 5:232
Roles/responsibilities of the paramedic, 1:81–98
citizen involvement in EMS, 1:91
community involvement, 1:90–91
continuing education, 1:98
documentation, 1:89
emergency response, 1:84
EMT code of ethics, 1:93. *See also* Ethics
hazmat incidents, 1:402–403

Oath of Geneva, 1:92
patient assessment, 1:85
patient management, 1:86–87
patient transfer, 1:89
personal/professional involvement, 1:91–92
preparation, 1:84
primary responsibilities, 1:83–90
professional attitudes, 1:93–94
professional attributes, 1:94–98
professional ethics, 1:92
professionalism, 1:92–98
rescue awareness and operations, 1:402–403
returning to service, 1:90
scene size-up, 1:84–85
support for primary care, 1:91
Rolling vehicles, 5:431
Rollover, 4:39
Rooting reflex, 1:512
Rope-sling slide, 4:392–393
ROSC, 3:212
Rotational impact, 4:36–38
Rotorcraft, 5:351. *See also* Air medical transport
Rough endoplasmic reticulum, 1:173
Rouleaux, 4:116
Round ligament, 3:696
Routes, 1:421–430
RSI, 4:329. *See* Rapid sequence intubation (RSI)
RSV, 3:635
Rubella, 1:25, 3:634–635
Rule of nines, 4:197–198, 5:129
Rule of palms, 4:198
Rules of evidence, 1:74
Rupture of the liver, 4:468

Rural EMS, 5:500–520
agricultural emergencies, 5:511–518
creative problem solving, 5:505–507
distance factor, 5:508–509
practicing, 5:502–507
quality considerations, 5:503
recreational emergencies, 5:518–520
special problems, 5:503–505
typical situations/decisions, 5:508–520
Rust out, 5:505
RV, 1:549, 3:12, 3:13
Ryan White Comprehensive AIDS Resources Emergency (CARE) Act, 1:30, 1:125, 3:613

SA node, 4:417
Sacral convexity, 4:348
Sacral nerves, 4:361
Sacral plexus, 3:277, 4:362
Sacral promontory, 4:355
Sacral spine, 4:355–356
Sacroiliac joint, 4:356
Sacrum, 4:347, 4:356
Saddle joints, 4:228
Safe driving, 1:108
Safe zone, 5:460
Safety officer (SO), 5:376
Safety procedures, 5:407–409
Salicylate poisoning treatment algorithm, 3:482
Salicylates, 1:321, 3:481
Saline lock, 1:456
Salivary glands, 2:80
Salt-poor albumin, 1:200, 1:433
Saltwater drowning, 3:569

Sampling error, 1:656
Saphenous nerve, 3:277
Saponification, 1:187
SARS, 1:25, 3:50–51, 3:626, 5:537
SB, 3:315
Scabies, 3:652–653
Scaffolding, 1:513
Scalds, 5:228
Scale, 2:37, 2:38
Scalp, 4:284
Scalp avulsion, 4:338
Scalp injury, 4:298–300
Scapula, 4:231–232
SCBA, 5:406
Scene-authority law, 5:366
Scene safety, 1:108–109, 2:190–194, 5:276–277, 5:317
Scene size-up
home care patient, 5:276
pediatric patients, 5:55, 5:57
Schizophrenia, 1:212, 3:669–670
School age, 1:517–518
physical examination, 2:169
School-age children, 5:49–50. *See also* Pediatrics
Sciatic nerve, 3:277
SCID, 1:274
Scissor gait, 5:255
SCIWORA, 4:374
Sclera, 4:295
Scoliosis, 4:375, 4:377
Scombroid (histamine) poisoning, 3:485
Scoop stretcher, 4:393
Scope of practice, 1:123
Scorpion stings, 3:492–493
Scrambling, 5:436
Scree, 5:436
Screening exam report, 2:176–178
Scrotal sac, 3:420
Scrotum, 3:420, 4:460
Scuba, 3:571

SD, 1:654, 1:655
Seat belts, 4:31
Sebaceous glands, 4:139
Sebum, 4:139
Second-degree burn, 4:196
Second-degree Mobitz I, 5:125
Second-degree Mobitz II, 5:127–128
Second messenger, 1:312
Secondary apnea, 5:5
Secondary collision, 4:30–31
Secondary contamination, 5:463
Secondary immune deficiencies, 1:273
Secondary immune response, 1:239
Secondary intention, 1:265
Secondary prevention, 1:105
Secondary response, 3:360
Secondary skin lesions, 2:58–59
Secondary Staging Area, 5:372
Secondary triage, 5:381
Secretion, 3:416
Secretory immune system, 1:248
Secretory vesicles, 1:173
Section chief, 5:375
Sector, 5:380
Secure attachment, 1:513
Sedation, 1:322
Sedative (induction) agents, 1:598
Sedative-hypnotic drugs, 5:205
Sedatives, 4:335–336
Seizure, 3:302–307
children, 5:113–114
elderly persons, 5:188
newborn, 5:31–32
Selective IgA deficiency, 1:273
Selective serotonin reuptake inhibitors (SSRIs), 1:327–328, 3:478

Selective serotonin reuptake inhibitors (SSRIs) poisoning treatment algorithm, 3:480
Self-adherent roller bandages, 4:159
Self-adhesion molecules, 1:252
Self-confidence, 1:96
Self-contained breathing apparatus (SCBA), 5:406
Self-motivation, 1:95, 5:322
Self-rescue techniques, 5:421
Selye, Hans, 1:275, 1:276
Semantic, 2:266
Semen, 3:420
Semi-decontaminated patients, 5:471
Semi-Fowler's position, 2:214
Semicircular canals, 4:293
Semilunar valves, 3:74
Seminal vesicle, 3:420
Semipermeable, 1:174
Sengstaken-Blakemore tube, 3:386
Senile dementia, 5:189
Senility, 5:189
Senior centers, 5:158
Senses
late adulthood, 1:523–524
toddlers/preschoolers, 1:515
Sensitization, 3:361
Sensorimotor evaluation, 3:288
Sensorineural deafness, 5:241
Sensorium, 5:270
Sensory aphasia, 5:245
Sensory impaired patients, 1:501–502
Sensory system, 2:161–162
Sepsis, 1:236
September 11 terrorist attacks, 1:72, 5:365

Septic arthritis, 4:247

Septic complications, 5:270–271

Septic shock, 1:223, 1:231–232, 4:119, 5:105–106

Septicemia, 1:236

Septum, 1:535

Sequestered cells, 1:271

Sequestration, 3:516

Seroconversion, 3:603

Serosa, 3:387

Serotonin, 1:257

Serotonin antagonists, 1:370

Serotonin syndrome, 3:479

Serous fluid, 4:154

Serous pericardium, 4:416

Serum, 1:382

Serum sickness, 1:270

Service quality, 1:74

Sesamoid bone, 4:227

Settlement, 1:123

Severe acute respiratory syndrome (SARS), 1:25, 3:50–51, 3:626, 5:537

Severe combined immune deficiencies (SCID), 1:274

Severe diffuse axonal injury, 4:306

Sexual assault, 3:707–709, 5:231–235

Sexual behavior, 1:379

Sexual organs, 4:459–460

Sexually attractive patient, 2:22

Sexually transmitted diseases (STDs), 3:646

Shaken baby syndrome, 5:229

Sharp objects, 5:431

Sharps container, 1:398

"Shattered Dreams," 4:16

Shear, 4:27

Shear points, 5:515

Shift work, 1:36–37

Shipping papers, 5:457

Shock, 1:213, 1:222, 4:108–130
  airway/breathing management, 4:123–124
  body's response to blood loss, 4:115–116
  capillary microcirculation, 4:116
  capillary washout, 4:117
  cardiogenic, 4:119–120
  cardiovascular system regulation, 4:113–115
  cellular ischemia, 4:116
  cellular metabolism, 4:108
  children, 5:103–107
  circulation, 4:110
  compensated, 4:117–118
  decompensated, 4:118
  defined, 4:86
  digestion, 4:110
  distributive, 4:119
  excretion, 4:110
  filtration, 4:110
  fluid resuscitation, 4:125
  focused history and physical exam, 4:121–123
  hemorrhage control, 4:124
  hormone production, 4:110
  hypovolemic, 4:119
  initial assessment, 4:120–121
  irreversible, 4:118
  isotonic fluid administration, 4:126
  neurogenic, 4:120
  obstructive, 4:119
  oxygen transport, 4:108–110
  PASG, 4:127–130
  pharmacological intervention, 4:130
  respiratory, 4:120
  scene size-up, 4:120
  temperature control, 4:127

Shock trauma resuscitation, 4:484–532
  air medical transport, 4:521–527
  airway, 4:497
  auscultation, 4:500
  body splinting, 4:510
  breathing, 4:497–498
  capillary refill, 4:528–529
  circulation, 4:498
  detailed physical exam, 4:501–504
  dispatch information, 4:490
  disposal of contaminated materials, 4:521
  flight-or-fight response, 4:511
  focused exam and history, 4:501
  general impression, 4:495–496
  geriatric patients, 4:517–519
  Glasgow Coma Scale, 4:505
  hazard identification, 4:492
  helicopter transport, 4:521–527
  hypoperfusion, 4:508
  hypotension, 4:508
  hypothermia, 4:509–510
  hypovolemia, 4:508
  injury prevention, 4:486–489
  inspection, 4:499–500
  interaction with other care providers, 4:519–520
  locate all patients, 4:493
  mechanism of injury analysis, 4:491–492
  mental status, 4:496–497
  noncritical patients, 4:511–512
  palpation, 4:500
  PASG, 4:527–528
  patient care refusal, 4:507
  pediatric patients, 4:512–517
  percussion, 4:500
  questioning, 4:499
  rapid isotonic infusion, 4:529
  rapid transport, 4:510–511
  rapid trauma assessment, 4:501
  resource needs determination, 4:493–494
  revised trauma score, 4:505, 4:506
  scene size-up, 4:490
  spinal precautions, 4:494–495
  standard precautions, 4:492–493
  transport decision, 4:506
  trauma assessment, 4:489–492
  trauma patient history, 4:504
  treat and release, 4:507
  vital signs, 4:505

Short haul, 5:440

Short spine board, 4:393–394

Shotgun, 4:68–69

Shotgun wounds, 4:420

Shoulder dystocia, 3:751

Shoulder girdle, 2:119

Shoulder girdle ligaments, 2:120

Shoulder injuries, 4:270–271

Shoulder muscles, 2:121

Shoulders, 2:116–122

Shunt, 5:138

Shy-Drager syndrome, 5:191

Sibling relationships, 1:516

Sick sinus syndrome, 3:112–113, 5:186

Sickle cell anemia, 3:534–535

Sickle cell trait, 3:534
Side effect, 1:314
SIDS, 5:130–131
Sigh reflex, 4:413
Sighing, 1:554
Sigmoid colon, 3:384
Silence, 2:19–20
Silent myocardial infarction, 5:183
Silo gas, 5:511
Silver fork deformity, 4:267
Simple diffusion, 3:417
Simple face mask, 1:634
Simple partial seizures, 3:304
Simple pneumothorax, 4:425–426
Simplex, 2:276
Single blinding, 1:651
Singular command, 5:371–372
Sinoatrial (SA) node, 4:417
Sinus arrest, 3:108–110
Sinus block, 3:110–111
Sinus bradycardia, 3:104–105, 3:106
Sinus dysrhythmia, 3:108
Sinus pause, 3:111
Sinus tachycardia, 3:105–107
Sinuses, 1:535
Sinusitis, 3:638
Siren, 5:346–347
Sitting posture, 1:23
Situational awareness, 5:370
Six rights of medication administration, 1:300–301, 1:395–396
Six-second method, 3:101
Skeletal muscle, 1:176
Skeletal muscle relaxants, 1:346
Skeletal organization, 4:230
Skeletal system, 1:178
Skin, 2:52–55, 4:185–187
Skull, 2:61, 2:63, 3:271
Skull fractures, 4:300–301

Slander, 1:131, 2:280, 2:302
SLE, 1:272
Sleep apnea, 5:284
Sleep deprivation, 1:37
Sling and swathe, 4:267
Slow-reacting substances of anaphylaxis (SRS-A), 1:257, 3:364
Slow-to-warm-up child, 1:514
Small cell carcinoma, 3:52
Small incidents, 5:377
Small intestine, 3:384, 3:400, 4:457
Small-volume nebulizer, 1:634
Smallpox, 5:538
Smith, Edwin, 1:51
Smoking, 3:37
Smooth endoplasmic reticulum, 1:173
Smooth muscle, 1:176, 1:538, 1:539, 3:7, 3:8
SMR, 4:376
Snakebites, 3:493–497
Sneezing, 1:554
Snoring, 1:555, 3:27
SO, 5:376
SOAP format, 2:305
Social clock, 1:521
Sociocultural, 3:664
Sodium, 4:214
Sodium (Na), 1:192
Sodium bicarbonate, 5:25, 5:89
Sodium channel blockers (class I), 1:351
Sodium nitroprusside, 1:358, 5:171
Sodium/potassium pump, 3:87
Soft and connective tissue injuries, 4:272–273
Soft palate, 1:612, 3:4
Soft splints, 4:257–258
Soft-tissue trauma, 4:134–181
    abdomen, 4:177
    abrasions, 4:144–145

amputations, 4:148, 4:172
ankle and foot, 4:171
assessment techniques, 4:164–165
associated injury, 4:157
avulsions, 4:147–148
blood vessels, 4:140
collagen synthesis, 4:151
compartment syndrome, 4:154–155, 4:156
contusions, 4:143–144
crush injuries, 4:144, 156
crush syndrome, 4:157–158, 4:173–175
delayed healing, 4:154
dermis, 4:139–140
detailed physical exam, 4:163–164
dressings/bandage, 4:158–160, 4:171
ear, 4:170
elbow and knee, 4:171
epidemiology, 4:138
epidermis, 4:139
epithelialization, 4:151
face, 4:169, 4:176
fasciae, 4:141
focused history and physical exam, 4:162–163
gangrene, 4:153
groin and hip, 4:170
hand and finger, 4:171
hematomas, 4:144
hemorrhage, 4:148–149
hemorrhage control, 4:165–168
hemostasis, 4:149
high-pressure tool injuries, 4:157
immobilization, 4:168–169
impaired hemostasis, 4:154
impaled objects, 4:146, 4:172–173
incisions, 4:146
infection, 4:151–153
infection injury, 4:158

inflammation, 4:150–151
initial assessment, 4:161–162
lacerations, 4:145–146
muscles, 4:141
neck, 4:170, 4:176, 4:177
neovascularization, 4:151
pain and edema control, 4:169
pressure injuries, 4:155
punctures, 4:146
rebleeding, 4:154
refer/release incidents, 4:178
scalp, 4:169
scene size-up, 4:161
shoulder, 4:170
sterility, 4:168
subcutaneous tissue, 4:140
tension lines, 4:142
tetanus, 4:153
thorax, 4:177
transport, 4:178
trunk, 4:170
Solid organ injury, 4:467
Solvent, 1:189
Somatic nervous system, 3:268
Somatic pain, 3:378–379
Somatoform disorders, 3:674–675
Somatostatin, 3:334
SOPs, 5:407
Soufflé cup, 1:409
Span of control, 5:369
Spasm, 4:241
Spasmodic croup, 5:96
Special needs children, 5:134–138
Special needs patients, 1:498–503
Special weapons and tactics (SWAT) team, 5:491
Specialty centers, 4:12
Specific gravity, 5:461, 5:531
Speech impairments, 5:245–246

Sperm cell, 3:419

Spermatozoa, 3:715

Sphenoid sinus, 3:6

Sphenoidal sinus, 3:4

Sphygmomanometer, 2:36

Spike, 1:435

Spina bifida (SB), 3:315, 5:258

Spinal accessory nerve, 4:290

Spinal alignment, 4:385–386

Spinal anatomy and physiology, 4:347–364

Spinal column, 2:134, 4:347

Spinal cord, 3:276, 3:278, 4:356–358

Spinal cord compression, 4:369

Spinal cord contusion, 4:369

Spinal cord hemorrhage, 4:369

Spinal cord injury without radiographic abnormality (SCIWORA), 4:374

Spinal cord syndromes, 4:370–371

Spinal curvatures, 2:134

Spinal disk disease, 2:132

Spinal meninges, 4:358–360

Spinal motion restriction (SMR), 4:376

Spinal nerve, 3:278

Spinal nerve plexuses, 4:362

Spinal nerves, 4:360–364

Spinal shock, 4:371

Spinal trauma, 4:344–403

assessment, 4:374–375

autonomic hyperreflexia syndrome, 4:372

axial stress, 4:366–367

blood supply to spine, 4:350

cervical collar application, 4:388

cervical spine, 4:351–352

coccygeal spine, 4:356

column injury, 4:368

cord injury, 4:368–370

diving injury immobilization, 4:397–398

final patient positioning, 4:395

helmet removal, 4:389–390

log roll, 4:391–392

long spine board, 4:395–397

lumbar spine, 4:354–355

manual cervical immobilization, 4:386–388

mechanisms of injury, 4:364–368

medications, 4:398–399

neurogenic shock, 4:372

orthopedic stretcher, 4:393

pediatric spinal injuries, 4:373–374

rapid extrication, 4:394–395

rapid trauma assessment, 4:379–383

rope-sling slide, 4:392–393

sacral spine, 4:355–356

scene size-up, 4:374–375

short spine board, 4:393–394

spinal alignment, 4:385–386

spinal cord, 4:356–358

spinal cord syndromes, 4:370–371

spinal meninges, 4:358–360

spinal nerves, 4:360–364

spinal shock, 4:371

standing takedown, 4:388–389

straddle slide, 4:392

thoracic spine, 4:352–354

transient syndromes, 4:372–373

vertebral column, 4:347–350

vest-type immobilization device, 4:393–394

vital signs, 4:384

Spine, 2:130–132, 2:134–136

Spinous process, 4:348

Spiral fracture, 4:244

Spleen, 3:384, 3:386, 4:458, 4:467

Splenic artery, 3:386

Splenic flexure, 3:400

Splinting devices, 4:256–262

SpO₂, 1:557–558

Spondylosis, 5:214

Spontaneous abortion, 3:728–729

Spontaneous pneumothorax, 3:57

Sports injuries, 4:54–55

Sports medicine, 1:11

Spotter, 5:343

Sprain, 4:241

SRS, 4:31–33, 5:431

SRS-A, 1:257, 3:364

SSM, 5:341

SSRIs, 1:327–328, 3:478

SSRIs antidepressant treatment algorithm, 3:480

ST segment, 3:95

ST-segment elevation myocardial infarction (STEMI), 5:188

Stable angina, 5:185

Staff functions, 5:375

Staging area, 5:372, 5:388

Staging officer, 5:388

Standard Competencies for EMS Personnel Responding to

Hazardous Materials Incidents, 5:450

Standard deviation (SD), 1:654, 1:655

Standard lung capacities, 4:412

Standard of care, 1:126

Standard operating procedures (SOPs), 5:407

Standard precautions, 1:24, 1:396, 2:188, 5:317

Standards, 5:366–368

Standing orders, 1:61, 2:250

Standing posture, 1:22

Standing takedown, 4:388–389

Staphylococcal enterotoxin, 5:533

Staphylococcal skin infections, 1:25

Starling mechanism, 1:214

Starling's law of the heart, 3:80, 4:87

START, 5:381

Startle reflex, 1:511

State court system, 1:122

State-level agencies, 1:59

Statewide EMS Technical Assessment Program, 1:54

Status asthmaticus, 3:45, 5:101

Status epilepticus, 3:306–307, 5:113

Statute of limitations, 1:128

STDs, 3:646

Stem cells, 1:245

STEMI, 5:188

Stenosis, 1:616

Sterile, 1:397

Sterile dressings, 4:159

Sterilization, 3:612

Sterilizing, 1:29

Sternal angle, 4:408

Sternal fracture/ dislocation, 4:423

Sternoclavicular dislocation, 4:444
Sternocleidomastoid muscles, 4:409
Sternum, 4:408
Stethoscope, 2:35
Stings, 3:488–493
Stock solution, 1:476
Stokes-Adams syndrome, 5:186
Stoma, 1:627, 5:135
Stomach, 3:384, 3:400, 4:456, 4:457
Straddle slide, 4:392
Strain, 4:241
Strainers, 5:420
Street equipment transportation, 5:442
Street gangs, 5:485–486
Stress, 1:35, 1:275
Stress and disease, 1:275–283
  cortisol, 1:278–279
  general adaptation syndrome, 1:275–276
  homeostasis, 1:276
  neuroendocrine regulation, 1:277–278
  psychological mediators and specificity, 1:276
  stress responses, 1:277–282
Stress management, 1:35–40, 1:108
Stress response, 1:36, 1:277
Stressor, 1:35, 1:275
Stretch, 4:26
Stretch receptors, 3:14
Stridor, 1:555, 2:90, 3:27
Stroke, 3:294–302, 5:187
Stroke volume, 1:213, 2:94, 3:80, 4:87
Structural collapses, 5:428–429
Structural lesions, 3:281
Structured concerns, 5:427
Study group, 1:651
Studying a Study and Testing a Test: How to Read the Medical Literature (Riegelman/Hirsch), 1:664
Stylet, 1:577
Subarachnoid hemorrhage, 3:297, 5:187
Subconjunctival hemorrhage, 4:315
Subcutaneous emphysema, 2:215, 3:25
Subcutaneous injection, 1:424–427
Subcutaneous tissue, 4:186
Subdural hematoma, 4:304
Subendocardial infarction, 3:235, 5:188
Subglottic, 4:196
Subluxation, 4:241–242
Sublingual, 1:400
Sublingual gland, 3:384
Submaxillary gland, 3:384
Submerged victims, 5:423
Submucosa, 3:387
Substance abuse, 3:499–506. *See also* Toxicology
  alcohol abuse, 3:503–506
  chronic alcohol ingestion, 3:504–506
  defined, 3:499
  drugs of abuse, 3:500–503
  drugs used for sexual purposes, 3:503
  fetal alcohol syndrome, 5:229, 5:251–252
  general alcoholic profile, 3:504
  geriatrics, 5:206–207
  in EMS, 1:21
  maternal drug abuse, 5:229
  withdrawal syndrome, 3:505
Substance-related disorders, 3:674
Subtle seizures, 5:32
Succinylcholine, 1:597, 5:83, 4:334–335
Sucking reflex, 1:512
Suction, 1:629
Suctioning, 1:629–631, 4:326
Suctioning catheters, 1:630
Sudden death, 3:209
Sudden infant death syndrome (SIDS), 5:130–131
Sudoriferous glands, 4:139
Suicidal patients, 3:452
Suicide, 3:679–680, 5:209–210
Sunburn, 4:196
Superficial burn, 4:196, 4:205
Superficial frostbite, 3:566
Superior articular facets, 4:348
Superior articular processes, 4:348
Superior gluteal nerves, 3:277
Superior lobe, 3:4
Superior turbinate, 3:6
Superior vena cava, 3:75, 3:77
Superior vena cava syndrome, 3:52
Supine hypotensive syndrome, 3:734–735, 4:461
Supplemental restraint systems (SRS), 4:31–33, 5:431
Suppository, 1:413
Supraclavicular nerve, 3:277
Supraglottic, 4:195
Supraspinous ligament, 4:350
Supraventricular tachycardia (SVT), 3:120–121, 5:108
Surface-absorbed toxins, 3:456
Surface absorption, 3:449
Surface water rescues, 5:416–425
Surfactant, 1:369, 3:9, 3:569
Surgically implanted medication delivery systems, 5:292
Surveillance, 4:6
Survival, 3:213
Suspensory ligament, 3:696
Sutures, 4:284
SVT, 3:120–121, 5:108
SWAT team, 5:491
Sympathetic nervous system, 1:339–346, 3:268, 4:86
Sympathetic postganglionic fibers, 1:340
Sympatholytics, 1:342
Sympathomimetics, 1:342, 5:168
Symphysis pubis, 3:696
Synapse, 1:333, 3:270
Synaptic signaling, 1:179
Synarthroses, 4:227
Synchronized cardioversion, 3:175–176
Synchronized cardioversion algorithm, 5:177
Syncope, 3:307, 5:185–186
Syncytium, 3:85
Synergism, 5:465
Synovial fluid, 4:230
Synovial joint, 2:110
Synovial joints, 4:227
Syphilis, 3:647–649
Syringe, 1:414–415
System status management (SSM), 5:341
Systematic sampling, 1:651
Systemic, 1:397

Systemic effects, 5:464
Systemic lupus
    erythematosus (SLE),
    1:272
Systole, 2:93, 3:79
Systolic blood pressure,
    2:44, 4:110

**T cell receptor (TCR),
    1:252**
T lymphocytes, 1:240,
    3:604
t test, 1:656
T wave, 3:94, 3:99
T_3, 3:332
T_4, 3:332
Tachycardia, 2:41, 3:23,
    3:101
  children, 5:108, 5:109
Tachycardia algorithm,
    3:119
Tachydysrhythmia, 3:104,
    5:108
Tachypnea, 2:42, 3:28,
    5:61
Tactical emergency
    medical service
    (TEMS), 5:480
Tactile fremitus, 3:25
Take-in equipment, 5:316
Tattoos, 5:486
TB, 3:622
TBW, 1:188
TCAs, 1:327–328
TCR, 1:252
Teachable moments,
    1:105
Teaching, 1:164
*Teaching Resource for
    Instructors in
    Prehospital Pediatrics
    (TRIPP)*, 5:44
Team leader, 5:314–315
Teamwork, 1:97
Teaspoon, 1:409
Technician level, 5:451
Teeth, 3:384
Teflon catheter, 1:440
Television, 1:517
Temperament, 1:514
Temperature, 1:475–476,
    2:47–48

Temperature/weather
    extremes, 5:441–442
Temporary cavity, 4:71
TEMS, 5:480
10-code, 2:266
Ten Commandments,
    1:153
Tenderness, 2:12
Tendonitis, 4:247
Tendons, 4:141, 4:238
Tenecteplase, 5:170
Tension lines, 4:142
Tension pneumothorax,
    1:583, 4:427–428,
    4:445–447
Teratogenic drugs, 1:302
Terminal-drop
    hypothesis, 1:524
Termination of action,
    1:316
Terminology, 2:268
  hazmat incidents,
    5:461–463
Terrorism, 5:450
Terrorist acts, 5:524–541
  biological agents,
    5:535–539
  biotoxins, 5:533
  chemical agents,
    5:530–535
  encephalitis-like agents,
    5:538
  explosive agents,
    5:527–528
  incapacitating agents,
    5:534
  nerve agents, 5:531–532
  nuclear detonation,
    5:528–530
  pneumonia-like agents,
    5:537–538
  pulmonary agents,
    5:533
  vesicants (blistering
    agents), 5:532
  WMDs, 5:526
Tertiary prevention,
    1:105
Testes, 3:336, 3:419, 4:460
Testicular torsion, 2:107
Testis, 3:420
Testosterone, 1:280

Tetanus, 3:606,
    3:643–644, 4:153
Tetralogy of Fallot, 5:8
Thalamus, 3:273, 3:274,
    3:276, 4:288
Theophylline, 3:483–484
Therapeutic abortion,
    3:729
Therapeutic
    communications,
    1:487–503
  basic elements,
    1:489–491
  children, 1:499–501
  compassionate touch,
    1:494
  elderly patients, 1:501
  eye contact, 1:494
  Hispanic families,
    1:501
  hostile/uncooperative
    patients, 1:503
  interview techniques,
    1:495–498
  nonverbal, 1:492–494
  professional behaviors,
    1:490–491
  sensory impaired
    patients, 1:501–502
  special needs patients,
    1:498–503
  techniques, 1:492–503
  transferring patient
    care, 1:503
  trust/rapport, 1:490
Therapeutic index, 1:316,
    3:476
Therapy regulators, 1:633
Thermal burns,
    4:187–189, 200–211
Thermal gradient, 3:548
Thermogenesis, 3:548
Thermolysis, 3:548–549
Thermoreceptors, 3:550
Thermoregulation,
    3:549–551
Thermoregulatory
    thermogenesis, 3:548
Thiamine, 4:337
Thiazides, 1:354
Third-degree AV block,
    5:129–130

Third-degree burn, 4:197
Third-party payers, 1:76
Thoracic aorta, 3:75
Thoracic convexity, 4:348
Thoracic duct, 4:414
Thoracic inlet, 4:408
Thoracic nerves, 3:277,
    4:361
Thoracic skeleton,
    4:407–408
Thoracic spin, 4:352–354
Thoracic trauma,
    4:404–451
  assessment, 4:438–443
  blunt cardiac injury,
    4:431–432, 4:447
  blunt trauma,
    4:418–419
  blunt trauma
    assessment, 4:441
  bronchi, 4:410
  cardiovascular
    inquiries, 4:430–435
  chest wall contusion,
    4:420
  chest wall injuries,
    4:420–424
  commotio cordis, 4:432
  diaphragm, 4:409
  esophagus, 4:417
  flail chest, 4:423–424,
    4:444–445
  great vessels, 4:417
  heart, 4:415–417
  hemothorax, 4:428–429,
    4:447
  lung volumes,
    4:411–412
  lungs, 4:410
  mediastinum, 4:414
  musculature,
    4:409–410
  myocardial
    aneurysm/rupture,
    4:434
  patho pearls, 4:437
  penetrating trauma,
    4:419–420, 4:421
  penetrating trauma
    assessment, 4:441–442
  pericardial tamponade,
    4:432–434, 4:447

Thoracic trauma, (contd.)
pneumothorax. See
Pneumothorax
pulmonary contusion,
4:429–430
pulmonary injuries,
4:425–430
rapid trauma
assessment, 4:438–440
Thoracic trauma, (contd.)
respiratory control,
4:412–414
rib fracture, 4:421–423;
4:444
scene size-up, 4:438
sternal fracture/
dislocation, 4:423
sternoclavicular
dislocation, 4:444
thoracic skeleton,
4:407–408
tracheobronchial injury,
4:436, 4:448
trachea, 4:410
traumatic asphyxia,
4:437, 4:448
traumatic dissection of
aorta, 4:434–435,
4:448
traumatic esophageal
rupture, 4:436
traumatic
rupture/perforation of
diaphragm, 4:435–436
Thoracic vertebrae,
4:347, 4:354
Thoracoabdominal
pump, 4:112
Thorax, 2:86, 4:75, 4:408
Threatened abortion,
3:728
Threshold limit
value/ceiling level
(TLV-CL), 5:463
Threshold limit
value/short-term
exposure limit
(TLV/STEL), 5:463
Threshold limit value/
time weighted average
(TLV/TWA), 5:463
Thrill, 2:95

Thrombocyte, 1:174,
1:198, 3:520
Thrombocytopenia,
3:520, 3:538
Thrombocytosis, 3:520,
3:538
Thrombolytics, 1:362
Thrombophlebitis, 1:450
Thrombosis, 3:523
Thrombotic strokes,
3:296
Thrombus, 1:451
Thymosin, 3:333
Thymus gland, 3:333
Thyroid cartilage, 1:534,
1:536, 1:617, 3:5
Thyroid gland,
1:373–374,1:534,
1:612, 1:617, 3:5,
3:332
Thyroid stimulating
hormone (TSH),
3:332
Thyrotoxic crisis,
3:348–349
Thyrotoxicosis, 3:347,
5:35
Thyroxine (T$_4$), 3:332
TIA, 3:299–300, 5:164
Tibia, 1:467, 4:234
Tibial fracture, 4:266
Tidal volume, 1:548, 2:44,
3:12–13, 4:411
Tiered response, 1:50
Tiered response system,
5:342
Tilt test, 4:103
Time management, 1:96
Tinnitus, 2:17, 5:167
Tissue, 1:176
Tissue-specific antigens,
1:269
Tissue-specific reactions,
1:269
TLV-CL, 5:463
TLV/STEL, 5:463
TLV/TWA, 5:463
TNKase, 5:170
Tocolysis, 3:737
Toddlers, 1:514–517,
5:48–49. See also
Pediatrics

physical examination,
2:168
Tolerance, 3:499
Tone, 4:239
Tongue, 1:534, 1:549, 3:5,
3:384
Tonic-clonic seizure,
3:303
Tonic phase, 3:303
Tonic seizures, 5:32
Tonicity, 1:200
Tonsils/adenoids, 1:534,
3:5
Topical anesthetic spray,
4:337
Topical medications,
1:399
Torsades de pointes,
5:141–142
Tort law, 1:122
Total body water (TBW),
1:188
Total downtime, 3:212
Total lung capacity,
1:548, 3:13, 4:412
Touch pad, 2:280
Tourniquet, 4:93
Toxic/explosive
chemicals, 5:427
Toxic inhalation, 3:53,
4:195
Toxic-metabolic states,
3:281
Toxic syndromes,
3:458–459
Toxicological
emergencies,
5:201–206
Toxicology, 3:444–499
acetaminophen,
3:481–482
carbon monoxide,
3:457–458
cardiac medications,
3:471–473
caustic substances,
3:473–474
ciguatera poisoning,
3:498–499
contaminated food,
3:485–486
cyanide, 3:468–471

defined, 3:447
epidemiology,
3:447–448
hydrocarbons,
3:475–476
hydrofluoric acid,
3:474–475
ingested toxins,
3:453–455
inhaled toxins,
3:455–456
injected toxins,
3:487–499
insect bites/stings,
3:488–493
lithium, 3:479–481
MAO inhibitors,
3:477–478
marine animal
injection, 3:497–498
metals, 3:482–485
newer antidepressants,
3:478–479
patient assessment/
management,
3:450–453
poison control centers,
3:448
poisonous
plants/mushrooms,
3:486–487
salicylates, 3:481
snakebites,
3:493–497
surface-absorbed
toxins, 3:456
theophylline,
3:483–484
toxic exposure routes,
3:448–450
toxic syndromes,
3:458–459
tricyclic
antidepressants,
3:476–477
Toxidrome, 3:457
Toxins, 1:235, 3:359,
3:447
tPA, 5:170
Trachea, 1:534, 1:536,
1:538, 1:617, 3:4, 3:5,
3:7, 3:384, 4:410

Tracheal cartilages, 1:536, 1:538, 3:7
Tracheal deviation, 3:25
Tracheal tugging, 3:22
Tracheobronchial injury, 4:436, 4:448
Tracheobronchial suctioning, 1:631
Tracheobronchial tree, 4:406
Tracheostomy, 5:135, 5:286
Tracheostomy tubes, 5:135
Tracrium, 1:597, 4:335
Traction splint, 4:258–259, 4:260
Traffic congestion, 5:341–342
Traffic hazards, 5:429–430
Training, 5:451
Trajectory, 4:63
Transcutaneous cardiac pacing, 3:176–179
Transdermal, 1:399
Transfusion, 1:199–200, 1:274, 4:509
Transfusion reactions, 3:526
Transient hypertension, 3:733
Transient ischemic attack (TIA), 3:299–300, 5:164
Transient quadriplegia, 4:372
Transitional fibers, 5:123
Transmural infarction, 3:234, 5:187
Transplantation, 1:274
Transport, 1:58, 1:87, 1:138
  neonates, 5:26
  pediatric patients, 5:55
  street equipment, 5:442
Transportation, 5:452
Transportation unit supervisor, 5:388–389
Transposition of the great vessels, 5:8, 5:9
Transverse cervical nerve, 3:277

Transverse colon, 3:384, 3:400
Transverse foramen, 4:351
Transverse fracture, 4:244
Transverse processes, 4:348
Trauma, 1:53
  abdominal. See Abdominal trauma
  blunt. See Blunt trauma
  burns. See Burns
  decision to transport, 4:14–15
  defined, 4:3
  evaluation, 4:9
  facial. See Head, facial and neck trauma
  Golden Period, 4:13–14
  head. See Head, facial and neck trauma
  hemorrhage. See Hemorrhage
  implementation, 4:9
  index of suspicion, 4:13
  injury prevention, 4:15–16
  intervention development, 4:8
  mechanism of injury analysis, 4:12–13
  musculoskeletal. See Musculoskeletal trauma
  penetrating. See Penetrating trauma
  QI, 4:16–17
  resuscitation. See Shock trauma resuscitation
  risk analysis, 4:6–8
  shock. See Shock
  soft-tissue. See Soft-tissue trauma
  spinal. See Spinal trauma
  surveillance, 4:6
  thoracic. See Thoracic trauma
  trauma registry, 4:16
Trauma care system, 4:9
Trauma Care Systems Planning and

Development Act of 1990, 4:9
Trauma center, 1:55
Trauma center designation, 4:10–12
Trauma patient, 2:211–221
Trauma patient intubation, 1:593
Trauma registry, 4:16
Trauma system quality improvement (QI), 4:16–17
Trauma triage criteria, 4:12
TraumaDEX, 4:105
Traumatic asphyxia, 4:437, 4:448
Traumatic brain injury, 5:126–127
Traumatic dissection of aorta, 4:434–435, 4:448
Traumatic esophageal rupture, 4:436
Traumatic rupture/perforation of diaphragm, 4:435–436
Treat and release, 1:88, 4:507
Treatment unit leader, 5:387
Trench foot, 3:567
Triage, 1:53, 5:380
Triage group supervisor, 5:380
Triage officer, 5:370
Triage tags, 2:310
Trial, 1:123
Trial courts, 1:122
Triangular bandage, 4:160
Triaxial joints, 4:228
Trichinosis, 3:600
Trichomoniasis, 3:650–651
Trichothecene mycotoxins, 5:533
Tricuspid valve, 3:74, 3:77
Tricyclic antidepressant poisoning treatment algorithm, 3:477

Tricyclic antidepressants, 3:476–477
Tricyclic antidepressants (TCAs), 1:327–328
Trigeminal nerve, 2:149, 4:290
Triiodothyronine (T$_3$), 3:332
Trimester, 3:719
Triple blinding, 1:651
TRIPP, 5:44
Trocar, 1:466
Trochlear nerve, 2:148, 4:290
Trophoblasts, 1:252
Troponin, 5:195
True posterior infarct, 3:240
Trunking, 2:277
Trust, 1:490
Trust vs. mistrust, 1:513
TSH, 3:332
Tuberculosis (TB), 1:381, 3:622
Tubing, 1:436
Tunica adventitia, 3:79, 4:88
Tunica intima, 3:77, 4:88
Tunica media, 3:77–79, 4:88
Turbinates, 3:5
Turgor, 1:190, 2:54, 5:271
Turnover, 1:276
Two-pillow orthopnea, 5:184
2:1 AV block, 5:128–129
2,3-bisphosphoglycerate (2,3-BPG), 3:515
12-lead angles, 3:226
12-lead ECG, 3:230, 3:231
Tylenol, 5:206
Type I ambulance, 1:69, 1:70, 5:337, 5:338
Type I diabetes mellitus, 1:210, 1:374–375, 3:340
Type I error rate, 1:652
Type I (IgE) reactions, 1:268–269
Type I second-degree AV block, 5:125–126

Type II ambulance, 1:69, 1:70, 5:337, 5:338
Type II diabetes mellitus, 1:208, 1:210, 1:374–375, 3:340–341
Type II error rate, 1:652
Type II (tissue-specific) reactions, 1:269
Type II second-degree AV block, 5:127–128
Type III ambulance, 1:69, 1:70, 5:337, 5:338
Type III (immune-complex-mediated) reactions, 1:269–270
Type IV (cell-mediated issue) reactions, 1:270

U wave, 3:94
UHF, 2:266
Ulcerative colitis, 3:392–394
Ulna, 4:232, 4:267
Ulnar nerve, 3:277
Ultrahigh frequency (UHF), 2:266
Ultraviolet keratitis, 4:196
Umbilical cord, 3:715, 3:716
  cutting, 5:13–14
Umbilical vein, 5:22–24
UN number, 5:454
Unblinded study, 1:651
Uncooperative patients, 1:503, 5:312–313
Unfertilized ovum, 3:715
Unified command, 5:372
Unintentional injury, 1:104
Unipolar frame traction splint, 4:260
Unipolar limb leads, 3:92, 3:224
Unit, 1:476
United States Fire Protection

Administration (USFPA), 3:596
United States Pharmacopeia, 1:296
Universal precautions (UP), 1:24, 2:188
Universalizability test, 1:158
Unresponsive medical patient, 2:230–231
Unstable angina, 5:185
UP, 1:24, 2:188
Up-and-over pathway, 4:34
Up-regulation, 1:313
Upper airway anatomy, 1:534–537, 3:5–7
Upper airway obstruction, 1:549, 3:34–35
Upper esophageal sphincter, 1:612
Upper extremity, 4:231–232
Upper gastrointestinal bleeding, 3:384–386
Upper gastrointestinal diseases, 3:383–391
Upper GI bleed, 5:193
Upper respiratory infection, 3:45–48
Urea, 3:413
Uremia, 3:431
Ureter, 3:419, 4:459
Urethra, 3:414, 3:419, 3:420, 3:695, 3:696, 4:459
Urethral opening, 3:694
Uricosuric drugs, 1:381
Urinary bladder, 3:414, 3:419, 3:420, 3:696, 4:459
Urinary stasis, 3:439
Urinary system, 2:100, 3:413, 4:458–459
  musculoskeletal system, 3:717–718
  pregnancy, 3:717–718
Urinary tract devices, 5:294

Urinary tract infections (UTIs), 3:439–441, 5:199
Urine, 3:413
Urology, 3:413
Urology and nephrology, 3:410–441
  acute renal failure, 3:426–429
  anatomy/physiology, 3:414–421
  chronic renal failure, 3:430–435
  epididymis and vas deferens, 3:420
  kidneys, 3:414–419
  pathophysiology, 3:421–426
  patient assessment/ management, 3:422–426
  penis, 3:420–421
  priapism, 3:438
  prostate gland, 3:420
  renal calculi, 3:435–438
  testes, 3:419–420
  ureters, 3:419
  urethra, 3:419
  urinary bladder, 3:419
  urinary tract infection, 3:439–441
Urosepsis, 5:199, 5:200
Urostomy, 5:294
Urticaria, 3:366
USFPA, 3:596
Uterine cavity, 3:715
Uterine fundus, 3:715
Uterine inversion, 3:754
Uterine rupture, 3:753–754
Uterine stimulants/relaxants, 1:378
Uterus, 3:695–697, 3:696, 3:715, 4:460
UTIs, 3:439–441, 5:199
Uvula, 1:534, 1:612, 3:5

V$_A$, 1:548
V$_{A-min}$, 1:548

VA, 5:157
Vaccine, 1:382
Vacutainer, 1:462
VADs, 5:291
Vagal maneuvers, 3:166
Vagal response, 5:18
Vagina, 3:695, 3:696, 3:715, 4:460
Vaginal entrance (introitus), 3:694
Vaginal orifice, 3:696
Vagus nerve, 2:152, 3:82, 4:113, 4:290, 4:414
Valium, 4:273, 4:335
Vallecula, 1:534, 1:536, 3:5
Valsalva maneuver, 5:166, 5:186
Valves of the heart, 3:76
Vapor density, 5:461
Vapor pressure, 5:461
Variance, 1:654, 4:655
Varicella, 1:25, 3:627
Varicella zoster virus (VZV), 1:236, 3:627
Varicose veins, 3:218
Varicosities, 5:186
Vas deferens, 3:420
Vascular access children, 5:85
Vascular access devices (VADs), 5:291
Vascular phase, 4:90
Vascular skin lesions, 2:55
Vasculitis, 3:217
Vasodepressor syncope, 5:185
Vasomotor center, 4:113
Vasopressin, 1:197, 5:169
Vasopressors, 3:369
Vasospastic angina, 5:185
Vasovagal syncope, 5:186
Vastus lateralis, 1:427
Vector, 3:227
Vecuronium, 1:597, 4:335
VEE, 5:538
Vehicle rescues, 5:429–436
Vehicle stabilization equipment, 5:435
Vehicular collisions, 4:28
  analysis, 4:39–40

Vehicular mortality, 4:41
Vein, 3:416, 4:89
Velocity, 4:24
Venezuelan equine encephalitis (VEE), 5:538
Venous access device, 1:458
Venous blood sampling, 1:461–465
Venous constricting band, 1:441
Venous system, 3:79
Ventilation, 1:541, 1:635–639. *See also* Airway management
defined, 3:10
neonates, 5:20–22
Ventral root, 3:278
Ventricular aneurysm, 5:188
Ventricular ectopic, 5:137
Ventricular enlargement, 3:255
Ventricular escape beat, 5:135–136
Ventricular fibrillation, 5:110, 5:142
Ventricular septal defect (VSD), 5:8
Ventricular syncytium, 3:85
Ventricular tachycardia (VT), 5:140–142
Ventricular tachycardia with a pulse, 5:108
Venturi mask, 1:634
Venule, 3:4
Verbal de-escalation, 3:684–685
Versed, 4:336
Vertebra, 4:347
Vertebra prominens, 4:351
Vertebral arch, 4:348
Vertebral artery, 3:276
Vertebral body, 3:278, 4:348
Vertebral column, 4:347–350
Vertebral foramen, 4:348

Vertebrobasilar system, 3:275
Vertigo, 4:293, 5:188
Very high altitude, 3:578
Very high frequency (VHF), 2:282
Very low-density lipoproteins (VLDLs), 1:362
Vesicants (blistering agents), 5:532
Vesicles, 1:175
Vesicular follicle, 3:715
Vest-type immobilization device, 4:393–394
Vestibular fold, 1:536
Vestibule, 3:7, 3:694
Veterans Administration (VA), 5:157
VHF, 2:282, 5:538
Vials, 1:416–1:418
Violent street incidents, 5:484–486
Viral hemorrhagic fever (VHF), 5:538
Virulence, 3:602
Viruses, 1:236, 3:598–599
Visceral pain, 3:378, 3:421
Visceral pericardium, 3:74
Visual acuity wall chart/card, 2:63
Visual field abnormalities, 2:69
Vital capacity, 3:13, 4:412
Vital signs, 1:510, 2:40–48, 4:514
children, 5:62, 5:68–69
head trauma, 4:324
infants, 1:509
late adulthood, 1:522
neonates, 5:20
nervous system assessment, 3:289–290
newborn, 5:20
pediatric patients, 2:172, 5:62, 5:68–69
respiratory system assessment, 3:27–28
shock trauma resuscitation, 4:505

spinal trauma, 4:384
Vitamins, 1:385
Vitreous humor, 4:294
VLDLs, 1:362
V_{min}, 1:548
Vocal cords, 1:534, 1:536, 3:5
Voice production disorders, 5:245–246
Volatility, 5:531
Voltage, 4:189
Volume expanders, 5:25
Volume on hand, 1:477
Volvulus, 3:399
Vomer, 4:291
Vomiting
children, 5:115–116
newborn, 5:34
Von Willebrand's disease, 3:539–540
VSD, 5:8
VT, 5:140–142
Vulva, 3:694
VZV, 1:236, 3:627

Wandering atrial pacemaker, 3:113–114
Warm (control) zone, 5:460
Warm (yellow) zone, 5:461
Warning placard, 5:452
Washout, 4:117
Waste removal, 1:218
Water, 1:188–191
Water rescues, 5:416–425
Water solubility, 5:461
Water temperature, 5:417–418
Watercraft crashes, 4:44
"Weak and dizzy," 3:310
Weapons of mass destruction (WMDs), 5:450, 5:453, 5:526
Weather/temperature extremes, 5:441–442
Weight conversion, 1:475
Weiner, A. S., 3:525
Well-being of paramedic, 1:14–43
back safety, 1:21–23

basic physical fitness, 1:17–23
death and dying, 1:31–35
equipment decontamination, 1:28–31
habits/addictions, 1:20–21
infectious diseases, 1:24–28, 1:25
interpersonal relations, 1:41
mental health services, 1:40
nutrition, 1:18–20
personal protection from disease, 1:24–31
roadway safety, 1:41–43
safety considerations, 1:41–43
stress/stress management, 1:35–40
warning signs of excessive stress, 1:38
Wenckebach, 5:125
Wernicke's syndrome, 3:294
Wet dressings, 4:159
Wet drowning, 3:568
Wet gangrene, 1:187
Wheezing, 1:555, 2:90, 3:27
Whispered pectoriloquy, 2:91
White blood cells, 1:198, 3:516–520
White matter, 4:358
"White Paper, The," 1:53
Whole bowel irrigation, 3:452
Whooping cough, 1:25
Wilderness protection, 5:406
Wind Chill Index, 3:560
Window phase, 3:603
Windshield survey, 5:369
Wiskott-Aldrich syndrome, 1:273
Withdrawal, 3:499, 3:505

Withdrawal syndrome, 3:505

WMDs, 5:450, 5:453, 5:526

Wolff-Parkinson-White (WPW) syndrome, 5:150–151

Work-induced thermogenesis, 3:548

Workplace hazards, 1:111

WPW syndrome, 5:150–151

Wrap points, 5:514

Wrist, 2:112

Wrist injury, 4:272

Written communication, 2:267–268

X-rays, 4:193

Xiphisternal joint, 4:408

Xiphoid process, 4:408

Yaw, 4:65

Years of productive life, 1:104

Yellow bone marrow, 4:227

Yellow treatment unit, 5:387

Yellow zone, 5:461

Zeolite, 4:105

Zollinger-Ellison syndrome, 3:391

Zone of coagulation, 4:188

Zone of hyperemia, 4:188

Zone of stasis, 4:188

Zygoma, 4:290

Zygomatic bone, 4:291